Virtually Safe Cigarettes

Reviving an Opportunity Once Tragically Rejected

Virtually Safe Cigarettes

Reviving an Opportunity Once Tragically Rejected

Gio Batta Gori
Health Policy Center, Bethesda, Maryland, USA

IOS
Press

Ohmsha

Amsterdam • Berlin • Oxford • Tokyo • Washington, DC

ISBN 1 58603 057 4 (IOS Press)
ISBN 4 274 90357 5 C3047 (Ohmsha)
Library of Congress Catalog Card Number: 00-102068

Publisher
IOS Press
Nieuwe Hemweg 6B
1013 BG Amsterdam
The Netherlands
fax: +31 20 620 3419
e-mail: order@iospress.nl

Distributor in the UK and Ireland
IOS Press/Lavis Marketing
73 Lime Walk
Headington
Oxford OX3 7AD
England
fax: +44 1865 75 0079

Distributor in the USA and Canada
IOS Press, Inc.
5795-G Burke Centre Parkway
Burke, VA 22015
USA
fax: +1 703 323 3668
e-mail: iosbooks@iospress.com

Distributor in Germany
IOS Press
Spandauer Strasse 2
D-10178 Berlin
Germany
fax: +49 30 242 3113

Distributor in Japan
Ohmsha, Ltd.
3-1 Kanda Nishiki-cho
Chiyoda-ku, Tokyo 101
Japan
fax: +81 3 3233 2426

LEGAL NOTICE
The publisher is not responsible for the use which might be made of the following information.

PRINTED IN THE UNITED STATES OF AMERICA

To the memory of Ernst Wynder, my friend.
We shared the conviction that less hazardous cigarettes
are of paramount interest in public health.

The Brown and Williamson Tobacco Corporation contributed to the funding of this book. The views expressed here are solely those of the author. Special thanks to Harcourt Inc. for permission to utilize in chapter two excerpts from an earlier paper by the author, which appeared in Regulatory Toxicology and Pharmacology 21:281-295, 1995. Also special thanks to John Wiley & Sons Ltd. for permission to utilize in chapter six excerpts from an earlier paper by the author, which appeared in Human Psychopharmacology 11:s33-s38, 1996.

Contents

Contents

x

Preface

By now it should be obvious that the goal of a smoke-free America by the year 2000 has been a chimera. Cigarettes are risky but still wanted and legal, American smokers still count around 50 million, and the recent settlement of Tobacco and the States ensures a vigorous cigarette market. Could the world do without tobacco and cigarettes? Of course it could and likely it should, but not for a long time to come.

That smokers will be around was clearly in the mind of senior managers at the National Cancer Institute in the late '60s, when they decided to set up the Smoking and Health Program to develop less hazardous cigarettes. Assisted by scores of experts, the Program provided a quantum jump in what was available in the open literature about how cigarettes are made, and why and how people smoke them.

Within 10 years the conceptual framework and some promising technologies for less hazardous cigarettes had been broadly defined, but they were not to be. Realistic policies were discarded abruptly in 1978, when the goal of abolition was officially embraced. To be sure, antismoking education and other measures have been massively successful in persuading some 50 million Americans and countless others around the world to quit smoking, but much more could have been achieved. Far from having been effective, abolitionist policies led to a major public health miscalculation, for they have opposed relentlessly any message that would encourage smokers to moderation, and any cigarette improvements of explicit health benefit—improvements that could have saved lives.

Calling cigarettes virtually safe or less hazardous is as calling a glass half full or half empty, and both perceptions reflect the plain epidemiologic reality that the risks of smoking are reduced if the amount of smoke inhaled is reduced. Still, for the last 20 years the hopes of reviving an interest in improved cigarettes progressively weakened. Until now, that is, as the settlement between Tobacco and the States raises inevitably the same moral obligation the National Cancer Institute accepted 30 years ago: how to protect millions who will continue to smoke.

In telling here why less hazardous cigarettes again should be a compelling issue, I explore some of the reasons, incentives, and modalities for their justification and introduction. There will be also a brief review of the National Cancer Institute's Smoking and Health Program, linking past achievements with present opportunities. I have chosen a simplified language and style to make the book accessible to a wider audience. Only a few sections required a more technical presentation, and the overall aim has been to use concepts that are sufficiently explicit to show why improved cigarettes are feasible. For ease of style, text references have been limited mostly to the essential.

More information about the achievements of the Smoking and Health Program is given in the Appendices, derived directly from the annual reports and other documents of the Program. Space limitations do not permit a full account of the Program's activities, but the information provided clearly shows how extensive the research has been. A bibliography of the Program's publications will help readers who may be interested in the original reports and in more technical details.

Considerably more work is needed to address the manufacture

of cigarettes that are not only less hazardous but also acceptable. Smokers are known to be faithful to their brands and tastes, but they can change in time. For one, today's average smoker is satisfied by cigarettes that yield smokes about twice as diluted as the smokes from cigarettes of 15 years ago. The road to improvement will be gradual, lest smokers might be driven to seek traditional cigarettes that an illegal trade would provide only too willingly. All the same, smokers could become interested in changing more rapidly if the health benefits of new cigarettes were officially endorsed. With this in mind, I shall also explore the prospects for an oversight authority that could independently judge the relative merits of emerging improvements.

Official acceptance of less hazardous cigarettes may not come easy, as it would mean a radical about-face that entrenched abolitionists would find unwelcome. They might object that such cigarettes could discourage some smokers who think of quitting, and encourage some nonsmokers to smoke. Yet these enticements could involve no more than a small minority, if at all real. They would be insignificant when measured against the unprecedented opportunity for saving countless lives among to the over 1 billion smokers worldwide. Zealous but patently ineffective presumptions should not stand in the way—not in an America that prides itself in teaching the world about the evils of intolerance.

Bethesda, Maryland
May 2000

Introduction

Given all that has been said and done about tobacco being public-health enemy number one, why is it that tobacco and cigarettes have not been made illegal? Why look for improved cigarettes when no cigarettes at all would be the ideal solution? Simply stated, the first reason is that over 1 billion smokers around the world insist on smoking, no matter what (*World Bank, 1999*). Even in advanced countries that have been saturated with anti-smoking messages, many smokers have decided the risk is worth taking. Europe and North America alone are home to over 150 million smokers.

The next obvious reason is that there is money in cigarettes, not only for farmers and the cigarette industry but much more for an assorted hierarchy of governments ranging from local municipalities to states and sovereign countries. Indeed, understanding the underlaying crisscrossing of financial interests is absolutely essential if one is to understand the social and political dynamics of the tobacco saga. To wit, the tobacco industry undoubtedly rakes in handsome profits, but few realize that the industry is a relatively minor taker. It is not common knowledge that governments have a long history of profiting much more than the industry from the taxation of tobacco, and without lifting as much as a finger, without a drop of sweat, and totally immune from collateral liabilities.

Governments would like to extract even more from the trade but there is a glitch: further increases of taxation historically have produced diminishing returns, for they increase the incentives of an opportunistic illegal market. In the end, levels of taxation must be finely tuned to balance maximum revenue and a marginal black market.

Governments have been addicted to tobacco revenues for centuries, which points to still another reason for last year's American settlement between many States and Big Tobacco. Remember the settlement, the one that will protect the industry from some liabilities in exchange for penalties that are to offset the costs of treating tobacco-linked diseases, or so the spin goes. Yet, the settlement also guarantees a continuing and greater inflow of tobacco taxes to public treasuries—an inflow that would have been very much imperiled, had antismokers been successful in banning legal cigarettes and thus in promoting an illegal trade. At the very least, the settlement very much depends on a continuing and successful tobacco economy, and implicitly recognizes the legal status of cigarettes for a long foreseeable future.

So it is that cigarettes are here to stay because too many voters indulge in and value the habit, tobacco taxation significantly contributes to public coffers that politicians manipulate, and there is only too real a danger of an uncontrollable black market. A further but perhaps no less important reason is a muted but widely held belief that a good part of the charges officially leveled against tobacco might have been inflated often beyond credibility.

Still, what counts is that smokers are here to stay—a fact of life that makes the case for improving cigarettes self-evident and the obvious moral thing to do. Are improvements possible, and what direction should they take?

The search for improved or less hazardous cigarettes gained

momentum in the late '50s with the first systematic epidemiologic studies on smoking and health. Those early studies, and all similar studies that followed, clearly reported that the risks decrease as the amount of tobacco smoked decreases, usually measured as the number of cigarettes smoked daily. Risks also decrease if smokers inhale less intensely, thus providing added evidence that risks would be smaller as the amount inhaled, namely the dose, becomes smaller. The initial response of public health policy was to encourage the development and marketing of cigarettes that would deliver less smoke, on the assumption that smokers of such cigarettes would inhale less.

The move marked the beginning of the grading of cigarettes on the basis of tar and nicotine yields, a practice that continues today even though it was clear at inception—as it is today—that the practice was a stopgap measure for want of better methods to determine actual smoker intake. The reason is that the grading calls for cigarettes to be smoked by a machine that takes puffs of fixed duration and volume, and at fixed intervals. By contrast, individual smokers use infinite variations of puff volume from time to time, and after puffing they also inhale with infinite variations of intensity. On these grounds, no smoking machine could ever be relied upon to measure how much smoke smokers actually intake. Nevertheless, the grading of cigarette yields by a standard smoking machine became rapidly popular, blissfully unconcerned that smokers' behavior does not agree with mechanical standards.

At the same time, extensive chemical analysis over several years had begun to discover upward of 6,000 components of smoke, making it also clear that not all components of smoke are equally toxic. Notably, the first U.S. Surgeon General's report on smoking of 1964 came to the conclusion that nicotine was probably not toxic at the levels inhaled by smokers, with the implication that the source of the primary pharmacologic reward to smokers was not of immediate concern. In the words of the U.S. Surgeon General: "There is no acceptable evidence that prolonged exposure to nicotine creates either dangerous functional changes of an objective nature or degenerative diseases . . . The fact that the over-all death rates of pipe and cigar smokers show little if any increase over non-smokers is very difficult to reconcile with a concept of high nicotine toxicity . . . . [I]t follows logically that the apparent increase in morbidity and mortality among cigarette smokers relates to exposure to substances in smoke other than nicotine." (*U.S. Surgeon General, 1964, p. 74*).

These findings made it possible to think that certain undesirable components of smoke could be removed by adding filters to cigarettes, a move that met with lasting commercial success and with some indication of reduced risk. Later on, other approaches would attempt to modify the tobacco in cigarettes, although it soon became clear that this was to be an undertaking of major proportions because of the extreme physical and chemical complexity of tobacco, of the combustion process, and of smoke itself.

Meanwhile, from the mid '50s researchers were successful in producing experimental skin tumors in mice either by the application of concentrated solutions of smoke tar—which includes the somewhat solid, as distinguished from the gaseous components of smoke—or by the application of selected tar components. The procedure came to be seen as offering the possibility of testing whether cigarette modifications could result in biological improvements. Spurred by these combined concepts and opportunities, research began in earnest to test whether specific carcinogens—substances that may cause cancer—could be selectively removed from smoke by certain additives or by otherwise modifying the tobacco in cigarettes. Many scientists joined in this effort including those from the tobacco industry. Indeed, later disclosures have shown that the industry's research at that time was intense, although not more successful than what was independently published in the open literature.

To accelerate the progress of improvement, the National

Cancer Institute stepped in with its own research and development program in 1968. The Smoking and Health Program (SHP) recruited an advisory committee, the Tobacco Working Group, that included top academic and government researchers in the field, as well as the research directors of the major U. S. cigarettes manufacturers. The program also availed itself of a vast network of consultants both from the U. S. and other countries (*See Appendix C*).

Initially, the major concern of the SHP was about the cancer-causing properties of smoke—i.e. the carcinogenicity or tumorigenicity of smoke. Testing in humans would have been both unethical and too time-consuming and as a remedy the SHP decided to adopt the only standardized test in animals available at that time, namely skin painting of smoke tar in mice. The procedure entailed collecting tar from modified smokes and painting it repeatedly on the shaved backs of mice to determine how fast and how severely tumors could be produced. Over some 5 years the method was applied to test the carcinogenic potential of tars from more than 150 differently modified cigarettes—modifications involving the tobacco itself, tobacco fractions such as leafs and stems, the paper wrapper of the cigarette, filters, adding or removing nicotine, additives and design changes that could affect the combustion of the cigarette, as well as tobacco substitutes (*See Appendices A and B*).

The point was to find whether modifications could both reduce the amount of tar produced per cigarette and also result in tars that would be less carcinogenic on an equal weight basis. Extensive prior understanding of the carcinogenic properties of polycyclic aromatic hydrocarbons and other coal tar components had raised hopes that undesirable substances could be selectively removed from tobacco smoke. In practice, trials were unable to show how specific smoke constituents could be selectively and substantially reduced. At the same time, tests demonstrated that the tar yield of cigarettes could be much reduced by using certain tobacco substitutes and cigarette modifications. Similarly, the carcinogenic potential of the tars on the skin of mice could also be reduced, although it remained unclear which specific changes in smoke and tar composition might have been responsible. The common penalty of these reductions was a noticeable drop in flavor and acceptability, which prompted an added research investment in remedial flavors.

Shortly after its beginning, the SHP began receiving additional support from the National Heart, Lung, and Blood Institute. This move augmented the scope of action of the program by extending its interests to cardiovascular and respiratory issues and to the pharmacologic and behavioral aspects of smoking. These new directions required mechanistic studies that only direct smoke inhalation procedures could answer.

Several animal inhalation test methods were developed, and analytical procedures were perfected to determine precisely how much nicotine and other smoke components smokers actually inhaled. Research in and out of the Program advanced on similar lines and began offering conclusive proof of what everyone had suspected, namely that the machine yields of tar and nicotine—which rated cigarettes for the market—bore only a vanishing relationship to the amount of smoke that smokers actually inhaled (*Russell et al., 1980; Hill & Marquardt, 1980*).

It is well known that the motivations of smokers extend to a variety of taste, esthetic, and behavioral incentives, of which the pharmacologic rewards of nicotine are by far the most significant. For nicotine alone it became apparent—with some exception for extremely low yield cigarettes—that smokers in general manage to utilize an average of about 1 mg of nicotine from cigarettes of any brand, regardless of the machine yields on the standard FTC smoking machine. Thus, the stage was being set for a shift of research emphasis toward understanding the effects of nicotine and of other major smoke components.

Spurred by these developments, from the mid '70s the SHP began large inhalation experiments in animals aimed at obtaining conclusive evidence about the precise roles of nicotine, carbon monoxide, and other smoke constituents. This research had been well underway for over 4 years, when the advent of a new secretary at the U.S. Department of Health, Education, and Welfare marked an abrupt change of policy. With support and pressure from a growing coalition of antismoking advocates, a crusade took over that sought the outright abolition of smoking. It held that a single puff of smoke was too much, and could not tolerate encouraging smokers to moderation. The new motto was that no cigarette—no matter how modified—should be allowed, and the professed aim of the crusade was a smoke-free America by the year 2000. Any and all efforts to develop improved cigarettes were summarily terminated, the Tobacco Working Group was disbanded, promising experiments were cut off before they could be completed, and the Smoking and Health Program came to an untimely end.

There could be no question that education and other efforts against smoking have been vastly successful in persuading millions of smokers to quit and in discouraging others from smoking. Countless premature deaths may have been prevented by these efforts. Still, while abolition could have been an ideal long term goal, its intransigent application has had undesirable effects.

America is not smoke-free by the year 2000, as could have been predicted, and it may come to pass that the blind inflexibility of abolition will be a cause of lasting regret. Indeed, the 20 year long opposition to moderation and to the introduction of even partially less hazardous cigarettes out to count for a sizable fraction of premature deaths among smokers who did not quit.

It is worth dwelling for a moment on this point. At about the time the SHP was disbanded, the major official compendium of the epidemiology on which antismokers rested their case was the U.S. Surgeon General's report on smoking and health of 1979 (*U.S. Surgeon General, 1979*). The compendium was repeated essentially unchanged in 1989 and is still quoted today (*U.S. Surgeon General, 1989*). At page 5-13, the 1979 report lists the major studies that show how lung cancer risk changes in relation to number of cigarettes smoked per day. The list is reproduced here in Table 1, where the studies show that smokers of 2 packs of cigarettes per day have over 4 times a greater risk of lung cancer as smokers of 1/2 pack per day. The U.S. Surgeon General's 1979 report also lists similar dose-response gradients for other diseases associated with cigarette smoking, and for overall mortality as well. Tables at pages 3-9 and 3-10 of the same report actually show that current smokers of less than 1 pack of cigarettes per day suffered less diseases and were generally healthier than nonsmokers—all the more remarkable because the studies quoted refer to smokers of traditional high-yield cigarettes marketed before 1960.

The standard claim of antismokers has been and still is that cigarettes cause some 450,000 premature deaths a year in the U.S. alone. Therefore, according to the dose and risk differentials as in Table 1, abolitionist policies could have been responsible for several million premature U.S. deaths since 1979, when they brought to an end federal and industrial efforts toward developing less hazardous cigarettes. Clearly, the number of premature deaths could be magnified many fold when projected worldwide, if indeed the number of premature deaths attributed to smoking is what it is claimed to be.

A conference on less hazardous cigarettes was organized at the end of 1979 at the Bambury Center of the Cold Spring Harbor Laboratory in Long Island, NY, under the auspices of Nobelist Dr. James Watson of DNA fame, who at that time was a member of the National Cancer Advisory Board of the National Cancer Institute (*Gori & Bock, 1980*). The conference provided a timely and comprehensive summary of the state-of-the-art on cigarette safety at the end of the '70s, setting the stage for future developments. It reviewed and clarified the means by which cigarette technology could reduce the amount of smoke and tar produced by cigarettes, and confirmed the safety and the central importance of nicotine—indicating that the future of less hazardous cigarettes was to be in the direction of smokes containing sufficient nicotine and eventually no undesirable components.

Table 1. Lung cancer mortality ratios for males, by current number of cigarettes smoked per day, from selected prospective studies. From the U.S. Surgeon General Report of 1979. p. 5–13.

	Cigarettes smoked per day	Mortality ratios
A.C.S. 25 states	Nonsmoker	1.00
	1–9	4.62
	10–19	8.62
	20–39	14.69
	40+	18.77
British doctors	Nonsmoker	1.00
	1–14	7.80
	15–24	12.70
	25+	25.10
Swedish males	Nonsmoker	1.00
	1–7	2.30
	8–15	8.80
	16+	13.90
Japanese males	Nonsmoker	1.00
	1–9	1.90
	10–14	3.52
	15–24	4.11
	25–49	4.57
	50+	5.78

That message was particularly convincing to the R. J. Reynolds Tobacco Company that first engaged in a costly and bold attempt to produce a credible model of a less hazardous cigarette. This novelty yielded smoke by heating rather than burning tobacco and therefore avoided the production of undesirable components, and was a leap forward from basic design concepts framed more that two decades earlier by Sir Charles Ellis of the British American Tobacco Company in England (*Ellis et al., 1967*). Marketed as the Premier™ brand, the prototype turned out to be not especially appealing to smokers who could find preferred choices in the market, but the greater blow to this valiant effort came from the opposition of anti-smoking forces that viewed less hazardous cigarettes as a serious threat to their goal of abolition at any cost.

Other cigarette manufacturers were waiting in the wings for the outcome of the R. J. Reynolds market trial, and were soon discouraged from attempting to produce and market cigarettes that could be presented as being less hazardous. In fact, all manufacturers have engaged in substantial research towards improved cigarettes and have introduced changes over the years, but those changes were and to this day still are not permitted to be presented to smokers as health related (*Fairclough, 2000*). What counts, however, is that numerous patents have been secured by all manufacturers. Many of these patents are probably of the sterile ground-stalking sort that industries use as pre-emptive devices, but many are applicable—at least in principle—to reduced hazard, and could be the launching grounds for new and intensified development.

The reality is that opportunities for product modifications were much restricted for a cigarette industry under siege. During the '80s and '90s cigarettes continued to be marketed on the basis of the FTC machine ratings of tar and nicotine yields, with improvements that marked a modest but general reduction of tar yields compared to nicotine yields. During that time official policy and advocacy groups have continued to be adamantly opposed to the introduction of less hazardous cigarettes and have effectively discouraged any explicit movement of the industry in this direction. Yet, by the end of the '90s things began to change. In essence, the settlement between the tobacco industry and the States is a *de facto* rejection of abolitionist policies and opens new opportunities for the introduction of improved cigarettes.

In self-interest, both the cigarette industry and the States should soon discover the moral obligation and the advantages of developing reduced-risk cigarettes, on the grounds that the settlement is predicated on a continuing market. This time the State Attorney Generals and other parties to the settlement should not wait 20 years, just to be confronted with the awful responsibility of not having acted soon enough to prevent what by their own assertions could be millions of premature deaths. The prospects for improvements are excellent, for there is a store of information that should make this goal fairly soon attainable.

Later on we shall consider in more detail why the introduction of less hazardous cigarettes must happen as a gradual process of departure from conventional products, lest too rapid a change may drive smokers to rely on traditional cigarettes that an illegal market would be very much ready to supply. The speed of transition would depend both on the pace of technological advances and on how soon smokers would adapt to changes in the acceptability and presentation of cigarettes.

Smokers would naturally change more readily if the health benefits of new cigarettes were endorsed by some independent authority, most likely an official oversight agency. Still, an initial incentive and a benchmark of desirable change could be the changing of the grading of cigarettes away from simple tar and nicotine yields, and in favor of a grading based on the tar to nicotine ratios of cigarette smokes. The reason is that smokers obtain whatever nicotine they need from any but the extremely low yield cigarettes—as we shall see later—and thus would be able to inhale proportionately less tar from smokes with a low tar to nicotine ratio.

Although other aspects of smoke and smoking would be meaningful in the evaluation of safety, an initial move toward a simple grading so defined would begin to educate and direct smokers to the right choices, and will spur manufacturers generally in the right directions. In the end, conceivably within a decade, virtually safe cigarettes will contain sufficient nicotine, buffers to limit irritation, some safe flavors and fragrances, and will likely require grading by more complex criteria. Based on the experience of the Smoking and Health Program of the National Cancer Institute, a public effort in this direction may conservatively cost 200 to 300 million dollars a year at most: a sum that would be a minor fraction of the several billion dollars in annual tax revenues from tobacco. It is high time to move on, much has to be done and any delay could continue to compromise the welfare of millions of smokers. Sinners they may be in the eyes of some, but is that a fair reason not to help them, especially since they foot the bill?

Cigarettes at the Third Millennium

Many would find it appealing to incinerate tobacco into the ashes of history, but realities seem to dispose otherwise. A tobacco settlement with the States has come to pass because the prospect of a sudden death of the industry, at the hands of overwhelming court actions, portends the emergence of an underground market to fill the daily demand of over 50 million American voters, who will keep smoking no matter what. A collapse of federal and local tax revenues could have followed, with a surge in crime, police costs, and social ills. Legal cigarettes are here to stay. Still, the settlement raises profound ethical questions because of the unresolved contrast between the principled aims of antismokers and the settlement's implicit dependence on a robust tobacco market.

As a political instrument, the settlement is questionable because it does not address public health issues adequately. However, it is apparent that it could acquire a moral face if it should revive and make prominent a mandate for the rapid development of less hazardous cigarettes, as recommended by the original draft settlement that failed in the 1988 Congress. This provision would accommodate traditional antismokers' concerns—albeit with needed concessions on their part—and is eminently feasible. Here, a grasp of the settlement's underpinning would seem desirable, as we embark to transmogrify what may look as a sow's ear into that silken purse.

THE SMOKERS

It is a tribute to the success of antismoking efforts that some 50 million American smokers did quit from the '70s on. However, the proportion of adult smokers in the U.S. population has remained virtually unchanged since the early '80s, with their numbers hovering around 50 million. Although disputed and peculiar, their reasons for smoking are many. Gone, perhaps, is the elegant trendiness once associated with smoking, although esthetic and tactile features undoubtedly add to its appeal. More to the point, research has confirmed the versatile pharmacology of nicotine in producing either arousal or relaxation—contrasting results that make smoking an adaptable experience with immediate rewards. Research also confirms that smokers are well aware of and actually overstate the risks of smoking (*Viscusi, 1990, 1992*). However, rewards obviously counterbalance the remote prospects of later disease and loss of longevity that so many studies and public health messages have pointed out.

The rewards of smoking are the main reason for the disappointment of antismoking efforts, despite more attempts to emarginate smokers with claims of passive smoking hazards and of addiction, and despite drives to prevent kids from smoking. The proportion of teenagers experimenting with cigarettes has been impervious to antismoking messages (*Luik, 1994*), and has remained unchanged for decades around 80%, with about 30% of them eventually becoming smokers even in countries that prohibit advertising.

Cultural and legal restrictions to passive smoking exposure have had no substantial impact on cigarette sales or number of smokers, while the assertion that nicotine is as addictive as crack cocaine has not been convincing. Official tallies show that some 50 million Americans did quit smoking on their own, and there is clearly addiction and addiction. Smokers do not lose their minds under the influence, do not terrorize with crime, engage in bizarre or dangerous behavior, become asocial, or destroy families (*Kassel, 1997; Warburton, 1992; Jarvik, 1991; Wonnacott et al., 1989*). By all accounts, their mood, behavior, performance, and sociality improve when they smoke. So, what gives?

Much as many may not like it, smokers are here to stay. At the same time, it is apparent that antismoking campaigns have had other indirect effects of dramatic consequence. They may have met resistance in persuading kids not to smoke and smokers to quit, but they have conquered public opinion with high powered publicity, they have influenced cultural values, and have opened the gates to the flood of legal actions that led parties to the settlement table.

A Flood of Legal Actions

By mid 1997 over 700 suits had been filed against the cigarette industry, up from some two dozen on file until two years earlier. The suits had been organized by a nationwide network of tort lawyers who had learned the ropes in previous campaigns on asbestos, pedicle screws, breast implants, and assorted products. Still, in the past the tobacco industry had been successful in persuading juries that the hazards of smoking had been so commonly known that there could be no claim of having been tricked into a dangerous habit.

This time, however, tort lawyers fixed the game by crafting and managing to pass legislation that would exclude most defense arguments, and by persuading the courts to accept certain allegations as established facts rather than as contentious issues. For instance, major claims represented that smokers are an economic burden to society and especially to nonsmokers, while ignoring several studies published by the prestigious Congressional Research Services of the Library of Congress, the Journal of the American Medical Association, and the New England Journal of Medicine—studies that document the net overall contribution of smokers to the economy and public treasuries (*Gravelle & Zimmermann, 1984; Werner, 1987; Manning et al., 1989; Barendregt et al., 1997*).

Such a positive ledger has several reasons. The diseases linked to smoking usually occur late in life, they are brief and not as costly as other conditions of senility, and smokers who may die sooner would reduce the social costs of pensions. It may sound hard-hearted, but from an economic point of view the argument is faultless and incontrovertible: in the social economy context smokers contribute and have always contributed more than they received.

Still, courts have been persuaded to declare this evidence inadmissible, increasing the risk that the industry could be subject to verdicts requiring payments of hundreds of millions of dollars, if not billions, in multiple jurisdictions. Squeezed to this point, the tobacco industry was heading to collapse, if it were not for the very coalition of plaintiff lawyers who could see the unhappy consequences of putting the tobacco industry out of existence. Hence, for these and other reasons, nearly three years ago a settlement was drafted and later presented to Congress, seeking liability relief for the industry in consideration of annual penalties. Eventually a divided Congress missed the opportunity for a federal settlement and paved the way for the settlement later negotiated by the States.

Although the settlement used the arguments of antismokers as a background, antismokers themselves were marginalized on account of their own long-standing prohibitionist policies. Here was a proposal that could become law, and would allow Tobacco to ransom its survival by a vast payment of money to settle certain claims: surely a heretical overture for an antismoking coalition that had spent years cultivating the high ethics of saving lives and kids, and of a smoke-free America by the year 2000. Objections were heard from antismoking ramparts, but soon it became clear that a settlement had the strongest pragmatic endorsements and would likely endure any assault. Short of leaving themselves out in the cold and irrelevant, antismokers had no choice but to join as the lesser partners at the settlement table.

With the settlement, more jockeying can be expected for the allocation of revenues among the States, and for defining how those moneys would be spent (*Fairclough, 1999*). Just recently the federal government has renewed its interest for a larger share of the tobacco trade, and has filed a lawsuit angling for a $25 billion a year package in addition to what the states already won (*St. Cloud & Fairclough, 1999; Jenkins, 1999, 2000*). Still, the addition of a new federal load to the States' settlement tax burden may break the proverbial camel's back, as it will likely provide an even more irresistible incentive to illegal trade, which could collapse the domestic tobacco industry, dry up tax revenues, expand crime . . . .

THE MENACE OF ILLEGAL TRADE

Any standard marine container can be filled with more than a million packs of cigarettes, and could be smuggled anywhere around the globe for a few thousand dollars. Once landed, it can be fitted to any 18 wheeler and moved anywhere in the U.S., in a matter of hours and in virtual anonymity. Keeping in mind that the production cost of a pack of cigarettes is less than $0.30, a tax burden that pushes the price to $4.50 per pack represents a potential profit of some $4 million per trailer—a transaction that can be completed in no time and repeated at will against a daily U.S. demand in excess of 1 billion cigarettes. Distribution and smuggling would be a piece of cake so long as cigarettes are legally sold and smoked, and while the underground retains traditional influence on the waterfront. Many aspiring entrepreneurs might think the potential rewards are worth the risk of ending deep in New York or Los Angeles harbor with a newly set pair of concrete boots.

This scenario is not a figment of imagination but the recent experience of Canadians and Swedes, which forced their governments to roll back unrealistic tax hikes that cut cigarette tax revenues mercilessly. With the price of a cigarette pack now approaching $5.00 in California alone, policing a U.S. market of over 1 billion cigarettes a day would be a nightmarish proposition for any law-enforcement agency. In fact, interstate smuggling has been and is a substantial and continuing business in the direction of high-tax locations such as Alaska and other states, and it is only kept from expanding by the fine tuning of federal, state, and local levies. When all chips are down, realistic taxation is the single efficient moderator of illegal trade and the guarantor of mounting tax receipts (*Newman, 1999*).

The force of this issue becomes clearer when realizing that tobacco taxation has been for time immemorial a noticeable source of federal funds and a major source of state and local revenues. Figures show that for 1996 alone the combined profits of the U.S. tobacco industry were around $6 billion, while the combined federal, state, and local tax revenues were in excess of $15 billion (*TI, 1977*). Presently, under the settlement terms the industry's profits are much reduced but the comparative ratio of public revenues is many fold greater than in 1996. Assorted governments are addicted to this easy mountain of cash, and are by far the largest beneficiaries of tobacco profits year after year, enough to make one wonder who has been and is effectively running the tobacco business in America. Indeed, it could be fairly argued that big Tobacco in the U.S. is *de facto* a nationalized industry, and has been such for many decades (*Jenkins, 2000*).

Then again, and after all rhetoric is exhausted, the first issue for a successful settlement is about the size of a tax capable of securing a stable equilibrium among all forces and expectations involved. If the federal government were to obtain a substantial settlement in addition to the one negotiated by the states, the combined penalties would require levies several fold above the current levels, and would induce irresistible incentives to an illegal trade.

In prior negotiations, Congress seemed assured that American smokers would accept taxes leading to a price around $3.50 a pack, but at that and higher prices how many smokers would "quit" and disappear from official tallies, only to be served by a cheaper underground ready for incredible profits? Could the government of a free country consider placing cost-effective and socially acceptable police detail at every cigarette retailer? Besides, only a paltry fraction of these penalties could come from industry's profits, and most will have to be shelled out by smokers. What is the legality and fairness of squeezing smokers who already pay in more than they receive from public treasuries? These and other questions would have to be resolved before any talk of how much additional federal penalties could be extracted. Yet such issues have received hardly serious consideration.

The picture currently arranged for public consumption still shows an abolitionist crusade bent to wipe out tobacco on health and moral grounds, an industry with a heavy conscience and an even worse image, and some 50 million American smokers branded as hapless addicted pariahs. What the picture does not show is the legal *leger-de-main* and the tortured accounting by which smokers have been made responsible for vast social costs and liable for exorbitant fines and lawyers' fees (*Bork, 1999*). To clinch it, some of the media have been retained to persuade America that the settlement is to redress hideous wrongs and to prevent future ones. Does it make sense?

Hardly so, or at least not yet. Undeniably, the settlement depends on the profitable survival of the evil industry, and the expectation that some 50 million Americans will dutifully continue to puff cigarettes and pay huge penalties. Have we changed the old song and dance about those dreadful cigarettes? Would the money go for public benefit or for some special interests? More at large, could something desirable lay hidden in what is bound to appear as a cynical story?

It could, and it all hinges on provisions laid out in the original settlement's draft considered by the 1997–98 Congress, which encouraged the development of less hazardous cigarettes. Because hostility to tobacco is motivated by the attributed health hazards, there could be light at the end of the tunnel if virtually safe cigarettes could come to dominate the market. If that should happen, then things would change substantially: perhaps the settlement would have had a moral face and purpose, and most of its sins might be forgiven. Are such cigarettes possible?

THE CASE FOR LESS HAZARDOUS CIGARETTES

According to antismoking wisdom a safe cigarette is one that is not lit, but it was not always so. From the late '60s and for a decade, the National Cancer Institute spent over $50 million in the Smoking and Health Program with the aim of developing less hazardous cigarettes.

More of this Program later, but its justification—fully vindicated in hindsight—was that smokers would continue to smoke against all dire warnings. The Program's hopes stood on two observations that are still valid today. One is that the risks of smoking decrease as the number of cigarettes smoked (the dose) decreases, and the other is that some components of smoke are toxic, but others—notably nicotine—may not be so in the amounts experienced by smokers. Therefore, an improved cigarette would reduce the amount of smoke inhaled, and would supply a smoke with fewer or no undesirable substances.

The National Cancer Institute's Program encouraged existing trends toward cigarettes of low yield but, more importantly, it contributed pivotal research and methods in defining smoke components and in understanding how and why people smoke. Toward the end of the '70s the Program was entering a more advanced and definitive phase, when it was shut down by antismokers who had come to run what was then the Department of Health, Education, and Welfare, and for whom nothing short of abolition was enough.

Still, the Program offered immediate incentives and at least one major manufacturer—the R.J. Reynolds Tobacco Company—tried marketing a credibly improved brand in the late '80s, only to be rebuffed with swift official opposition. The reaction discouraged further attempts until the tentative introduction in the late '90s of a second generation version of the original brand by the R.J. Reynolds Company and of a new brand by Philip Morris, both of radical design and of very limited appeal to smokers. In any event, the industry continued intensive research documented by scores of patents potentially applicable to less hazardous approaches. Such a technical legacy holds immediate promise if renewed efforts were to be encouraged, although one cannot help wondering—as noted before—what potential health benefits might have been lost in twenty years of forcible neglect at the hands of official abolitionist intransigence.

What would a less hazardous cigarette or a virtually safe one look like? The central role of nicotine in smoking is confirmed beyond doubt: cigarettes without nicotine fail to interest experienced smokers and beginners alike, as the marketing of a virtually nicotine-free cigarette by the Philip Morris Company has shown. The safety of nicotine at the doses experienced by smokers was first pointed out in the original U.S. Surgeon General report on smoking of 1964, which stated that "the low mortality ratios of pipe and cigar smokers, indicate that the chronic toxicity of nicotine in quantities absorbed from smoking and other methods of tobacco use is very low and probably does not represent an important health hazard" (*U.S. Surgeon General, 1964*).

This conclusion has been confirmed with increasing evidence, notably by the official Independent Committee on Smoking and Health in England, and by various researches (*Froggatt, 1988; Wald et al., 1981*). In the U.S., the Food and Drug Administration (FDA) now permits the free sale without prescription of nicotine patches and gums that contain more nicotine than a pack of cigarettes—devices that are commonplace and prescribed by doctors to 15 year old youngsters. Lately, the FDA has even permitted nicotine inhalers designed to compete with cigarettes, and there is now a legal international market of nicotine products in open competition with tobacco (*Werner et al., 1997*).

21

Smokers, of course, do not smoke for nicotine alone but also for other components that contribute to aroma and flavor, and that moderate the otherwise irritating impact of nicotine. Details would soon get arcane—and more of them later—but it is certain that cigarettes progressively less problematic from a health point of view can be made available. Naturally, they would require novel manufacturing methods and considerable research and testing to satisfy the public oversight of a regulatory agency, perhaps the FDA, if Congress should give that agency the necessary authority (*Supreme Court, 2000*).

As of the latter, the failed settlement draft considered by Congress in 1998 was assigning a paradoxical regulatory task to the FDA, asking the agency to enforce a reduction of nicotine to levels that presumably prevent addiction. Still, as also noted before, nicotine could not compare with hard drugs, and the charge of addiction could not stand separate from that of the long-term health risks attributed to smoking. But what if the risks of improved cigarettes were reduced to the level of soft drinks, hamburgers, candy, or whole milk? Under these circumstances the charge of addiction would become irrelevant, and would free the development of less hazardous cigarettes that may deliver enough nicotine and fewer or no undesirable components, and that could eliminate the annoyance of second hand smoke as an added bonus.

Thus, if a more promising picture is to emerge, official policy would have to install a cigarette oversight authority fully and openly aware that nicotine is not the problem in smoking. To do otherwise would be to persist in a profound misunderstanding of how cigarettes are made and used, and would paralyze any attempt to improve cigarettes.

A scenario of virtually safe cigarettes might likely raise novel problems. Innovative technical solutions for improved cigarettes may not be confined to the tobacco industry, and the pharmaceutical industry already has staked claims. Nothing would prevent other entrepreneurs from getting into the game and to establish a plurality of manufacturers. When that might happen, the traditional industry tied to current settlements may no longer be capable of meeting its obligations. At the same time, virtually safe cigarettes may render irrelevant certain current policies and settlements—a prospect unwelcome to assorted beneficiaries. But why should smokers' taxes go for roadwork and other general revenue projects unrelated to health (*Fairclough, 1999; Timberg, 1999; Jenkins, 1999, 2000*), when smokers already contribute to public coffers more than they receive?

Still, at the start it is traditional antismokers who should find ways to fulfill long-standing principles more efficiently. It is high time to abandon the zealous intransigence that made them irrelevant in the settlement games, that has blinded them to real opportunities, and that has made their abolitionist stance accountable for a multitude of preventable deaths. This awful responsibility negates any argument that less hazardous cigarettes might entice some smokers not to quit, and some nonsmokers to smoke. There should be incentives, not obstacles to innovation, and antismokers could have important roles in overseeing the gradual development of improved cigarettes for the benefit of the 50 million Americans who wish to smoke, and for untold more smokers worldwide.

As always, the excellent should not be the enemy of the good, because the alternative is not a pretty one. Without provisions to actively encourage better products—and by any sober and realistic appraisal—current settlements offer perverse incentives for a status quo tied to a market of traditionally hazardous cigarettes. Adding an exceedingly onerous tax burden will further deteriorate public health by inevitably fostering a black market that couldn't care less of improving cigarettes. Such a prospect of big time trouble is hardly in keeping with the image America likes to portray to the world: an exemplar society of freedom, fairness, justice, and enlightenment. At the threshold of a third millennium, America should rise to the occasion.

The Epidemiologic Evidence for Less Hazardous Cigarettes

The justification for less hazardous or virtually safe cigarettes derives directly from epidemiologic studies. All studies that have linked cigarette smoking with various diseases have also noted that the risks increase with the number of cigarettes smoked daily, with the intensity of inhalation, with how much of a cigarette is smoked, whether the cigarettes is filtered or not, and with other features that define the amount, i.e. the dose, of smoke inhaled. All studies show a sharp drop in risk as the dose inhaled decreases (*U.S. Surgeon General, 1964, 1979, 1989*).

Moreover, epidemiologic studies allow to calculate a dose that is compatible with virtually no discernible risk, namely a threshold dose at or below which risk is not significant (*Gori, 1976; Gori & Mantel, 1991*). Persons who inhale a daily equivalent to 3–4 cigarettes may not attain lung cancer risks significantly different from those of non-smokers as Tables 2, 3, and 4 show. Data in the Tables are obtained by statistical regression of epidemiologic dose-response data and are given as the upper limits of 95% confidence intervals whose lower limits are null risk values, according to the common procedure of regulatory practice (*Gori, 1976; Gori & Mantel, 1991; Gaylor et al., 1997*).

Table 2. Maximum levels of daily cigarette consumption at which lung cancer risk in male smokers may not be significantly increased from the risk of non-smokers (*from Gori & Mantel, 1991*).

Reference	Max. Cigarettes/day
British Doctors*	6.3
Swedish Men**	3.9
ACS 9 States***	5.4
ACS 25 States**	0.9
U.S. Veterans***	0.6
Canadian Veterans***	1.6
Japanese Men**	3.1
California Men***	· 7.0

*Doll and Peto, 1978
**U.S. Surgeon General, 1979. page 5-13 table 2.
***U.S. Surgeon General, 1982. page 38 table 6.

Table 3. Maximum levels of daily cigarette consumption at which risk for coronary heart disease mortality in male smokers may not be significantly increased from the risk of non-smokers, based on epidemiologic data (*from Gori & Mantel, 1991*).*

Reference	Max. Cigarettes/day
U.S. Veterans	1.5
ACS 9 States	2.5
Japanese Men	4.0
Canadian Veterans	4.5
British Physicians	4.5
Swedish Men	2.5
California Men	3.0
Swiss Physicians	3.0

*Epidemiologic data from U.S. Surgeon General, 1983, p. 118.

Table 4. Maximum levels of daily cigarette consumption at which risk for respiratory disease mortality in male smokers may not be significantly increased from the risk of non-smokers, based on epidemiologic data (*from Gori & Mantel, 1991*).*

Reference	Max. Cigarettes/day
Chronic Bronchitis	
U.S. Veterans	5.5
Canadian Veterans	2.6
Emphysema	
U.S. Veterans	2.2
Canadian Veterans	2.7
California Men	5.5
Bronchitis and Emphysema	
British Physicians	3.0

*Epidemiologic data from U.S. Surgeon General, 1984, p. 202.

It could be argued that this reasoning may be invalid if smokers of 3–4 cigarettes daily are atypical and may not inhale. This objection falls, however, when realizing that the threshold values of Tables 2, 3 and 4 come not from observations in light smokers alone, but are statistical extrapolations determined by the continuum of smoking intensity observations, from the highest to the lowest. Those values are valid derivations defined by the composite risk function of smokers at all levels of daily cigarette consumption (*Gori & Mantel, 1991*).

In any event, and besides it being obvious, multiple scientific reports sustain the reduction of risk to minimal or negligible levels as the amount of smoke inhaled decreases. Because the issue is important in considering less hazardous cigarettes, the next few pages review the most significant of those reports in a language that is often technical and that some might find obscure. Readers interested only at-large in the subject may safely skip to the next chapter.

No-effect observations at comparatively high doses are also routinely reported in experimental animal exposures to whole smoke or its fractions (*IARC, 1986*), and are also directly observable in epidemiologic studies. For instance, a compendium of 34 year follow-up data recently published for the Framingham study—the longest and most closely monitored epidemiologic study of its kind in the United States, which followed every aspect of the lives of several thousand people in that community—reports that adjusted lung cancer rates were not elevated for smokers of 1–10 cigarettes/day below age 65 (*Freund et al, 1993*). Similarly, the British Doctors study in England is widely regarded as the best continuing study and perhaps the best in the world. In that study, lung cancer mortality rates were the same in nonsmokers and in smokers of 1–14 cigarettes/day. Mortality from all diseases was actually slightly lower in smokers of 1–14 cigarettes/day than in non-smokers (*Doll et al., 1980*). To these reports one should add the evidence that moderate pipe and cigar smoking are not associated with increased risks of lung cancer and other diseases (*U.S. Surgeon General, 1964*).

It is also of interest that the studies listed in Tables 2, 3, and 4 pertain to smokers of pre-1960 cigarettes with average tar yields well over 25 milligrams per cigarette, nearly twice as much as the average for current cigarettes. Conceivably, the lower current cigarettes yields could make today's thresholds even higher than those listed in Tables 2, 3, and 4.

Direct epidemiologic evidence for no-observable-adverse-effect-levels (NOAELs) or thresholds for coronary heart disease (CHD) is even more impressive and direct, to the point of requiring no extrapolation. The prospective Framingham study report states: "For all CHD a clear relationship exist only for younger men. Women may have a slightly increased risk below age 65, while no relationship is seen for men or women past age 65" (*Freund et al., 1993*). However, for any smokers of 1–10 cigarettes/day the age adjusted rates are generally below the rates of nonsmokers. Age adjusted rates are also unchanged for lung cancer in any smokers of 1–10 cigarettes/day below age 65. These reports are consonant with previous reports from the

Framingham trial (*Kannel et al., 1987*).

The British Doctors study reported on mortality rates in female British doctors after 22 years of observation (*Doll et al., 1980*). There was no increase in mortality rates at any level of daily cigarette consumption for pulmonary heart disease. For ischemic heart disease and lung cancer, mortality rates were the same in nonsmokers and in smokers of 1–14 cigarettes/day. Mortality for all diseases was actually slightly lower in smokers of 1–14 cigarettes/day than in non-smokers.

For male British doctors, mortality rates in the group smoking 1–14 cigarettes/day were slightly elevated after 20 years of observation (*Doll & Peto, 1976*). However, extrapolation from dose/response functions, as shown above, indicates that mortality for cardiovascular diseases would not be elevated for smokers inhaling an evenly dispersed daily dose equivalent to 4–5 pre-1960 cigarettes (*Gori, 1976; Gori & Mantel, 1991*).

A large cohort study of white women in Maryland reported threshold effects (*Bush & Comstock, 1983*). The Western Collaborative Group Study also reported clear threshold values, especially after adjustment for type A personality confounding (*Jenkins et al., 1968*). Moreover, many studies would have likely reported threshold values if their lowest exposure category had been 10 or less cigarettes/day (*Oliver, 1974; PPRG, 1978; Rosenberg et al., 1985*).

To these reports one should add the generally accepted evidence that moderate pipe and cigar smoking are not associated with increased risks of lung cancer, cardiovascular, and respiratory illnesses. On this basis, the first U.S. Surgeon General's report on smoking and health, and others, concluded that nicotine and carbon monoxide are unlikely to have adverse cardiovascular effects, since their blood levels are quite similar in cigarette, pipe, and cigar smokers (*U.S. Surgeon General, 1964; Wald et al., 1981*). In regard to nicotine, this conclusion was also echoed officially by the Independent Scientific Committee on Smoking and Health of the United Kingdom (*Froggatt, 1988*).

The evidence of NOAEL thresholds for active smoking is not

confined to epidemiologic studies: it is also generally apparent in studies of the biomarkers and risk factors that are thought to have a pathognomic role. Indeed, thresholds should also be viewed in the context of the obvious resistance and defenses that humans must develop against xenobiotics from a variety of sources, and against the inevitable background of DNA damage from natural metabolic functions that cause an average of 10,000 measurable DNA modification events per hour in each mammalian cell (*Billen, 1990; Ames & Gold, 1991*).

It has been suggested that mutagens and carcinogens may have a role in the initiation and pathogenesis of CHDs. In this context, the meaning of the mutagenicity associated with smoking remains speculative. Extensive studies by the National Toxicology Program and other researchers have failed to validate mutagenicity as a predictor of carcinogenicity in animal bioassays or in man (*Ashby & Tennant, 1991; Zeiger et al., 1990; Tennant, 1988; IARC, 1987; USEPA, 1986; OECD, 1984*). Studies have also shown that the mutagenicity of smoker's urine is elevated only in smokers of over 10 cigarettes/day, offering other evidence of a threshold effect (*van Doorn et al., 1967; Mohtashamipur et al., 1985*). More recent studies report that—although mutagenic—cigarette smoking may actually protect against additional genotoxic insults (*Oesch et al., 1994*).

A review by the International Agency for Research on Cancer listed 10 studies that could not find differences in sister chromatid exchange (SCE) frequencies in peripheral lymphocytes of smokers and non-smokers, while studies reporting a dose/response gradient were consistent with a NOAEL threshold for smoking less than 10 cigarettes/day (*IARC, 1986, pp. 191–192*).

Following nuclease P1 enrichment techniques, DNA adducts were detected in oral tissues, but the adduct burden in smokers of 1–10 cigarettes/day was not different from the burden in nonsmokers, giving another confirmation of threshold (*Jones et al., 1993*).

Hypotheses have proposed that increased blood clotting

capacity may explain the association of heavy smoking and cardiovascular events. However, the Framingham study reports an absence of cardiovascular risks for smokers of 1–10 cigarettes/day, consonant with an immaterial change in mean fibrinogen (about 1%) in smokers of less than 1 pack of cigarettes/day (*Kannel et al., 1987*). It has been suggested that two eicosanoids, prostacyclin and thromboxane A2 are altered in smokers, but studies indicate no change in smokers of less than 10–15 cigarettes/day (*Wennmalm et al., 1991*).

A study of 51,723 participants of community-based cholesterol screening clinics in 10 U.S. cities found no association between active smoking and plasma cholesterol levels in men and women over age 60, and no elevation of plasma cholesterol for younger subjects smoking less than 10 cigarettes/day (*Muscat et al., 1991*).

These considerations tell that the active smoking of less than 10 cigarettes/day is unlikely to adversely influence lipidemic CHD risk factors. As such, they support the notion of NOAELs for active smoking and cardiovascular diseases. In fact, the National Cholesterol Education Program only lists smoking of over 10 cigarettes/day as a possible risk factor (*NCEP, 1988*).

Compromised ventilatory function has been suggested as a possible risk factor for CHDs, however there is evidence for respiratory NOAELs in the reported associations with active smoking. Early reports of forced respiratory volume (FEV1) and forced vital capacity (FVC) deficits in smokers are still compatible with NOAEL thresholds below 10 cigarettes/day (*Dockery et al., 1988; Sorlie et al., 1986*).

A threshold effect at some 10 cigarettes/day was also reported for emphysema in asthmatic patients (*Kondoh et al., 1990*). Elastin peptide concentration in circulation has been suggested as a marker of lung elastin degradation and thus of emphysematous changes. A recent study found no correlation between elastin peptide concentration and smoking (*Frette et al., 1994*). Another study found that severity of microscopic emphysema did not

31

increase with daily cigarette consumption (*Gillooly & Lamb, 1993*).

The possible effects of carbon monoxide (CO) on the cardiovascular system are largely based on inferences from dated claims (*Aronow, 1978*). In general, such claims held that 1–2% CO concentrations trigger angina episodes, even though they are close to typical background ambient concentrations. Such claims have been difficult to accept because most epidemiologic studies of active smoking report no-effect thresholds for angina at well over 10 cigarettes smoked per day, as noted above. Over the years Aronow's claims have been criticized as suffering from a number of technical and design problems (*Sheps et al., 1987*).

The National Academy of Sciences had this to say: "There were some subjective elements in the evaluation of these patients, and the physician conducting these tests was aware of the test conditions, i.e., smoking or not, and ventilated or not. Consequently, the findings of this study, in the absence of a true double-blind approach, require verification by other research workers" (*NAS, 1986*).

In regard to the possible aggravation of angina by CO, a National Academy report and EPA regulations consider that such effects may occur at carboxyhemoglobin (COHb) blood concentrations above 3% (*NAS, 1986 p.261; USEPA, 1984*). Because this is a risk management figure with an ample safety margin, the true threshold would be substantially higher. In any event, a 3% COHb level is seldom reached even in heavy smokers (*NAS, 1986; IARC, 1986; Jarvis et al., 1983*). Moreover, the first U.S. Surgeon General's report found no adverse cardiovascular effects in moderate pipe and cigar smokers despite CO exposures similar to or higher than those of cigarette smokers (*U.S. Surgeon General, 1964*).

The evidence for no-effect-thresholds is even more clamorous in the case of overall morbidity, which refers to the frequency of disease and disability for smokers and nonsmokers while they are alive. The 1979 U.S. Surgeon General's report on smoking and health in the U.S. reports that overall and specific morbidity *was considerably reduced* in smokers of fewer than 20 cigarettes per day, a finding confirmed by official U.S. studies by the National Center for Health Statistics, and by a more recent official survey of the Health Department of Australia (*Wilson, 1967; U.S. Surgeon General, 1979, pp. 3–9, 3–10; Australian Bureau of Statistics, 1994*). As an aside, it is interesting to speculate about the reasons for the puzzling official reluctance to encourage reports on this topic, especially because clear and strong evidence has been officially available at least since 1965.

The intransigent opinion enforced by public authorities in the United States has been to deny that safe threshold doses exist, especially for any agent or situation suspected of causing cancer. This opinion is a matter of dogma and without factual support, because no-effect thresholds of exposure must exist or else no one could survive without cancer and other diseases. In any event, and without conceding to this opinion, it should still be transparent that reducing doses of smoke intake could reduce the risks of smoking to levels that are a fraction of the average risks reported by epidemiologic studies of smoking and disease.

Hence the twin concepts of moderation in smoking and of less hazardous cigarettes cannot escape in any consideration of public health opportunities. Yet, both a message of moderation and the encouragement of better cigarettes have been strenuously opposed by the abolitionist antismoking crusade, despite the tragic ineffectiveness of its policies. Even if less hazardous cigarettes may not completely eliminate the risks of smoking, it is clear they could come very near to achieving that goal. The numbers of premature deaths that could be spared is potentially so large as to dwarf the preventive projections of the Environmental Protection Agency and the Food and Drug Administration, which together might hypothetically prevent a few thousand premature deaths a year at best (*Gough, 1990*). Thus, a philosophy of moderation and of less hazardous or virtually safe cigarettes is undoubtedly a much closer and compassionate approach to the reality of human frailties and needs. As such, it has an excellent prospect of becoming a major contribution to public health.

CHAPTER THREE

How Cigarettes Are Made and Work

This section cannot be a comprehensive characterization of the science and technology about the tobacco plant and related agricultural practices, the curing of tobacco leaves, and the design and the engineering of cigarettes—all matters that are treated in greater detail in more technical literature (*Davis & Nielsen, 1999*). Here, a thumbnail review is provided to cover what is needed to understand the manifold complexities of what appears as a deceptively simple device, and the opportunities for the development of less hazardous cigarettes.

THE TOBACCO PLANT

Tobacco belongs to the *Solanaceae* family and is closely related to potatoes, tomatoes, peppers, eggplants, and the night-shade (*Atropa belladonna*), all of which contain varying measures of nicotine. The genus of tobacco is *Nicotiana*, of which the most common variety is *N. tabacum*. The plant presents a stalk 5 to 7 feet tall, around which broad leaves grow: larger at the ground and generally smaller towards the top. Among components and features that contribute to the aromatic and stimulant properties of smoke, the most significant is the alkaloid nicotine. Other alkaloids are present in the tobacco plant, but none approach the importance of nicotine, which remains the principal agent for the pharmacologic and physiologic rewards of smoking (*Tso, 1999*).

From the point of view of the plant, nicotine is an effective pesticide. Its concentration in *N. tabacum* varies up to some 5% in the higher leaves on the stalk, and gradually lower below. The average nicotine content of traditional commercial leaf is in the order of 2%. Higher maximum concentrations can be obtained by selection or cultivation practices, but they are progressively toxic to the plant itself, and result in plants that are smaller and stunted. Moreover, nicotine concentrations much above 3% in cigarette tobacco result in smokes that are irritant and unpleasant.

The harvested green leaves are first dried according to either of two distinct processes: air drying and flue-curing. The former involves hanging the whole plant or its leaves in open-air but covered barns until dry. It results in leaves that are dark in color after undergoing a series of fermentations that have changed their chemical composition: the most significant change being a major loss of sugars. The scarcity of sugars contributes to relatively more alkaline and harsher-feeling smokes from air cured leaves, the most common of which are the Burley, Maryland, and cigar leaf varieties.

The flue-curing process utilizes enclosed barns wherein a source of heat dries the harvested leaves far more quickly than in the air-drying process, thus preventing fermentation and the loss of many leaf components. The process actually increases the relative concentration of reducing sugars, and leaf so treated generates relatively more acidic and milder-feeling smokes. Flue-cured tobacco includes most commonly the Virginia, Carolina, and Georgia leaf varieties.

In general, subtle changes in the acidity of the smoke change the physical conditions of nicotine and its interaction with irritation receptors in the mouth and throat: harshness becoming more pronounced as smoke becomes more alkaline. Later on, the importance of this issue will be considered in more detail.

After curing, all leaf still produces unsuitable smokes and needs to undergo an aging process. It usually entails tight packing in wooden containers (hogsheads), which are kept in controlled atmosphere storage for up to 3 years. During that time additional slow fermentations and other changes occur, resulting in finished leaf ready for cigarette manufacture. One advantage of the multi-annual curing process is the availability of large stores of aged tobacco. Those stores afford manufacturers the latitude of overcoming year-to-year variations in leaf quality and composition, and in attaining a degree of product uniformity (*Tso, 1999*).

Possible tobacco modifications toward less hazardous cigarettes include changes in the chemical and structural nature of the leaf, which are obtained by genetic or agricultural means, by solvent extraction of selected components, by physical expansion of the leaf matrix to increase its volume but not its weight, and by transformation of the leaf and leaf parts with paper-making processes that permit the removal of selected components and the inclusion of functional additives.

THE PROCESSING OF TOBACCO INTO CIGARETTES

In the United States, American cigarette manufacturers buy virtually all tobaccos grown in the country. Thus, American cigarettes are manufactured from a blend of all leaf varieties grown in the United States, plus around 10% of some aromatic air-dried leaf varieties from the Middle East. After blending, aged leaf is conditioned to an appropriate moisture content and is shredded in narrow strips. Processing of tobacco generates considerable leaf fragments—known as fines—which are transformed into what is known as reconstituted tobacco sheet by methods and machinery close to those of paper-making (*Norman, 1999*).

Some components that could be altered during this transformation, including nicotine, are extracted from the fines before paper-making operations, and then added back to the finished product. Inert diluents such as clays may be added to the sheet as fillers or extenders. Usually the process requires high temperatures similar to those encountered in food-processing. These temperatures induce well-known flavor-enhancing Maillard reactions between sugars and nitrogen-containing compounds—reactions that can be promoted by the addition of small quantities of ammonium salts and/or ammonia, analogous to standard procedures in food processing, the roasting of coffee, and so on. Reconstituted tobacco sheets are then treated as regular leaf, shredded, and added to cigarette blends in amounts that usually do not exceed 15–20% (*Norman, 1999; Fisher, 1999*).

Subtle differences in the proportions of leaf varieties and reconstituted tobacco characterize the blend compositions of different cigarette brands.

Traditional additives to these blends include humectants to prevent excessive drying of cigarettes upon storage (usually glycerol), various amounts of reducing sugars (usually glucose or fructose), and proprietary fragrance compositions that further differentiate brand characteristics.

CIGARETTE STRUCTURE

Final blends formulated for individual brands are fed to cigarette-making machines that channel blends into the cylindrical shapes of cigarettes, wrapped in paper, with or without a filter tip at one end. Cigarettes are then packaged in packs of usually twenty units, ten packs per carton, sixty cartons per case, ready for shipment.

The paper that wraps a cigarette can have different porosity or permeability to air, which can affect the amount of air that is drawn in, and that mixes with and dilutes smoke during puffing of a lit cigarette. Because they affect the influx of air and oxygen, the porosity and combustibility of paper can also affect the burning characteristics of cigarettes. Filters of different efficiency also affect the ease of flow, the pressure drop within the cigarette, the amount and velocity of air influx, and thus the combustion process itself. Similarly, most modern cigarettes are provided with a series of tiny radial holes along the circumference of the filter end, away from the mouthpiece. These ventilation holes allow air to be drawn in and to be mixed with the smoke as the lit cigarette is puffed, also contributing to modulate the combustion process and to diluting the smoke (*Norman, 1999*).

Today, cigarette paper, filters, ventilation holes, and reconstituted tobacco are by far the major factors that contribute to differentiate commercial cigarette brands, as these characteristics affect the combustion process and hence the composition of the smoke, the dilution of the smoke with air and hence the density of the smoke and its taste and harshness, the ease by which puffs are drawn, and the number of puffs that can be obtained from a cigarette, also depending on how fast it will burn. Still, despite subtle differences the actual tobacco blend compositions of American cigarettes is similar. Virtually all American cigarettes contain somewhat less that 1 gr of tobacco each, which translates into a uniform content of somewhat less than 20 mg of nicotine per cigarette, regardless of brand.

CIGARETTE COMBUSTION AND SMOKE FORMATION

When a cigarette is first lit, a burning zone is established that usually takes the shape of a conical coal with the apex pointing away from the cigarette. This burning cone has roughly 3 layers: the outermost is ash, the center one is the burning coal proper, and the last one is made up of the first layer of tobacco that begins to be transformed and burned by the heat of the coal. Usually, the paper wrapper of the cigarette burns up to the level of the burning coal proper, leaving a narrow gap between the circumference of the paper and that of the coal itself. When the cigarette is puffed, air is drawn in through that gap and supplies oxygen to the burning coal which is induced to advance further into the cigarette, and to burn more tobacco and more paper with each subsequent puff. The coal also advances by smoldering between puffs, albeit at much reduced speed and while producing what is known as side-stream smoke (*Baker, 1999*).

The temperature of the burning coal is about 800–900 Centigrades when puffed, and falls to some 600–500 Centigrades between puffs. During puffs, air that is drawn around the coal carries the coal's heat toward the unburnt tobacco in a plume of temperature that cools very rapidly. At some 10 millimeters behind the burning coal the temperature is essentially the same as outside the cigarette. Yet, it is in those 10 millimeters that smoke generates through very complex chemical and physical events that are only partially understood.

Essentially, smoke is the product of the incomplete combustion of tobacco through processes of pyrolysis and distillation that vaporize materials at the high temperatures immediately behind the burning cone. These vapors soon recondense in a fog of microscopic droplets that are entrained in the rapidly cooling air-stream flowing through the cigarette, eventually exiting as smoke at the filter end.

Of the components of tobacco, those that vaporize at the lowest temperatures have the better chance of surviving intact in the smoke itself, while other materials will increasingly experience more and more severe transformation as their volatility decreases. Thus, flavors and nicotine usually survive substantially intact and transfer well into smoke, but cellulose, waxes, proteins, sugars, and other substances undergo dramatic transformations. Materials that cannot burn end up in ashes.

The smoke itself is made up of a gas phase in which billions of very small droplets are suspended. The droplets make up the particle phase of smoke, which eventually is reduced to what is commonly known as tar. The amount of smoke delivered by a cigarette will depend on how the cigarette is smoked, namely on the number of puffs taken and the volume and duration of the puffs. A standard testing procedure was adopted over 30 years ago by the Federal Trade Commission (FTC) and adopted fairly uniformly around the world (*FTC, 1966*).

The procedure entails the smoking of cigarettes on machines that take one puff of 35 milliliters volume and two second duration every minute, until cigarettes are consumed. The smoke thus generated is passed through a filter pad where the retained particulate can be weighted to yield the amount of tar produced. The tar weight can be expressed as either wet or dry, the latter after eliminating the entrained water. Nicotine transfers in smoke within the tar particles and is likewise retained in the filter, and can be weighted separately. It has always been understood that the yields of tar and nicotine measured by the FTC method are specific to the method and cannot represent actual yields to individual smokers who exhibit changing patterns of puff volume, duration, and frequency (*FTC, 1966*).

Over 4000 components of cigarette smoke have been identified, many of them with known carcinogenic or otherwise toxic properties when considered individually (*Baker, 1999*). Still, the relatively low concentration of most components and the likely presence of competitive suppressing interactions end up giving a very low immediate or short-term toxicity to smoke. Leading investigators have concluded that cigarette smoke acts more as a promoter of cancer and other negative effects, which become apparent only after chronic exposure to smoke over several decades (*Doll, 1978; Doll & Peto, 1978; Klawanski & Fox, 1984; Altshuler, 1989; Albert, 1989*).

Hope had been raised that the best known carcinogens and other toxicants present in smoke could be selectively removed in an attempt to reduce the chronic effects of exposure. Some reductions have been achieved, but their benefits have remained prospective because some specific reductions are usually accompanied by the increase of other problematic components. Continuing research in this direction is bound to be fruitful, and there is recent indication that at least tobacco related nitrosamines might be amenable to substantial selective removal (*O'Donnell & Williams, 1998*).

CHAPTER FOUR

Developing Less Hazardous Cigarettes at The National Cancer Institute

The accumulation of epidemiologic reports about the risks of smoking was peaking by the mid 50's, but it elicited mixed reactions from the public health establishment of the time. The official position was cautious and unwilling to precipitate what appeared as premature control measures. Mutually reinforcing considerations for this caution were a perceived absence of scientific objectivity in the epidemiologic reports, a reluctance to impose policies not objectively justified, and a culture that embraced a tradition of tobacco use as an expression of high fashion.

Dr. Alexander Gilliam was head of epidemiologic research at the National Cancer Institute and was openly discounting the causal roles of reported smoking risks (*Gilliam, 1954*). He was steeped in the experimental tradition of infectious diseases and was skeptical of the new techniques that characterized the epidemiologic studies of cancer, cardiovascular, and other multifactorial diseases.

Unlike infections—caused by specific bacteria, viruses, parasites, and other necessary causes—multifactorial diseases are associated statistically with many risk factors, none of which appear to be necessary or sufficient causes of the diseases.

Generally speaking, the epidemiologic investigations of multifactorial diseases are unable to disentangle the complex causal networks of such diseases, and cannot approach their study in the controlled experimental framework that scientific testing requires. Those investigations were and are still characterized as being observational, in the sense that they lack the randomized structure of proper test and control comparisons, and are not sustained by the experimental verification of specific causes.

It is of note that the controversy about the evidentiary meaning of multifactorial epidemiology has not subsided and continues to this day, when leading epidemiologists candidly agree about the seemingly insurmountable obstacles plaguing their discipline (*Taubes, 1995*). These difficulties have been best and succinctly described by Sir Richard Doll, arguably a dean of modern epidemiology, who wrote with his colleague Richard Peto:

"[E]pidemiological observations...have serious disadvantages... [T]hey can seldom be made according to the strict requirements of experimental science and therefore may be open to a variety of interpretations. A particular factor may be associated with some disease merely because of its association with some other factor that causes the disease, or the association may be an artifact due to some systematic bias in the information collection...

[I]t is commonly, but mistakenly, supposed that multiple regression, logistic regression, or various forms of standardization can routinely be used to answer the question: 'Is the correlation of exposure (E) with disease (D) due merely to a common correlation of both with some confounding factor (or factors) (C)?... Moreover, it is obvious that multiple regression cannot correct for important variables that have not been recorded at all...

[T]hese disadvantages limit the value of observations in humans, but...until we know exactly how cancer is caused and how some factors are able to modify the effects of others, the need to observe imaginatively what actually happens to various different categories of people will remain" (*Doll & Peto, 1981, page 1218*).

Of course, the need to investigate the causes of human diseases was and still is pressing. Yet, in the late '50s most health officials were more of a traditional and sober scientific persuasion than interventionist advocates. They would not hesitate to endorse coercive public action to control the well-known causes of cholera, typhus, yellow fever, polio, malaria, and other infections, but were reluctant to issue public warnings and lifestyle prescriptions on the basis of "imaginative" interpretations of statistical constructs that were lacking proper scientific corroboration.

Over time, albeit with persistent controversy, the concept of multifactorial causation found its way in public health, along with profound changes in the cultural perceptions of what are the acceptable limits of official intervention. Today, a relaxed concept of causation is the basis for most regulatory action in health, safety, and the environment. Its use is sustained not by scientific arguments but by judgments and considerations about collective prudence that current public health administrators feel entitled to define. By contrast, public opinion and public health officials in the '50s still felt that prudence was a private matter of individual choice, and that public intervention required some objective justification.

At that time, the scientific reserve of Dr. Gilliam was shared and enhanced by the influence of prominent pathologists at the National Cancer Institute, Drs. Harold Stewart and Wilhelm Hueper, who together were reluctant to propose public health action in smoking and health, on account of what they saw as weak causal evidence (*Garnett, 1998*). Dr. James Shannon, director of the National Institutes of Health, was himself extremely cautious in endorsing causal roles to cigarette smoking and in proposing public health action (*Breslow et al. 1978, vol. 2, pp. 609–613*).

At higher policy levels, during a 1957 hearing the Surgeon

General Leroy Burney and the director of the National Cancer Institute, Dr. John Heller, told Congress they could not see compelling scientific or policy reasons for public health warning messages and other federal interventions in the matter of tobacco smoking (*Burney & Heller, 1957*). Undoubtedly, their positions reflected the mood of that time, when cigarettes were still highlights of fashion in a sympathetic culture that traced its origins to the singular role of tobacco as the economic engine of America's early centuries. A long tradition of popular lore had been that smoking might comport some health risk, but no substantial scientific reports had raised concern that cigarettes might be a defective product.

Eventually, a more proactive role was assumed by the subsequent Surgeon General, Dr. Luther Terry. With encouragement and assistance from the American Cancer Society and other advocacy organizations, Dr. Terry succeeded in motivating the national media in shaping a more public role for the office of the Surgeon General, and was instrumental in producing the famous 1964 report that marked a watershed in public policy and action in smoking and health (*Brandt, 1990; Parascandola, 1997*).

Still, the compilers of the 1964 report were uneasy about direct assertions of causation and took care to warn that: "[s]tatistical methods cannot establish proof of a causal relationship in an association. The causal significance of an association is a matter of judgment which goes beyond any statement of statistical probability" (*U.S. Surgeon General, 1964, p. 20*). In essence it was an admission that the report's conclusions were the consensual judgment of a committee rather than based on independent scientific evidence. Parallel developments also took place in England at about the same time, and similar policy positions on both sides of the Atlantic became mutually reinforcing. These policies inaugurated a dialectical/consensual approach to the resolution of causality issues that to this day pervades risk assessment practices in public health and regulation throughout the western world. So far the practice has survived repeated challenges, although many commentators have continued to voice concern about the apparent inversion of roles, whereby policy speaks to science (*Berridge, 1999; Wildavsky, 1995; Collingridge & Reeve, 1986*).

In the wake of this 1964 landmark report, top officials at the National Cancer Institute (NCI) confronted the need of addressing cigarette smoking and lung cancer. Their actions also reflected the mood of the time, when about half of the adult and voting population of the United States were smokers, and there were still lingering questions over the interpretation of epidemiologic reports about the risks of smoking. At that time abolitionist ideas were not credible because most people had close memories of the alcohol prohibition catastrophe of a few decades earlier, and everyone was persuaded that people would continue to smoke despite all warnings. What is more, most decision-makers in high public health positions were smokers (*Wynder, 1997*).

Encouraged by the universal observation that the risk of smoking was proportional to the dose inhaled, the NCI under the direction of Dr. Kenneth Endicott saw the opportunity of a research program to investigate the development of less hazardous cigarettes. In mid 1968 the NCI Smoking and Health Program was formally chartered after extensive consultation and the broad approval of Dr. James Shannon, director of the National Institutes of Health, and of the directors of the National Heart, Lung, and Blood Institute, and of the National Institute of Environmental Health Sciences. Consensus also came from the Office of the Secretary of the Department of Health, Education, and Welfare.

Initial plans were set by a selected group of scientists at the Institute who were familiar with experimental carcinogenesis, following observations that cancer could be produced in animals by the administration of certain substances, that the cancer response was roughly proportional to the dose applied, and that different substances had different potencies of cancer induction. Attempts to produce cancer in animals by the administration of whole smoke by inhalation had not been successful, but test methods had been developed by painting tar solutions on the dorsal skin of mice, where tumors could eventually arise. Thus, skin painting of tars in mice was considered to be a useful screening test, especially since prior experience had already concluded that virtually all carcinogenic principles of cigarette smoke were confined to the smoke's particulate or tar, rather than to the gas phase (*U.S. Surgeon General, 1964; IARC, 1986*).

On the strength of this initial assessment, the NCI management decided it would be reasonable to test whether specific cigarette modifications could result in lower tar production, and in tars that had lower capacity to induce tumors in experimental animals. Much hope was given initially to the possibility of selectively removing specific smoke components. Other considerations were that modified cigarettes should maintain certain traditional characteristics that would make them acceptable to smokers, such as overall appearance, burning and smoldering rates, resistance to puff drawing, and the like.

At that time, no one outside of the cigarette industry had a good idea of what making cigarettes was all about, and it became apparent that a successful program would have to rely on the cooperation of industry experts. The tobacco industry had an obvious interest in developing less hazardous cigarettes that could be commercially successful, and although not apparent at that time, most manufacturers had run considerable research in this direction, but were concerned that open efforts to improve cigarettes could encourage litigation. Thus, the industry proved very much willing to cooperate with a project run by the NCI, and the research directors of the main American cigarette manufacturers joined the advisory committee to the NCI's Smoking and Health Program, known as the Tobacco Working Group (TWG).

This advisory committee included a majority of scientists from

Table 5. Scientists who served on the Tobacco Working Group

1968–70	Carl G. Baker, National Cancer Institute
1972–75	William W. Bates, Liggett & Myers Tobacco Company
1977–77	Sam P. Battista, Arthur D. Little, Inc.
1968–77	Fred G. Bock, Roswell Park Memorial Institute
1968–73	Roswell K. Boutwell, University of Wisconsin
1968–70	Hans L. Falk, National Institute of Environmental Health Sciences
1973–77	Alfred Fishman, Hospital of the University of Pennsylvania
1974–75	Jean D. Gibbons, University of Alabama
1969–77	Gio B. Gori, National Cancer Institute
1972–77	Michael R. Guerin, Oak Ridge National Laboratory
1974–77	Ian Higgins, University of Michigan
1973–75	Dietrich Hoffmann, American Health Foundation
1972–77	Ivor W. Hughes, Brown & Williamson Tobacco Company
1968–76	Charles J. Kensler, Arthur D. Little, Inc.
1968–69	Paul Kotin, National Institute of Environmental Health Sciences
1973–77	Henry C. McGill, University of Texas
1969–77	Gardner C. McMillan, National Heart, Lung and Blood Institute
1968–70	Ian A. Mitchell, Office of the Secretary, Department of Health, Education, and Welfare.
1972–77	Thomas B. Owen, National Cancer Institute
1976–77	Alan Rodgman, R. J. Reynolds Tobacco Company
1968–74	Umberto Saffiotti, National Cancer Institute
1968–74	Marvin A. Schneiderman, National Cancer Institute
1976–77	Robert B. Seligman, Philip Morris Tobacco Company
1972–74	Irving J. Selikoff, Mt. Sinai School of Medicine
1968–76	Murray Senkus, R. J. Reynolds Tobacco Company
1974–75	Philippe Shubik, Eppley Institute for Research in Cancer
1968–77	Alexander W. Spears, Lorillard Tobacco Company
1968–69	Jesse L. Steinfeld, National Cancer Institute
1968–77	T. C. Tso, Agricultural Research Service, U.S. Department of Agriculture
1968–74	Benjamin L. Van Duuren, New York University
1968–76	Helmut Wakeham, Philip Morris Tobacco Company
1968–73	Ernst L. Wynder, American Health Foundation

the NCI, from the National Heart, Lung, and Blood Institute, from the National Institute of Environmental Health Sciences, from the Secretary's Office of the Department of Health, Education, and Welfare (DHEW), from the Department of Agriculture, and from academic institutions. Members who served on the TWG over the years are listed in Table 5. Dr. Carl Baker, then director of NCI's Etiology Division and shortly after director of the Institute, was the first chairman of the TWG. Among other duties, I was first assigned as executive secretary to the committee, and became its chairman and director of the Smoking and Health Program in 1969, when actual operations began.

The range of the affiliations and of the scientific interests of TWG members attests to the broad support of the Smoking and Health Program within the U.S. Department of Health, Education, and Welfare, and to the notable intellectual and scientific resources the program enjoyed. While the TWG defined the scientific and technical directions, the Smoking and Health Program also required and received supervision and annual approval from the National Cancer Advisory Board that had general oversight of the National Cancer Institute, and from the President's Cancer Panel reporting directly to the President of the United States (*NCI, 1968–80*). In addition, the affiliation with the National Heart, Lung, and Blood Institute required supervision and approvals from the National Advisory Board of that Institute. From time to time, the program was also presented and discussed at Congressional hearings, and received the frequent attention of national and international media.

During its first year, the TWG concentrated on becoming acquainted with the cigarette-making processes and with deciding what modifications could be initially addressed. Funds were set aside for the program and laboratories were identified that could produce tar from modified cigarettes, that could characterize cigarettes and the tars by chemical analysis, that could execute the skin painting tests in mice, that could analyze the results by histopathology, and that could produce statistical analyses of the data. A reference cigarette was also identified and produced in sufficient quantities at the University of Kentucky, so that research results could be compared against a uniform standard.

There were four sets of experimental cigarettes produced and tested between 1970 and 1977, and they are listed in Appendix B. These 150 or so modifications covered various aspects of cigarette design, tobacco varieties and modifications, additives, reconstituted tobacco, and tobacco substitutes. All cigarettes were produced without charge by various cigarette manufacturers, adding up to over 70 million pieces. The tar from these cigarettes was produced with the aid of newly designed machines capable of smoking several thousand cigarettes per hour. The smokes of experimental cigarettes were extensively analyzed and characterized by a special unit at Oak Ridge National Laboratories under the direction of Dr. Michael Guerin. Testing the tumor-inducing potency (tumorigenicity or carcinogenicity) of experimental tars was conducted on over 40,000 mice at various laboratories. Additional research and quality control were provided by Drs. Ernst Wynder and Dietrich Hoffmann at the American Health Foundation in New York, at Arthur D. Little Laboratories in Cambridge, Massachusetts, under the direction of Dr. Charles Kensler, and at the U.S. Department of Agriculture under the direction of Dr. T.C. Tso.

Despite many efforts and the extensive assistance of affiliated research teams, a substantial selective removal of undesirable components from tobacco smoke proved unattainable in practice. More generically, however, the results made it clear that modifications could attain variations of tar tumorigenicity in the order of 20–30% and even greater, as for instance in the case of experimental cigarettes made from tobacco leaf stems, and from artificial tobacco substitutes. Still, most experimental cigarettes were radical departures from what could be considered functional cigarettes. In general, cigarettes modifications were specifically designed to determine the effects of certain components and design characteristics, and their results could not be readily or easily translated into actual products.

Many modifications were dramatically successful in reducing the amount of tar that could be produced from a cigarette, some yielding as much as 95% less tar than the standard reference cigarette (*SHP, 1976a, 1976b, 1977, 1979*). Together, these experiments provided valuable information about the methods for modifying and reducing the amount of tar delivered by cigarettes, although limitations in transferring those findings to practice encouraged the exploration of other opportunities.

The NCI efforts and interests were soon expanded by those of the National Heart, Lung, and Blood Institute (NHLBI) that provided additional funds and expertise. With this partnership, the NCI's interests were focusing on cancer, and those of the NHLBI were to address those aspects of smoking that might be responsible for cardiovascular and respiratory risks. Of principal interest were tars and their components, nicotine, carbon monoxide, nitrogen oxides, and a few other. Their precursors in tobacco—from seeds to processed blends—and in cigarette components and design were the primary targets of new cigarette modifications.

The combined interest of the two Institutes addressed the development of animal models that could test whole smoke by inhalation, as the only way to study cardiovascular and respiratory effects, and early precursor changes of cancer interest. Various efforts explored the possibility of such models in mice, rats, hamsters, dogs, and primates. They were supported by the parallel development of accessory analytical tools, notably those for the detection of the extremely low levels of nicotine in the blood of smokers and experimental animals.

It was common understanding at the time that nicotine had a central role in smoking, and that less hazardous cigarettes could not be acceptable without nicotine being present. In fact, by 1976 the NCI's Smoking and Health Program had already conducted clinical trials where a nicotine aerosol administered to smokers was shown to reduce dramatically the smokers' interest in cigarettes (*SHP, 1979*). In addition, the epidemiologic record indicated that nicotine may not have significant adverse effects, as had been noted in the original 1964 U.S. Surgeon General Report on smoking, which had concluded that :

"There is no acceptable evidence that prolonged exposure to nicotine creates either dangerous functional changes of an objective nature or degenerative diseases . . . The fact that the over-all death rates of pipe and cigar smokers show little if any increase over non-smokers is very difficult to reconcile with a concept of high nicotine toxicity . . . . [I]t follows logically that the apparent increase in morbidity and mortality among cigarette smokers relates to exposure to substances in smoke other than nicotine" (*U.S. Surgeon General, 1964, p. 74*).

These considerations were the subject of discussions in the early '70s within the Smoking and Health Program, and helped to formulate a concept of less hazardous cigarettes that would retain sufficient nicotine but that would reduce tar and other components. In fact, this concept and some of the lessons learned from the testing of modified cigarettes already were soon being translated into several "lite" cigarette brands that began to appear on the market by the mid '70s.

At the same time it was apparent that available epidemiologic reports reflected the effects of smoke as a whole, namely of the peculiar synergistic or antagonistic interactions of its traditional components. Thus, it became of concern that substantial modifications of cigarettes might bring about novel chemical and biological interactions, possibly with toxic modes unknown in the smokes of traditional cigarettes.

This concern made it imperative to investigate the potential adverse effects of the modification of nicotine levels in cigarettes and in smoke in relation to parallel modifications of tobacco and cigarette design that might reduce tar and other components. Of all inhalation tests under development, the one in beagles turned out to be most suited for these investigations (*SHP, 1975*). The procedure had been planned jointly with the National Heart, Lung, and Blood Institute and with assistance from top experts in the United States. It demanded meticulous preparatory work for several years, especially in the design and standardization of the necessary smoking machines and of the exposure conditions.

The SHP also began producing quantities of cigarettes that would yield the same amount of tar but different amounts of nicotine, prepared by removing from or adding nicotine to a standard tobacco blend, and by utilizing agronomically selected high nicotine tobacco varieties (*Tso, 1972; SHP, 1979*). Eventually, several large inhalation studies were underway by 1975, with the aim of testing the effects of changing levels of nicotine, carbon monoxide, and nitrogen oxides. This new and advanced stage of research of the SHP had all the promise of success, and the program was broadly admired and praised. In 1976, the director of the SHP received the Public Health Service Superior Service Award on account of the notable achievements of the Program. Activities were due to continue well if it had not been for the sudden policy reversals that took place in mid-1977 at the Department of Health, Education, and Welfare (DHEW), the head agency of the NCI, the NHLBI, and the Smoking and Health Program.

With the advent of the Carter Administration, the DHEW policy toward smoking changed from a pragmatic, multifaceted approach cognizant that large numbers of Americans would continue to smoke despite all warnings, to an abolitionist policy of intransigence aiming at the forcible eradication of cigarettes and tobacco products in general. This policy maintained that any and all cigarettes were unsafe, and found incompatible any and all efforts to develop less hazardous cigarettes. As a result, all research efforts in this direction were canceled.

By the end of 1979 virtually all SHP activities toward the development of less hazardous cigarettes were halted, funds were withdrawn, research programs were terminated before completion, staff was removed or reassigned. The loss of several promising inhalation studies that had been set up at great effort and expense was especially lamentable. Only one of those studies was ever completed, although its conclusions were not published. Not surprisingly, those conclusions were in sharp contrast with the new policy at DHEW. The completed study was the result of a major collaboration with the National Heart, Lung, and Blood Institute, and was set to test the effects of tar, nicotine, and carbon monoxide levels in various combinations of intensity, coupled with a high cholesterol diet known to induce atherosclerosis in the test beagles. At the end of two years of testing the final report of the study concluded:

"An inhalation study was performed to determine whether chronic exposure to cigarette smoke—whether enriched with carbon monoxide or not, and containing high and low levels of nicotine—would contribute to the atherosclerotic process in beagle dogs during a period of up to two years duration, during which they were fed exclusively on a high cholesterol, high fat, low essential fatty acids atherogenic diet. A total 204 permanently tracheostomized male beagles were placed on this diet for four weeks and then started on six differential treatments. Six groups of 34 dogs were randomly formed as follows:

Variable	Group1	Group2	Group3	Group4	Group5	Group6
Nicotine	None	Low	High	Low	High	None
Carbon monoxide	Low	Low	Low	High*	High*	High*

* Carbon monoxide added to each puff.

By any criteria evaluated, Group 1 dogs were the most severely affected by the atherosclerotic process and Group 5 the least . . . . The results appear to be indicative of a possible protective effect from cigarette smoking and or CO inhalation than of an atherogenic effect" (*Hazleton, 1980*).

Of course, this was a well-run experiment but also a single episode that would have required replication and evaluation against other parallel ongoing experiments—experiments that unfortunately were canceled before completion. Nevertheless, its results are indicative of the insights that this type of research likely would have produced, and in many ways could be interpreted as being curiously in line with the epidemiologic reports of no-effect thresholds or even reduction of certain risks in moderate smokers, as presented here earlier. The study certainly did not add to the concern that nicotine and carbon monoxide would be dangerous components of smoke from improved cigarettes, at least at the levels tested. Still, the chances of further clarification were negated by the new abolitionist policies.

The Smoking and Health Program was dismantled with the loss of several million dollars in canceled ongoing research, and of major opportunities to understand the pathogenesis of smoking related diseases and of the processes that could lead to less hazardous cigarettes. Yet, in some 12 years the program left a legacy of opportunities and knowledge on which new efforts could be grafted once new opportunities could arise (*Appendix A; Gori & Boch, 1980*). The major achievements of the SHP were as follows:

- The central role of nicotine in tobacco smoke was confirmed. Clinical trials did show that administration of nicotine aerosols reduced smokers' demand for cigarettes. In animal tests, the uptake of a nicotine aerosol was shown to be independent of aerosol pH, in a 5 to 9 range of pH values (*SHP, 1979*).

- Initial tests in humans and animals strongly indicated that less hazardous cigarettes should maintain sufficient nicotine, while reducing tar and other components (*Gori, 1980*).

- Methods were developed for the precise determination of nicotine and cotinine in blood of experimental animals and of smokers (*ADL, 1974, SHP, 1979*).

- The technology was developed for adjusting nicotine levels and nicotine/tar yields in cigarettes through breeding of new tobacco varieties, tobacco extraction, substitution techniques, re-blending of the tobacco, and filtration and smoke dilution devices (*SHP, 1979*)

- Several types of cigarette filters were tested for their effectiveness in reducing tumorigenic and adverse respiratory characteristics of cigarette smoke. These tests resulted in specific recommendations for improved cigarette filters. Air dilution filters were especially effective in reducing the tumorigenicity of smoke (*ADL, 1976; SHP, 1976c*).

- Over 150 experimental cigarettes were produced, many of which were made with tobacco selectively stripped of its components. Several of these variants yielded drastically reduced amounts of tar. Skin painting tests in mice showed that the tumorigenic potency of these tars was often reduced (*SHP, 1976a,1976b, 1977, 1979; Appendix B*).

- It was shown that certain cigarette modifications were likely to be unproductive or even undesirable (*SHP, 1976a,1976b, 1977, 1979; Appendix B*).

- It was possible to produce cigarettes that contained virtually no tobacco, and that yielded minimal amounts of tar of reduced tumorigenic potency (*SHP, 1979; Appendix B*).

- Profiles of cigarette flavor acceptability characteristics had been defined and methodologies for returning flavor additives to stripped tobacco were explored, thus indicating possible ways to make less hazardous cigarettes acceptable to smokers (*ADL, 1979; Cain, 1980*).

- Modifications that increased the burning rate of cigarettes were positively correlated with reduced tumorigenicity of smoke (*SHP, 1979*).

- Mouse skin painting experiments did show that solvent extraction of reconstituted tobacco sheets with water or a combination of solvents did reduce tumorigenic components of cigarette smoke (*SHP, 1976a, 1976b, 1977, 1979; Appendix B*).

• The addition of clays and other inert diluents to reconstituted tobacco sheets reduced the tumorigenic potency of smoke (*SHP, 1979*).

• Fertilizers, pesticides, and suckering agents applied to tobacco did not affect the tumorigenicity of smoke (*SHP, 1979*).

• In collaboration with Dr. T. C. Tso of the Plant Science Research Division of the U.S. Department of Agriculture, the Smoking and Health Program also helped advance novel agronomic and tobacco treatment techniques that were promising for less hazardous cigarettes. Several post-harvest processes were tested that might bypass tobacco curing and aging, and reduce undesirable smoke components. The breeding of new tobacco varieties eventually led to commercial leaf cultivars that yielded increased nicotine, and that could be directly utilized in the production of improved cigarettes with low tar to nicotine ratios (*Tso & Chaplin, 1977*).

CHAPTER FIVE

Less Hazardous Cigarettes and the Tobacco Industry

Although the Smoking and Health Program's efforts toward less hazardous cigarettes had been abruptly and prematurely halted, they left a legacy of opportunities that the cigarette industry was cautiously willing to explore. In the quest for such cigarettes the Smoking and Health Program had identified essentially two basic approaches: top-down and bottom-up. The former would gradually strip tobacco and smoke of precursors and components that may be undesirable. The latter implied a start from scratch, where a suitable smoke might be produced by adding desirable or necessary components to an artificial aerosol that would act as a carrier.

Still, the political situation had become more complex. In addition to the continuing concern of possible legal challenges that the explicit marketing of less hazardous cigarettes might encourage, the industry was now facing the new official abolitionist policy of the U.S. Department of Health, Education, and Welfare, allied to the militant intransigence of diverse antismoking interests. How would this powerful coalition react to the introduction of cigarettes that could be presented with the explicit message of being less hazardous?

As described before, the question was eventually tested by the

R.J. Reynolds Company, with the introduction in 1988 of a completely new cigarette design that utilized a radical bottom-up approach. Branded as the Premier™ cigarette, it took off from concepts patented over 20 years earlier by Sir Charles Ellis of the British American Tobacco Company in England (*Ellis et al., 1967*). Still, the development of Premier™ had required many years of clever work by a team under the direction of the visionary Dr. G. Robert Di Marco, and after large capital investments in the necessary research and the unique machinery that manufactured the new devices.

The Premier™ design differed fundamentally from traditional cigarettes. Although the device looked and felt externally as a cigarette, it would not burn and be consumed as conventional cigarettes did. At one end it had a mouthpiece but essentially no filter, at the other end it had a plug of a combustible carbonaceous mixture that when lit in a conventional way would keep burning for about 10 minutes and would provide peaks of high temperature when forcibly oxygenated during puffs. This heating plug was encased in a cylindrical metal capsule that contained a reservoir filled with a solution of nicotine and fragrances—the latter to be vaporized by the heat source during the high temperature peaks induced by puffing. Following the capsule, the cigarette was filled with a conventional tobacco blend intended to impart tobacco flavors to the warm aerosol flowing through during puffs.

The cigarette had passed an extensive battery of toxicological tests, and was delivering a smoke quite unlike that of any conventional cigarettes (*RJR, 1988*). Other than for its novelty, it was apparent that Premier™ could not be an immediate hit with smokers, most of whom might only gradually gain interest in its new taste. Yet, what killed the prospects of this cigarette—and of future improvements—was not so much the reluctance of smokers, but rather the aggressive opposition of antismoking forces that saw the device as a menace to their abolitionist crusade, and threatened to have Premier™ regulated by the U.S.

Food and Drug Administration—a regulation that would have been automatically triggered if health-related claims were made, and that would have ended all market prospects. At that time, the threat was enough to discourage other cigarette manufacturers from attempting to introduce similarly less hazardous products, although most producers were ready to introduce devices that could compete with Premier™. Eventually, an improved version of Premier™ (the Eclipse™ brand) and a new device by Philip Morris (the Accord™ device) were quietly market tested in the late '90s. They have been largely unnoticed because of persistent problems of acceptability, but also because their explicit presentation as less hazardous would not have been permitted (*Fairclough, 2000*).

At the same time, gradually most manufacturers had been exploring and introducing some desirable changes, albeit without explicit claims of reduced risk—notably a progressive selection of tobacco leaf that could yield more nicotine and less tars and thus make their products less hazardous. All along, an intriguing record of patents indicates that most manufacturers had done considerable research. Not all patents were transformable into viable technology and many were of the usual ground-staking kind aimed simply at preempting encroachments, but together they indicate that the tobacco industry had been ready to do much more if the official policy climate had been permissive.

As noted before, the stubborn political impediments raised on various fronts against the early introduction of less hazardous cigarettes must be counted as a tragically missed opportunity of potentially vast public health consequences. The senselessness of this opposition is the more puzzling because it has been and still is enforced by those who should know, for they are the same who claim that smoking kills nearly half a million Americans every year. That claim is primarily based on epidemiologic evidence, the same evidence that clearly shows—as we have seen—that risk is reduced if dose or exposure is reduced.

It should not be possible to be or to have been blind to the incontrovertible epidemiologic message that a reduced intensity of smoking means a substantially reduced risk. That message did show and still shows that a moderation of intake could reduce traditional risks by more than 75%, even without admitting the likelihood of no-risk thresholds. It should be a foregone conclusion that many lives were thus lost to an intransigent antismoking crusade in the last quarter of this century. Who should bear witness to this tragedy?

Although a principled antismoking crusade has met with undeniable and considerable success, it has fallen much short of its goal of a smoke-free America by the year 2000. This failure is underlined by the settlement between the tobacco industry and the States, which recognizes and depends on the continuing presence of a multitude of smokers. The settlement, though, would be just as remiss as abolitionist miscalculations if it did not aggressively address the risk-reducing opportunities of less hazardous cigarettes, and better sooner than later.

In principle, what is first needed is a rehabilitation of nicotine. The grotesque portrayal of nicotine as the equivalent of heroin or crack cocaine must be reversed, and its reality as a harmless and effective stimulant should be reinstated. Finally, once less hazardous cigarettes are available, smokers should be made aware of their potential benefits. Regulators and the market should offer incentives for reduced risk products, thus encouraging a race toward cigarettes of lower and lower risk.

CHAPTER SIX

Nicotine,
The Wronged Stimulant

The antismoking crusade was ready to grasp anything that could demonize smoking, and in 1988 the U.S. Surgeon General declared on his own authority that smoking was an enslaving addiction, and that nicotine was a drug of abuse equal to crack cocaine. On its face the statement was and is preposterous, but the media loved its capacity to conjure anxieties and to foster allegations of dark conspiracies. In reality, claiming that nicotine is as addictive as crack cocaine required muddling and distorting the meaning of addiction, and upholding against all obvious evidence that the behavioral consequences of smoking and of addiction to hard drugs are one and the same.

What addiction is, whether addiction is a disease—and if so, what kind of disease—cannot be determined purely from a medical or behavioral angle, but rather from more basic considerations of language, given the surrounding instabilities of meaning and logic. In its basic use, the word "addiction" means a habit, an insistent way to keep doing things. In fact, this has been the meaning of the word down to this day when colloquially we describe people "addicted" to good deeds, to chocolate, to food, to sex, to the good life, as well as to gambling, alcohol, hard-drugs, and so on.

Such various attributions of "addiction" imply a continuum of valuations, from the laudable to the condemnable. In other words, addiction is not a quantal concept like black and white or being dead or alive: it rather represents a range of situations subject to different perceptions. More and more during the last decades in medical, behavioral, regulatory, and legal talk "addiction" has been assigned a pejorative meaning, usually identified with the abuse of psychotoxic substances. It is presented as a repetition of abuses that eventually cancel volition and personal responsibility, thus generating needed therapies and other interventions, and leading to social costs and crime. Official, social, and cultural sanctions have been assigned to this syndrome, even though official and professional interests have resisted a definition of precisely why and in whose eyes addiction becomes objectionable.

Today, when addiction becomes of medical or social interest it invariably carries the pejorative meaning of recurring uncontrollable excess. Because the word has moral implications and its attributes are prone to subjective valuation, some questions arise. For instance: who appraises addiction: the observer or the observed? Indeed, it matters if the claimant is an official authority, and if the people branded as addicted by such an external dogma may actually feel quite normal, as smokers generally do. Elementary fairness requires that when addiction is used to impose social labels and sanctions, it should be defined by objective attributes rather than arbitrary claims.

Fairness further requires these attributes not to be frivolous, thus exposing a second potential source of subjective valuation. It would not be sufficient to rely on the mere recurrences implied by addiction, nor on therapeutic outcomes in the subjects involved, nor on medical, physiologic, psychologic, or behavioral markers to which contrived ethical implications can be appended. A social language striving to be equitably normative should explicitly identify why, to whom, and by which standards individual addiction becomes objectionable and therefore subject to sanction.

"Uncontrollable excess" must be defined in the context of some repetitive action implied by addiction. However, recurrence may be a necessary but not a sufficient criterion because many actions in life are or must be highly repetitive—some actually carrying risks—without being defined as uncontrollable or addictive. Think, for instance, of keyboard work and metacarpal syndromes, tennis and tennis-elbows, sweets and tooth decay, over-eating and longevity loss, and so on.

Indeed, in ethical, social, and normative parlance "objectionable addiction" has been specifically restricted to conditions involving substance abuse. Therefore, considering the features of these conditions, forcible intervention seems justified when repetitive uncontrollable excess leads to objectionable ends such as loss of volition on account—for instance—of psychoactivity and withdrawal symptoms.

Still, in order to be problematic, psychoactivity should not be a simple pleasurable experience but must be deranged, while withdrawal must be objectively severe. We could propose, therefore, that addiction becomes objectionable when it implies severe withdrawal symptoms that are alleviated by renewing the intoxicating experience, triggering a repetition no longer controlled by personal volition. However, psychotoxicity alone may not qualify addiction because an occasional intoxication—by alcohol or psychoactive substances—does not materialize the recurring loss of volition leading to the repetitiveness of addiction.

In turn, the severity of withdrawal must be such that it compels repetition by any means. Thus, psychotoxicity, severe withdrawal, loss of personal volition, and uncontrollable repetition, seem collectively the necessary attributes if addiction is to merit social objection and sanction. These attributes span a domain of severity and thus require specific definition of the intensities above which social action is justified. Unfortunately, applicable metrics have not been defined and therefore the limits for defining addiction are expedient and opportunistic.

Scientists may use "addiction" without ethical implications—a value-neutral technical term defining tentative experimental models with behavioral and physiologic descriptors. Healing professions and authorities, on the other hand, often use *ad hoc* descriptors and pretensions of scientific objectivity in raising social, ethical, and legal objections to addiction.

In reality, among descriptors of addiction only psychotic intoxication may be an attribute that can be objectively measured. Severity of withdrawal and loss of personal volition are open-ended concepts, except at their maximum when they identify addiction to hard-drugs: the true standard of objectionable addiction. Yet, there has been reluctance—official and otherwise—to adopt the features of hard drug abuse as the legitimate benchmarks.

Behavioral and health scientists have attempted to seek objective markers for some attributes of addiction, but the results have not been persuasive. The World Health Organization (WHO) and others have struggled for 40 years with a model definition of addiction. In the 1957 WHO definition:

"Drug Addiction is a state of periodic or chronic intoxication produced by repeated consumption of a drug (natural or synthetic). Its characteristics include: (1) an overwhelming desire or need (compulsion) to continue taking the drug and to obtain it by any means; (2) a tendency to increase the dose; (3) a psychic (Psychological) and generally a physical dependence on the effects of the drug; (4) detrimental effect on the individual and on society" (*WHO, 1957*).

In the same 1957 report, WHO experts felt the need to distinguish addiction from habituation, the latter being thus defined:

"Drug Habituation (habit) is a condition resulting from the repeated consumption of a drug. Its characteristics include: (1) a desire (but not a compulsion) to continue taking the drug for the sense of well being it engenders; (2) little or no tendency to increase the dose; (3) some degree of psychic dependence on the effect of the drug, but absence of physical dependence and hence of an abstinence syndrome; (4) detrimental effect, if any, primarily on the individual" (*WHO, 1957*).

Because the subjective vagueness of these descriptors, WHO experts from 1964 to 1974 abandoned both concepts of addiction and habituation in favor of a unified concept of dependence:

"Drug Dependence. A state, psychic and sometimes also physical, resulting from the interaction between a living organism and a drug, characterized by behavioral and other responses that always include a compulsion to take the drug on a continuous or periodic basis in order to experience its psychic effects, and sometimes to avoid the discomfort of its absence" (*WHO, 1974*).

This earlier definition still did not satisfy, and dependence was defined in even vaguer terms in 1993:

"A cluster of physiological, behavioral and cognitive phenomena of variable intensity, in which the use of a psychoactive drug (or drugs) takes on a high priority. The necessary descriptive characteristics are a preoccupation with a desire to obtain and take the drug and persistent drug-seeking behavior . . . The existence of a state of dependence is not necessarily harmful in itself, but may lead to self-administration of the drug at dosage levels that produce deleterious physical or behavioral changes . . ." (*WHO, 1993*).

It is apparent that the experts became less and less comfortable with precise attributes and ended up with a definition lacking specificity. By declaring that ". . . a state of dependence is not necessarily harmful in itself . . ." the word "dependence" now seems to cover the same range of situations as the generic term of addiction, namely from the laudable to the objectionable.

Skeptics have surmised that this vagueness might have been designed to ease the inclusion of otherwise conjectural syndromes in medical costs reimbursement programs. More likely, it was the outcome of mounting semantic confusion fostered by multiple and competing professional interests, and by the resulting incapacity or unwillingness to identify objectively a specific scientific, medical, social, regulatory, and legal construct as objectionable addiction.

To make matters more complex, a hypothesis has been advanced that the definition of addiction should not place overwhelming responsibility on the substances abused, because many people use those substances sporadically and without being labeled as objectionably addicted. Others may chronically use the same substances for stress or pain relief, without consequences of objectionable addiction—for instance, the users of opiates and benzodiazepines for pain or mood control.

Despite the elastic vagueness of the words, only a small fraction of people seem to end up being classified as objectionably addicted, even though many substances that can be abused are easily available. Such a differential classification has suggested that what makes addicts are addiction-prone personalities—addiction being viewed as an endogenous attribute. In time, this hypothesis has invoked the concept of cognitive dissonance, negative socio-cultural influences, devastating family environments, and so on. Collectively, this implies a multifactorial causation for addiction, where the substances abused are no more than accessories.

In any event, the WHO expert definitions of addiction are unsatisfactory both in a semantic and scientific context. A certain routine is not necessarily objectionable if it should have pleasurable, euphoriant, or even hallucinogenic effects that reinforce a repetitive experience. It is not necessarily offensive if it should include the development of tolerance or assuefaction to a substance, as for the traditional use of alcoholic beverages as food or entertainment. Even the occasional drunkenness of otherwise sober individuals or the occasional experience with hard drugs seem to elicit hardly more than raised eyebrows. In such instances, the occasional loss of volition is not a controlling determinant of social disapproval. Indeed—excluding puritanical obsessions—ancient and current mores seem largely indifferent to the occasional intoxication of individuals.

Still, addiction as defined by simultaneous intoxication, severe withdrawal symptoms, loss of personal volition, and uncontrollable repetition is bound to create personal, social, and material concerns. Quantifiable attributes of psychotoxicity associated with hard drug abuse—the socially objectionable abuse—include states of altered consciousness, impaired reasoning and coordination, alterations of memory and concentration, judgment distortions, overpowering delusions and hallucinations. In the addict, the attraction dominates to the point that possession and use of the drug become obsessive and overcome all other values, resulting in multiple personality changes, loss of moral constraints, disregard of family ties and responsibilities, illegal activities, violence, criminality, and generally asocial behavior.

In such an addict, withdrawal usually is life-threatening and requires hospitalization. It is characterized by muscular disorders and nausea, seizures, rapidly changing blood pressure and body temperature, hallucinations, delusions, delirium, paranoid and suicidal moods. Mental faculties of reasoning and judgment may be impaired for months or years after the acute symptoms of withdrawal cease, often leading to irreversible dementia or psychotic conditions.

Clearly, these are not garden variety symptoms: their salient characteristics make them easy to describe and to quantify as to intensity and persistence. Yet we have seen how vague the medical and behavioral definitions of addiction have been made. Addiction has been defined in elastic terms, not in precisely quantifiable terms, although a legitimate and objective definition is likely possible. It would require adopting those intensities of attributes that characterize the classic addiction to hard drugs, although this has not happened and semantic ambiguities have been left festering and are ready-made for exploitation. Again, the clamorous example is the 1988 claim by the U.S. Surgeon

General that smokers are as addicted to cigarettes as others are to heroin and cocaine.

This incredible assertion defies common sense because the daily experience of everyone tells that smokers and hard-drug addicts are not the same people. The equivocation is apparent even if one were to adopt the loose definition of addiction advanced by the healing professions, as reviewed above. In fact, the World Health Organization has characterized smoking as a habit, not an "addiction," and even statements by previous U.S. Surgeon Generals in the U.S. also qualified smoking as a habit. For instance, the original 1964 U.S. Surgeon General's report reads:

"The tobacco habit should be characterized as an habituation rather than an addiction, in conformity with accepted World Health Organization definitions, since once established there is little tendency to increase the dose; psychic but not physical dependence is developed . . . No characteristic abstinence syndrome is developed upon withdrawal . . . Discontinuation of smoking . . . is accomplished best by reinforcing factors which interrupt the psychogenic drives" (*U.S. Surgeon General, 1964, p. 354*). "The overwhelming evidence points to the conclusion that smoking—its beginning, habituation, and occasional discontinuation—is to a large extent psychologically and socially determined" (*U.S. Surgeon General, 1964 p. 40*).

To smokers, smoking is pleasant in many ways and therefore it could be expected it to be mildly reinforcing as any pleasant experience tends to be. There is no good evidence of tolerance in smokers. A certain dose is gradually attained early when people start smoking, but it is not exceeded because it would make smoking unpleasant. Uncontrollable, compulsive use is not apparent in smokers: the U.S. Surgeon General acknowledges that over 40 million smokers quit on their own in the United States alone, in a climate where cigarettes are legally and readily available. The all important qualifier of psychotoxicity is absent in smokers, who actually display better intellectual performance when smoking. For several centuries now, many of the most brilliant intellects in the arts and sciences have been smokers. Finally, there is no evidence of physical dependence: withdrawal symptoms are usually absent, transient and mild at best, and less noticeable that the withdrawal symptoms experienced by people on strict diets. Jack Henningfield, a principal contributor to the U.S. Surgeon General's claim of smoking "addiction," himself wrote a few years ago:

"The following constraints and inconsistencies should be noted when considering the evidence for a tobacco withdrawal syndrome. First, a syndrome of reliable physiologic signs . . . has not been described. [W]ith the exception of the desire to smoke . . . other phenomena typically occur only in a fraction of all subjects abstinent from cigarettes .·. . For instance . . . weight gain, gastrointestinal disturbances, or anxiety may each occur in less than one third of all subjects; and up to one half of abstinent subjects may report no symptoms at all.

"The second major issue is that while tobacco withdrawal is commonly equated with nicotine withdrawal, there is little evidence that nicotine produces physiologic dependence . . . Administration of nicotine-receptor antagonists . . . has not been shown to evoke a withdrawal syndrome . . . [P]roviding abstinént smokers with a nicotine-containing chewing gum only partially attenuates physical complaints . . . [and] in animal studies, abrupt abstinence is not followed by . . . a withdrawal syndrome. These inconsistencies . . . impose constraints on the comparison . . . of tobacco withdrawal with that of withdrawal from opioids, sedatives, and ethanol . . . The relevance of this point goes beyond semantic issues of classification [because] when withdrawal is considered in the context of drug dependence it generally connotes a more narrowly specified set of conditions (viz. a reliable syndrome of behavioral and physiologic changes)" (*Henningfield, 1984. pp. 147–148*).

Such a statement amounts to an admission that—by comparison to withdrawal from hard-drug abuse—smoking withdrawal simply does not exist. Most smokers quit without consequence whatsoever. A few may experience some discomforts of craving that quickly disappear spontaneously or are curable by the mildest intervention. Severe cases are said to exist, but are undocumented in the scientific literature, even at the anecdotal level. If anything, it can be argued that at present smokers may be somewhat less comfortable about quitting because the addiction label and the proliferation of cessation clinics and devices makes them think that quitting has become a difficult ordeal—a concern also voiced by prominent antismokers (*Chapman, 1995*).

If smoking is an addiction it is of a mild and forgivable kind, and does not qualify as addiction to hard drugs. In fact, if persistent abuse of hard-drugs is the paradigm of addiction, then the use of the term in connection with smoking is improper, and generates a moral and normative confusion that is incompatible with a forthright public policy.

Lewis Carroll had Humpty Dumpty saying that: "When I use a word . . . it means just what I choose it to mean, neither more nor less" (*Carroll, p. 238*). If antismoking crusaders adopt the same presumption in labeling smoking as a social disease of addiction, then theirs is unquestionably a public disease of words. As used by antismoking crusaders, the term addiction becomes an abuse of language.

The artifice of labeling nicotine as a drug on the same level as crack cocaine is underscored by decisions of the U.S. Food and Drug Administration. The agency permits the free over-the-counter sales of nicotine patches and gums that contain more nicotine than a pack of cigarettes, and that are commonly prescribed for people of all ages—including children. It is hard to believe that the Food and Drug Administration would approve similar products containing cocaine.

That nicotine is not comparable to hard drugs of addiction has been further underscored by a recent decision of the U.S. Department of Justice. Since 1996, the Department had vigorously pursued a grand jury investigation to determine whether executives of top U.S. tobacco manufacturers had lied to Congress, as they did not concede that nicotine was as addictive as hard drugs, nor that the level of nicotine in cigarettes was being manipulated. During three years of a most probing investigation the grand jury could not reached an indictment and the Department quietly abandoned the case in late 1999 (*Davis & St. Cloud, 1999; St. Could & Fairclough, 1999; Meier & Johnston, 1999*).

No official apology or change-of-mind admissions are likely to be forthcoming, as they should. In the end, however, it is clear that a honest official position would be a return to the original 1964 U.S. Surgeon General report, which viewed smoking as an enticing habit offering many existential and coping rewards. The report also concluded that nicotine is a mild stimulant of no toxic concern at the doses experienced by smokers. In other words, the safety of nicotine depends on its dose, as with any substance that is potentially toxic. Thus, how much nicotine should be delivered by less hazardous cigarettes?

How Much Nicotine in Less Hazardous Cigarettes?

The answer to this question would come easy if we knew how much nicotine smokers obtain from cigarettes, since the U.S. Surgeon General had concluded in 1964 that such an amount was safe or at least unlikely to have discernible adverse effects (*U.S. Surgeon General, 1964*). The safety conditions of nicotine in cigarettes would be further clarified if the doses to smokers were comparable to the doses permitted by the Food and Drug Administration in the use of nicotine-delivering patches, gums, and inhalers.

From the late '70s on, new methodologies have permitted increasingly accurate measurements of nicotine levels in the blood of smokers. Those measurements are in consistent agreement that the average intake of smokers is around 1 mg of nicotine per cigarette, with a maximum that does not exceed about 2 mg per cigarette, and despite a nicotine content between 15 and 20 mg per cigarette (*Hill & Marquardt, 1980; Russell et al., 1980, 1986; Ebert et al., 1983; Benowitz et al., 1983, 1986; Gori & Lynch, 1985, 1986; Gori et al., 1986; Robinson et al., 1994; Davis et al., 1998*).

This maximum ceiling of intake is the consequence of nicotine effects that are known to become unpleasant to the point of discouraging smoking altogether if a certain dose is exceeded. It is also apparent that, although 1 mg may be the average intake, the actual intake per individual cigarette may vary at different times. One underlaying reason is that nicotine is rapidly transformed by normal metabolic processes that reduce by about 50% its concentration in blood with every succeeding hour. After a night sleep smokers are virtually depleted of nicotine and might tend to smoke their first morning cigarettes more aggressively.

Momentary stress and arousal may also contribute to higher intakes and doses, while relaxation may result in the opposite. Precisely how doses vary is not known, but they are certain to vary with different smokers, and even with the same smoker under different circumstances. From current knowledge it is likely that less hazardous cigarettes would have to be capable of delivering a maximum around 3 mg of nicotine in smoke, if they are to satisfy aggressive smoking for about 10 puffs.

Most smokers will use much less than this amount most of the time. In fact it is well known that smokers do not utilize efficiently all the nicotine present in cigarettes, when considering that traditional cigarettes contain an average of 15–20 mg of nicotine, of which only an average of 1 mg might be utilized. Less hazardous products, therefore, could contain lesser amounts of nicotine than current cigarettes, provided that nicotine is made available in a form that could be readily inhaled.

This suggests that nicotine in a less hazardous smoke should be presented in a rather acidified form to make it less irritant. In an acidic smoke nicotine is protonated, bound to other molecules, and less reactive. More of the nicotine exists as a reactive free base as the alkalinity increases, but an alkaline smoke increases the irritant effects of nicotine, favors mouth absorption, inhibits inhalation, subtracts nicotine from effective receptors, and makes cigarettes unacceptable to smokers. A relatively alkaline smoke increases what is known as the "kick" or impact of nicotine in the mouth and pharynx, but inhibits lung absorption. Thus, less hazardous cigarettes should make nicotine inhalation increasingly more efficient, as other undesirable components of smoke are gradually reduced or eliminated.

Realistically, less hazardous cigarettes will only be made available gradually. The reasons are that smokers would not readily accept smokes that depart drastically from traditional tastes, and unless gradually weaned they might turn to traditional cigarettes that a black market would gladly provide. Therefore, initial modifications will have to be in the top-down mode as discussed above—progressively removing undesirable precursors from traditional cigarette blends. Gradualism also would be consonant with the inevitable time needed to experiment and retool in manufacturing.

It is difficult to predict how long it will take to convert the market to a point where true less hazardous cigarettes might be almost exclusively demanded. The speed of conversion would depend on many issues, and it certainly could accelerate under appropriate incentives.

CHAPTER EIGHT

Incentives for
Less Hazardous Cigarettes

It would be easy to think of tax incentives and the like, but Americans truly love a race—and a race could be the trump card to jump-start the introduction of gradually improving cigarettes. We only have to look back at the competition that was ignited by the requirement to grade cigarette according to their tar and nicotine content, under procedures endorsed by the U.S. Federal Trade Commission (FTC). In less than 10 years the average yields were almost halved, and by the late '70s cigarettes were available that yielded less than 2 milligrams of tar on the FTC machine. With the right incentive, something similar could happen for less hazardous cigarettes. How should cigarettes be graded?

First, it will be necessary to admit that the ranking of cigarettes on the basis of tar and nicotine yields, obtained by a standard smoking machine, has led to an official consumer message that continues to be misleading to this day. Those yields are measured by an officially approved procedure, but smokers puff away quite unlike the government smoking machine. Unlike the machine, smokers also inhale at unequal intensities, and in so doing they put the lie to any pretension that the FTC machine—or any other such device—could predict actual intake.

With the advent of more precise analytical methods in the late '70s, several reports began to show that the blood levels of nicotine in smokers had marginal relation to the nicotine yield of cigarettes as measured by the FTC smoking machine. It was apparent that smokers of cigarettes of low FTC yield attained only marginally lower blood nicotine levels as smokers of high FTC yield cigarettes (*Hill & Marquardt, 1980; Russell et al., 1980, 1986; Ebert et al., 1983; Benowitz et al., 1983, 1986; Gori & Lynch, 1985, 1986; Gori et al., 1986; Robinson et al., 1994; Davis et al., 1998*).

As prior noted, studies did show that the average nicotine intake was about 1 mg per cigarette, regardless of the FTC yield. The obvious conclusion was that smokers of low FTC yield cigarettes would compensate upward by smoking cigarettes more aggressively than the smoking machine, while smokers of high yield cigarettes would compensate downward. The puzzling thing is that it was known since the beginning that the FTC method was an unreliable predictor of intake. The original FTC charter reads in part:

"No two human smokers smoke in the same way. No individual smoker always smokes in the same fashion. The speed at which one smokes varies both among smokers, and usually also varies with the same individual under different circumstances even within the same day. Some take long puffs (or draws)—some take short puffs. That variation affects the PM (PM = particulate matter) quantity in the smoke generated . . . .

"The . . . . method does not and cannot measure these many variations in human smoking habits. It does not measure PM or nicotine in the smoke generated while the cigarette is not being puffed. It does not measure all of the PM or nicotine in any cigarette, but only that in the smoke drawn in the standardized machine smoking according to the prescribed method" (*FTC, 1966*).

Inevitably, the unpredictable and obviously wide variation of puffing and inhalation intensities in different smokers—and in the same smoker at different times—make it impossible to think of a method that would be predictive of the quantity of tar and nicotine that any individual smoker might extract from any cigarette under any circumstance. Thus, what could be said about a reliable grading of cigarettes?

For an answer, it is important to realize that the purpose of a consumer message is to help smokers distinguish between brands and hopefully to select those that are less hazardous. To do so, the message only has to rank reliably the *relative expectations* of risk from different brands, thus escaping the impossible task of being specific about the *quantity* of smoke a smoker might obtain. With this in mind we should recall that smokers appear to smoke for nicotine satiation, up to a point where nicotine makes smoking unpleasant. The level of nicotine that induces satiation is not constant but varies with smokers, and even in the same smoker under different circumstances. Recall also that nicotine is not a safety concern at the doses inhaled by smokers *but tar is* (*U.S. Surgeon General, 1964; IARC, 1986*). It then follows that the hazard of cigarettes becomes more and more reduced as the yield of tar in smoke is progressively reduced, while the yield of nicotine is not change below a certain optimal level.

Therefore, less hazardous cigarettes—and any cigarette, for that matter—should be graded and ranked according to the tar to nicotine ratios of their smokes. On this basis, smokers will be able to select those brands that give them the less tar for the amount of nicotine they seek at any given time.

By a fortunate coincidence, the determination of tar to nicotine ratios of cigarettes does not require new methods or equipment. Experimental evidence shows that the tar to nicotine ratio of smoke is affected little by how a cigarette is smoked within the range of puffing kinetics that smokers are likely to display, the estimated variance being ± 10–15% (*Browne et al., 1980; Schlotzhauer & Chortyk, 183; Rickert et al., 1983*). Thus, whether a cigarette is puffed by a smoker or by the FTC smoking machine, the amounts of smoke generated may be different, but the mean tar to nicotine ratios will remain acceptably comparable. Such a correspondence indicates that the current analytical FTC method for cigarette testing can still be utilized for an improved cigarette classification and a more relevant consumer message. The difference would be in the presentation of the data, to be given not as direct analytical figures, but as the ratio of tar to nicotine yields.

Of course, there is tar and tar, and tar differences will be enhanced as cigarettes gradually improve by removing undesirable tar components and thus producing tars that are progressively less hazardous. In time, there would be ways to reduce aromatic hydrocarbons, tobacco-specific nitrosamines, heavy phenols and other undesirables and irritants now present in tars. Therefore, what could still be defined as tar in the future may have become progressively of lesser concern.

Still, the tar to nicotine ratio of FTC yields would be quite appropriate until tar compositions are substantially modified. When such modifications may become a reality, the grading of cigarettes will require added certifiable assurance that implications of reduced risk are trustworthy, to extend beyond the simple measurement of tar/nicotine ratios. Appropriate tests and representations will be needed, which raises the question of how to test for reduced risks, who should test, and who should certify the tests and their outcomes.

Testing for Assurance of Reduced Hazard

In time, as smoke modifications become more successful, a more complex evaluation of reduced risk will become necessary. For one thing, the modification of cigarettes may comport new treatments of tobacco, new materials and additives, new designs and processes that could reduce overall tar yield and composition while introducing unknown hazards. Today, that prospect is more than enough to require the intervention of some public oversight agency that could define what tests might be necessary and whether tests so performed might be successful. Such an agency would provide an independent and legal public warranty for modified products. What could be the scope of regulation?

In the practice of the United States and of the industrialized world, the safety of products is not tested in the absolute but always—and inevitably—in terms that are relative to the intended uses, to the available alternatives, and ultimately to the costs and benefits of uses. Nonetheless, safety and health statutes and regulations generally are written to imply the attainment of virtual safety, which in turn is made to appear as absolute safety in the messages that reach and persuade the public to feel safe.

However, the regulation of less hazardous cigarettes will have to rest on contrasting premises. It will have to begin by recognizing the necessity of gradual changes from traditional to progressively improved specimens, that is from certain levels of hazard to progressively lesser levels. This fundamental policy shift may not come easy, given the inflated and unrealistic safeguards that current public opinion has been persuaded to expect from official regulation. Yet it will have to be made, because it reflects the reality of the problem at hand.

Once such a basic change of premises is understood and translates into appropriate statutory language, an initial step would need to establish a point of departure, a benchmark against which to compare future improvements. Most likely that benchmark will be in the form of a reference cigarette. For years the University of Kentucky has provided a standard cigarette (the 1R1 standard) that has been used as a control in countless studies, including most of the experiments performed by the Smoking and Health Program of the National Cancer Institute. Among other advantages, using this cigarette as the initial standard would allow comparing new results with those of many prior experiences in risk reduction, and of using at least some test modalities that have already been designed to function well with the Kentucky reference cigarette.

There will be more basic ways of evaluating hazard reduction. The simplest and most obviously reliable is the attainment and recognition of an overall reduction of exposure and dose. The more complex and uncertain way is the evaluation of hazard after the reduction or elimination of undesirable smoke components. In a third way, as discussed previously, dose reduction could be evaluated by the reduction of tar/nicotine ratios of the smokes from modified cigarettes. This approach would be valid for initial cigarette modifications that approximately maintain the chemical configurations exemplified by the smoke of the Kentucky reference cigarette. It would not be valid, however, for evaluating radically different smokes coming from *ersatz* cigarettes of bottom-up design, or from substantial top-down modifications of traditional cigarettes. In those instances, judgments of reduced risk will be reached based on the reduction of undesirable smoke components and the results of biological and clinical tests.

In considering tests, it will be necessary to decide which endpoints to address and which tests could be appropriate. Testing for carcinogenicity may not be a realistic option because decades of attempts have generally failed to reliably cause lung cancer or other diseases in animals by smoke inhalation. Even chronic inhalation procedures that test smoke as a promoter of carcinogenesis—after the application of a positive carcinogen— would be of questionable value relative to real life smoking conditions. The old stand-by of the skin painting test in mice would be a surrogate of problematic relevance to whatever true carcinogenic mechanisms of smoke in human lungs, and would likely provide illusory signals of hazard differentials. What is more, all chronic tests would require inordinate time for completion, and would retard indefinitely any progress toward cigarettes of reduced risk.

Much useless work could be avoided by recognizing a crucial truth: namely the impossible task of looking for animal tests that could directly provide convincing results about the relative carcinogenic risk of different cigarettes smokes to humans. For a variety of biological reasons there are and likely could be no such tests, and it will be necessary to rely on indirect methods that may provide credible clues.

Thus, the groundwork for the evaluation of an improved smoke should be a thorough chemical characterization complemented by a detailed description of the modifications and processes employed. This information should provide a framework for a material comparison with the parallel construct of the standard reference cigarette. Biological tests might include a battery of genetic effects tests (mutagenicity, sister chromatid exchange, chromosomal aberrations, efficiency of repair, etc.), and short and medium term inhalation tests in animals that may uncover differential signals of cellular proliferation and differentiation, or inflammation. The latter could also monitor

85

biochemical parameters and metabolic endpoints, such as urine mutagenicity.

It would be essential to acknowledge that the baggage of plausible hints about cancer causation that has accumulated over the last few decades remains the only store of whatever imprecise understanding is available. By any sober reasoning, it can only provide an open judgment about increased or decreased hazard from any presumptive agent, in the face of persisting and multifactorial uncertainties about the individual or synergistic causal roles of specific agents and situations. Moreover the scope and intensity of any evaluation should be moderated by the realization that progressive improvements will be likely short lived. More so during the initial phases of development when the pace of new ideas could rapidly supersede existing models, and might restrict their market lifespan to less than one year.

Under the circumstances it is conceivable that certain models of modified cigarettes may receive rapid but time-limited approval, thus ensuring brief exposures and the minimization of possible misjudgments. Approvals for more extended periods may be considered for modifications that provide a clear warrant of reduced risk, until virtually safe models could be identified and made available.

There is another important consideration that would make the regulatory task much easier. It is that traditional precautionary principles apply in reverse to cigarettes, making it much easier to judge about the reduction of a known risk than to certify the probable absence of risk. And again, in evaluating cigarettes for reduced carcinogenic hazards the task could not be the customary one of determining the absence of risk, but rather one of reaching a judgment that a potential has been reduced.

Above all it will be important to keep in mind that only plausible judgments are possible in this regard, and that it should be improper to characterize those judgments as endorsed by objective scientific verification. Such a characterization would be illusory and arguably would amount to deceptive malpractice.

Still, judgments can and will be made, including binding regulatory ones. They will have a better chance of being just and acceptable if they were to be reached in a transparent, realistic, and public process of evaluation.

Similar considerations would apply to the assessment of reduced risk for cardiovascular and respiratory endpoints. The same animal inhalation tests used for the determination of cellular proliferation and differentiation could be adapted to provide cardiovascular and respiratory signals. It is also very much conceivable that crucial short-term tests related to cell proliferation/differentiation and to cardiovascular and respiratory endpoints could be performed in human volunteer smokers directly.

Functional respiration and cardiovascular tests, pulmonary lavages, bronchoscopy, biopsies and other clinical outcomes in tests of short and medium term duration in smokers might become the preferred and most relevant discriminants in reaching judgments of differential hazard. Ethical issues in the use of volunteer smokers would be largely resolved if the chemical characterization of smokes, the *in vitro* tests, and animal tests were performed before human testing could be allowed.

In all, there is little doubt that a suitable protocol of tests can be arrived at, capable of supporting a knowledgeable judgment. This possibility leads to the next issue, which is about who should determine the test protocol, who should perform the tests, and who should evaluate and certify the outcome of the tests.

Protocols for chemical characterization present no difficulties and have been well developed and standardized over the years. *In vitro* laboratory tests of genetic effects are also routine, but the true expertise for the critical inhalation tests of tobacco smoke is a specialized competence shared by less than a score of experts in the U.S., only a few of them in federal employ. Methods for clinical evaluations in human volunteers would be virtually routine.

At the same time a thorough understanding of the manufacturing processes of cigarettes would be incumbent on whichever official entity ends up with the task of supervising the certification of improved cigarettes—an understanding that for the moment is exclusive to the cigarette industry, and partially shared by a handful of outside people (*Davis & Nielsen, 1999*).

In the absence of this knowledge a cigarette regulator could not function without risking major blunders. As an example, it has been plainly obvious to anyone minimally informed that certain actions and pronouncements of the U.S. government in the last few years have been hastily put together without understanding the agronomic, engineering, pharmacologic, organoleptic, and marketing details of cigarettes. Doomed from their inception, those efforts have been an embarrassment of expenditures and failure. One can only think of the untenable addiction claims by the Food and Drug Administration and the U.S. Surgeon General, and the grasping naiveté of the failed federal settlement negotiations of 1998. An even more salient example is the ill conceived and recently abandoned 3 year grand jury investigation by the Justice Department, which could not prove that the tobacco industry conspired to mislead the public, regulators, and Congress about the health risks of smoking and the addictive properties of nicotine (*Davis & St. Cloud, 1999; St. Cloud & Fairclough, 1999; Meier & Johnston, 1999*).

Thus, and before any regulatory effort is considered, it would seem desirable to call for a fact-finding advisory conference of experts, to systematize a record of existing technical and scientific knowledge on which to build a meaningful battery of tests and their evaluation criteria. Preferably, the conference should include congressional staffers expert in regulatory policy, regulators from various agencies, academic and industry experts. To avoid possible conflict of interest it should be organized outside of a regulatory agency, and the National Institutes of Health or some University could provide a suitable venue. The conference also could prove very useful if it explored and recommended the most promising options about where and how to set up a regulatory body, and about suitable tests. At the beginning of 2000 and with the support of the Food and Drug Administration (FDA), the Institute of Medicine of the U.S. National Academy of Sciences has initiated a preliminary and rather limited inquiry in this direction, which might lead to useful insights if comprehensively expanded (*Institute of Medicine, 2000*).

In 1996 the FDA first staked a claim for the regulation of cigarettes, a move that had been promoted and endorsed by antismoking advocates and some policymakers. In the wake of protracted legal and political skirmishes the claim was eventually resolved by the Supreme Court in March 2000. The court decided that the FDA does not have the necessary authority to regulate cigarettes, which Congress alone would have to provide with a new or amended statute (*Supreme Court, 2000*). The reading of the Court appears to be in line with a statutory language and limitations that had been clear all the time. Until its 1996 claim, the FDA itself had repeatedly asserted it did not have authority to regulate cigarettes, but was forced to revert its long standing position by an activist commissioner and its counsels, apparently against the advice of senior career staff. In reality, previous FDA reservations were based on good reasons beyond statutory considerations, chiefly because the century old tradition of the agency has consistently aimed at providing public reassurance of virtual safety. Clearly the FDA would need new authority to turn this tradition on its head for the special task of regulating less hazardous cigarettes.

Besides, the agency would have to find remedy for a contradictory position in which it has put itself. On one hand it has declared that nicotine is as addictive as crack cocaine and that it would seek its elimination from cigarettes if given regulatory authority. On the other it permits the free over-the-counter sales of patches and chewing gums that contain more nicotine than a pack of cigarettes: products that amount to a legal, large, and growing nicotine market (*Werner et al., 1997*). If it were to regulate cigarettes, the agency would have to return to a proper posture of neutrality and not of advocacy, in an about-face that may prove difficult.

Thinking of other options, it would be necessary to select an agency that has statutory experience with the need to pass judgments about substances, devices, or situations that carry an intrinsic risk. The Occupational Health and Safety Administration may come to mind, although for obvious reason this agency would not make a suitable candidate. The Department of Agriculture (DoA) might offer a plausible venue. It has excellent technical and scientific experience with the tobacco plant and its curing and aging, up to the point when the finished agricultural product transfers to cigarette manufacturers. What DoA does not have is the clinical and testing expertise required for the supervision of less hazardous cigarettes, although the department could be assisted by other federal agencies, for instance the National Institutes of Health.

Regardless of administrative location, the unusual requirements for the regulation of cigarettes will call for an unusual solution. Most likely it would have to be a special-statute regulatory unit, assisted by an executive committee with membership from various federal agencies. The statute itself would have to endorse a policy of progressive risk reduction rather than a search for virtual safety. The committee would avail itself of external advice and expertise, and would issue regulatory guidelines for the tests to be performed. It would also define the criteria the committee would use in evaluating tests results. Tests could be performed at industry's expense by independent laboratories certified and supervised by the regulatory unit.

Whatever the solution, it should be made only after a comprehensive examination of what less hazardous cigarettes are all about, and with the explicit intent of encouraging rather the hampering their development. There should be clarity in this regard, and it should be justified by the certainty that available technology is capable of reducing cigarette hazards if it were allowed to proceed in certain directions—directions that have been so far denied because of genuine or affected ignorance, or because of unjustifiable intolerance.

Ignorance can be overcome with a modicum of effort. A more open understanding of cigarettes and of the human dimensions of smoking may help to move the public discourse beyond a persisting and illiberal abolitionist crusade. Looking back, so many disappointments in American history have been caused by a militant intolerance that still resonates in certain intrusive fringes of American society. As we stand at the threshold of a third millennium, it may be high time to grow up.

Epilogue

The world could certainly do and likely do better without tobacco and cigarettes, but not anytime soon. We live in an imperfect society of imperfect people, were imperfect solutions are the ones more likely to work. From any pragmatic public health perspective there could be no opposition to less hazardous cigarettes, because commanding realities invalidate opposing policies. What are these realities?

First are the 50 million Americans and over 1 billion other smokers worldwide who continue to smoke as a personal choice and despite all warnings. Contrary to wanton protestations, these people find value in smoking, their habit lacks behavioral or social consequences that are negative, and the issue of whether it qualifies as an addiction is ostensibly a manipulative cavil. Official U.S. and Australian surveys show that moderate smokers are generally healthier than nonsmokers. The life expectancy of smokers may be shorter by a few years, but as a group they remain productive voters well into retirement, and their numbers are legion.

The popularity of tobacco has made national and local governments dependent on tobacco taxes. The U.S. settlements show that assorted governments rake in by far the greatest profits from the tobacco trade, surpassing by many fold whatever profits the tobacco industry is allowed to make. In effect, the settlements and continuing litigation aim at maximizing revenue from the tobacco trade, limited only by the necessity to minimize incentives for a black market. They aim at barely ensuring the survival of the tobacco industry, whose profits are effectively regulated much as those of a nationalized public utility. If it were not for these reasons, cigarettes might have been made illegal long ago.

With this in mind, it should be clear that any tax and settlement levies imposed on cigarettes could not derive from the tobacco industry but will be penalties imposed on and paid directly by smokers, with the tobacco industry as the functional tax collector. Without entering into a discussion about the legal merits and fairness of those penalties, it is demonstrable beyond doubt that smokers are forced to shell out amounts of taxes vastly in excess of any services they may receive from public treasuries. As money is concerned, nonsmokers and America are and have been for decades in deep debt to smokers.

It also happens that the risks associated with smoking are real, but strongly dose dependent. The epidemiologic and research record shows that these risks could be reduced to fractions of their historic levels if modified cigarette smokes could minimize the inhalation of undesirable components. This approach could prevent millions of premature deaths, and the technologies to achieve such a goal need to be perfected but are entirely feasible. By any fair appraisal, these opportunities ought to prevail over the proven ineffectiveness of abolitionist policies. Thus, given the outstanding tax contribution of 50 million U.S. smokers, it would be callous and ungrateful if this opportunity were not pursued in America as a matter of national policy. This is the stark reality check. By comparison, Utopian and crusading quarrels cannot sound but hollow.

Text References

ADL (1974): Measurement of tobacco smoke components in human subjects. Report to the National Cancer Institute. Contract NO1-CP-33349. Arthur D. Little, Inc. Cambridge, MA.

————(1979): Development of a flavor system and nicotine mimic for acceptability to smokers of candidate potentially less hazardous cigarettes. Final Report. Contract ECI-SHP-75-116. Arthur D. Little, Inc. Cambridge, MA.

Albert R (1989): Carcinogen risk Assessment. Environ Health Perspect, 81:103-105.

Altshuler B (1989): Quantitative models for lung cancer induced by cigarette smoke. Environ Health Perspect, 81:107-108.

Ames BN, Gold LS (1991): Endogenous mutagens and the causes of aging and cancer. Mutat Res 250:3–16.

Aronow WS (1978): Effect of passive smoking on angina pectoris. New Eng J Med 299:21–24.

Ashby J, Tennant RW (1991): Definitive relationships between chemical structure, carcinogenicity, and mutagenicity for 301 chemicals tested by the U.S. NTP. Mutat Res 257:229–306.

Australian Bureau of Statistics (1994): 1989–90 National Health Survey: Lifestyles and Health Australia. Australian Bureau of Statistics. Canberra.

Baker RR (1999): Smoke chemistry. In: Davis L, Nielsen MT (Eds.) Tobacco. Production, chemistry and technology. Balckwell Science. Oxford.

Barendregt JJ, Bonneux L, van der Maas PJ (1997): The health care costs of smoking. N Engl J Med 337:1052–1057.

Benowitz NL. Et al. (1983): Smokers of low-yield cigarettes do not consume less nicotine. N Eng J Med 309:139–142.

Benowitz NL, Jacob P (1984): Daily intake of nicotine during cigarette smoking. Clin Pharmacol Ther 35:499–504.

Benowitz NL, et al. (1986): Reduced tar, nicotine, and carbon monoxide exposure while smoking ultralow – but not low-yield cigarettes. J Am Med Assoc 256:241–256.

Berridge V (1999): Passive smoking and its prehistory in Britain: policy speaks to science? Soc Sci & Med 49:1183–1195.

Billen D (1990): Spontaneous DNA damage and its significance for the "Negligible Dose" controversy in radiation protection. Radiat Res 124:242–245.

Bork RH (1999): Tobacco suit is the latest abuse of the rule of law. The Wall Street Journal, Thursday, September 23, 1999. P. A22.

Brandt AM (1990): The cigarette, risk, and the American culture. Daedalus, Fall 1990:155–176.

Breslow L et al. (1978): A history of cancer control in the United States, 1946–1971. 4 Vol. Department of Health, Education, and Welfare. Publication No. NIH 78-1516–19. National Cancer Institute, Bethesda, MD.

Browne CL, Keith CH, Allen RE (1980): The effect of filter ventilation on the yield and composition of mainstream and sidestream smokes. Beitr Tabacksforsh Internat 10:81–90.

Burney L, Heller J (1957): Testimony in: False and misleading advertising—Filter tip cigarettes. Hearings before a Subcommittee of the Committee on Government Operations. U.S. House of Representatives, 85th Congress, 1st session, July 18–26, 1957.

Bush TL, Comstock GW (1983): Smoking and cardiovascular mortality in women. Am J Epidemiol 118:480–488.

Cain WS (1980): Sensory attributes of cigarette smoking. In: Gori GB, Bock FG (Eds) A safe cigarette? Bambury report No. 3. Proceedings of a meeting held at the Bambury Center. Cold Spring Harbor Laboratory. Cold Spring Harbor, NY. pp. 239–250.

Carroll L: Alice in Wonderland and through the looking glass. Grosset & Dunlap Publishers.

CDC (1997): Cigarette smoking among adults—United States, 1995. Morbidity and Mortality Weekly Report 46:1217–1220. Center for Disease Control, Atlanta, GA.

——— (1998): State-specific prevalence among adults of current cigarette smoking and smokeless tobacco use and per capita tax-paid sales of cigarettes—United States. Morbidity and Mortality Weekly Report 47:922–926. Center for Disease Control, Atlanta. GA.

Chapman S (1995): Smokers: why do they start—and continue? World

Health Forum (WHO) 16:1–9.

Collingridge D, Reeve C, Eds. (1986): Science speaks to power. The role of experts in policy making. Frances Pinter, London.

Davis RA, Caldwell WS, Robinson JH, et al., A further study of FTC yield and nicotine absorption in smokers. Psychopharmacology 139:291–299, 1998.

Davis DL, Nielsen MT (Eds) (1999): Tobacco: production, chemistry and technology. Blackwell Science, London, 1999.

Davis A, St. Cloud D (1999): Justice agency winds down tobacco probe. The Wall Street Journal. March 11, 1999, p. A3.

Dockery DW, Speizer FE, Ferris BG, et al. (1988): Cumulative and reversible effects of lifetime smoking on simple tests of lung function in adults. Am Rev Respir Dis 137:286–292.

Doll R (1978): An epidemiologic perspective of the biology of cancer. Cancer Res, 38:3573-3583.

Doll R, Peto R (1978): Cigarette smoking and bronchial carcinoma: dose and time relationships among regular smokers and lifelong non-smokers. J Epidemiol Commun Health, 32:303-313.

Doll R, Peto R (1976): Mortality in relation to smoking: 20 years' observations on male British doctors. Br Med J 2:1525–1536.

Doll R, Gray R, Hafner B, et al. (1980): Mortality in relation to smoking: 22 years' observations on female British doctors. Br Med J 280:967–971.

Doll R, Peto R (1981): The causes of cancer. J Nat Cancer Inst 66:1192–1312.

Ebert RV, McNabb ME, McClusker KT, et al. (1983): Amount of nicotine and carbon monoxide inhaled by smokers of low-tar, low-nicotine cigarettes. J Am Med Ass 250:2840–2842.

Ellis CD, Cookham D, Hughes IW (1967): Smoking devices. U.S. Patent 3,356,094.

Fairclough G (2000): Reynolds says new cigarette may be safer. The Wall Street Journal, April 20, 2000, p. B16.

——— (1999): States plan assorted uses for tobacco settlement. The Wall Street Journal. August 24, 1999, p. A4.

Fisher P (1999): Tobacco blending. In: Davis L, Nielsen MT (Eds.) Tobacco. Production, chemistry and technology. Balckwell Science. Oxford.

Frette C, Wei SM, Neukirk F, et al. (1992): Relation of serum elastin peptide concentration to age, FEV1, smoking habits, alcohol consumption, and protease inhibitor phenotype: an epidemiologic study in working men. Thorax 47:937–942.

Freund KM, Belanger AJ, D'Agostino RB, et al. (1993): The health risks of smoking. The Framingham study: 34 years of follow-up. Ann Epidemiol

3:417–424.

Froggatt P, (1988): Fourth Report of the Independent Committee on Smoking & Health. Her Majesty's Stationery Office, London.

FTC (1966): Cigarettes and related matters. Method to be employed in determining tar and nicotine content. Supplemental observations following the November 30, 1966 hearing before the Federal Trade Commission. Federal Trade Commission, Washington, DC.

Garnett C (1998): Stetten fellow examines history of tobacco control at NIH. NIHAA Update. Newsletter of the NIH Alumni Association 10(2):14–15.

Gaylor DW, Axelrad JA, Brown RP, et al. (1997): Health risk assessment practices in the U.S. Food and Drug Administration. Regul Toxicol Pharmacol 26:307–321, 1997.

Gilliam AG (1954): Epidemiology in non-communicable diseases. Pub Health Reports 69:907–913.

Gillooly M, Lamb D (1993): Microscopic emphysema in relation to age and smoking habit. Thorax 48:491–495.

Gori GB (1976a): Low risk cigarettes: a prescription. Science 194:1243–1246.

——— (1976b): Approaches to the reduction of total particulate matter (TPM) in cigarette smoke. Pages 451–461 in E. L. Wynder, D. Hoffmann and G. B. Gori, eds. Smoking and Health I: Modifying the Risk for the Smoker. DHEW Publ. No. (NIH) 76–1221,. National Cancer Institute, Bethesda, MD.

——— (1980a): Less hazardous cigarettes: theory and practice. In: Gori GB, Bock FG (Eds). A safe cigarette? Bambury report No. 3. Proceedings of a meeting held at the Bambury Center. Cold Spring Harbor Laboratory. Cold Spring Harbor, NY pp. 261–279.

——— (1980b): A summary appraisal. In: Gori GB, Bock FG (Eds) A safe cigarette? Bambury report No. 3. Proceedings of a meeting held at the Bambury Center. Cold Spring Harbor Laboratory. Cold Spring Harbor, NY. pp. 353–359.

Gori GB, Battista SP, Thayer PS, Guerin MR, Lynch CJ (1975): Chemistry and in vitro bioassay of smoke from experimental filter cigarettes. Smoking and Health Program, National Cancer Institute, DHEW Publ. No. (NIH) 76–1076. National Cancer Institute, Bethesda, MD.

Gori GB, Benowitz NL, Lynch CJ (1986): Mouth versus deep airways absorption of nicotine in cigarette smokers. Pharmacol Biochem Behav 25:1181–1184.

Gori GB, Bock FG (Eds) (1980): A safe cigarette? Bambury report No. 3. Proceedings of a meeting held at the Bambury Center. Cold Spring Harbor Laboratory. Cold Spring Harbor, NY.

Gori GB, Lynch CJ (1985): Analytical cigarette yields as predictors of smoke bioavailability. Regul Toxicol Pharmacol 5:314–26.

Gori GB, Mantel N (1991): Mainstream and environmental tobacco smoke. Regul Toxicol Pharmacol 14:88–105.

Gough M (1990): How much cancer can EPA regulate away? Risk Anal 10:1–6.

Gravelle JG, Zimmermann D, (1994): Cigarette taxes to fund health care reform: An economic analysis. Congressional Research Services, The Library of Congress, Washington, DC.

Hammond EC (1980): The long-term benefits of reducing tar and nicotine in cigarettes. In: Gori GB, Bock FG (Eds) A safe cigarette? Bambury report No. 3. Proceedings of a meeting held at the Bambury Center. Cold Spring Harbor Laboratory. Cold Spring Harbor, NY. pp. 13–18.

Hazleton Inc., (1981): Final report. Inhalation bioassay of cigarette smoke in dogs. Effects of nicotine and carbon monoxide on atherogenesis. Project No. 976–904. Contract No. NCI-SHP-75-112, the National Cancer Institute, Smoking and Health Program. Hazleton Laboratories America Inc., Vienna, VA.

Henningfield, JE (1984): Behavioral pharmacology of cigarette smoking. In: Advances in behavioral pharmacology. Thompson T, Dews PB, Barrett JE, Eds., Academic Press, New York, 1984. pp. 147–148.

Hill P, Marquardt H, Plasma and urine changes after smoking different brands of cigarettes. Clin Pharmacol Ther 27:652–658, 1980.

IARC (1986): Tobacco smoking: Monographs on the evaluation of the carcinogenic risk of chemicals to humans, Vol 38. International Agency for Research on Cancer—World Health Organization, Lyon.

——— (1987): Overall evaluation of carcinogenicity: An updating of IARC Monographs Volumes 1 to 42. Supplement 7. International Agency for Research on Cancer—World Health Organization, Lyon.

Institute of Medicine (2000): Assessing the science base for tobacco harm reduction. Project BNBH-H-99-05-A. Institute of Medicine. National Academy of Sciences. Washington, DC.

Jarvis MJ, Russell MAH, Feyerabend C (1983): Absorption of nicotine and carbon monoxide from passive smoking under natural conditions of exposure. Thorax 38:829–833.

Jenkins HW (2000): Look who's falling in love with tort reform. The Wall Street Journal, April 26, 2000, p. A27.

——— (1999): Another tobacco lawsuit (yawn). The Wall Street Journal. September 29, 1999. P. A23.

Jenkins CD, Rosenman RH, Zyzanski SJ (1968): Cigarette smoking. The relationship to coronary heart disease and related risk factors in the Western

Collaborative Group Study. Circulation 38:1140–1155.

Jones NJ, McGregor AD, Waters R (1993): Detection of DNA adducts in human oral tissue: correlation of adduct levels with tobacco smoking and differential enhancement of adducts using the butanol extraction and nuclease P1 version of 32P postlabeling. Cancer Res 53:1522–1528.

Keith CH (1980): Physical methods for the modification of tobacco smoke. In: Gori GB, Bock FG (Eds) A safe cigarette? Bambury report No. 3. Proceedings of a meeting held at the Bambury Center. Cold Spring Harbor Laboratory. Cold Spring Harbor, NY. pp. 225–238.

Kannel WB, D'Agostino RB, Belanger AJ (1987): Fibrinogen, cigarette smoking, and risk of cardiovascular disease: Insights from the Framingham study. Am Heart J 113:1006–1010.

Kassel JD (1997): Smoking and attention: a review and reformulation of the stimulus-filter hypothesis. Clin Psychol Rev 17:451–478.

Klawansky S, Fox MS (1984): A growth rate distribution model for the age dependence of human cancer incidence: A proposed role for promotion in cancer of the lung and breast. J Theor Biol, 111:531-587.

Kondoh Y, Taniguchi H, Yokoyama S, et al. (1990): Emphysematous changes in chronic asthma in relation to cigarette smoking. Chest 97:845–849.

Luik JC (Ed.) (1994): Do tobacco advertising bans really work? A review of the evidence. The Niagara Institute. Niagara on the Lake, Ontario, Canada.

Manning WG, Keeler EB, Newhouse JP, et al. (1989): The taxes of sin. Do smokers and drinkers pay their way? J Am Med Ass 261:1604–1609.

Margetts BM, Jackson AA (1993): Interactions between people's diet and their smoking habits: the dietary and nutritional survey of British adults. Br Med J 307:1381–1384.

Meier B, Johnston D (1999): How inquiry into tobacco lost its steam. Criminal case ran out of time and energy. The New York Times, Sunday September 26, 1999. p. 1

Mohtashamipur E, Norpoth K, Lieder F (1985): Isolation of frameshift mutagens from smoker's urine: experiences with three concentration methods. Carcinogenesis 6:783–788.

Muscat JE, Harris RE, Haley NJ, et al. (1991): Cigarette smoking and plasma cholesterol. Am Heart J 121:141–147.

NAS, National Academy of Sciences (1983): Risk assessment in the Federal Government: managing the process. National Academy Press, Washington, DC.

NAS, National Research Council, National Academy of Sciences (1986): Environmental Tobacco Smoke: measuring exposures and assessing health effects. National Academy Press, Washington, DC.

NCEP (1988): Report of the National Cholesterol Education Program Expert Panel on detection, evaluation, and treatment of high blood cholesterol in adults. Arch Int Med 148:36–69.

NCI (1960–80): Minutes of the meetings of the National Cancer Advisory Board and of the President's Cancer Panel, 1968–80. National Cancer Institute, Bethesda, Maryland.

Newman A (1999): Smoke one for the tax man. The price of cigarettes is getting higher. Where does all the money go? New York Times Magazine. February 28, 1999, p. 21.

Norman A. (1999): Cigarette design and materials. In: Davis L, Nielsen MT (Eds.) Tobacco. Production, chemistry and technology. Balckwell Science. Oxford.

O'Donnell FE, Williams JR (1998): Tobacco related products. US Patent No. 5803081, September 8, 1998.

OECD (1984): The international expert group for hazard assessment of the OECD Chemical Program. Data interpretation guidelines for initial hazard assessment of chemicals. Organization for Economic Cooperation and Development, Paris.

Oesch F, Hengstler JG, Fuchs J (1994): Cigarette smoking protects mononuclear blood cells of carcinogen exposed workers from additional work exposure-induced DNA single strand breaks. Mutat Res 321:175–185.

Oliver MF (1974): Ischaemic heart disease in young women. Br Med J 4:253–259.

Parascandola J (1997): The surgeons general and smoking. Publ Health Reports 112:440–442.

PPRG, The Pooling Project Research Group (1978): Relationship of blood pressure, serum cholesterol, smoking habit, relative weight and ECG abnormalities to incidence of major coronary events: Final report of the Pooling Project. J Chronic Dis 31:201–306.

Rickert WS, Robinson JC, Young JC, et al. (1983): A comparison of the yields of tar, nicotine, and carbon monoxide of 36 brands of Canadian cigarettes tested under three conditions. Prev Med 12:682–694.

RJR, R.J. Reynolds Tobacco Company (1988): Chemical and biological studies on new cigarette prototypes that heat instead of burn tobacco. R.J. Reynolds Tobacco Company, Winston-Salem, NC.

Robinson JH, Caldwell WS, de Bethizy JD (1994): Nicotine uptake and metabolism in smokers. Rec Adv Tob Sci 20:5–31.

Rosenberg L, Kaufman DW, Helmrich SP, et al. (1985): Myocardial infarction and cigarette smoking in women younger than 50 years of age. J Am Med Ass 253:2965–2969.

Russell MA, Jarvis M, Iyer R, et al. (1980): Relation of nicotine yield of cigarettes to blood nicotine concentration in smokers. Br Med J 280:972–976.

Russell MAH, et al. (1986): Reduction of tar, nicotine, and carbon monoxide intake in low tar smokers. J Epidemiol Community Health 40:80–85.

Samfield M (1980): Research and manufacturing in the U.S. cigarette industry. Lockwood Publishing Co. New York, NY.

Selke WA (1980): Reconstituted tobacco sheet. In: Gori GB, Bock FG (Eds) A safe cigarette? Bambury report No. 3. Proceedings of a meeting held at the Bambury Center. Cold Spring Harbor Laboratory. Cold Spring Harbor, NY. pp. 205–214.

Sheps DS, Adams KF, Bromberg PA (1987): Lack of effect of low levels of carboxyhemoglobin on cardiovascular function in patients with ischemic heart disease. Arch Environ Health 42:108–116.

Schlotzhauer WS, Chortyk OT (1983): Effects of varied smoking machine parameters on deliveries of total particulate matter and selected smoke constituents from ultra-low-tar cigarettes. J Anal Toxicol 7:92–95.

SHP (1975): Proceedings of the tobacco smoke inhalation workshop on experimental methods in smoking and health research. Smoking and Health Program, National Cancer Institute. Gori, GB (ed.) DHEW Publ. No. (NIH) 75-906. National Cancer Institute, Bethesda, MD.

——— (1976a): Toward less hazardous cigarettes, Report No. 1: The first set of experimental cigarettes. Smoking and Health Program, National Cancer Institute. Gori GB (ed.) DHEW Publ. No. (NIH) 76-905. National Cancer Institute, Bethesda, MD.

——— (1976b): Toward less hazardous cigarettes, Report No. 2: The second set of experimental cigarettes. Smoking and Health Program, National Cancer Institute. Gori GB (ed.) DHEW Publ. No. (NIH) 76-1111. National Cancer Institute, Bethesda, MD.

——— (1976c): Chemistry and in vivo bioassay of smoke from experimental filter cigarettes. Gori GB (Ed). Smoking and Health Program. The National Cancer Institute, Bethesda, Maryland.

——— (1977): Toward less hazardous cigarettes, Report No. 3: The third set of experimental cigarettes. Smoking and Health Program, National Cancer Institute. Gori GB (ed.) DHEW Pub. No. (NIH) 77-1280. National Cancer Institute, Bethesda, MD.

——— (1978): An operational manual for the Beagle dog inhalation model. Gori GB (ed.) Smoking and Health Program. National Cancer Institute, Bethesda, MD.

——— (1979): The fourth set of experimental cigarettes. Smoking and Health Program. The National Cancer Institute, Bethesda, Maryland.

Sorlie P, Lakatos E, Kannel WB, et al. (1987): Influence of cigarette smoking on lung function at baseline and at follow-up in 14 years: the Framingham study. J Chronic Dis 40:849–856.

St. Cloud D, Fairclough G (1999): U.S. Sues tobacco makers in massive case. Clinton seeks the recovery of over $20 billion spent a year on sick smokers. The Wall Street Journal. Thursday, September 23, 1999. p. A3.

Supreme Court (2000): Food and Drug Administration, et al., petitioners v. Brown & Williamson Tobacco Corporation et al. On writ of certiorari to the United States Court of Appeals for the Fourth Circuit. No. 98-1152. March 21, 2000. The U.S. Supreme Court, Washington, DC.

Taubes G (1995): Epidemiology faces its limits. Science 269:164–169.

Tennant RW (1988): Relationship between in vitro genetic toxicity and carcinogenicity studies in animals. Ann NY Acad Sci 534:127–132.

TI, The Tobacco Institute (1997): The tax burden of tobacco. Historical compilation. Volume 31, 1996. The Tobacco Institute. Washington, DC.

Timberg C (1999): Virginia road plan relies on tobacco. The Washington Post. August 13, 1999, p. 1.

Tso TC (1972): Physiology and biochemistry of tobacco plants. Dowden, Hutchinson & Ross, Stroudsburg, PA 18360.

Tso TC , Chaplin JF (1977): Simple correlation and multiple regression among leaf characteristics, smoke components and biological responses of bright tobaccos. USDA Technical Bulletin No. 1551.

Tso TC (1980): Modification through agricultural techniques for developing a safer tobacco. In: Gori GB, Bock FG (Eds) A safe cigarette? Bambury report No. 3. Proceedings of a meeting held at the Bambury Center. Cold Spring Harbor Laboratory. Cold Spring Harbor, NY. pp. 181–190.

Tso TC (1999): Seed to smoke. In: Davis L, Nielsen MT (Eds.) Tobacco. Production, chemistry and technology. Balckwell Science. Oxford.

USEPA (1984): U.S. Environmental Protection Agency. Revised evaluation of the health effects associated with carbon monoxide exposure: An addendum to the 1979 EPA air quality criteria document for carbon monoxide. Publication No. EPA-600/8-83-033F. USEPA, Washington, DC.

U.S. Surgeon General (1964): Smoking and health. Report of the advisory committee to the Surgeon General of the Public Health Service. U.S. Department of Health, Education, and Welfare. Public Health Service Publication No.1103., Washington, DC.

——— (1979): Smoking and health: A report of the Surgeon General. DHEW publication No. (PHS):79-50066. Department of Health Education and Welfare, Washington, DC.

——— (1982): The health consequences of smoking: Cancer. A report of the Surgeon General. U.S. Department of Health and Human Services. Office on Smoking and Health, Rockville, MD.

——— (1993): The health consequences of smoking: Cardiovascular diseases.

A report of the Surgeon general. U.S. Department of Health and Human Services, Washington, DC.

—— (1984): The health consequences of smoking: Chronic obstructive lung diseases. A report of the Surgeon General. U.S. Department of Health and Human Services, Washington, DC.

—— (1988): The health consequences of smoking: Nicotine addiction. Report of the Surgeon General. U.S. Department of Health and Human Services. Public Health Service. Publication No. 88-8406. Washington, DC.

—— (1989): Reducing the health consequences of smoking: 25 years of progress. A report of the Surgeon General. DHHS publication No. CDC 89-8411. U.S. Department of Health and Human Services. Public Health Service. Center for Disease Control. Atlanta, GA.

van Doorn R, Bos RP, Leijdekkers CM, et al. (1979): Thioether concentration and mutagenicity of urine from cigarette smokers. Int Arch Occup Environ Health 43:159–166.

Van Duuren BL (1980): Carcinogens, cocarcinogens and tumor inhibitors in cigarette smoke condensate. In: Gori GB, Bock FG (Eds) A safe cigarette? Bambury report No. 3. Proceedings of a meeting held at the Bambury Center. Cold Spring Harbor Laboratory. Cold Spring Harbor, NY. pp. 105–112.

Viscusi WK (1990): Do smokers underestimate risk? J Polit Econ 98:1253–1260.

—— (1992): Smoking: Making the risky decision. Oxford University Press, New York.

Wald NJ, Idle M, Boreham J, et al. (1981): Serum cotinine levels in pipe smokers: evidence against nicotine as cause of coronary heart disease. Lancet October 10:775–777.

Warburton DM (1992): Nicotine as a cognitive enhancer. Prog Nauropsychopharm Biol Psychiat 16:181–191.

Wennmalm A, Benthin G, et al. (1991): Relation between tobacco use and urinary excretion of Thromboxane A2 and Prostacyclin metabolites in young men. Circulation 83:1698–1704.

Werner KE (1987): Health and economic implications of a tobacco-free society. J Am Med A ss 258:2080–2086.

Werner KE, Slade J, Sweanor DT (1997): The emerging market for long-term nicotine maintenance. J Am Med Ass 278:1087–1092.

WHO, World Health Organization (1957): Expert Committee on addiction-producing drugs. Seventh report. World Health Organization, Geneva.

—— (1974): Expert Committee on drug dependence. Twentieth report. World Health Organization, Geneva.

—— (1993): Expert Committee on drug dependence. Twentyeighth report. World Health Organization, Geneva.

Wildavsky A (1995): But is it true? A citizen's guide to environmental health and safety issues. Harvard University Press, Cambridge, MA.

Wilson RW (1967): Cigarette smoking and health characteristics. United States—July 1964–June 1965. Public Health Service, National Center for Health Statistics, Series 10, No 34. Public Health Service Publication No. 1000. U.S. Department of Health, Education and Welfare, Washington, DC.

Wonnacott S, Russell MA, Stolerman IP (1989): Nicotine psychopharma-cology: molecular, cellular & behavioural aspects. Oxford University Press. Oxford.

World Bank (1999): Curbing the epidemic. Governments and the economics of tobacco control. The World Bank, Washington, D.C.

Wynder EL (1997): Tobacco as a cause of lung cancer: Some reflections. Am J Epidemiol 146:687–694.

Zeiger E, Haseman JK, Shelby MD, et al. (1990): Evaluation of four in vitro genetic toxicity tests for predicting rodent carcinogenicity: confirmation of earlier results with 41 additional chemicals. Envir Molecul Mutagen Supp. 18:1–14.

APPENDIX A

Aims and Accomplishments of the Smoking and Health Program, 1968–1979

The overall goal of the National Cancer Institute's Smoking and Health Program (SHP)—carried out with the advice of the Tobacco Working Group and in coordination with the National Heart, Lung, and Blood Institute, and the United States Department of Agriculture—was the reduction of the morbidity and mortality associated with cigarette smoking. In achieving this goal, the SHP directed its efforts to the following objectives:

1. Development of methods for the pharmacologic understanding of smoking.

2. Identification of the hazardous components of tobacco products and the development of methods for minimizing or eliminating these components from cigarettes acceptable to smokers.

In fulfilling its mission, the SHP carried on a coordinated, broadly based research effort from 1968 to 1979. Projects have included: studies of smoking patterns and preferences in humans; pharmacologic studies; cigarette design and manufacturing modifications; analytical chemical studies; development of animal and human tests; and testing of modified cigarettes in animals. The SHP also sponsored epidemiologic studies and

107

studies into smoking cessation methodologies. Here, however, only studies and results related to the development of less hazardous cigarettes are reported, mainly reflecting the more detailed accounts given in the annual reports of the SHP. The latter are listed in Appendix D among other publications of the Program.

PHARMACOLOGIC STUDIES

The SHP recognized that nicotine plays an important role in controlling smoking behavior. Consequently, pharmacologic studies were directed at elucidating the potential role of nicotine in less hazardous cigarettes, and pharmacologic intervention was considered as a possible approach for changing smoking behavior. Research focused on determining the pharmacokinetics of nicotine, and in evaluating whether nicotine aerosols might be able to match the rewards of smoking. Major achievements were as follows:

- A study tested the use of a nicotine aerosol in dogs. When 80 mg/ml unbuffered nicotine aerosols were administered by inhalation to anesthetized dogs, blood nicotine values of as high as 750 ng/ml were obtained with a 30 minute period.

- With assistance from the National Bureau of Standards, tests investigated the influence of pH and nicotine concentration levels on aerosol particle size distribution. A series of solutions containing 30, 60, and 90 mg /ml of nicotine, each at three pH levels of 5.5, 7.0, and 9.0, were studied. Analysis indicated that solution pH or nicotine concentration had little influence on aerosol particle size distribution under test conditions.

- The effect of aerosol pH on nicotine uptake was studied by inhalation in beagle dogs. Analysis did show that the rate of pulmonary uptake is independent of acidity/basicity in the range of pH 5 to 9. This was the first study on record to examine the effect of pH on pulmonary uptake of nicotine.

- Commercial aerosol generation devices were tested at the National Bureau of Standards to determine if they could be used for nicotine aerosol bioassays. Available devices were found of use and produced 95% or more of respirable particles in the range below 2 microns in diameter.

- Two clinical trials used nicotine in aerosol form as a substitute for smoking. It was learned that nicotine can be taken into the bloodstream in concentrations comparable to those obtained from the average cigarette. The aerosols could be used over a prolonged period of time without noticeable toxic or harmful effects. A number of individuals maintained high cotinine (the principal nicotine metabolite) levels throughout the trial. Most participants showed a sharp drop in cigarette consumption.

Cigarette Modifications

With a view to make cigarettes less hazardous, initially the SHP focused on the possibility of altering the composition of tobacco smoke and the concentration of undesirable components, by using different filters, by varying the porosity or composition of the cigarette paper, by using specialized tobacco transformations and extractions, by using non-tobacco substitutes, and by altering tobacco curing and agronomic practices. Some 150 cigarette modifications tested are listed in Appendix B. A critical aspect of the problem was to make less hazardous cigarettes acceptable to smokers, thus requiring the development of flavor additives for modified cigarettes. Major program achievements were as follows:

- Progress was made in identifying the weakly acidic cocarcinogens in cigarette smoke, which were thought to be major contributors to the overall tumorigenic activity of cigarette smoke. New cocarcinogens were also identified in the neutral fraction of cigarette smoke condensates.

- A number of nitrosamines and nitrosamides present in smoke have been identified as organ-specific carcinogens in animal tests. Three nonvolatile, tobacco specific nitrosamines, including N'-nitrosonornicotine, N'-nitrosoanatabine, and NNK (4-(N-methyl-N-nitrosamino) -1-(3-pyridyl)-1-butanone), were tested for mutagenicity as well as for carcinogenicity. NNK ranked highest in activity and induced primarily hepatomas in rats.

- New methods have-been developed for the determination of nicotine and cotinine levels in physiological fluids and for the determination of nitrogen oxides in smoke.

- Profiles of cigarette flavor acceptability characteristics have been defined and methodology for returning flavor additives to stripped tobacco has been developed. These advances could make it possible to design potentially less hazardous smoking products that are flavor-acceptable to the smoker.

- The technology was developed for adjusting nicotine levels and nicotine/tar yields in cigarettes through tobacco extraction, substitution techniques, reblending of the tobacco, reconstituted tobacco sheet processes, filtration, and smoke dilution devices.

- Homogenized leaf curing followed by a reconstitution process was found to enable the selective removal of some tobacco components which may contribute to the hazards of smoking. Newly developed crystallization process allowed the selective removal of protein fractions, and thus to reduce the levels of combustion products such as hydrogen cyanide and aza-arenes in smoke.

- Several types of cigarette filters were tested for their effectiveness in reducing the tumorigenic, cytotoxic, ciliatoxic, and alveolar macrophage inhibitory characteristics of cigarette smoke. These bioassays resulted in recommendations for improved cigarette filters.

- More than 150 different experimental cigarettes have been tested for tumorigenicity on mouse skin. The results yielded valuable information concerning properties of cigarettes which contribute to the tumorigenicity of cigarette smoke condensates (aka tars).

- A study defined the pharmacokinetics of carbon monoxide, nicotine, and the primary nicotine metabolite, cotinine, in the beagle dog model. The study provided a basis for definition of dose levels for inhalation tests in animals and man.

Experimental Cigarettes Tested by the Smoking and Health Program

Experience since the early fifties had indicated that certain modifications of cigarettes can affect the chemical composition and the specific carcinogenic activity of the resulting smoke and condensate. Some of these findings were consistent enough to allow a degree of predictability in planning experimental cigarette modifications.

Initially, the assessment of pertinent literature and consultation with domestic and foreign experts led the Tobacco Working Group and the Smoking and Health Program (SHP) of the National Cancer Institute to formulate a set of promising cigarette models. In time, these models evolved in a series of four sets of experimental cigarettes that were sequentially formulated and tested. Tables 1 to 4 provide a complete list of experimental cigarettes of the SHP.

Experimental cigarettes were all compared to the same standard cigarette provided by the University of Kentucky (The 1R1 cigarette). For each series, a Standard Experimental Blend (SEB) was formulated as the basic blend to be modified. The SEBs of the different series were manufactured to be substantially comparable. All cigarettes underwent extensive chemical characterization of their fabrication materials and of the produced smokes.

Experimental cigarettes were smoked on standard smoking machines to yield smoke condensate (tar), in quantities sufficient for chronic bioassays in mice. Mice were painted with tar solutions on the shaved skin of their backs for lifetime, and lesions were visually noted and examined histopathologically. The number and grade of malignancy of lesions, and the time it took for their appearance were used to compare the specific tumorigenicity of tars from different experimental cigarettes.

In addition, the tumorigenic activity of smoke condensates were correlated with cigarette characteristics, tobacco modifications and processes, and with the levels of specific smoke components, in an effort to pinpoint the most promising directions of change.

Over 70,000,000 experimental cigarettes have been manufactured for use by the Smoking and Health Program. The studies that utilized these cigarettes investigated the contribution of different variables to mouse skin tumorigenicity and other biologic endpoints, the tendency of human smokers to compensate, the effect of flavor additives on acceptability, and the respiratory and cardiovascular effects of smoke inhalation in animal models.

MOUSE SKIN TUMORIGENICITY ASSAYS

A series of four experiments tested the contribution by a variety of cigarette properties to the tumorigenicity of cigarette smoke condensate on mouse skin. More than 150 different types of experimental cigarettes were manufactured for this purpose, and a complete list appears at the end of this section. The smoke generated by each cigarette was collected, condensed, and the tumorigenic potency of the resultant cigarette smoke condensate or tar was assayed by daily application to mouse skin.

Two standard cigarette types were adopted as a basis of comparison in each series of experimental cigarettes. The first was the 1R1 cigarette developed by the University of Kentucky in the early 1960s and subsequently used in many studies as a standard control cigarette. The second was a standard experimental blend (SEB) designed to represent the tobacco composition of the average American cigarette marketed in 1970. Although SEBs for different series were made from different tobacco crops, the same blend composition was used for each of the four series of experiments.

Series I of Experimental Cigarettes

Starting with the first experimental series in 1969, the Tobacco Working Group recommended 21 modifications of the SEB I as the experimental variants, as follows:

- Variation of paper porosity, which affects the aeration of the burning zone and therefore the oxygenation and the temperature conditions determining pyrolysis and distillation.

- Variation of the width of tobacco cut, which may affect the aeration of the cigarette.

- Concentration of nitrate, which would favor combustion, but may also affect formation of nitrogen oxides and nitrosamines.

- Various fractions of the SEB I blend, such as leaves only and stems only, to determine the relative contribution of different blend fractions.

- Reconstituted Tobacco Sheets (RTS), where the SEB I blend was transformed into processed tobacco sheets by various techniques similar to paper making. The characteristics of the sheets are determined by their final density, the removal of certain tobacco components, or the addition of non-tobacco fractions. These modifications in turn determine the amount of tobacco used per cigarette and allow removal of tobacco components or addition of inert tobacco diluents. All of these changes affect the aeration, pyrolysis, and distillation, and eventually the chemistry and biologic activity of the resulting smoke.

These modifications produced the following:

- Reconstituted tobacco sheets (RTS) in general resulted in condensates less tumorigenic than the SEB I. The condensate activity did not appear to be affected by the relative density of the RTS, but was affected by the removal of certain tobacco fractions or the addition of diluent additives, according to specific manufacturing methods.

- High paper porosity decreased the tumorigenic activity of condensate on mouse skin.

- The addition of nitrate to the SEB I (doubling the total nitrate present) failed to reduce the condensate tumorigenicity for mouse skin, contrary to previous reports. However, in this test the relative concentrations of nitrate in control and test cigarettes may not have been not sufficiently different to modify the tumorigenicity of condensates.

- Different shred widths of tobacco failed to affect the tumorigenicity of SEB I condensate for mouse skin.

- Cigarettes made solely of tobacco stems produced condensates of the lowest tumorigenic activity for mouse skin. Stems differ in many ways from whole tobacco and their composition provided guidelines for further tobacco modifications.

- The relative concentration of nicotine, either in the tobacco or in the condensate, correlated with the condensate tumorigenic activity for mouse skin. It was unclear whether nicotine itself is tumorigenic or co-tumorigenic, or merely an indicator of other tumorigens, the concentration of which may naturally parallel that of nicotine.

Series II of Experimental Cigarettes

The second cigarette experiment began in 1972, based on results from the first experiment and added agronomic considerations.

The University of Kentucky 1R1 and the SEB I were used as references. The SEB II had the same blend composition as the SEB I but was produced from a different leaf crop and by a different manufacturer. Experimental variables in this second experiment consisted of:

- Tobacco processing to affect the packing density (the amount of tobacco per cigarette and thus the amount of tar and nicotine yield), and the aeration of the burning zone (thus the oxygenation and temperature of the burning process).

- Tobacco from plants with both normal and low nicotine content, to compare possible nicotine tumorigenicity.

- Concentration of fertilizer (nitrogen), to determine whether high or normal fertilization leads to condensates of different tumorigenicity.

- Tobacco leaf processing, to determine whether plants treated with fatty alcohol produce leaves with greater tumorigenic capacities than those of leaves from hand-suckered plants. (Note: Suckering refers to the practice of removing the tobacco plant inflorescence to increase leaf growth. Removal can be by hand of by the application of certain fatty alcohols.)

- Non-tobacco cigarettes, to compare the tumorigenicity of artificial tobacco substitutes (ATSs) with that of SEB II.

These modifications produced the following:

- The low nicotine/normal fertilizer, and low nicotine/high fertilizer blends showed significantly lower tumorigenicity than the normal nicotine/normal fertilizer blends. However, there were no significant differences between the low nicotine/normal fertilizer and low nicotine/high fertilizer blends.

- The Reynolds puffed, Philip Morris expanded, and freeze-dried SEB II blends showed no significant differences among themselves. The Philip Morris expanded and freeze-dried SEB II blends showed significantly lower condensate tumorigenicity than SEB II. (Note: Puffing or expanding are two processes that increase the volume of tobacco leaf without increasing its weight.)

- Two artificial tobacco substitutes (ATS) tested showed a wide range of response when unblended, specifically the lowest and highest condensate tumorigenicity, the latter being comparable to 1R1 and SEB blends. Blends of these materials with SEB II were not significantly different from SEB II alone. Condensates from cigarettes made entirely of these materials were physically different from tobacco condensates and were not homogeneous. The results required further exploration before conclusions could be drawn concerning the value of ATSs.

- Smoke condensates from plants treated with any amounts of fatty alcohol and hand-suckered plants showed no significant differences in tumorigenicity among themselves or from the SEB II.

- The results of correlation analyses of several constituents of tobacco leaf and condensates of the second cigarette series complement those of the first series. Nicotine and condensate yields were highly correlated with tumorigenic activity on mouse skin. Static burn rate was negatively correlated with tumorigenic activity. Since static burn rate can affect the chemical composition of the smoke, this may be an indication that a fast burning rate is a characteristic of reduced hazard. Other compounds negatively correlated with tumorigenicity in both experiments were acetaldehyde, formaldehyde, NOx, CO, and acrolein. Positively correlated with tumorigenicity were total phenolics in the leaf, water content of cigarette, and benz[a]anthracene in the condensate. These data by no means prove that any condensate constituents are causative agents in tumorigenesis. These constituents may only be indicators of some other factor affecting tumorigenicity. The results did, however, provide clues about the design of new experimental variables.

Series III of Experimental Cigarettes

The Third series of experimental cigarettes took off from the results of the first two series. The University of Kentucky 1R1, the SEB I, and the SEB II were used as references. The SEB III had the same blend composition as the SEB I and SEB II, but was produced from a different leaf crop and by a different manufacturer. Experimental variables in this second experiment consisted of:

- Paper porosity was varied. A special paper was also tested.

- The role of sugars, humectants, flavorings, and additives was examined.

- Several dilution filters were tested in cigarettes wrapped in paper of varying porosity's. A permanganate filter was tested, with a cellulose acetate filter as a control.

- Further tests were performed on cigarettes made of artificial tobacco substitutes, that were wrapped in papers of varying porosities, both with and without dilution filters.

These modifications produced the following:

- Comparisons among the additive variables indicate that magnesium nitrate reduced the tumorigenicity of cigarette condensate.

- Neither sugar nor humectant affected the tumorigenicity at the lower (12.5 mg) dose levels of tar application on mouse skin. They could have contributed tumorigenicity at higher dose levels. Powdered cocoa increased tumorigenicity at all dose levels.

- Dilution filters proved effective in reducing tumorigenicity. Neither the permanganate filter nor the cellulose acetate filter reduced tumorigenicity.

- There were no significant differences among the paper porosity variables or between these variables and SEB III.

- Two artificial tobacco substitutes (ATS-A and ATS-B) were included in this experiment. The ATS-A cigarette was exceptionally effective in reducing cigarette tumorigenicity, whereas the ATS-B cigarette fared poorly in the tests. Experimental difficulties arose with ATS-B regarding the solvent used in the second and third experiments.

Series IV of Experimental Cigarettes

The fourth series of experimental cigarettes was influenced by the three previous series. The University of Kentucky 1R1, the SEB I, the SEB II, and the SEB III were used as references. The SEB IV had the same blend composition as the previous SEBs, but was produced from a different leaf crop and by a different manufacturer. Experimental variables in this fourth experiment were as follows:

- Different processes of reconstituted tobacco sheet were tested, and especially the effects of inorganic fillers on both the chemistry and the biological activity of the resulting smoke condensates.

- Nicotine extraction methods were examined to understand further the relationship between nicotine and mouse skin tumorigenesis, as well as the impact of extraction on biological activity.

- Levels of tobacco leaf waxes were tested for their relationship to tumorigenicity.

- Special papers, additives, and processed smoking materials were studied.

- Cigarettes were treated with pesticides, to ascertain their impact on the chemical and biological activity of the condensates, as well as the mobility of the pesticide itself.

These modifications produced the following:

- Overall, Bright tobacco variants produced condensates slightly less tumorigenic than Burley tobacco variants, although Bright and Burley variants were comparable in terms of chemical analysis.

- One of the reconstituted tobacco cigarettes (10% cellulose fiber additive, nicotine added back in the form of nicotine citrate) resulted in less tumorigenic condensate Otherwise, both the paper and slurry reconstitution processes resulted in tumorigenicity either comparable to or significantly higher than the SEB IV. (Note: Paper and slurry are two different processes to obtain reconstituted tobacco sheets.)

- No significant tumorigenic differences were observed between cigarettes made from pesticide-treated and pesticide-free tobacco.

- Cigarettes made from expanded stems of tobacco leaf were significantly less tumorigenic than the SEB IV.

- A positive correlation was observed between nicotine yield and biological response. However, because of variations in other condensate yields, it was not clear that the correlation implies a causal relationship.

- Results from the fourth experimental cigarette series corroborated earlier findings that, in reducing mouse skin tumorigenicity, the preferred paper porosity should allow an air-flow of approximately 60 cm./min.

1. List of Series I Experimental Cigarettes

1 University of Kentucky Reference (1R1)
2 SEB I
3 SEB I, High porosity citrate paper (Schweitzer #505) (48 cm/min)

4 SEB I, Low porosity phosphate paper (Ecusta Reference A of Schweitzer Regular Verge) (11 cm/min)

5 SEB I, Nitrates added as KNO3, to 2x natural level of SEB I.

6 SEB I, cut coarse (20 cuts/in)

7 SEB I, cut fine (60 cuts/in)

8 SEB I, with low porosity phosphate paper and coarse cut (combination of codes 4&6)

9 SEB, I, with high porosity citrate paper and high nitrate content (combination of codes 3&5)

10 SEB I, Laminae only (only leaves of the formula used)

11 SEB I, Flue-cured Laminae only (only flue-cured leaves of formula used)

12 SEB I, Burley laminae only (only Burley leaves used)

13 SEB I, Stems only (only flue-cured and Burley stems used, rolled and cut)

14 SEB I, Stems only, made into RTS by Schweitzer paper process

15 SEB I, Stems and fines only, made into RTS by AMF slurry process

16 RTS of whole SEB I by Schweitzer paper process, no additives, medium density

17 RTS of whole SEB I by Schweitzer paper process, 7.5% wood pulp added, low density

18 RTS of whole SEB I by Schweitzer paper process, 7.5% wood pulp added, medium density

19 RTS of whole SEB I by Schweitzer paper process, 7.5% wood pulp added, high density

20 RTS of whole SEB I by AMF slurry process, no additives, medium density

21 RTS of whole SEB I by AMF slurry process, additives*, low density

22 RTS of whole SEB I by AMF slurry process, additives*, medium density

23 RTS of whole SEB I by AMF slurry process, additives*,

high density

*Additives were:

Glycerin 2.81%
Invert sugar. 5.31%
Methocel 7.35%
Refined unbleached sulfite pulp 4.59%
Ethylhydroxyethyl cellulose 1.84%

2. List of Series II Experimental Cigarettes

1 University of Kentucky Reference (1R1)
2 SEB I
3 SEB II
4 SEB II
5 SEB II
6 SEB II
7 ATS-A, 100%
8 ATS-A, 50% & SEB 11, 50%
9 RJ Reynolds puffed SEB II
10 Philip Morris expanded SEB II
11 Freeze-dried SEB II
12 Straight Burley, normal nicotine, normal nitrogen fertiliza-
    tion *(NN)
13 Straight Burley, low nicotine, normal nitrogen fertilization
    (LN)
14 Straight Burley, low nicotine, high nitrogen fertilization
    *(LH)
15 Straight flue-cured, normal nicotine, normal nitrogen fertil-
    ization (NN)
16 Straight flue-cured, low nicotine, normal nitrogen fertiliza-
    tion (LN)
17 Straight flue-cured, low nicotine, high nitrogen fertilization
    (LH)
18 Blend 3 parts flue-cured, I part Burley (NN)
19 Blend 3 parts flue-cured, 1 part Burley (LN)
20 Blend 3 parts flue-cured, 1 part Burley (LH)
21 Hand suckered (no suckering chemicals used)

22 Fatty-alcohol—normal
23 Fatty-alcohol—100x.
24 ATS-B straight (100%)
25 ATS-B, 50% & SEB 11, 50%

*Normal Nicotine variety, NC95. Low Nicotine variety, LN90. Normal Nitrogen rate, 61lb/acre High Nitrogen rate, 100lb/acre
Note: ATS = Artificial Tobacco Substitute

3. List of Series III Experimental Cigarettes

1 University of Kentucky Reference (1R1)
2 SEB I
3 SEB I
4 SEB III
5 SEB III
6 SEB III
7 SEB III
8 SEB III
9 SEB III (Schweitzer paper 489-14; Low porosity) (5cm/min)
10 SEB III (Verge 55 paper-high porosity) (60 cm/min)
11 SEB III (Schweitzer perforated paper-very high porosity) (100 m/min)
12 SEB III No sugar, with humectant
13 SEB III With sugar, no humectant
14 SEB III With 1% cocoa, no sugar, no humectant
15 SEB III No sugar, no humectant (no casing)
16 SEB III With L&M additive #1 (Magnesium Nitrate, 5.72%)
17 SEB III With L&M additive #2 (Zinc Oxide, 7.09%)
18 SEB III With L&M additive #3 (Magnesium Nitrate, 5.61%, Zinc oxide, 6.96%)
19 SEB III Burley Blend, cased with sugar, no humectant
20 SEB III Burley Blend, cased with sugar, no humectant
21 SEB III Burley Blend, no casing (no sugar)
22 SEB III With dilution filter

23 SEB III With dilution filter and Schweitzer perforated paper (100 cm/min)
24 SEB III With cellulose acetate filter
25 SEB III With Permanganate filter
26 ATS-A, 30% & SEB 111, 70%, plus flavor
27 ATS-A, 3.0% & SEB 111, 70%, plus flavor
28 ATS-B, 100% (old material, old dyes)
29 ATS-B, 100% (new material, no dyes)
30 ATS-B, 100% (old material, no dyes)
31 ATS-B (old material, no dyes) 50% & SEB 111, 50% (casing applied to tobacco portion only)
32 SEB III
33 ATS-A, 30% & SEB 111, 70% plus flavor with Verge 60cm/sec paper
34 ATS-A, 50% & SEB 111, 50% (casing applied to tobacco portion only)
35 ATS-B, 100% (old material, new dyes)
36 ATS-B, 100% (new material, new dyes)

Note:
　　ATS-A = Artificial Tobacco Substitute A
　　ATS-B = Artificial Tobacco Substitute B

4. List of Series IV Experimental Cigarettes

1 University of Kentucky Reference (1R1)
1A SEB III
2 SEB IV
3 SEB IV
4 SEB IV
5 SEB IV
6 SEB IV, RTS, PJS paper process, no additives
7 SEB IV, RTS, PJS paper process, 10% additives (cellulose fiber)
8 SEB IV, RTS, PJS paper process, 10% additives (cellulose fiber), no return of water soluble substances
9 SEB IV, RTS, PJS paper process, 10% additives (cellulose

fiber), nicotine reduced by proprietary process

10 SEB IV, RTS, PJS paper process, 10% additives (cellulose fiber), nicotine reduced and added back in form of nicotine citrate to level of Code 32, SEB IV

11 SEB IV, RTS, AMF slurry process, no additives except 2.8% glycerin, 5.31% invert sugar

12 SEB IV, RTS, AMF slurry process, 13% additives (see Note 1)

13 SEB IV, RTS, AMF slurry process, 13% additives plus 6% pH adjustment (see Note 2)

14 SEB IV, RTS, AMF slurry process, extracted with hexane-isopropyl alcohol azeotrope, 13% additives (see Note 1)

15 SEB IV, RTS, AMF slurry process, extracted with isopropyl alcohol water azeotrope, 13% additives (see Note 1)

16 SEB IV, RTS, PJS paper process, 10% additives (cellulose fiber), waxy substances reduced

17 SEB IV, RTS, AMF slurry process 57%, plus 30% calcium carbonate, plus Note 1

18 SEB IV, RTS, AMF slurry process 27%, plus 60% calcium carbonate, plus Note 1

19 SEB IV, RTS, AMF slurry process 27%, extracted with iso-propyl alcohol-water azeotrope, plus 60% calcium carbonate, plus Note 1

20 SEB IV, RTS, PJS paper process, 10% additives (cellulose fiber), plus 25% inorganic fillers (calcium carbonate 18%, clay 7%)

21 SEB IV, RTS, PJS paper process, 10% additives (cellulose fiber) Hydrogen peroxide treated

22 SEB IV expanded stems, 100'.

23 SEB IV expanded stems 50%, SEB IV 50%

25 SEB IV, 70%, Ecusta material 30%

27 SEB IV nicotine removed

28 SEB IV nicotine at 0.5 mg/cig.

29 SEB IV nicotine at 1.0 mg/cig.

30 SEB IV nicotine at 1.5 mg/cig.

31 Burley leaf with full return of stem
32 Burley leaf RTS, AMF slurry process, 15% additives (see Note 3)
33 Burley HLC RTS, AMF slurry process, 15% additives (see Note 3)
34 Bright leaf with full return of stems
35 Bright leaf RTS, AMF slurry process, 15% additives (see Note 3)
36 Bright HLC RTS, AMF slurry process, 15% additives (see Note 3)
37 Pesticide free tobacco
38 Pesticide treated tobacco
39 SEB IV, treated with PMO (1.5% by weight)
40 SEB IV, with special 100cm/min paper

Note 1. Additives:
    Refined Unbleached Sulfite Pulp 6.05%
    Galacto-Mannan Gums 5.85%
    Cellulose Ether Gums 0.52%
    Dialdehyde Crosslinker 0.58%
    Total 13.00%
Note 2. Additives: Same as Note 1, plus
    Sodium Hydroxide 3.20%
    Citric Acid 2.80%
    Total 6.00%
Note 3. Additives:
    Refined Unbleached Sulfite Pulp 6.25%
    Triethylene Glycol 2.25%
    Galacto-Mannan Gums 4.48%
    Cellulose Ether Gums 1.42%
    Dialdehyde Crosslinker 0.60%
    Total 15.00%

RTS = Reconstituted Tobacco Sheet
PJS = Peter J. Schweitzer Inc.
AMF = AMF, Inc.
HLC = Homogenized Leaf Cured

CIGARETTES FOR INHALATION STUDIES

A total of 4,200,000 cigarettes were manufactured for use in several studies of the effects of co-varying the concentrations of tar, nicotine, and carbon monoxide on the development of pulmonary and cardiovascular diseases in various animal models. Experiments were designed to last from 2 to 5 years and were well underway by the end of 1979, when they were suddenly terminated before completion by the National Cancer Institute. Several million dollars of research investments were lost, as well as the promise of definitive insight about the contribution of smoking to cancer, cardiovascular and respiratory diseases. Of these studies only one was completed, but its publication was suppressed. A summary of its results is reported at page 55 of this volume.

List of Smoking and Health Program Consultants

Dr. Peter Abbrecht, University of Michigan
Dr. Fawky Abdallah, Imperial Tobacco Limited
Dr. Paul Allen, University of Delaware
Dr. Alan Armitage, Council for Tobacco Research, London
Dr. Mark Armstrong, University of Texas
Dr. James Atkins, University of Texas
Dr. Oscar Auerbach, Veterans Administration Hospital, New Jersey
Dr. Donald Austin, California Tumor Registry
Dr. John Bailar, National Cancer Institute
Dr. James Bain, Emory University
Dr. Carl G. Baker, National Cancer Institute
Dr. J. Barnhart, University of California
Dr. David Bates, University of British Columbia
Dr. William W. Bates, Liggett & Myers Tobacco Company
Dr. Mario Battigelli, University of North Carolina
Dr. Sam Battista, Arthur D. Little, Inc.
Dr. C. Becker, Cornell University
Dr. John F. Benner, University of Kentucky
Dr. John Berg, Colorado Regional Cancer Registry
Dr. Vernon Bishop, University of Texas
Dr. Henry Blackburn, University of Minnesota
Dr. William Blot, National Cancer Institute
Dr. Donald M. Blount, National Heart, Lung and Blood Institute
Dr. Edwin Boatman, University of Washington
Dr. Fred G. Bock, Roswell Park Memorial Institute

Dr. Roswell K. Boutwell, University of Wisconsin
Dr. Edward Bresnick, Medical College of Georgia
Dr. Kenneth Brinkhous, University of North Carolina
Dr. Stuart Brooks, Ohio State University
Dr. Charles C. Brown, National Cancer Institute
Dr. Roy Brown, Mt. Sinai School of Medicine
Dr. Bill Bullock, Bowman Gray School of Medicine
Dr. John Caton, Oak Ridge National Laboratories
Dr. Ercole Cavalieri, University of Nebraska
Dr. James F. Chaplin, U.S. Department of Agriculture
Dr. O.T. Chortyk, Richard B. Russell Research Center
Dr. Thomas B. Clarkson, Bowman-Gray School of Medicine
Dr. Philip T. Cole, University of Alabama
Dr. Richard Corlett, University of Washington
Dr. Pelayo Correa, Louisiana State University Medical Center
Dr. Morton J. Cowan, National Heart, Lung and Blood Institute
Dr. John Craighead, University of Vermont
Dr. Sidney Cutler, Georgetown University School of Medicine
Dr. Gerald Deneau, University of California School of Medicine
Dr. Louis Diamond, University of Kentucky
Sir Richard Doll, University of Oxford
Dr. Edward F. Domino, University of Michigan
Dr. Grace M. Donnelly, University of Kentucky
Dr. John Edward Dunn, California Department of Public Health
Dr. John T. Edsall, Harvard University
Dr. Gerald F. Egan, Exxon Corporation
Dr. L. Engelking, University of Florida
Dr. Ronald Estabrook, University of Texas
Dr. Hans L. Falk, National Institute of Environmental Health Sciences
Dr. Alfred Fishman, Hospital of the University of Pennsylvania
Dr. Robert Forster, Hospital of the University of Pennsylvania
Dr. Bernard Fox, National Cancer Institute
Dr. F. John Francis, University of Massachusetts
Dr. Joseph F. Fraumeni, Jr., National Cancer Institute
Dr. Perry J. Gehring, Dow Chemical Company
Dr. Jean D. Gibbons, University of Alabama
Dr. Gerald Goeringer, Georgetown University Medical School
Dr. Saxon Graham, SUNY-Downstate Medical Center
Dr. Michael R. Guerin, Oak Ridge National Laboratories
Mr. William Haenszel, Illinois Cancer Council
Mr. Howard M. Halter, AMF Incorporated

Dr. E. Cuyler Hammond, American Cancer Society
Dr. Naomi Harley, New York University Medical Center
Dr. John Hayes, Mallory Institute
Dr. Harry W. Hays, U.S. Department of Agriculture
Dr. S. Hecht, American Health Foundation
Dr. Allen Heim, National Cancer Institute
Dr. John Heller, National Cancer Institute
Dr. J. Alan Herd, New England Primate Center
Dr. Ian Higgins, University of Michigan
Dr. Marcus E. Hobbs, Duke University
Dr. Dietrich Hoffmann, American Health Foundation
Dr. Daniel Horn, National Clearinghouse for Smoking and Health
Dr. Evan C. Horning, Baylor College of Medicine
Dr. I.W. Hughes, Brown and Williamson Tobacco Corporation
Dr. Robert E. Hyatt, Mayo Clinic
Dr. Ronald H. Ingram, Peter Bent Brigham Hospital
Dr. Thomas N. James, University of Alabama Medical Center
Dr. Murray E. Jarvik, VA Brentwood Hospital
Dr. Harold A. Kahn, Johns Hopkins University
Dr. Morley Kare, Monell Chemical Senses Center
Dr. Charles H. Keith, Celenese Fibers Company
Dr. Kenneth Keller, North Carolina State University
Dr. Ann Kennedy, Harvard School of Public Health
Dr. Charles J. Kensler, Arthur D. Little, Inc.
Mr. Robert L. Kersey, Liggett and Myers Tobacco Company
Dr. Irving Kessler, University of Maryland School of Medicine
Dr. Charles Key, New Mexico Tumor Registry
Dr. Jerome Kleinerman, St. Luke's Hospital
Dr. Francis Klocke, Buffalo General Hospital
Dr. George B. Koelle, University of Pennsylvania School of Medicine
Dr. Bruce Kottke, Mayo Clinic
Dr. B.K. Krotoszynski, I I I Research Institute
Dr. H. Kubota, Oak Ridge National Laboratories
Dr. Marvin Kuschner, State University of New York
Dr. Louis Lasagna, University of Rochester
Mr. Thomas Lee, National Bureau of Standards
Dr. S. Lehrer, Tulane Medical Center
Dr. Claude J. Lenfant, National Heart, Lung and Blood Institute
Dr. Morton Levin, Johns Hopkins University
Dr. William Lijinsky, Oak Ridge National Laboratory
Mr. Clifford Lilly, Philip Morris, U.S.A.

Dr. Jorge Litvak, Pan American Health Organization
Dr. Jonn P. Long, University of Iowa
Dr. Joseph Lyon, University of Utah
Dr. Harold N. MacFarland, Gulf Oil Corporation
Dr. Mahley, National Heart, Lung and Blood Institute
Dr. Owen Maller, U.S. Army R&D Command
Dr. A. Marchok, Oak Ridge National Laboratory
Dr. Charles Mattina, Peter J. Schweitzer Inc.
Dr. Bruce McCullough, Southwest Foundation for Research and Education
Dr. Daniel McGee, National Heart, Lung and Blood Institute
Dr. Henry McGill, Jr., University of Texas
Dr. C.A. McMahan, University of Texas
Dr. Gardner C. McMillan, National Heart, Lung and Blood Institute
Dr. Harold Menkes, Johns Hopkins University
Dr. Sanford A. Miller, Massachusetts Institute of Technology
Dr. Ralph Mitchell, Battelle Memorial Institute
Dr. E.L. Moore, U.S. Department of Agriculture
Dr. William Moorman, National Institute for Occupational Safety and
  Health
Dr. Gerald P. Morie, Tennessee Eastman Company
Dr. Kenneth Moser, University Hospital of San Diego County
Dr. Jay Moskowitz, National Heart, Lung and Blood Institute
Dr. Robert Murphy, University of Colorado Medical School
Dr. Paul Nettesheim, Oak Ridge National Laboratories
Dr. Mark Nickerson, McGill University
Dr. Thomas Osdene, Philip Morris, U.S.A.
Dr. Clifford H. Patrick, National Institute on Aging
Dr. Philip Pratt, Duke University Medical Center
Dr. Osgood D. Priddle, Bausch and Lomb
Dr. James R. Prine, Los Alamos Scientific Laboratory
Dr. Roger L. Priore, Roswell Park Memorial Institute
Dr. Donald F. Proctor, Johns Hopkins School of Hygiene
Dr. Duane W. Proppe, University of Texas
Dr. Russell Prough, University of Texas
Dr. K. Pump, University of British Columbia
Dr. Gunter Rathkamp, Waters Mestenick, G.m.b.H.
Dr. William Reece, Iowa State University
Dr. William K. Riker, University of Oregon Medical School
Dr. W.E. Rinehart, Bio/Dynamic, Inc.
Dr. Abel L. Robertson, Jr., Case Western Reserve University
Dr. John Rockett, National Bureau of Standards

Dr. Alan Rodgman, R.J. Reynolds Tobacco Company
Dr. M.A.H. Russell, University of London
Dr. Geno Saccomanno, St. Mary's and V.A. Hospitals
Dr. Umberto Saffiotti, National Cancer Institute
Dr. Richard St. Clair, Bowman Gray University
Dr. J.M. Salhany, University of Nebraska
Dr. Irwin Schmeltz, American Health Foundation
Dr. Marvin A. Schneiderman, National Cancer Institute
Dr. Frederick Schultz, Lorillard Research Center
Dr. Robert B. Seligman, Philip Morris, U.S.A.
Dr. Irving J. Selikoff, Mt. Sinai School of Medicine
Dr. William Selke, Kimberly-Clark Corporation
Dr. Murray Senkus, R.J. Reynolds Tobacco Company
Dr. Michael B. Shimkin, University of California
Dr. Robert Sparks, Kellogg Foundation
Dr. A.W. Spears, Lorillard Research Center
Dr. Reuel Stallones, University of Texas School of Public Health
Dr. Mearl F. Stanton, National Cancer Institute
Dr. Jesse L. Steinfeld, National Cancer Institute
Dr. G.W. Stokes, University of Kentucky
Dr. James R. Stokely, Oak Ridge National Laboratories
Dr. Jack T. Strong, Louisiana State University
Dr. Martin Summerfield, Princeton University
Dr. Philip S. Thayer, Arthur D. Little, Inc.
Dr. Wilbur Thomas, Albany Medical College
Dr. Bela Toth, University of Nebraska
Dr. Richard E. Tracy, Louisiana State University
Dr. T.C. Tso, U.S. Department of Agriculture
Dr. Walter S. Tyler, University of California
Dr. Mayo Uziel, Oak Ridge National Laboratories
Dr. Benjamin L. Van Duuren, New York University
Dr. Steven Vatner, New England Primate Center
Dr. Helmut Wakeham, Philip Morris, U.S.A.
Dr. Lee Wattenberg, University of Minnesota
Dr. Elizabeth Weisburger, National Cancer Institute
Dr. Edward R. White, Armed Forces Institute of Pathology
Dr. R. Wilson, Washington State University
Dr. Harry C. Wong, Howard University
Dr. Otto Wong, Georgetown University
Dr. John Wyatt, University of Kentucky
Dr. Ernst L. Wynder, American Health Foundation

Dr. Stanley Yamashiro, University of Southern California
Dr. Donovan Yeates, New York University
Dr. Raymond Yesner, Veterans Administration Hospital, Connecticut

APPENDIX D

Publications of Studies Funded by the Smoking and Health Program

Adir, J., R. P. Miller and K. S. Rotenberg. 1976. Disposition of nicotine in the rat after intravenous administration. Res. Commun. Chem. Pathol. Pharmacol. 13:173.

Anonymous, 1979. The Fourth Series of Experimental Cigarettes. Smoking and Health Program. The National Cancer Institute.

Auerbach, O. 1979. Natural history of carcinoma of the lung. "Pulmonary diseases." (A.P. Fishman, ed.) McGraw Hill Book Co., N. Y., vol. 2, Ch. 126, pp. 1388–1396.

Auerbach, O., L. Garfinkel and V. R. Parks. 1979. Scar cancer of the lung. Cancer 43:636–642.

Auerbach, O., E. C. Hammond and L. Garfinkel. 1979, Changes in bronchial epithelium in relation to cigarette smoking, 1955–1960 vs. 1970–1977. New Eng. J. Med. 300:381–386.

Auerbach, O., G. Saccomanno, R. D. Brown and L. Garfinkel. 1978 Histologic Findings in the Tracheobronchial Tree of Uranium Miners and Nonminers with Lung Cancer. Cancer 42:483–489.

Battista, S. P. 1976. Cilia toxic components. Pages 517–534 in E. L. Wynder, D. Hoffmann and G. B. Gori, eds. Smoking and Health I :Modifying the Risk for the Smoker. DHEW Pub. No. (NIH) 76-1221, U.S. Government Printing Office, Washington, D.C.

Battista, S. P., I. A. Blieden, S. H. Loring and J. M. Drazen. 1975. Implantation of retrograde catheters in closed chest dogs by laparotomy/bronchoscopy. Fed. Proc. 33:569. (abstr.)

Battista, S. P., G. B. Gori, M. R. Guerin and C. J. Kensler. 1973. A new system for quantitatively exposing laboratory animals by direct inhalation.

Arch. Environ. Health 27:376.

Battista, S. P., P. Mione, A. Lapey, G. Gori and W. Metcher. 1980. Role of clotting factor(s) in the ciliastasis induced by animal, human and cystic fibrosis serum. Arch. of Environ. Health. 35:239–246

Bayne, C. K. 1979. A probability prediction model of mouse skin tumors based on chemical components of cigarette smoke condensates. ORNL/TM-7037, available from NTIS, Springfield, VA 22161.

Benedict, W. F., M. Karon and R. E. Kouri. 1973. Malignant transformation produced by cytosine arabinoside. Pediatr. Res. 7:310.

Benedict, W. F. and R. E. Kouri. 1973. The relationship between 1-D-arabinofuranosylcytosine (Ara-C) transformation and chromosomal changes in hamster fetal cells. Genetics 74:195–205.

Benedict, W. F., N. Rucker, J. Faust and R. E. Kouri. 1975. Malignant transformation of mouse cells by cigarette smoke condensate. Cancer Res. 35:857–860.

Benedict, W. F., N. Rucker, C. Mark and R. E. Kouri. 1975. Correlation between the balance of specific chromosomes and the expression of malignancy in hamster cells. J. Natl. Cancer Inst. 54:157–162.

Bock, F. G. and G. B. Gori. 1978. Sebaceous gland suppression activity of experimental cigarette smoke condensates. Proceedings of the Sixth Annual Meeting of the American Association for cancer Research 19:43 (Abstract).

Bock, F. G. and T. C. Tso. 1976. Chemical and biological identification of tumorigenic components of tobacco. Pages 161–174 in E. L. Wynder, D. Hoffmann and G. B. Gori, eds. Smoking and Health I: Modifying the Risk for the Smoker. DHEW Pub. No. (NIH) 76-1221, U.S. Government Printing Office, Washington, D.C.

———. 1976. Tumor promoting activity of agriculture chemicals. Pages 175–190 in E. L. Wynder, D. Hoffmann, and G. B. Gori, eds. Smoking and Health I: Modifying the Risk for the Smoker. DHEW Pub. No. (NIH) 76-1221, U.S. Government Printing Office, Washington, D.C.

Brunnemann, K. D., J. D. Adams, D. P. S. Ho and D. Hoffmann. 1977. The influence of tobacco smoke on indoor atmospheres II. Volatile and tobacco-specific nitrosamines in main and sidestream smoke and their contribution to indoor pollution. Proc. 4th Joint Conf. on Sensing on Environ. Pollutants, New Orleans, LA., pages 876–880.

Brunnemann, K. D. and D. Hoffmann. 1974. Chemical studies on tobacco smoke. XXIV. Quantitative method for carbon monoxide and carbon dioxide in cigarette and cigar smoke. J. Chromatogr. Sci. 12:70–75.

———. 1974. Chemical studies on tobacco smoke XXXIV. Gas chromatographic determination of ammonia in cigarette and cigar smoke. J. Chromatogr. Sci. 13:159–163.

———. 1975. Chemical Studies on tobacco smoke. XXXIV. Gas chromatographic determination of ammonia in cigarette and cigar smoke. J. Chromatogr. Sci. 13:159–163.

———. 1978. Chemical studies on tobacco smoke LIX. Analysis of volatile nitrosamines in tobacco smoke and polluted indoor environments. IARC Sci. Publ. No. 19, pages 343–356.

Brunnemann, K.D., D. Hoffmann, E. L. Wynder and G. B. Gori. 1976. Chemical studies on tobacco smoke. XXXVII. Determination of tar, nicotine and carbon monoxide in cigarette smoke. A comparison of international smoking conditions. Pages 441–449 in E. L. Wynder, D. Hoffmann and G. B. Gori, eds. Smoking and Health I: Modifying the Risk for the Smoker. DHEW Pub. No. (NIH) 76-1221, U. S. Government Printing Office, Washington, D.C.

Brunnemann, K. D., H. C. Lee and D. Hoffmann. 1975. Catechols in tobacco smoke: quantitative analysis and precursors. Paper presented at the 29th Tobacco Chemists' Research Conference, College Park, MD., October 8–10.

———. 1976. Chemical studies on tobacco smoke. XLVIII. On the quantitative analysis of catechols and their reduction. Anal. Lett. 9:939–955.

Brunnemann, K. D., G. Stahnke and D. Hoffmann. 1978. Chemical studies on tobacco smoke LXI. Volatile pyridines: Quantitative analysis in mainstream and sidestream smoke of cigarettes and cigars. Anal. Lett. All 7:545–560.

Brunnemann, K. D., L. Yu and D. Hoffmann. 1972. Assessment of carcinogenic volatile N-nitrosamines in tobacco and in mainstream and sidestream smoke from cigarettes. Cancer Res. 37:3218–3222.

———. 1977. Chemical studies on tobacco smoke. XLIX. Gas chromatographic determination of hydrogen cyanide and cyanogen in tobacco smoke. J. Anal. Toxicol.1:38–42.

Burke, N.D., R.T. Mayer and R.E. Kouri. 1977. 3-Methylcholanthrene-Induced monooxygenase (0-deethylation) Activity of Human Lymphocytes. Cancer Res: 37(2): 460–463.

Burton, D., 1975. Guidelines for establishing a smoking program. Paper presented at the Third World Conference on Smoking and Health, New York, N.Y., June 2–5.

Busbee, D. L., D. Colvin, I. E. Muijsson, F. Rose and E. T. Cantrell. 1975. Aryl hydrocarbon hydroxylase induction in the amphibian, Ambystoma tigrinum. Comp. Biochem. Physiol. 50:33.

Busbee, D. L., C. R. Shaw and E. T. Cantrell. 1972. Aryl hydro-carbon hydroxylase induction in human leukocytes. Science 178: 315–316.

Cantrell, E., M. Abreu and D. Busbee. 1976. A simple assay for aryl hydrocarbon hydroxylase in cultured human lymphocytes. Biochem. Biophys. Res. Commun. 70(2):474–479.

Cantrell, E., M. Abreu-Greenberg and D. Busbee. 1975. Metabolism of diphenyloxazole by cultured human lymphocytes. Pager presented at the Gulf Coast Molecular Biology Conference, January 1975. (abstr.)

Cantrell, E., M. Abreu-Greenberg and D. Busbee. 1975. Metabolism of PPO by mouse liver microsomes. Life Sci. 17:317.

―――. 1976. Diphenyl-oxazole as an inducer and substrate for aryl hydrocarbon hydroxylase. Texas J. Sci., Spec. Publ. 1:125.

Cantrell, E., M. Abreu-Greenberg, D. Busbee and J. Guyden 1976. Metabolism of 3H-diphenyloxazole by cultured human lymphocytes. Fed Proc 35:253.

Cantrell, E., M. Abreu-Greenberg, J. Guyden and D. Busbee. 1975. Metabolism of diphenyloxazole (PPO) by mouse liver microsomes. Life Sci. 17:317.

Cantrell, E. and E. Bresnick. 1972. Benzopyrene hydroxylase activity in isolated parenchymal and nonparenchymal cells of rat liver. J. Cell Biol. 52:316–321.

Cantrell, E. and D. Busbee. 1972. Benzopyrene hydroxylase in circulating leukocytes after exposure to polycyclic hydrocarbons. Paper presented at the Fifth International Congress of Pharmacology.

Cantrell, E., D. Busbee, G. Warr and R. Martin. 1973. Induction of aryl hydrocarbon hydroxylase in human lymphocytes and pulmonary alveolar macrophages—a comparison. Life Sci. 13:1649–1654.

Cantrell, E., R. Martin, G. Warr, D. Busbee, G. Kellerman and C. Shaw. 1973. Induction of aryl hydrocarbon hydroxylase in human pulmonary alveolar macrophages by cigarette smoking. Trans. Assoc. Am. Physicians 86:121–130.

Carmella, S., S. S. Hecht and D. Hoffmann. 1979. Quantitative analysis of alkyl-2-hydroxy-2-cyclopenten-1-ones in tobacco smoke. Presented at the 33rd Tobacco Chemists' Research Conference, Lexington, KY, October 29–31.

Carter, H. W., J. M. Frasca and O. Auerbach. 1976. Morphologic changes produced in the distal respiratory system of smoking dogs: A correlative optical, transmission and scanning electron microscopy study. Proceedings 9th Annual SEM Symposium, Toronto, Canada, 1976. Proceedings of Workshop on Advances in Biomedical Applications of the SEM, IIT Research Institute, Chicago, April 1976, Part V:225–232.

Caton, J. E., M. P. Maskarinec and G. M. Henderson. 1979. Separation and determination of harmane and nonharmane by liquid chromatographic techniques. Presented at the 33rd Tobacco Chemists' Research Conference, Lexington, KY, October 29–31.

Caton, J. E., J. R. Stokely and M. R. Guerin. 1975. Depletion of constituents in contained smoke aerosols for inhalation exposure dosimetry. Paper presented at the 29th Tobacco Chemists' Research Conference, College Park, MD., October 8–10.

Chen, C. B., S. S. Hecht and D. Hoffmann. 1978. A study of chemical carcinogenesis II. Metabolic A -hydroxylation of tobacco specific carcinogen N''-nitrosonornicotine. Cancer Res. 38:3639–3645.

Clark, R. 1974. The "I can't" resistance to quitting smoking. Intl. Ment. Health News Letter 16:9–10.

Coomes, M., I. Muijsson, E. Cantrell and D. Busbee. 1975. Induction of 16-a hydroxylase in cultured lymphocytes. Paper presented at the Gulf Coast Molecular Biology Conference, January. (abstr.)

———. 1976. 16-a Hydroxylase in cultured human lymphocytes. Texas J. Sci. Spec. Publ. 1:92.

Coomes, M., I. Muijsson, W. Mason, E. Cantrell, D. Anderson and D. Busbee. 1976. Aryl hydrocarbon hydroxylase and 16-a hydroxylase in the cultured human lymphocyte system. Biochem. Genet. 14:671–685.

Craig, D. K., A. P. Wehner and W. G. Morrow. 1972. The generation and characterization of a respirable aerosol of chrysotile asbestos for chronic inhalation studies. Am. Ind. Hyg. Assoc. J. 33:283–292.

Dagle, G. E., K. E. McDonald and L. 6. Smith. 1975. Pulmonary carcinogenesis in rats with cigarette smoke condensate and beeswax pellets: preliminary results. Paper presented at the American College of Veterinary Pathologists, Respiratory Pathology Subgroup, December 5.

Dalbey, R. 0 Griesemer, I. Rubin and W. Maddox. 1976. Tobacco smoke inhalation studies in rats. Toxicol. Appl. Pharmacol. 37:557–569.

Decker, J. R., P. J. Hoff and R. D. Phillips. 1976. Automated rodent respiratory monitor and histogram computer—a preliminary report. Biomed. Sci. Instrum. 12:7–13.

Demoise, C. F.* R. E. Kouri and C. E. Whitmire. 1974. Cell-mediated immunity after intratracheal exposure to 3-methylcholanthrene and its relationship to tumor transplant growth in C3H/F Mai mice. Page 72 in E. Karbe and J. F. Park, eds. Experimental Lung Cancer. Springer-Verlag, New York.

DeVera, N., I. Schmeltz, S. S. Hecht and D. Hoffmann. 1979. Moderately polar non-P.A.H. neutral components in cigarette smoke. Presented at the 33rd Tobacco Chemists' Research Conference, Lexington, KY, October 29–31.

Diamond, L. 1976. Bioassaying candidate less-hazardous cigarettes: methods for early detection of peripheral airway dysfunction. Pages 433–439 in E. L. Wynder, D. Hoffman, and G. B. Gori, eds. Smoking and Health I: Modifying the Risk for the Smoker. DHEW Pub. No. (NIH) 76-1221, U.S. Government Printing Office, Washington, D.C.

Dong, M., I. Schmeltz and D. Hoffman. 1978. Purification of quinolines for bioassay by preparative high pressure liquid chromatography. J. Chromatogr. 150:269–272.

Dong, M., I. Schmeltz, E. Jacobs and D. Hoffmann. 1978. Chemical studies on tobacco smoke LV. Aza-Arenes in tobacco smoke. J. Anal. Toxicol. 2:21–25.

Dong, M., I. Schmeltz, E. LaVoie and D. Hoffmann. 1978. Aza-Arenes in the Respiratory Environment: Analysis and Assays for Mutagenicity in "Carcinogenesis-A Comprehensive Survey." (R. W. Jones and R. I. Freudenthal, eds.) Raven Press, New York. 3:97–108.

Drath, D., P. Davies, M. Karnovsky and G. Huber. 1978. The effect of tobacco smoke inhalation on the pulmonary alveolar macrophage (PAM). J. of Reticuloendothelial Soc. 23:49i.

Drath, D., M. Karnovsky and G. Huber. 1979. Tobacco smoke: Effects on pulmonary host defense. Inflammation. 3(3):281–8.

Enjeti, Suresh, B. Hazelwood, S. Permutt, H. Menkes and P. Terry. 1978. Pulmonary function in young smokers: Male-female differences. Am. Rev. Resp. Dis. 118:667–676.

Gargus, J. L., J. J. Gart, R. P. Kwapien and G. B. Gori. 1973. Replicate control values in large-scale mouse dermal bioassays of tobacco smoke condensates. Toxicol. Appl. Pharmacol. 25:487.

Gori, G. B. 1975. Artificial tobacco substitutes. J. Am. Med. Assoc. 234:489–490.

———., (ed.) 1975. Proceedings of the Tobacco Smoke Inhalation Workshop on Experimental Methods in Smoking and Health Research. DHEW Publ. No. (NIH) 75-906.

———. 1976. Low-risk cigarettes: a prescription. Science 194:1243–1246.

———. 1976. Approaches to the reduction of total particulate matter (TPM) in cigarette smoke. Pages 451–461 in E. L. Wynder, D. Hoffmann and G. B. Gori, eds. Smoking and Health I: Modifying the Risk for the Smoker. DHEW Publ. No. (NIH) 76-1221, U.S. Government Printing Office, Washington, D.C.

———., (ed.) 1976. Toward Less Hazardous Cigarettes, Report No. 1: The First Set of Experimental Cigarettes. DHEW Publ. No. (NIH) 76-905, U.S. Government Printing Office, Washington, D. C.

———., (ed.) 1976. Toward Less Hazardous Cigarettes, Report No. 2: The Second Set of Experimental Cigarettes. DHEW Publ. No. (NIH) 76-

1111, U.S. Government Printing Office, Washington, D.C.

————., (ed.) 1977. Toward Less Hazardous Cigarettes, Report No. 3: The Third Set of Experimental Cigarettes. DHEW Pub. No. (NIH) 77-1280.

————., (ed.). 1979. Toward Less Hazardous Cigarettes, Report No. 4: The Fourth Set of Experimental Cigarettes. The National Cancer Institute, Bethesda, MD.

————., (ed.) 1978. An Operational Manual for the Beagle Dog Inhalation Model. Smoking and Health Program, National Cancer Institute. Bethesda, MD.

————., (ed.). Proceedings of the tobacco smoke inhalation workshop on bioassay models and inhalation toxicology. U.S. DHEW, PHS, NIH, NCI. DHEW Pub. No. (NIH) , U.S. Government Printing Office, Washington, D. C.

————. 1980. Less Hazardous Cigarettes. In: A safe cigarette? Gori GB, Boch FG (Eds.) Cold Spring Harbor Laboratory, Cold Spring Harbor, N.Y.

Gori, G. B., S. P. Battista, P. S. Thayer, M. R. Guerin and C. J. Lynch. 1975. Chemistry and in vitro bioassay of smoke from experimental filter cigarettes. Smoking and Health Program, National Cancer Institute, DHEW Publ. No. (NIH) 76-1076, U.S. Government Printing Office, Washington, D.C.

Gori, G. B. and C. J. Lynch. 1978. Toward Less Hazardous Cigarettes. J. Am. Med. Assoc. 240:1255–1259.

Gori, G. B. and B. J. Richter. 1978. Macroeconomics of Disease Prevention in the United States. Science. 200:1124–1130.

Gottung, P. W. 1978. Combustion Characteristics of Low-Tar Reduced Hazard Cigarettes with Interpretations Based on Porous Reactor Theory. M.S.W. Thesis, Princeton University, Princeton, NJ.

Gray, J. C., S. D. Kung and S. G. Wildman. 1978. Polypeptide chains of the large and small subunits of fraction I protein from tobacco. Arch. Biochem. Biophys. 185(l):272–281.

Griest, W. H. and M. Guerin. 1977. Influence of Tobacco Type on Smoke Composition. Recent Advances in Tobacco Science. 3:121.

Griest, W. H., M. R. Guerin, R. B. Quincy and H. Kubota. 1977. "Chemical Characterization of Experimental Cigarettes and Cigarette Smoke condensates in the Third Cigarette Experiment," in Report No. 3, Toward Less Hazardous Cigarettes, The Third Set of Experimental Cigarettes. Gio B. Gori, ed. DHEW Publication No. (NIH) 77-1280.

Griest, W. H., H. Kubota and M. R. Guerin. 1975. Resolution of poly-nuclear aromatic hydrocarbons by packed column GLC. Anal. Lett. 8:949.

Griest, W. H., R. Quincy and M. R. Guerin. 1977. Selected constituents in the smoke of domestic low tar cigarettes. ORNL/TM-6144/P1. Available from NTIS, Springfield, VA 22161.

Guerin, M. R. 1971. Tobacco Smoke Analysis Program Progress Report for the period ending 1 July, 1971. ORNL-4435, Oak Ridge, TN.

———. 1976. Chemical characterization of experimental cigarettes and cigarette smoke condensate. Pages 60–84 in Toward Less Hazardous Cigarettes, Report No. I: The First Set of Experimental Cigarettes. Smoking and Health Program, National Cancer Institute. DHEW Pub. No. (NIH) 76-905, U.S. Government Printing Office, Washington, D.C.

———. 1976. Chemical characterization of experimental cigarettes and cigarette smoke condensate. Pages 33–55 in Toward Less Hazardous Cigarettes, Report No. 2: The Second Set of Experimental Cigarettes. Smoking and Health Pro ram, National Cancer Institute. DHEW Pub. No. (NIH) 761111.

———. 1976. Discussion—identification of carcinogens, tumor promoters and cocarcinogens in tobacco smoke. Pages 155–159 in E. L. Wynder, D. Hoffmann, and G. B. Gori, eds. Smoking and Health I: Modifying the Risk for the Smoker. DHEW Pub. No. (NIH) 76-1221, U.S. Government Printing Office, Washington, D. C.

———. 1979. Chemical composition of cigarette smoke. In: A safe cigarette? Gori GB, Boch FG (Eds.) Banbury report No. 3, Cold Spring Harbor Laboratory, New York.

Guerin, M. R., C. H. Ho, I. B. Rubin, W. H. Griest and H. Kubota. 1975. Chemical fractionation and multicomponent gas chromatographic analysis of coal-derived liquids. Paper presented at CONFAB-75, Fossil Fuel Chemistry and Energy, Laramie, Wyo., July 22–26.

Guerin, M. R., W. L. Maddox and J. R. Stokely. 1975. Tobacco smoke inhalation exposure: concepts and devices. Pages 31–44 in Proceedings of the Tobacco Smoke Inhalation Workshop on Experimental Methods in Smoking and Health Research. DHEW Pub. No. (NIH) 75-906, U.S. Government Printing Office, Washington, D.C.

Guerin, M. R. and P. Nettesheim. 1972. Tobacco smoke chemistry and i halation bioassay methodologies. Paper presented at the Carcinogenesis Collaborative Conference, San Antonio, Tex., October 2–4.

———. 1973. Tobacco Smoke Research Program Progress Report. ORNL-4879, Oak Ridge, TN.

———. 1975. ORNL Tobacco Smoke Research Program Summary Report. ORNL-5008. Oak Ridge, TN.

Guerin, M. R. and G. Olerich. 1972. Quantitative utility of the trimethylsilylation of smoke condensate and particulate matter. Paper presented at the CORESTA/TCRC Joint Conference, Williamsburg, Va., October

22–28.

———. 1976. Direct gas chromatographic determination of catechol in cigarette smoke. Tob. Sci. XX:19–21.

Guerin, M. R., G. Olerich and A. D. Horton. 1974. Routine gas chromatographic component profiling of cigarette smoke for the identification of biologically significant constituents. J. Chromatogro. Sci. 12:385–391.

Guerin, M. R., G. Olerich and R. B. Quincy. 1974. Multialiquot determination of phenol, cresols, glycerol, catechol, nicotine, and free fatty acids. Paper presented at the 28th Tobacco Chemists' Research Conference, Raleigh, N.C., October 28–30.

Guerin, M. R., G. Olerich and W. T. Rainey. 1974. Gas chromatographic determination of non-volatile fatty acids in cigarette smoke. Anal. Chem. 46:761–763.

Guerin, M. R. and W. O. Shults. 1971. Tobacco Smoke Analysis Program Progress Report for the period ending September 1, 1970. ORNL-4642.

Haq, M. Z., S. J. Rose, L. R. Deiderich and A. R. Patel. 1974. Identification and quantitative measurement of some N-heterocyclics in marijuana smoke condensates. Anal. Chem. 46:1781.

Harley, N., B. S. Cohen and T. C. Tso. 1978. p0210 in Tobacco. Presented at the Symposium on Public Health Aspects of Radioactivity in Consumer Products, Atlanta, Georgia, Feb. 1977. Symposium Summaries, published by the Nuclear Regulatory Commission. Washington, DC.

Hayashi, M., G. Sornberger and G. Huber. 1978. Differential sexual response in the mucus composition of tracheal goblet cells and gland following experimental exposure to tobacco smoke. Proceedings of the XIII World Conference on Diseases of the Chest.

———. 1978. Differential response in the male and female tracheal epithelium following exposure to tobacco smoke. Chest Apr. 73(4): 515-8.

———. 1979. Morphometric analyses of tracheal gland secretion and hypertrophy in male and female rats after experimental exposure to tobacco smoke. Am. Rev. Respir. Dis. Jan. 119 (1): 67–73.

Hecht, S. S., W. E. Bondinell and D. Hoffmann. 1974. Chemical studies on tobacco smoke. XXIX. Chrysene and methylchrysenes: presence in tobacco and carcinogenicity. J. Natl. Cancer Inst. 53:1121–1133.

Hecht, S. S., S. Carmella and D. Hoffmann. 1973. Chemical studies on tobacco smoke LIV. Determination of hydroxybenzyl alcohols and hydroxyphenyl ethanols in tobacco and tobacco smoke. J. Anal. Toxicol. 2:56–59.

Hecht, S. S., D. H. Chen, D. M. Dong, R. M. Ornaf, D. Hoffmann and T. C. Tso. 1977. Chemical studies on tobacco smoke. LI. Studies on non-volatile nitrosamines in tobacco. Beitr. Tabakforsch. 9:1–6.

Hecht, S. S., C. B. Chen, N. Hirota, R. M. Ornaf, T. C. Tso and D. Hoffmann. 1978. A study of tobacco carcinogenesis XVI. Tobacco specific nitrosamines: Formation from nicotine in vitro and during tobacco curing and carcinogenicity in strain A mice. J. Natl. Cancer Inst. 60:319–824.

Hecht, S. S., C. B. Chen and D. Hoffmann. Tobacco specific nitrosamines: Occurrence, formation, carcinogenicity and metabolism. Acc.Chem. Res. 12:92–98.

Hecht, S. S., C. B. Chen, G. D. McCoy and D. Hoffmann. 1978. A study of tobacco carcinogenesis XVII. Tobacco specific nitrosamines: Occurrence, carcinogenicity and metabolism. Proc. 8th Northeastern Regional Mtg. Am. Chem. Soc. Symp. on Nitrosamines. Ser. 101:125–152.

Hecht, S. S., C. B. Chen, R. M. Ornaf, D. Hoffmann and T. C. Tso. 1978. Chemical studies on tobacco smoke. LVI. Tobacco specific nitrosamines: Origins, carcinogenicity and metabolism. In "Environmental Aspects of N-nitroso Compounds," Lyon, IARC Scientific Publ. No. 19:395–413.

Hecht, S. S., C. B. Chen, R. M. Ornaf, E. Jacobs, J. D. Adams and D. Hoffmann. 1978. Chemical studies on tobacco smoke LVII. Reaction of nicotine and sodium nitrite: Formation of nitrosamines and fragmentation of the pyrrolidine ring. J. Org. Chem. 43:72–76.

Hecht, S. S., E. LaVoie and D. Hoffmann. 1978. A study of chemical carcinogenesis 13. Structure-activity relationships in polynuclear aromatic hydrocarbons. Proc. of the Lawrence Berkeley Laboratory Conference on Carbonaceous Particles in the Atmosphere. (T. Novakov, ed.) Nat]. Techn. Inform. Serv., U. S. Dept. Commerce, Springfield, VA, 177–186.

Hecht, S. S., R. M. Ornaf and D. Hoffmann. 1975. Chemical studies on tobacco smoke. XXXIII. N'-nitrosonornicotine in tobacco. Analysis of possible contributing factors in biological implications. J. Natl. Cancer Inst. 54:1237–1244.

———. 1975. Chemical studies on tobacco smoke. XLI. Quantitative determination of the carcinogen N'-nitrosonornicotine in tobacco, using high-speed liquid chromatography. Anal. Chem. 47:2046–2048.

———., I. Schmeltz and D. Hoffmann. 1977. Chemical studies on tobacco smoke. LVIII. Nitrogenous compounds in cigarette smoke and their possible precursors. Rec. Adv. Tob. Sci. 3:59–63.

Hecht, S. S., I. Schmeltz, D. Hoffmann and E. L. Wynder. 1976. Chemical Studies on tobacco smoke. XL. Identification of carcinogens in tobacco. Pages 125–145 in E. L. Wynder, D. Hoffmann and G. B. Gori, eds. Smoking and Health I: Modifying the Risk for the Smoker. OHEW Publ. No. (NIH) 76-1221, U.S. Government Printing Office, Washington, D.C

Hecht, S. S., R. Thorne, R. R. Maronpot and D. Hoffmann. 1975. A study of tobacco carcinogenesis. XIII. Tumor promoting subfractions of the weakly acidic fraction. J. Natl. Cancer Inst. 55:1329.

Hecht, S. S., T. C. Tso and D. Hoffmann. 1976. Selective reduction of tumorigenicity of tobacco smoke. IV. Approaches to the reduction of nitrosamines and aromatic amines. Pages 535–545 in E. L. Wynder, D. Hoffmann and G. B. Gori, eds. Smoking and Health I: Modifying the Risk for the Smoker. DHEW Publ. No. (NIH) 76-1221, U.S. Government Printing Office, Washington, D.C.

Higgins, C. E., J. R. Stokely and M. R. Guerin. 1975. Organic gas phase composition of contained smoke aerosols used for inhalation testing. Paper presented at the 29th Tobacco Chemists' Research Conference, College Park, MD., October 8–10.

Higgins, C. E., J. R. Stokely, M. R. Guerin and T. L. Roberts. 1974. Applications of "blind assay" methodology to organic gas phase constituents in tobacco smoke. Paper presented at the 28th Tobacco Chemists' Research Conference, Raleigh, N.C., October 28–30.

Higgins, I. T. T. 1976. Relative risks of various tobacco usages for emphysema and/or chronic bronchitis. Pages 389–405 in E. L. Wynder, D. Hoffmann, and G. B. Gori, eds. Smoking and Health I: Modifying the Risk for the Smoker. DHEW Pub. No. (NIH) 76-1221, U.S. Government Printing Office, Washington, D.C.

Hilfrich, J., S. S. Hecht and D. Hoffmann. 1977. A study of tobacco carcinogenesis. XV. Effects of N'-Nitrosonornicotine and N'-Nitrosoanabasine in Syrian golden hamsters. Cancer Letter. 2:169–176.

Hilfrich, J., I. Schmeltz and D. Hoffmann. 1978. Effects of N'-nitrosodiethanolamine and 1,1-diethanol-hydrazine in Syrian Golden Hamsters. Cancer Lett. 4:55–60.

Hill, P. 1976. Nicotine: an etiological factor for heart disease. Pages 313–319 in E. L. Wynder, D. Hoffmann, and G. B. Gori, eds. Smoking and Health I: Modifying the Risk for the Smoker. DHEW Pub. No. (NIH) 76-1221, U.S. Government Printing Office, Washington, D.C.

Hill, P. and E. L. Wynder. 1974. Smoking and cardiovascular disease. Effect of nicotine on the serum epinephrine and corticoids. Am. Heart J. 87:491–496.

Hinds, W. K. 1978. Size characteristics of cigarette smoke. American Ind. Hyg. Assoc. J. 39:48–54.

Hirota, N. 1979. Intranuclear rodlets in undifferentiated carcinomas of salivary glands in strain A mice in a study involving a tobacco-specific nitrosamine (NNN). Cancer Lett. 6:365–369.

Ho, C.-h, W. H. Griest and M. Guerin. 1976. Application of the blind assay to biological activity and tobacco smoke terpenes. Anal. Chem. 48:2223.

Hoffmann, D. 1972. Benzo(I)pyrene in polluted air. Prev. Med. 1:450–451.

Hoffmann, D., W. E. Bondinell and E. L. Wynder. 1974. On the carcinogenicity of methylchrysenes. Science 183:215–216.

Hoffmann, D., J. D. Adams, K. D. Brunnemann and S. S. Hecht. 1979. Chemical studies on tobacco smoke LXII. Assessment of tobacco specific NI-nitrosamines in tobacco products. Cancer Res. 39:2505–2509.

Hoffmann, D., J. D. Adams and E. L. Wynder. 1979. Chemical studies on tobacco smoke XLV. Formation and analysis of carbon monoxide in cigarette mainstream and sidestream smoke. Prev. Med. 8:344–350.

Hoffmann, D., K. D. Brunnemann and G. B. Gori. 1975. Chromatographic determination of vinyl chloride in tobacco smoke. Presented at the 29th Tobacco Chemists' Research Conference, College Park, Md., October 8–10.

Hoffmann, D., K. D. Brunnemann, G. B. Gori and E. L. Wynder. 1975. On the carcinogenicity of marijuana smoke. Page 63 in V. C. Runeckles, ed. Recent Advances in Phytochemistry, Vol. I. Plenum Publishing Corp., New York.

Hoffmann, D., K. D. Brunnemann, 1. Schmeltz and E. L. Wynder. 1978. Trace analysis in respiratory carcinogenesis. Proc. 9th Materials Res. Symp., Gaithersburg, Md.

———. 1979. Trace analysis in respiratory carcinogenesis. "Trace Organic Analysis: A New Frontier in Analytical Chemistry" (H. S. Hertz and S. N. Chester, eds.) Natl. Bureau of Standards Special Publ. No. 519, U. S. Government Printing Office (No. 003-003-02054-1), Washington, D. C., pp. 131–141.

Hoffmann, D., M. Dong and S. S. Hecht. 1977. Origin in tobacco smoke of N'-nitrosonornicotine, a tobacco-specific carcinogen: Brief communication. J. Natl. Cancer Inst. 58:1841–1844.

Hoffmann, D., S. S. Hecht, R. M. Ornaf and E. L. Wynder. 1974. Chemical studies on tobacco smoke. XXX. N-nitrosonornicotine in tobacco. Science 186:265–267.

Hoffmann, D., S. S. Hecht, 1. Schmeltz and E. L. Wynder. 1975. New separation techniques for classes of smoke compounds. Paper presented at the 29th Tobacco Chemists' Research Conference, College Park, Md., October 8–10.

Hoffmann, D., S. S. Hecht and E. L. Wynder. 1979. The role of polynuclear aromatic hydrocarbons in tobacco carcinogenesis. Presented at the "Polycyclic Aromatic Hydrocarbons Conference" of the Verein Deutscher Ingenieure, Hanover, Federal Republic of Germany, Sept. 18–21.

Hoffmann, D. and V. Mazzola. 1970. Chemical studies on tobacco smoke. XI. Dibenzofurans in cigarette smoke. Beitr. Tabakforsch. 5:183–188.

Hoffmann, D., C. Patrianakos, K. D. Brunnemann and G. B. Gori. 1976. Chromatographic determination of vinyl chloride in tobacco smoke. Anal.

Chem. 48:47–50.

Hoffmann, D., R. Raineri, S. S. Hecht, R. R. Maronpot and E. L. Wynder. 1975. A study of tobacco carcinogenesis. XIV. On the carcinogenicity of N'-nitrosonornicotine and N'-nitrosoanabasine. J. Natl. Cancer Inst. 55:977–981.

Hoffmann, D. and G. Rathkamp. 1970. Chemical studies on tobacco smoke. X. Quantitative determination of 1-alkylindoles in cigarette smoke. Anal. Chem. 42:366–370.

———. 1970. Chemical studies on tobacco smoke. XII. Quantitative determination of nitrobenzenes in cigarette smoke. Anal. Chem. 42:1643–1647.

Hoffmann, D. and G. Rathkamp. 1972. Chemical studies on tobacco smoke. XIV. Quantitative determination of fluorenes in cigarette smoke and their formation by pyrosyntheses. Anal. Chem. 44:899–904.

Hoffmann, D., G. Rathkamp, K.D. Brunnemann and E.L. Wynder. 1973. Chemical studies on tobacco smoke. XXII. On the profile analysis of tobacco smoke. Sci. Total Environ. 2: 157–171.

Hoffmann, D., G. Rathkamp and Y. Y. Liu. 1974. Chemical studies on tobacco smoke. XXVI. On the isolation and identification of volatile and non-volatile N-nitrosamines and hydrazines in cigarette smoke. Int. Agency Res. Cancer Monogr. 9:155–165.

Hoffmann, D., G. Rathkamp, S. Nesnow and E. L. Wynder. 1972. Chemical studies on tobacco smoke. XVI. Fluoranthenes: quantitative determination in cigarette smoke, formation by pyrolysis, and tumor-initiating activity. J Natl. Cancer Inst. 49:1165–1175.

Hoffmann, D., A. Rivenson, S. S. Hecht, J. Hilfrich, N. Kobayashi and E. L. Wynder. Model studies in tobacco carcinogenesis with the Syrian Golden Hamster. Prog. Explt. Tumor Res. 24:370–390.

Hoffmann, D., L. D. Sanghvi, and E. L. Wynder. 1974. Chemical studies on tobacco smoke. XXVIII. Comparative analysis of bidi and cigarette smoke. Int. J. Cancer 14:49–53.

Hoffmann, D., I. Schmeltz, S. S. Hecht and E. L. Wynder. 1976. On the identification of carcinogens, tumor promoters and cocarcinogens in tobacco smoke. Pages 125–145 in E. L. Wynder, D. Hoffmann, and G. B. Gori, eds. Smoking and Health I: Modifying the Risk for the Smoker. DHEW Pub. No. (NIH) 76-1221, U.S. Government Printing Office, Washington, D.C.

———. 1978. Polynuclear aromatic hydrocarbons in tobacco carcinogenesis. In Polycyclic hydrocarbons and Cancer. Chemistry, Molecular Biology and Environment. H. Gelboin and P. O. Tso, eds. Academic Press. 1:85–117.

———. 1978. Volatile Carcinogens: Occurrence, formation and analysis. In Detection and Prevention of Cancer: Part 1, Marcel Decker, New York,

NY. 2:1943–1959.

Hoffmann, D. and E. L. Wynder. 1970. Chamber development and aerosol dispersion. Pages 173–191. In:Hanna HG, et al., (Eds.) Inhalation Carcinogenesis. U.S. Atomic Energy Commission, Washington, D.C.

———. 1971. A study of tobacco carcinogenesis. XI. Tumor initiators, tumor accelerators, and tumor promoting activity of condensate fractions. Cancer 27:848–864.

———. 1972. Selective reduction of tumorigenicity of tobacco smoke. II. Experimental approaches. J. Natl. Cancer Inst. 48:1855–18bd.

———. 1972. Chemical studies on tobacco smoke. XV. Chemical composition and tumorigenicity of tobacco smoke. Pages 123–147 . In: Schmeltz L (Ed.) The Chemistry of Tobacco and Tobacco Smoke. Plenum Press, New York.

———, 1972. Chemical studies on tobacco smoke. XVIII. Smoke of cigarettes and little cigars. An analytical comparison. Science 178:1197–1199.

Hoffmann, ed. 1974. Proceedings of the International Symposium on Identification and Measurements of Environmental Pollutants. Campbell Printing, Ottawa, Canada, (National Research Council of Canada).

Hoffmann, D. and E. L. Wynder. 1974. Positive controls in environmental respiratory carcinogenesis. Pages 35–39 in L. Goldberg, ed. Carcinogenic Testing of Chemicals. CRC Press, Cleveland, Ohio.

———. 1975. The carcinogenic fractions of cigarette smoke (review). Paper presented at the Workshop on the Significance of Po210 in Tobacco and Tobacco Smoke. Smoking and Health Program, National Cancer Institute, Bethesda, MD. August 25.

———. 1976. Environmental respiratory carcinogenesis. In:Searle CE (Ed.) On chemical carcinogens. ACS Monograph 173. American Chemical Society, Washington, D.C., pp. 324–365.

———. 1976. Selective reduction of tumorigenicity of tobacco smoke. III. The reduction of polynuclear aromatic hydrocarbons in cigarette smoke. Pages 495–504 in E. L. Wynder, D. Hoffmann, and G. B. Gori, eds. Smoking and Health I: Modifying the Risk for the Smoker. DHEW Publ. No. (NIH)76-1221, U.S. Government Printing Office, Washington, D.C.

———. 1976. Smoking and occupational cancer. Prev. Med. 5:245–261.

———. 1978. Identification and reduction of carcinogens in the respiratory environment. Zentralbl. Bakt. Hyg. 1. Abt. Orig. B. 166:113–135.

Holmberg, R. W., J. R. Stokely and M. R. Guerin. 1975. electron microscope measurement of methyl cyanoacrylate fixed tobacco smoke particles: application to inhalation exposure systems. Paper presented at the 29th Tobacco Chemists' Research Conference, College Park, Md., October 8–10.

Horton, A. D., R. F. Apple, A. S. Meyer and M. R. Guerin. 1976. A puff-averaging analytical cigarette smoking device. Tob. Sci. XX:22–24.

Horton, A. D. and M. R. Guerin. 1972. Quantitative gas chromatographic determination of smoke components using the sulfur-specific photometric detector. Paper presented at the CORESTA/TCRC Joint Conference, Williamsburg, Va., October 22–28.

————. 1973. Chemical characterization of a little cigar. Paper presented at the Cigar Research Council Seminar, University of Maryland, College Park, Md., February 7–9.

————. 1974. Determination of acetaldehyde and acrolein in the gas phase of cigarette smoke using cryothermal gas chromatography. Tob. Sci. 18:19–22.

————. 1974. Gas-solid chromatographic determination of carbon monoxide and carbon dioxide in cigarette smoke. J. Assoc. Offic. Anal. Chem. 57:1.

————. 1974. Quantitative determination of sulfur compounds in the gas phase of cigarette smoke. J. Chromatogr. 90:63.

Horton, A. D., M. R. Guerin and G. Olerich. 1971. Sulfur-containing compounds in the gas phase of cigarette smoke. Paper presented at the 25th Tobacco Chemists' Research Conference, Louisville, Ky., October 6–8.

Horton, A. D., M. R. Guerin, J. R. Stokely and A. S. Meyer. 1973. Determination of nitrogen-containing components in the gas phase of cigarette smoke by use of the Coulson electrolytic conductivity detector. Paper presented at the 27th Tobacco Chemists' Research Conference, Winston-Salem, NC, October 3–5.

Horton, A. D., J. R. Stokely and M. R. Guerin. 1974. Gas chromatographic determination of nitric oxide (NO) in cigarette smoke. Anal. Lett. 7:177–195.

Hu, M. W., W. E. Bondinell and D. Hoffmann. 1974. Chemical studies on tobacco smoke. XXIII. Synthesis of carbon-14 labeled myosmine, nornicotine, and N'-nitrosonornicotine. J. Labeled Compd. 10:79–88.

Innerarity, C. L., A. H. Lyter, L. T. Innerarity and A. R. Patel. 1974. Analytical studies on the polyphenolic content of tobacco from NCI experimental cigarettes. Paper presented at the 23th Tobacco Chemists' Research Conference, Raleigh, NC, October 28–30.

Jenkins, R. A., J. E. Caton, M. P. Ilaskarinec, T. M. Gayle and M. R. Guerin. 1979. Analytical and instrumental support of the NCI tobacco smoke inhalation bioassays. National Cancer Institute Smoking & Health Program Contractors' Conference, Savannah, GA, March 11–14.

Jenkins, R. A. and T. M. Gayle. 1979. An instrumental inhaled smoke dosimeter for the quantitative characterization of aerosol exposures. Presented at the 19th Annual Harford Life Sciences Symposium, Richland, WA, October 22–24.

Jenkins, R. A. and B. E. Gill. 1978. Procedures for the determination of nitric oxide and nitrogen dioxide in cigarette smoke by chemiluminescent analysis. Presented at the 32rd Tobacco Chemists' Research Conference, Montreal, Quebec, Canada, October 30–November 1, 1978.

Jenkins, R. A., R. B. Quincy and M. R. Guerin. 1979. Carbon monoxide deliveries of commercial cigarettes: relationship to other smoke constituents. Presented at the 33rd Tobacco Chemists' Research Conference, Lexington, KY, October 29–31.

———. 1977. Selected constituents in the smokes of U.S. commercial cigarettes: tar, nicotine, carbon monoxide and carbon dioxide. ORNL/TMI-b870. Oak Ridge, TN.

———. 1979. Selected constituents in the smokes of foreign commercial cigarettes: tar, nicotine, carbon monoxide and carbon dioxide. ORNL/TM-0869. Oak Ridge, TN.

Jenkins, R. A., R. B. Quincy, M. R. Guerin and M. P. Maskarinec. 1979. Analytical chemistry development and support for the NCI S&HP. National Cancer Institute Smoking & Health Program Contractors' Meeting, Savannah, GA, March 11–14.

Kellerman, G., E. Cantrell and C. R. Shaw. 1973. Variations in extent of aryl hydrocarbon hydroxylase induction in cultured human lymphocytes. Cancer Res. 33:1654–1656. Kendrick, J., P. Nettesheim, M. Guerin, J. Caton, W.

Kendrick, J., P. Nettesheim and A. S. Hammons. 1974. Tumor Induction in tracheal grafts: a new experimental model for respiratory carcinogenesis studies. J. Natl. Cancer Inst. 52:1317–1325.

Kendrick, J., I. B. Kobayashi, N., D. Hoffmann and E. L. Wynder. 1974. A Study Of tobacco carcinogenesis. XII. Epithelial changes induced in the upper respiratory tracts of Syrian golden hamsters by cigarette smoke. J. Natl. Cancer Inst. 53:1085–1089.

Kouri, R. E., C. F. Demoise and C. E. Whitmire. 1974. The significance of the aryl hydrocarbon hydroxylase enzyme systems in the selection of model systems for respiratory carcinogenesis. In: Karbe E, Park JF (Eds.) Experimental Lung Cancer. Springer-Verlag, New York. p. 48.

Kouri, R. E. 1978. Relationship between levels of aryl hydrocarbon hydroxylase activity and susceptibility of 3-methylcholanthrene and benzo(a)pyrene-induced cancers in inbred strains of mice. In: Freudenthal R, Jones P (Eds.) Polynuclear Aromatic Hydrocarbons. Academic Press. P.139.

Kouri, R.E., R. L. Imblum, R.G. Sosnowski, D.J. Slomiany and G.E. McKinney. 1979. Parameters influencing quantitation of 3-methylcholanthrene-induced aryl hydrocarbon hydroxylase activity in cultured human lymphocytes. J. Environ Pathol Toxicol. Mar–Apr. 2(4): 1079–98.

Kouri, R. E., R. Kiefer and E. M. Zimmerman. 1974. Hydrocarbon metabolizing activity of various mammalian cells in culture. In vitro 10:18–25.

Kouri, R.E., S.A. Kurtz, P.J. Price, W.F. Benedict. 1975. 1-Beta-D-arabino-furanoxylcytosine-induced malignant transformation of hamster and rat cells in culture. Cancer Res. 35(9): 2413–2419.

Kouri, R. E., H. Ratrie, S. A. Atlas, A. Niwa and D. W. Nebert. 1974. Aryl hydrocarbon hydroxylase induction in human lymphocyte cultures by 2,3,7,8-tetrachlorodibenzo-p-dioxin. Life Sci. 15:1585–1595.

Kouri, R. E., H. Ratrie and C. E. Whitmire. 1973. Evidence for genetic relationship between susceptibility to 3-methylcholanthrene induced subcutaneous tumors and inducibility of aryl hydrocarbon hydroxylase. J. Natl. Cancer Inst. 51:197–200.

———. 1974. Genetic control of susceptibility to cancers induced by 3-methylcholanthrene. In :Proceedings of the XI International Cancer Congress.p.77.

———. 1974. Genetic control of susceptibility to 3-methylcholanthrene-induced subcutaneous sarcomas. Int. J. Cancer 13:714–720.

Kouri, R. E., T. Rude, P. E. Thomas and C. E. Whitmire. 1976. Studies on pulmonary aryl hydrocarbon hydroxylase activity in inbred strains of mice. Chem. Biol. Interactions 13:317–331.

Kouri, R. E., R. A. Salerno and C. E. Whitmire. 1973. Relationships between aryl hydrocarbon hydroxylase inducibility and sensitivity to chemically-induced subcutaneous sarcomas in various strains of mice. J. Natl. Cancer Inst. 50:363–368.

Kouri, R.E., C. E. Whitmire and W. F. Benedict. 1975. In vivo and in vitro effects of cigarette smoke condensate fractions. Am. Assoc. Cancer Res. 16:173.

Kubota, H. 1975. Analysis of cigarette tobacco smokes and condensates. Oak Ridge Associated Universities Lectures. Tennessee State University, Nashville, Tenn., Jan. 17, and Georgia State University, Atlanta, Ga., May 22.

Kubota, H., W. H. Griest and M. R. Guerin. 1976. Determination of carcinogens in tobacco smoke and coal-derived samples. Pages 281–289 in D. D. Hemphill, ed. Proceedings of the 9th Annual Conference on Trace Substances in Environmental Health, June 9–12, 1975. University of Missouri, Columbia.

Kubota, H., M. R. Guerin and J. A. Carter. 1972. Inorganic analytical methods of tobacco smoke analysis—a comparative study. Paper presented at the CORESTA/TCRC Joint Conference, Williamsburg, Va., October 22–28.

Kubota, H., M. R. Guerin and C. A. Pritchard. 1971. Polar apiezons for the gas chromatographic determination of phenanthrene and benzo(a)anthracene in smoke condensates. Paper presented at the 25th Tobacco Chemists' Research Conference, Louisville, Ky., October 6–8.

Kuehl, T., C. Chappell, M. Tuttle and W. Rogers. 1979. Maternal cigarette smoking effects on fetal growth in the baboon, Papio cynocephalus. Paper presented to the Texas Branch of the American Association of Laboratory Animal Science, College Station, Texas, May.

Kung, S. D. and T. C. Tso. 1977. Amino acid composition and nutritional value of fraction 1 and fraction 2 proteins from different species of nicotiana. Paper presented at the 1977 Annual Meeting of the Phytochemical Society of North America, August 1977.

————. 1978. Tobacco as a potential food source and smoke material II. Soluble protein content, extraction and amino acid composition. J. of Food Sci. 43:1844–1848.

LaVoie, E., V. Bedenko, N. Hirota, S. S. Hecht and D. Hoffmann. 1979. A comparison of the mutagenicity, tumor initiating activity and complete carcinogenicity of polynuclear aromatic hydrocarbons. Presented at the 3rd Symp. on Polynuclear Aromatic Hydrocarbons; Ann Arbor Sci. Press, 705–721.

Liu, Y. Y. and D. Hoffmann. 1973. Chemical studies on tobacco smoke. XIX. Quantitative determination of maleic hydrazine in cigarette smoke. Anal. Chem. 45:2270–2273.

Liu, Y. Y., 1. Schmeltz and D. Hoffmann. 1974. Chemical studies on tobacco smoke. XXVII. Quantitative analysis of hydrazine in tobacco and cigarette smoke. Anal. Chem. 46:885–899.

Loscutoff, S. M., J. Decker, G. Larson and G. Preecs. 1975. Closing volume measurements in smoking dogs. Physiol. 18:298. (abstr.)

Lubet, R. A., D. Q. Brown and R. E. Kouri. 1973. The role of 3-OH-benzo(a)pyrene in mediating benzo(a)pyrene-induced cytotoxicity and transformation in cell culture. Res. Commun. Chem. Pathol. Pharmacol. 6:929–942.

Lynch, C. J. and G. B. Gori. 1980. Non-detectable risk levels in cigarette smoking. Proc. of Conference on Less Hazardous Cigarettes. Banbury Report 3, Banbury Center, Cold Spring Harbor Laboratory, Cold Spring Harbor, NY.

Lynch, C. J. and M. W. Layard. 1976. Development of a less hazardous cigarette. Presented at the 9th International Biometric Conference. Boston, Mass.

Lynch, C. J. and R. J. Thomas. 1977. Some statistical considerations in international epidemiology. Studies of tobacco-related diseases. Paper presented at the Joint Statistical Meeting of the American Statistical Association and the Biometric Society.

Lynch, C. J. and W. W. Yu. 1979. Fourth cigarette experimental survival curves based on histopathologically verified tumors. Enviro Control, Inc., Rockville, MD.

———. 1979. Fourth cigarette experiment life tables based on histopathology. Enviro Control, Inc., Rockville, MD.

Maddox, W. L. and G. W. Allin. 1975. Improved exposure devices, Pages 59–61 in M. R. Guerin and P. Nettesheim, ed. ORNL Tobacco Smoke Research Program. Summary report. ORNL-5008. NTIS, Springfield, Va.

Maddox, W. L. and M. R. Guerin. 1972. High speed photometric analyzer in the tobacco sciences. Paper presented at the CORESTA/TCRC Joint Conference, Williamsburg, Va., October 22–28.

Maddox, W. L. , M. R. Guerin, G. Kendrick, D. A. Creasia, P. Nettesheim, W. E. Dalbey and J. R. Stokely. 1978. A tobacco smoke inhalation exposure device for rodents. Arch Environ Health 33:64.

Maddox, W. L. and G. Mamantov. 1977. Analysis of cigarette smoke by Fourier transform infrared spectroscopy. Anal. Chem. 49:331.

Maddox, W. L., R. B. Quincy, H. H. Ross, G. Olerich and M. R. Guerin. 1971. Carbon-14 and neutron irradiated cigarettes for animal lung deposition experiments. Paper presented at the 25th Tobacco Chemists' Research Conference, Louisville, Ky., October 6–8.

Manning, D. L., M. P. Maskarinec and R. W. Harvey. 1979. High performance liquid chromatographic studies of ion molecular weight carbonyl compounds in tobacco smoke. Presented at the 33rd Tobacco Chemists' Research Conference, Lexington, KY, October 29–31.

Marquardt, H., A. Bendich, F. S. Phillips and D. Hoffmann. 1971. Binding of (G-3 H) -7,12-dimethylbenz(a)anthracene to DNA of normal and of rapidly dividing hepatic cells in rats. Chem. Biol. Interactions. 3:1–11.

Maskarinec, M. P. and M. R. Guerin. 1979. Preparations of glass capillary columns for the gas chromatographic analysis of tobacco smoke constituents. Presented at the 33rd Tobacco Chemists' Research Conference, Lexington, KY, October 29–31.

Maskarinec, M. P., R. W. Harvey and J. E. Caton. 1978. A novel method for the isolation and quantitative analysis of nicotine and cotinine in biological fluids. J. Anal. Toxicol. 2:124–126.

———. 1978. Rapid, Quantitative determination of nicotine by high pressure liquid chromatography. Presented at the 32nd Tobacco Chemists' Research Conference, Montreal, Quebec, October 30–November 1.

Mason, W.L., I.E. Muijsson-Arnold, M. McKenzie, E.T. Cantrell and D.L. Busbee. 1978. Steroid hydroxylase induction in cultured human lymphocytes: effects of the menstrual cycle. Steroids. Jan. 31(l): 1–7.

McGill, H., A. Coleho and W. Rogers. 1977. Screening non-human primates for models of cardiopulmonary disease. Paper presented at the Inaugural meeting of the American Primatological Society.

McGill, H. and W. Rogers. 1979. The baboon as a model for cigarette smoking. Symposium on the use of nonhuman primates in cardiovascular disease. San Antonio, Texas, February.

McGill, H., W. Rogers, D. Johnson and R. Wilbur. 1973. Cigarette smoking baboons: demonstration of feasibility. Proceedings of the Society for Experimental Biology and Medicine. 157:672–676.

McGill, H., W. Rogers., M. Montiel and C. McMahan. 1978. Responses of baboon to cigarette smoking. Abstracts of the 32nd Annual Meeting, Council on Arteriosclerosis, American Heart Association, November.

McLemore, T., R. Martin, D. Busbee, R. Richie, R. Springer, K. Toppell, and E. Cantrell. 1979. Aryl hydrocarbon hydroxylase activity in pulmonary macrophages and lymphocytes from lung cancer and non-cancer patients. Cancer Res. 37:1175–1186.

Menkes, H.A., S. Permutt and B.H. Cohen. 1979. Patterns of pulmonary function abnormalities in high risk groups. Pages 301–302 in P.T. Macklem and S. Permutt, eds. The Lung in Transition Between Health and Disease. Marcel Dekker, New York.

Menkes, H., and P.B. Terry, S. Permutt, and B. Cohen. Pulmonary function and risk for obstructive lung disease. In J. Dosman and D. Cotton, eds. Proceedings of the International Symposium on Grain Dust and Health: Occupational Pulmonary Disease. Focus on Grain Dust and Health. Academic Press, New York.

Miller, R. P., J. Adir, and K. S. Rotenberg. 1975. Pharmacokinetics of intravenous nicotine in rats. The Pharmacologist 17: 193.

Morosco, G. J. and G. C. Goeringer. 1979. Determination of pancreatic elastase and serum alpha-anti-trypsin in dogs exposed to cigarette smoke. Federation Proc. 38:583.

———. 1979. Pancreatic elastase and serum alpha,-antitrypsin levels in beagle dogs smoking high and low nicotine cigarettes: Possible mechanism of pancreatic cancer in cigarette smokers. J. of Toxicol. and Environ. Health. 5:879–890.

Muijsson, I., M. Coomes, E. Cantrell, O. Anderson, and D. Busbee. 1975. The induction of 16(a)hydroxylase in cultured human lymphocytes. Biochem. Genet. 13:501.

Mushinski, M. H. and S. D. Stellman. 1978. Impact of new smoking trends on women's occupational health. Prev. Med. 7:349–365.

Nebert, D. W., W. F. Benedict, and R. E. Kouri. 1974. Aromatic hydrocarbon produced tumorigenesis and the genetic differences in aryl hydrocarbon hydroxylase induction. Pages 271–288 in P. Tso and J. DePaola, eds. Chemical Carcinogenesis, Part A. Marcel Dekker, New York.

Nebert, D. W., R. E. Kouri, H. Yagi, D. M. Serina, and A. R. Boobis. Genetic differences in benzo(a)pyrene carcinogenic index in vivo and in mouse cytochrome 4-450-mediated benzo(a)pyrene metabolite binding to DN in vitro. In R. Snyder and N. Koscis, eds. Reactive intermediates. Plenum Press, New York.

Nettesheim, P., M. R. Guerin, J. Kendrick, J. Caton, W. Dalbey and R. Griesemer. 1977. Acute and chronic inhalation in rats. In E. L. Wynder, D. Hoffmann, and G. B. Gori, eds. Proceedings of 3rd World Conf. Smoking and Health Vol. II. DHEW Pub. No. (NIH) 77-1413.

Nettesheim, P., M. R. Guerin, J. Kendrick, I. Rubin, J. Stokely, D. Creasia, W. Maddox and J. E. Caton. 1975. Control and maximization of tobacco smoke dose in chronic animal studies. Pages 17–26 in Proceedings of the Tobacco Smoke Inhalation Workshop on Experimental Methods in Smoking and Health Research. DHEW Pub. No. (NIH) 75-906. U.S. Government Printing Office, Washington, D. C.

Nightingale, T. E., H. Y. C. Wong and C. Fransinel. 1979. Dose-response effect of cigarette smoking on plasma nicotine and cotinine levels of dogs. Federation Proc. 38:583.

Page, B. F. J. 1974. The continuous measurement of C-14 activity in circulating blood by liquid scintillation counting. Pages 273–278 in M. A. Crook and P. Johnson, eds. Liquid Scintillation Counting, Vol. 3, Heyden, London.

Page, B. F. J. and M. W. Baines. 1974. The continuous monitoring of C-14 activity in blood. Int. J. Appl. Radiat. Isotopes 25:45.

Page, B. F. J., B. Woolsgrove, L. F. Charseaud and R. Binns. 1973. Use of radioactive tracer techniques in investigations associated with cigarette smoking. Ann. Occup. Hyg. 16:409–416.

Park, J. F., E. B. Howard, B. O. Stuart, A. P. Wehner and J. V. Dilley. 1970. Cocarcinogenic studies in pulmonary carcinogenesis. Pages 417–432 in P. Nettesheim, M. G. Hanna, Jr. and J. W. Deatherage, Jr., eds. Morphology of Experimental Respiratory Carcinogenesis. AEC Symposium Series 21, NTIS, Springfield, Va.

Patel, A. R. 1976. Preparation and monitoring of cigarette smoke condensate samples 1. Smoking and Health Program, National Cancer Institute. OHEW Pub. No. (NIH) 76-905. U.S. Government Printing Office, Washington, D.C.

Patel, A. R. and G. B. Gori. 1975. Preparation and monitoring of marijuana smoke condensate samples. Bull. Narc. 27:47.

Patel, A. R., M. X. Haq, C. L. Innerarity, L. T. Innerarity and K. Weissgraber. 1974. Fractionation studies of smoke condensate samples from Kentucky reference cigarettes. Tob. Sci. 18:58.

Patrianakos, C. and D. Hoffmann. 1979. Chemical studies on tobacco smoke. LXIV. On the analysis of aromatic amines in cigarette smoke. J. Anal. Toxicol. 3:150–154.

Permutt, S. and H.A. Menkes. 1979. Spirometry: Analysis of forced expiration within the time domain. Pages 113–152 in P.T. Macklem and S. Permutt, eds. The Lung in Transition Between Health and Disease. Marcel Dekker, New York.

Piade, J. J., J. O. Adams and D. Hoffmann. 1979. Alkaloids and nonvolatile N-nitrosamines of tobacco and smoke of dark cigarettes. Presented at the 33rd Tobacco Chemists' Research Conference, Lexington, KY, October 29–31.

Pochay, V. E., R. Y. H. Wong, B. E. Glennon and G. L. Huber. 1978. Intestinal parasites of the white Carneau pigeon. American Association of Laboratory Animal Science. Proceedings of the 29th Annual Session. (abstr.).

Prough, R. A., R. L. Imblum and R. E. Kouri. 1976. NADH-cytochrome c reductase activity in cultured human lymphocytes: similarity to the liver microsomal NADH-cytochrome b5 reductase and cytochrome b5 enzyme system. Arch. Biochem. Biophys. 176:119–126.

Rathkamp, G. and D. Hoffmann. 1970. Chemical studies on tobacco smoke. XIII. Inhibition of the pyrosynthesis of several selective smoke constituents. Beitr. Tabakforsch. 5:302–306.

Rathkamp, G., T. C. Tso and D. Hoffmann. 1973. Chemical studies on tobacco smoke. XX. Smoke analysis of cigarettes made from bright tobaccos differing in variety and stalk positions. Bietr. Tabakforsch. 7:179–189.

Rivenson, A., T. Ohmori, S. S. Hecht and D. Hoffmann. 1979. Organotropic carcinogenicity of tobacco specific N-nitrosamines. Presented at the 5th Meeting of the European Association for Cancer Research in Vienna, September 9–12.

Roehrs, J., W. Rogers, B. McCullough and W. Johanson. 1978. Airway function in smoking baboons. Amer. Rev. of Res. Dis. 117:256. (abstr.).

Rogers, W. 1977. The effect of cigarette type on blood carbon monoxide levels: studies with the cigarette smoking baboon. Amer. Rev. of Res. Dis. 115:158.

————., 1979. Animal models of smoke inhalation. Paper presented at National Heart, Lung and Blood Institute Conference on the influence of smoking on cardiovascular disease. San Antonio, Texas, January.

Rogers, W. and D. Johnson. 1978. Effects of cigarette nicotine content on smoking behavior urinary cotinine output in cigarette smoking baboons. Paper presented to Amer. Soc. of Primatologists. September.

Rogers, W. and M. Tuttle. 1979. Neonatal behavior responses in baboons. Paper presented to Animal Behavior Society. New Orleans, Louisiana, June.

Rotenberg, K. S., R. P. Miller and J. Adir. 1975. Pharmacokenetics of intravenous nicotine in rats at various doses. Paper presented at the Annual Meeting of the American Academy of Pharmaceutical Sciences, Atlanta, Ga. (abstr.).

Rubin, 1. B. 1973. A simplified method for the determination of labeled alkane hydrocarbons in mammalian tissue and blood after exposure to radiolabeled cigarette smoke. Anal. Lett. 6:387.

Rubin, D. A. Creasia, W. L. Maddox, M. R. Guerin and P. Nettesheim. 1976. Respiratory tract deposition of smoke particles using a nasal by-pass device. Arch. Environ. Health. 31:131–135.

Rubin, I. B., B. E. Gill, M. R. Guerin, J. Kendrick and P. Nettesheim. 1978. Correlation of respiratory parameters in hamsters with the lung deposition of radiolabeled cigarette smoke. Environ. Res. 16:70–76.

Sanders, C. L., T. A. Jackson, R. R. Adee, C. J. Powers and A. P. Wehner. 1971. Distribution of inhaled metal oxide particles in pulmonary alveoli. AMA Arch. Intern. Med. 127:1085–1089.

Sandusky, H. W. 1976. A computer-simulated cigarette model for use in the development of less hazardous cigarettes. P11D. thesis, Princeton University, Princeton, NJ.

Sandusky, H. W., T. j. Ohlemiller and M. Summerfield. 1977. Beitrage zur Tabakforschung, Band 9, Heft 3. October, pages 117–125.

Schechtman, L.M., S. Beard, C. Oivels, R. Joslekar, D. Slomiany. 1978. Simultaneous determination of the cytotoxic, mutagenic and transforming activities of benzo(a)pyrene (BP) metabolically activated in vitro (meeting abstract). Proc Am Assoc Cancer Res. 19:142.

Schmeltz, I., K. D. Brunnemann and D. Hoffmann. 1978. Analytical methods for polynuclear hydrocarbons. In "Detection and Prevention of Cancer." Part 1, Marcel Decker. 2:1973–1992.

Schmeltz, I. S., K. G. Chiong and D. Hoffmann. 1973. On the formation and analysis of ethyl carbamate in tobacco and tobacco smoke. J. Anal. Toxicol. 2:265–268.

Schmeltz, I. and D. Hoffmann. 1976. Formation of polynuclear,aromatic hydrocarbons from combustion of organic matter. Pages 225–239 In: L. Freudenthal and P. W. Jones, eds. Polynuclear aromatic hydrocarbons: Chemistry, metabolism, and carcinogenesis. Raven Press. New York, NY.

————. 1976. The physiochemical nature of cigarette smoke. Pages 13–34 in

E. L. Wynder, D. Hoffmann and G. B. Gori, eds. Smoking and Health I: Modifying the Risk for the Smoker. DHEW Pub. No. (NIH) 76-1221, U.S. Government Printing Office, Washington, D. C.

Schmeltz, I. and D. Hoffmann. 1977. Chemical studies on tobacco smoke L. Nitrogen-containing compounds in tobacco and tobacco smoke. Chem. Rev. 77:295–311.

Schmeltz, I., D. Hoffmann and E. L. Wynder. 1975. Chemical studies on tobacco smoke. XXXII. Toxic and tumorigenic agents in tobacco smoke: analytical methods and modes of origin. Pages 281–295 in Proceedings of 8th Annual Conference on Trace Substances in Environmental Health, Columbia, MO. (June 11–13, 1974).

————.* 1975. The influence of tobacco smoke on indoor atmospheres. I. An overview. Prev. Med. 4:66–82.

Schmeltz, I., J. Tosk, H. Hilfrich, N. Hirota, D. Hoffmann and E. L. Wynder. 1978. Bioassays of napthalene and alkylnaphthalenes for cocarcinogenic activity. Relation to tobacco carcinogenesis. "Carcinogenesis-A Comprehensive Survey" (R.W. Jones and R.I. Freudenthal, eds.) Raven Press, New York. 3:47–60.

Schmeltz, I., J. Tosk and D. Hoffmann. 1975. Naphthalenes in cigarette smoke: analysis and formation paper presented at the 29th Tobacco Chemists' Research Conference, College Park, Md., October 8–10.

————. 1976. Formation and determination of naphthalenes in cigarette smoke. Anal. Chem. 48:645–650.

Schmeltz, I., J. Tosk, G. Jacobs and D. Hoffmann. 1977. Chemical studies on tobacco smoke. XXXV. The redox potential and quinone content of cigarette smoke. Anal. Chem. 49:1924–1929.

Schmeltz, I., A. Wenger, D. Hoffmann and T. C. Tso. 1978. Chemical studies on tobacco smoke. LIII. Use of radioactive tobacco isolates for studying the formation of smoke components. J. Agriculture and Food Chemistry. 26:234–239.

————. 1979. Chemical studies on tobacco smoke LXIII. On the fate of nicotine during pyrolysis and in a burning cigarette. J. Agr. Food Chem. 27:602–608.

Schneider, S., B. McCullough, N. Greene and W. Rogers. 1978. Bronchoalveolar lavage in the assessment of pulmonary immune parameters in the normal and smoking baboon. Paper presented to American Soc. of Primatologists, September.

————. 1979. Phagocytic and cytotoxic capacity of bronchoalveolar macrophages in the normal and smoking baboon. Paper presented to American Society of Microbiology. Houston, Texas, December, 1978. Texas Journal of Science 32:196.

Schottenfeld, D., R. C. Gantt and E. L. Wynder. 1974. The role of alcohol and tobacco in multiple primary cancers of the upper digestive system, larynx and lung: a prospective study. Prev. Med. 3:277–293.

Segal, A., C. Katz and B. L. Van Duuren. 1971. Structure and tumor-promoting activity of anthralin (1,8-dihydroxy-9-anthrone) and related compounds. J. Med. Chem. 14:1152–1154.

Shewchuk, L. A. 1975. Experiences of the American Health Foundation Smoking Cessation Programs. Paper presented at the American Lung Association Conference on Smoking, Atlanta, Ga.

————. 1975. Problems of high-risk populations and high-risk non-responders: smoking behavior. Page 93 in J. W. Cullen, B. H. Fox and R. N. Ison, eds. Cancer: the behavioral dimensions. Raven Press, New York.

Shewchuk, L. A., A. R. Jaffin, R. R. Clark, O. Burton, M. Forman and R. Oubren. 1977. Preliminary observations on an intervention program for heavy smokers. Int. J. Addict. 12:323–336.

Sivak, A. and B. L. Van Duuren. 1967. Effects of tumor initiators and promotors in cell culture systems. Page 61 in Abstracts, 58th Annual Meeting of the American Association of Cancer Research, Chicago, Ill.

————. 1967. Phenotypic expression of transformation: induction in cell culture by a phorbol ester. Science 157:1443–1444.

————. 1968. Studies with carcinogens and tumor-promoting agents in cell culture. Exp. Cell Res. 49:572–583.

————. 1969. Cell culture models for tumor promotion. Page 28 in Proceedings 20th Annual Meeting of the Tissue Culture Association, Detroit, Mich.

————. 1970. A cell culture system for the assessment of tumor-promoting activity. J. Natl. Cancer Inst. 44:1091–1097.

Smith, P., F. Stitik, J. Smith, R. Rosenthal and H. Menkes. 1979. Tantalum inhalation and airway responses. Thorax 34: 486–492.

Stokely, J. R. and M. R. Guerin. 1973. Chemical characterization of tobacco smoke in an intermittent animal exposure device. Paper presented at the 27th Tobacco Chemists' Research Conference, Winston-Salem, NC.

Stokely, J. R., J. H. Moneyhun and M. R. Guerin. 1975. Chemical indicators and methods for determination of tobacco smoke concentrations in inhalation exposure systems. Paper presented at the 29th Tobacco Chemists' Research Conference, College Park, MD.

Thomas, P. E., R. E. Kouri and J. J. Hutton. 1973. The genetics of aryl hydrocarbon hydroxylase induction in mice: a single gene difference between C57BL/6 and DBA/2J. Biochem. Genet. 6:157–168.

Tso, T. C. 1977. Tobacco and tobacco smoke. In: N. Childers and G. Russo, eds. Nightshade crops and health problems. Horticultural Publications,

Somerset Press, Inc., Sommerfield, NJ, pp. 42–93.

———. 1977. Tobacco as potential food source and smoke material. Beitr. Tabakforsch. 9:63–66.

Tso, T. C. and J. F. Chaplin. 1977. Simple correlation and multiple regression among leaf characteristics, smoke components and biological responses of bright tobaccos. USDA Technical Bulletin No. 1551.

Tso, T. C. and H. Chu. 1977. The fate of fatty compounds and surfactants used as sucker-control of agents on field tobacco. Beitr. Tabakforsch. 9:58–62.

Tso, T. C. and G. B. Gori. 1975. Leaf quality and usability theoretical model 1. Pages 258–275 in Chemical Marketing and Economics. American Chemical Society, Philadelphia, Pa.

———. 1975. Leaf quality and usability theoretical model 1. Beitr. Tabakforsch. 8:167–173.

Tso, T. C., G. B. Gori and D. Hoffmann. 1976. Reduction of nicotine and tar in tobacco and cigarettes through agricultural techniques. Pages 35–48 in E. L. Wynder, D. Hoffmann and G. B. Gori, eds. Smoking and Health I: Modifying the Risk for the Smoker. DHEW Pub. No. (NIH) 76-1221, U.S. Government Printing Office, Washington, D. C.

Tso, T. C., G. Rathkamp and D. Hoffmann. 1973. Chemical studies on tobacco smoke. XXI. Correlation and multiple regression among selected cigarette smoke constituents and leaf characteristics of Bright tobacco. Beitr. Tabakforsch. 7:190–194.

U.S. Department of Health, Education and Welfare. 1973. Adult Use of Tobacco. 1970. National Clearinghouse for Smoking and Health, Washington, D. C.

Van Duuren, B. L. 1966. The fluorescence of tobacco coumarins, hydroxyflavones and related compounds. Page 63 in Abstracts, 4th International Tobacco Scientific Congress, Athens, Greece.

———. 1968. Tobacco carcinogenesis. Cancer Res. 28:2357–2362.

———. Tumor-promoting agents in two-stage carcinogenesis. Pages 31–68. In F. Homburger, (Ed.) Progress in Experimental Tumor Research, Vol. II. Hafner Publishing Co., Inc., New York.

Van Duuren, B. L., T. Blazej, B. J. Goldschmidt, C. Katz, S. Melchionne and A. Sivak. 1971. Cocarcinogenesis studies on mouse skin and inhibition of tumor induction. J. Natl. Cancer Inst. 46:1039–1044.

Van Duuren, B. L., M. Conklin, G. C. Lavers and A. Segal. 1967. Synthesis of laurate esters of pyrogallol and related phenols. J. Chem. Soc., Section C (London): 588–590.

Van Duuren, B. L. and B. M. Goldschmidt. 1976. Cocarcinogenic and tumor-promoting agents in tobacco carcinogenesis. J. Natl. Cancer Inst.

56:1237–1242.

Van Duuren, B. L., C. Katz and B. M. Goldschmidt. 1973. Brief communication: cocarcinogenic agents in tobacco carcinogenesis. J. Natl. Cancer Inst. 51:703–705.

Van Duuren, B. L., A. Sivak, B. M. Goldschmidt, C. Katz and S. Melchionne. 1970. Initiating activity of aromatic hydrocarbons in two-stage carcinogenesis. J. Natl. Cancer Inst. 44:1167–1173.

Van Duuren, B. L., A. Sivak, B. M. Goldschmidt and C. Katz. 1971. Tobacco carcinogenesis: cocarcinogens, promoting and inhibitory agents. Page 2 in Proceedings 62nd Annual Meeting of the American Association of Cancer Research, Chicago.

Van Duuren, B. L., A. Sivak, C. Katz and S. Melchionne. 1971. Cigarette smoke carcinogenesis: importance of tumor promoters. J. Natl. Cancer Inst. 47:235–240.

Van Duuren, B. L., A. Sivak and L. Langseth. 1967. The tumor promoting activity of tobacco leaf extract and whole cigarette tar. Brit. J. Cancer 21:46.0–463.

Van Duuren, B. L., A. Sivak, L. Langseth, B. M. Goldschmidt and A. Segal. 1968. Initiators and promoters in tobacco carcinogenesis. (Paper presented at the World Conference on Smoking and Health, New York, September 11–13, 1967.) Natl. Cancer Inst. Monogr. No. 28:173–180.

Van Duuren, B. L., A. Sivak, S. Melchionne and C. Katz. 1970. Initiating activity of weak carcinogens in two-stage carcinogenesis on mouse skin. Page 39 in Proceedings of the 10th International Cancer Congress, Houston.

Van Duuren, B. L., A. Sivak, A. Segal, et al. 1973. Dose-response studies with a pure cancer-promoting agent, phorbol myristate acetate. Cancer Res. 33:2166.

Van Duuren, B. L., A. Sivak, A. Segal, L. Orris and L. Langseth. 1966. The tumor-promoting agents of tobacco and tobacco smoke condensate. J. Natl. Cancer Inst. 37:519–526.

Veal, J. T. and G. E. Dagle. 1976. Evaluation of beeswax-tri-caprylin vehicle for pulmonary carcinogenesis studies. Toxicol. Appl. Pharmacol. 35:157–164.

Wehner, A. P. 1977. Inhalation experiments with air pollutants in rodents, No. 103. In: Second Congress of International Society for Aerosols in Medicine, Warsaw, Poland. April 20–22. (abstr.).

Wehner, A. P. R. H. Busch and R. J. Olson. 1974. Effect of chronic exposure to cigarette smoke on tumor incidence in the Syrian golden hamster. Pages 360–368 in Experimental Lung Cancer. Springer-Verlag, New York.

———. 1976. Effects of diethylnitrosamine and cigarette smoke in hamsters.

J. Natl. Cancer Inst. 56:749–756.

Wehner, A. P., R. H. Busch, R. J. Olson and D. K. Craig. 1975. Chronic inhalation of asbestos and cigarette smoke by hamsters. Environ. Res. 10:368–383.

———. 1975. Chronic inhalation of nickel oxide and cigarette smoke by hamsters. Am. Ind. Hyg. Assoc. J. 36:801–810.

———. 1977. Chronic inhalation of cobalt oxide and cigarette smoke by hamsters. Am Ind. Hyg. Assoc. J. 38:338–346.

Wehner, A. P. and O. K. Craig. 1972. Toxicology of inhaled NiO and CoO in Syrian golden hamsters. Am Ind. Hyg. Assoc. J. 33:146–155.

Wehner, A. P., O. K. Craig and B. O. Stuart. 1972. An aerosol exposure system for chronic inhalation studies with rodents. Am. Ind. Hyg. Assoc. J. 33:483–487.

Wehner, A. P., R. J. Olson and R. H. Busch. 1976. Increased life span and decreased body weight in cigarette-smoke-exposed hamsters. Arch. Environ. Health. 31:146–153.

Wehner, A. P., B. O. Stuart and C. L. Sanders. 1979. Inhalation studies with Syrian golden hamsters. Prog. Exp. Tumor Res., Vol. 24, pp 177–198.

Wehner, A. P., et al. 1974. Investigation of Cocarcinogenicity of Asbestos, Cobalt Oxide (CoO), Nickel Oxide (NiO), Diethylnitrosamine and cigarette smoke. Final report to National Cancer Institute, Bethesda, Md., Battelle-Northwest, Richland, Washington.

———., et al. 1967. The Measurement of Cigarette Smoke Deposited in Dogs by a Method Simulating Human Smoking. Technical Report SNP 1-95 to Council for Tobacco Research, New York, NY., Battelle-Northwest, Richland, Wa.

Whitlock, J. P., H. L. Cooper and H. V. Gelboin. 1972. Aryl hydrocarbon (benzopyrene) hydroxylase as stimulated in human lymphocytes by mitogens and benz(a)anthracene. Science 177:618–619.

Whitmire, C. E., C. F. Demoise and R. E. Kouri. 1974. The role of the hose in the development of in vivo models for carcinogenesis studies. Page 20 in E. Karbe and J. F. Park, eds. Experimental Lung Cancer. Springer-Verlag, New York.

Wong, R. Y. H., V. E. Pochay, B. E. Glennon, J. W. Shea and G. L. Huber. 1978. Some normal hematological values of the white carneau pigeon. American Association of Laboratory Animal Science, proceedings of the 29th Annual Session. #61. (abstr.)

Wynder, E. L. 1971. Etiological aspects of squamous cancers of the head and neck. J. Am. Med. Assoc. 215:452–453.

———. 1972. Etiology of lung cancer. Reflections on two decades of research. Cancer 30:1332–1333.

———. 1974. Working groups in cancer etiology. Cancer Res. 34:1516–1518.

———. 1975. Towards the prevention of larynx cancer. Laryngoscope. 85(7):1190–1196.

———. 1975. Guest editorial: The tenth anniversary of the Surgeon General's report on smoking and health: Have we made any progress? J. Natl. Cancer Inst. 54:533–534.

———. 1975. Towards reducing tobacco-related cancers. "Cancer epidemiology, environmental factors," Proc. XI Intl. Cancer Congress, Florence, 1974, Excerpta Medica 3:138–143.

———. 1975. An epidemiological evaluation of the causes of cancer of the pancreas. Cancer Res. 35:2228–2232.

———. 1977. Cultural and behavioral aspects of risk factors: Society's obligation. J. Environ. Pathol. Toxicol. 1:11–18.

———. 1977. Epidemiology and prevention of cancer: A question of scientific and economic priorities. Nature 268:284.

———. 1977. Research on smoking behavior: Interrelationships of smoking to other variables and preventive approaches. Natl. Inst. Drug Abuse Res. Monogr. 17:67–95.

———. 1977. Toward the prevention of cancer. Cancer Bull. 29:186–191.

———. 1978. Environmental Carcinogenesis. Clinical Bulletin. 8:3–9.

———. 1978. The epidemiology of cancers of the upper alimentary and upper respiratory tracts. Laryngoscope 88:50–51.

Wynder, E. L., L. S. Covey and K. Mabuchi. 1973. Lung cancer in women: present and future trends. J. Natl. Cancer Inst. 51:391–401.

———. 1974. Current smoking habits by selected background variables: their effect on future trends in tobacco-related diseases. Am. J. Epidemiol. 100:168–177.

Wynder, E. L., L. S. Covey, K. Mabuchi and M. H. Mushinski. 1975. Towards the prevention of cancer of the larynx. Laryngoscope. 85:1190–1196.

———. 1976. Environmental factors in cancer of the larynx. A second look. Cancer 38:1591–1601.

Wynder, E. L. and R. Goldsmith. 1977. The epidemiology of bladder cancer: A second look. Cancer. 40:1246–1268.

Wynder, E. L. and G. B. Gori. 1977. Contribution of the environment to cancer incidence: an epidemiologic exercise. J. Natl. Cancer Inst. 58:825–832.

Wynder, E. L. and S. S. Hecht, eds. 1976. "Lung Cancer." UICC Techn. Report Series Vol. 25, Geneva, International Union Against Cancer, page 170.

Wynder, E. L. and D. Hoffmann. 1970. The epidermis and the respiratory tract as bioassay systems in tobacco carcinogenesis. Brit. J. Cancer. 24:547–579.

Wynder, E. L. and D. Hoffmann. 1972. Carcinogens in the air. Pages 118–138 in proceedings of the 24th Annual Symposium on Fundamental Cancer Research, Houston.

———. 1972. Less harmful ways of smoking. J. Natl. Cancer Inst. 48:1749–1758.

Wynder, E. L. and D. Hoffmann. 1975. The tenth anniversary of the Surgeon General's report on smoking and health: Have we made any progress (Guest Editorial). J. Natl. Cancer Inst. 54:533–534.

———. 1976. Tobacco and tobacco smoke. Sem. Oncol. 3:5–15.

Wynder, E. L. and D. Hoffmann. 1979. Smoking and Health: Pathogenic and preventive considerations. Bull. Schweizer Akademic Med. Wissenschaften 35:83–98.

Wynder, E. L. and D. Hoffmann. 1979. Tobacco and health: Societal challenge. New Eng. J. Med. 300:894–903.

Wynder, E. L., D. Hoffmann and P. Ashwanden, eds. 1972. Less harmful ways of smoking. (Proceedings of a Workshop of the Second World Conference on Smoking and Health, London, September 20–24, 1971.) J. Natl. Cancer Inst. 48:1739–1891.

Wynder, E. L., D. Hoffmann, P. Chan and B. Reddy. 1975. Interdisciplinary and experimental approaches: Metabolic epidemiology in "Persons at High Risk of Cancer, An Approach to Cancer Etiology and Control, pp. 485–501, (J. F. Fraumeni, ed.). Academic Press, New York.

Wynder, E. L., D. Hoffmann and G. B. Gori, eds. 1976. Smoking and Health 1: Modifying the Risk for the Smoker. DHEW Pub. No. (NIH) 76–1221, U.S. Government Printing Office, Washington, D.C.

Wynder, E. L., D. Hoffmann, G. D. McCoy, L. A. Cohen and B. S. Reddy. 1978. Tumor promotion and cocarcinogenesis as related to man and his environment. In Carcinogenesis—A Comprehensive Survey. "Mechanisms of Tumor Promotion and Cocarcinogenesis." (T. J. Slaga, A. Sivak and R. K. Boutwell, eds.) Raven Press, New York. 2:59–77.

Wynder, E. L. and K. Mabuchi. 1972. Etiological and preventive aspects of human cancer. Prev. Med. 1:300–334.

———. 1972. Lung cancer in cigar and pipe smokers. Prev. Med. 1:529–542.

———. 1973. Etiological and environmental factors. J. Am. Med. Assoc. 226:1546–1548.

———. 1974. Some reflections on the epidemiology of lung cancer. Pages 146–151 in C. Maltoni, ed. Proceedings of the Second International Symposium of Cancer Detection and Prevention, Bologna, Italy. Excerpta, Amsterdam.

Wynder, E. L., K. Mabuchi and E. J. Beattie, Jr. 1970. The epidemiology of lung cancer. Recent trends. J. Am. Med. Assoc. 213:2221–2228.

Wynder, E. L., K. Mabuchi and D. Hoffmann. 1975. Tobacco. Pages 102–125 in D. Schottenfeld, ed. Cancer Epidemiology and Prevention. Charles C. Thomas Publisher, Springfield, IL.

Wynder, E. L., K. Mabuchi, N. Maruchi and J. G. Fortner. 1973. A case-control study of cancer of the pancreas. Cancer 31:641–648.

———. 1973. Epidemiology of cancer of the pancreas. J. Natl. Cancer Inst. 50:645–667.

Wynder, E. L., K. Mabuchi and W. F. Whitmore, Jr. 1974. Epidemiology of adenocarcinoma of the kidney. J. Natl. Cancer Inst. 53:1619–1634.

Wynder, E. L. and M. H. Mushinski. 1979. The epidemiology of smoking and the development of lung and bladder cancer. Paper presented at Conference on Smoking and Disease, Celle, Germany.

Wynder, E. L., M. Mushinski and J. C. Spivak. 1977. Tobacco and alcohol consumption in relation to the development of multiple primary cancers. Cancer 40:1872–1878.

Wynder, E. L., M. Mushinski and S. Stellman. 1976. The epidemiology of the less harmful cigarette. Pages 1–12 in E. L. Wynder, D. Hoffmann and G. B. Gori, ed. Smoking and Health I: Modifying the Risk for the Smoker. DHEW Pub. No. (NIH) 76-1221, U.S. Government Printing Office, Washington, D.C.

Wynder, E. L. and P. Peacock. 1974. Commentary: The practice of disease prevention. J. Am. Med. Assoc. 229:1743.

Wynder, E. L. and S. D. Stellman. 1977. Comparative epidemiology of tobacco-related cancers. Cancer 37:4608–4622.

———. 1979. "The impact of long-term filter cigarette usage on lung and larynx cancer risk: A case control study." J. Natl. Cancer Inst. 62:471–477.

Zeldes, S. G. and A. D. Horton. 1973. "Trapping and Determination of Labile Compounds in the Gas Phase of Cigarette Smoke." Anal. Chem. 50:779.

Zimmerman, E. M., R. E. Kouri, K. Higuchi, F. Laird and A. E. Freeman. 1975. Uptake metabolism and persistence of 3-methylcholanthrene in rat embryo cells infected with murine leukemia virus. Cancer Res. 35:139–143.

Zwicker, G.M. R.E. Filipy, J.F. Park, S.M. Loscutoff, H.A. Rasan and D.L. Stevens. 1978. Clinical and Pathological effects of Cigarette Smoke Exposure in Beagle Dogs. Arch Pathol. Lab. Med. Dec. 102(12): 623–8.

DATE DUE

DEMCO 38-296

Praise for *The Great Influenza*

"Monumental . . . powerfully intelligent . . . unflinching . . . Barry's book is not just a masterful narrative of the events of 1918 but also an authoritative and disturbing morality tale of science, politics and culture. . . . One of the strengths of Barry's book is that it goes well beyond medical facts and figures. . . . [It is] a sweeping style that consistently focuses on real human beings, and he cares deeply and unapologetically about morality and politics. . . . Barry has done a remarkable service in writing *The Great Influenza*."
—*Chicago Tribune*

"Here is a writer of distinction with a deep philosophical underpinning. . . . I loved the range of this book, how it directs a searchlight on science and scientists and gives us so much more than its title. We have no cold statistics to pore over, no tables of case fatalities. Instead, we are entering the forgotten world of personalities of medical science . . . compelling and brilliant."
—*Journal of the American Medical Association* (JAMA)

"Sometimes the book reads like a detective novel; other times it reads like science fiction. . . . A fascinating and frightening account of sickness, fear, stupidity, scientific exploration, and occasional heroism. . . . If this book were merely about the causes and effects of the 1918 influenza pandemic, it would be an engrossing tale, but the story encompasses much more. . . . Ultimately, Barry brings his narrative into the present with provocative implications."
—*The Charlotte Observer*

"Immensely readable . . . a multistranded narrative account of the most devastating pandemic the world has ever known, as well as a history of twentieth-century science and medicine . . . He describes how the influenza virus attacks the body with a clarity that lays the conceptual groundwork for much that would ensue. . . . And as a piece of social history, *The Great Influenza* is invaluable. It shows the courage and cowardice of individuals under great pressure; it shows how institutions, captive to the ethics of the time, can rise to the occasion or abjectly fall. . . . It's a lesson to ponder in our times."
—*The Seattle Times*

"Magisterial . . . evocative . . . unusual literary panache . . . impressively up-to-date understanding . . . very artfully constructed [with phrases] repeated like Wagner's leitmotifs . . . The fact is that flu is one of the most formidable infections confronting humankind. The virus mutates constantly as it circulates among birds, pigs, and human beings, so each new flu season now challenges experts . . . His message for our time is clear."
—*The New York Review of Books*

"Compelling and timely."
—*The Boston Globe*

"Barry writes like an angel. . . . Through a vision of the scientists of the day he brings back the tension and excitement, the despair and the sorrow . . . yes I have indulged myself and read the book twice. . . . Barry's writing . . . manage[s] to capture the science of virology. . . . This book is a wake-up call."
—*Nature*

"Hypnotizing, horrifying, almost incomprehensible . . . energetic, lucid prose . . . His important story stands solidly and eloquently on its own as a work of history and a cautionary tale."
—*The Providence Journal*

"History brilliantly written . . . *The Great Influenza* is a masterpiece."
—*Baton Rouge Advocate*

"A medical thriller . . . It combines popular history and popular science in a way that reminds one of David McCullough's great books on the Johnstown flood and the building of the Panama Canal and the Brooklyn Bridge. *The Great Influenza* might be the most interesting such concoction since . . . well, since the same author's *Rising Tide: The Great Mississippi Flood of 1927 and How It Changed America.*" —*Arkansas Times*

"What distinguishes Mr. Barry's account is its thoroughness and the writer's command of both the science and the politics that conspired to spread the disease . . . compelling . . . The storytelling is vivid . . . masterly detail."
—*The Dallas Morning News*

"Majestic, spellbinding treatment of a mass killer . . . With the same terrorizing flair of Richard Preston's *Hot Zone*, the author follows the disease . . . as if from Weegee's camera." —*Kirkus Reviews* (starred review)

"Barry puts the pandemic into a context of medical, national, and world history. . . . His well-researched and well-written account raises the obvious question: Could it happen again? And the answer is: Of course it could."
—*Los Angeles Times*

"Barry provides enormous insight into the very nature of science . . . *The Great Influenza* is a must read for its unnerving relevance to today's scientific challenges of emerging and reemerging infectious diseases and the society's tragic confrontations with war and terrorism . . . alarming similarities to today . . . gripping."
—Ronald Atlas, former president of the American Society of Microbiology, *ASM News*

"Terrifying . . . The lessons of 1918 couldn't be more relevant."
—*Newsweek*

"An enthralling symphony of a book, whose every page compels."
—*Booklist* (starred review)

PENGUIN BOOKS

THE GREAT INFLUENZA

John M. Barry is the author of four previous books: *Rising Tide: The Great Mississippi Flood of 1927 and How It Changed America; Power Plays: Politics, Football, and Other Blood Sports; The Transformed Cell: Unlocking the Mysteries of Cancer* (cowritten with Steven Rosenberg); and *The Ambition and the Power: A True Story of Washington.* He lives in New Orleans and Washington, D.C.

THE GREAT

INFLUENZA

The Epic Story of the
Deadliest Plague in History

JOHN M. BARRY

PENGUIN BOOKS

PENGUIN BOOKS

Published by the Penguin Group

Penguin Group (USA) Inc., 375 Hudson Street, New York, New York 10014, U.S.A.

Penguin Group (Canada), 90 Eglinton Avenue East, Suite 700, Toronto,
Ontario, Canada M4P 2Y3 (a division of Pearson Penguin Canada Inc.)

Penguin Books Ltd, 80 Strand, London WC2R 0RL, England

Penguin Ireland, 25 St Stephen's Green, Dublin 2, Ireland (a division of Penguin Books Ltd)

Penguin Group (Australia), 250 Camberwell Road, Camberwell,
Victoria 3124, Australia (a division of Pearson Australia Group Pty Ltd)

Penguin Books India Pvt Ltd, 11 Community Centre, Panchsheel Park, New Delhi – 110 017, India

Penguin Books (NZ), cnr Airborne and Rosedale Roads, Albany,
Auckland 1310, New Zealand (a division of Pearson New Zealand Ltd)

Penguin Books (South Africa) (Pty) Ltd, 24 Sturdee Avenue, Rosebank,
Johannesburg 2196, South Africa

Penguin Books Ltd, Registered Offices:
80 Strand, London WC2R 0RL, England

First published in the United States of America by Viking Penguin,
a member of Penguin Group (USA) Inc. 2004
First published in Penguin Books 2005
This edition with a new afterword published in Penguin Books 2005

10 9 8 7 6 5 4 3 2 1

Photograph credits appear on page 547.

THE LIBRARY OF CONGRESS HAS CATALOGED THE HARDCOVER EDITION AS FOLLOWS:
Barry, John M.
The great influenza : the epic story of the deadliest plague in history / John M. Barry.
p.   cm.
Includes bibliographical references and index.
ISBN 0-670-89473-7 (hc.)
ISBN 0 14 30.3649 1 (pbk.)
1. Influenza—History—20th century.   I. Title.
RC150.4.B37 2004
614.5'18'09041—dc22   2003057646

Printed in the United States of America
Set in Minion
Designed by Francesca Belanger

To my darling Anne

and to the spirit that was Paul Lewis

Contents

THE GREAT INFLUENZA

PROLOGUE

THE GREAT WAR had brought Paul Lewis into the navy in 1918 as a lieutenant commander, but he never seemed quite at ease when in his uniform. It never seemed to fit quite right, or to sit quite right, and he was often flustered and failed to respond properly when sailors saluted him.

Yet he was every bit a warrior, and he hunted death.

When he found it he confronted it, challenged it, tried to pin it in place like a lepidopterist pinning down a butterfly, so he could then dissect it piece by piece, analyze it, and find a way to confound it. He did so often enough that the risks he took became routine.

Still, death had never appeared to him as it did now, in mid-September 1918. Row after row of men confronted him in the hospital ward, many of them bloody and dying in some new and awful way.

He had been called here to solve a mystery that dumbfounded the clinicians. For Lewis was a scientist. Although a physician he had never practiced on a patient. Instead, a member of the very first generation of American medical scientists, he had spent his life in the laboratory. He had already built an extraordinary career, an international reputation, and he was still young enough to be seen as just coming into his prime.

A decade earlier, working with his mentor at the Rockefeller Institute in New York City, he had proved that a virus caused polio, a discovery still considered a landmark achievement in the history of virology. He had then developed a vaccine that protected monkeys from polio with nearly 100 percent effectiveness.

That and other successes had won him the position of founding head of the Henry Phipps Institute, a research institute associated with the University of Pennsylvania, and in 1917 he had been chosen for the great honor of giving the annual Harvey Lecture. It seemed only the first of many honors that would come his way. Today, the children of two prominent scientists who knew him then and who crossed paths with many Nobel laureates say their fathers each told them that Lewis was the smartest man they had ever met.

The clinicians now looked to him to explain the violent symptoms these sailors presented. The blood that covered so many of them did not come from wounds, at least not from steel or explosives that had torn away limbs. Most of the blood had come from nosebleeds. A few sailors had coughed the blood up. Others had bled from their ears. Some coughed so hard that autopsies would later show they had torn apart abdominal muscles and rib cartilage. And many of the men writhed in agony or delirium; nearly all those able to communicate complained of headache, as if someone were hammering a wedge into their skulls just behind the eyes, and body aches so intense they felt like bones breaking. A few were vomiting. Finally the skin of some of the sailors had turned unusual colors; some showed just a tinge of blue around their lips or fingertips, but a few looked so dark one could not tell easily if they were Caucasian or Negro. They looked almost black.

Only once had Lewis seen a disease that in any way resembled this. Two months earlier, members of the crew of a British ship had been taken by ambulance from a sealed dock to another Philadelphia hospital and placed in isolation. There many of that crew had died. At autopsy their lungs had resembled those of men who had died from poison gas or pneumonic plague, a more virulent form of bubonic plague.

Whatever those crewmen had had, it had not spread. No one else had gotten sick.

But the men in the wards now not only puzzled Lewis. They had to have chilled him with fear also, fear both for himself and and for what this disease could do. For whatever was attacking these sailors was not only spreading, it was spreading explosively.

And it was spreading despite a well-planned, concerted effort to contain it. This same disease had erupted ten days earlier at a navy facility in Boston. Lieutenant Commander Milton Rosenau at the Chelsea Naval Hospital there had certainly communicated to Lewis, whom he knew well, about it. Rosenau too was a scientist who had chosen to leave a Harvard professorship for the navy when the United States entered the war, and his textbook on public health was called "The Bible" by both army and navy military doctors.

Philadelphia navy authorities had taken Rosenau's warnings seriously, especially since a detachment of sailors had just arrived from Boston, and they had made preparations to isolate any ill sailors should an outbreak occur. They had been confident that isolation would control it.

Yet four days after that Boston detachment arrived, nineteen sailors in Philadelphia were hospitalized with what looked like the same disease. Despite their immediate isolation and that of everyone with whom they had had contact, eighty-seven sailors were hospitalized the next day. They and their contacts were again isolated. But two days later, six hundred men were hospitalized with this strange disease. The hospital ran out of empty beds, and hospital staff began falling ill. The navy then began sending hundreds more sick sailors to a civilian hospital. And sailors and civilian workers were moving constantly between the city and navy facilities, as they had in Boston. Meanwhile, personnel from Boston, and now Philadelphia, had been and were being sent throughout the country as well.

That had to chill Lewis, too.

Lewis had visited the first patients, taken blood, urine, and sputum samples, done nasal washings, and swabbed their throats. Then he had come back again to repeat the process of collecting samples and to study the symptoms for any further clues. In his laboratory he and everyone under him poured their energies into growing and identifying whatever pathogen was making the men sick. He needed to find the pathogen. He needed to find the cause of the disease. And even more he needed to make a curative serum or a preventive vaccine.

Lewis loved the laboratory more than he loved anyone or anything. His work space was crammed; it looked like a thicket of icicles—test tubes in racks, stacked petri dishes, pipettes—but it warmed him, gave him as much and perhaps more comfort than did his home and family. But he did not love working like this. The pressure to find an answer did not bother him; much of his polio research had been conducted in the midst of an epidemic so extreme that New York City had required people to obtain passes to travel. What did bother him was the need to abandon good science. To succeed in preparing either a vaccine or serum, he would have to make a series of guesses based on at best inconclusive results, and each guess would have to be right.

He had already made one guess. If he did not yet know precisely what caused the disease, nor how or whether he could prevent it or cure it, he believed he knew what the disease was.

He believed it was influenza, although an influenza unlike any known before.

Lewis was correct. In 1918 an influenza virus emerged—probably in the United States—that would spread around the world, and one of its earliest appearances in lethal form came in Philadelphia. Before that worldwide pandemic faded away in 1920, it would kill more people than any other outbreak of disease in human history. Plague in the 1300s killed a far larger proportion of the population—more than one-quarter of Europe—but in raw numbers influenza killed more than plague then, more than AIDS today.

The lowest estimate of the pandemic's worldwide death toll is twenty-one million, in a world with a population less than one-third today's. That estimate comes from a contemporary study of the disease and newspapers have often cited it since, but it is almost certainly wrong. Epidemiologists today estimate that influenza likely caused at least fifty million deaths worldwide, and possibly as many as one hundred million.

Yet even that number understates the horror of the disease, a horror contained in other data. Normally influenza chiefly kills the elderly and infants, but in the 1918 pandemic roughly half of those who died were young men and women in the prime of their life, in their twenties and thirties. Harvey Cushing, then a brilliant young surgeon who would go on to great fame—and who himself fell desperately ill with influenza and never fully recovered from what was likely a complication—would call these victims "doubly dead in that they died so young."

One cannot know with certainty, but if the upper estimate of the death toll is true as many as 8 to 10 percent of all young adults then living may have been killed by the virus.

And they died with extraordinary ferocity and speed. Although the influenza pandemic stretched over two years, perhaps two-thirds of the deaths occurred in a period of twenty-four weeks, and more than half of those deaths occurred in even less time, from mid-September to early December 1918. Influenza killed more people in a year than the Black Death of the Middle Ages killed in a century; it killed more people in twenty-four weeks than AIDS has killed in twenty-four years.

The influenza pandemic resembled both of those scourges in other ways also. Like AIDS, it killed those with the most to live for. And as priests had done in the bubonic plague, in 1918, even in Philadelphia, as modern a city as existed in the world, priests would drive horse-drawn wagons down the streets, calling upon those behind doors shut tight in terror to bring out their dead.

Yet the story of the 1918 influenza virus is not simply one of havoc, death, and desolation, of a society fighting a war against nature superimposed on a war against another human society.

It is also a story of science, of discovery, of how one thinks, and of how one changes the way one thinks, of how amidst near-utter chaos a few men sought the coolness of contemplation, the utter calm that precedes not philosophizing but grim, determined action.

For the influenza pandemic that erupted in 1918 was the first great collision between nature and modern science. It was the first great collision between a natural force and a society that included individuals who refused either to submit to that force or to simply call upon divine intervention to save themselves from it, individuals who instead were determined to confront this force directly, with a developing technology and with their minds.

In the United States, the story is particularly one of a handful of extraordinary people, of whom Paul Lewis is one. These were men and some very few women who, far from being backward, had already developed the fundamental science upon which much of today's medicine is based. They had already developed vaccines and antitoxins and techniques still in use. They had already pushed, in some cases, close to the edge of knowledge today.

In a way, these researchers had spent much of their lives preparing for the confrontation that occurred in 1918 not only in general but, for a few of them at least, quite specifically. In every war in American history so far, disease had killed more soldiers than combat. In many wars throughout history war had spread disease. The leaders of American research had anticipated that a major epidemic of some kind would erupt during the Great War. They had prepared for it as much as it was possible to prepare. Then they waited for it to strike.

The story, however, begins earlier. Before medicine could confront this disease with any promise of effect, it had to become scientific. It had to be revolutionized.

Medicine is not yet and may never be fully a science—the idiosyncrasies, physical and otherwise, of individual patients and doctors may prevent that—but, up to a few decades before World War I, the practice of medicine had remained quite literally almost unchanged from the time of Hippocrates more than two thousand years earlier. Then, in Europe first, medical science changed and, finally, the practice of medicine changed.

But even after European medicine changed, medicine in the United States did not. In research and education especially, American medicine lagged far behind, and that made practice lag as well.

While for decades European medical schools had, for example, required students to have a solid background in chemistry, biology, and other sciences, as late as 1900, it was more difficult to get into a respectable American college than into an American medical school. At least one hundred U.S. medical schools would accept any man—but not woman—willing to pay tuition; at most 20 percent of the schools required even a high school diploma for admission—much less any academic training in science—and only a single medical school required its students to have a college degree. Nor, once students entered, did American schools necessarily make up for any lack of scientific background. Many schools bestowed a medical degree upon students who simply attended lectures and passed examinations; in some, students could fail several courses, never touch a single patient, and still get a medical degree.

Not until late—very late—in the nineteenth century, did a virtual handful of leaders of American medical science begin to plan a revolution that transformed American medicine from the most backward in the developed world into the best in the world.

William James, who was a friend of—and whose son would work for—several of these men, wrote that the collecting of a critical mass of men of genius could make a whole civilization "vibrate and shake." These men intended to, and would, shake the world.

To do so required not only intelligence and training but real courage, the courage to relinquish all support and all authority. Or perhaps it required only recklessness.

In *Faust*, Goethe wrote,

> 'Tis writ, "In the beginning was the Word."
> I Pause, to wonder what is here inferred.
> The Word I cannot set supremely high:
> A new translation I will try.
> I read, if by the spirit, I am taught,
> This sense, "In the beginning was the Thought...."

Upon "the Word" rested authority, stability, and law; "the Thought" roiled and ripped apart and created—without knowledge or concern of what it would create.

Shortly before the Great War began, the men who so wanted to transform American medicine succeeded. They created a system that could produce people capable of thinking in a new way, capable of challenging the natural order. They, together with the first generation of scientists they had trained—Paul Lewis and his few peers—formed a cadre who stood on alert, hoping against but expecting and preparing for the eruption of an epidemic.

When it came, they placed their lives in the path of the disease and applied all their knowledge and powers to defeat it. As it overwhelmed them, they concentrated on constructing the body of knowledge necessary to eventually triumph. For the scientific knowledge that ultimately came out of the influenza pandemic pointed directly—and still points—to much that lies in medicine's future.

Part I
THE WARRIORS

CHAPTER ONE

O N SEPTEMBER 12, 1876, the crowd overflowing the auditorium of Baltimore's Academy of Music was in a mood of hopeful excitement, but excitement without frivolity. Indeed, despite an unusual number of women in attendance, many of them from the uppermost reaches of local society, a reporter noted, "There was no display of dress or fashion." For this occasion had serious purpose. It was to mark the launching of the Johns Hopkins University, an institution whose leaders intended not simply to found a new university but to change all of American education; indeed, they sought considerably more than that. They planned to change the way in which Americans tried to understand and grapple with nature. The keynote speaker, the English scientist Thomas H. Huxley, personified their goals.

The import was not lost on the nation. Many newspapers, including the *New York Times,* had reporters covering this event. After it, they would print Huxley's address in full.

For the nation was then, as it so often has been, at war with itself; in fact it was engaged in different wars simultaneously, each being waged on several fronts, wars that ran along the fault lines of modern America.

One involved expansion and race. In the Dakotas, George Armstrong Custer had just led the Seventh Cavalry to its destruction at the hands of primitive savages resisting encroachment of the white man. The day Huxley spoke, the front page of the *Washington Star* reported that "the hostile Sioux, well fed and well armed" had just carried out "a massacre of miners."

In the South a far more important but equally savage war was being waged as white Democrats sought "redemption" from Reconstruction in anticipation of the presidential election. Throughout the South "rifle clubs," "saber clubs," and "rifle teams" of former Confederates were being organized into infantry and cavalry units. Already accounts of intimidation, beatings, whippings, and murder directed against Republicans and blacks had surfaced. After the murder of three hundred black men in a single Mississippi county, one man, convinced that words from the Democrats' own mouths would convince the world of their design, pleaded with the *New York Times,* "For God's sake publish the testimony of the Democrats before the Grand Jury."

Voting returns had already begun to come in—there was no single national election day—and two months later Democrat Samuel Tilden would win the popular vote by a comfortable margin. But he would never take office as president. Instead the Republican secretary of war would threaten to "force a reversal" of the vote, federal troops with fixed bayonets would patrol Washington, and southerners would talk of reigniting the Civil War. That crisis would ultimately be resolved through an extra-constitutional special committee and a political understanding: Republicans would discard the voting returns of three states—Louisiana, Florida, South Carolina—and seize a single disputed electoral vote in Oregon to keep the presidency in the person of Rutherford B. Hayes. But they also would withdraw all federal troops from the South and cease intervening in southern affairs, leaving the Negroes there to fend for themselves.

The war involving the Hopkins was more muted but no less profound. The outcome would help define one element of the character of the nation: the extent to which the nation would accept or reject modern science and, to a lesser degree, how secular it would become, how godly it would remain.

Precisely at 11:00 A.M., a procession of people advanced upon the stage. First came Daniel Coit Gilman, president of the Hopkins, and on his arm was Huxley. Following in single file came the governor, the mayor, and other notables. As they took their seats the conversations in the audience quickly died away, replaced by expectancy of a kind of declaration of war.

Of medium height and middle age—though he already had iron-gray hair and nearly white whiskers—and possessed of what was described as "a pleasant face," Huxley did not look the warrior. But he had a warrior's ruthlessness. His dicta included the pronouncement: "The foundation of morality is to have done, once and for all, with lying." A brilliant scientist, later president of the Royal Society, he advised investigators, "Sit down before a fact as a little child, be prepared to give up every preconceived notion. Follow humbly wherever and to whatever abysses nature leads, or you shall learn nothing." He also believed that learning had purpose, stating, "The great end of life is not knowledge but action."

To act upon the world himself, he became a proselytizer for faith in human reason. By 1876 he had become the world's foremost advocate of the theory of evolution and of science itself. Indeed, H. L. Mencken said that "it was he, more than any other man, who worked that great change in human thought which marked the Nineteenth Century." Now President Gilman gave a brief and simple introduction. Then Professor Huxley began to speak.

Normally he lectured on evolution, but today he was speaking on a subject of even greater magnitude. He was speaking about the process of intellectual inquiry. The Hopkins was to be unlike any other university in America. Aiming almost exclusively at the education of graduate students and the furtherance of science, it was intended by its trustees to rival not Harvard or Yale—neither of them considered worthy of emulation—but the greatest institutions of Europe, and particularly Germany. Perhaps only in the United States, a nation ever in the act of creating itself, could such an institution come into existence both so fully formed in concept and already so renowned, even before the foundation of a single building had been laid.

"His voice was low, clear and distinct," reported one listener. "The audience paid the closest attention to every word which fell from the lecturer's lips, occasionally manifesting their approval by applause." Said another, "Professor Huxley's method is slow, precise, and clear, and he guards the positions which he takes with astuteness and ability. He does not utter anything in the reckless fashion which conviction sometimes countenances and excuses, but rather with the deliberation that research and close inquiry foster."

Huxley commended the bold goals of the Hopkins, expounded upon his own theories of education—theories that soon informed those of

William James and John Dewey—and extolled the fact that the existence
of the Hopkins meant "finally, that neither political nor ecclesiastical sec-
tarianism" would interfere with the pursuit of the truth.

In truth, Huxley's speech, read a century and a quarter later, seems
remarkably tame. Yet Huxley and the entire ceremony left an impression
in the country deep enough that Gilman would spend years trying to
edge away from it, even while simultaneously trying to fulfill the goals
Huxley applauded.

For the ceremony's most significant word was one not spoken: not a
single participant uttered the word "God" or made any reference to the
Almighty. This spectacular omission scandalized those who worried
about or rejected a mechanistic and necessarily godless view of the universe. And it came in an era in which American universities had nearly
two hundred endowed chairs of theology and fewer than five in medicine, an era in which the president of Drew University had said that, after
much study and experience, he had concluded that only ministers of the
Gospel should be college professors.

The omission also served as a declaration: the Hopkins would pursue
the truth, no matter to what abyss it led.

In no area did the truth threaten so much as in the study of life. In no
area did the United States lag behind the rest of the world so much as in
its study of the life sciences and medicine. And in that area in particular
the influence of the Hopkins would be immense.

By 1918, as America marched into war, the nation had come not only
to rely upon the changes wrought largely, though certainly not entirely,
by men associated with the Hopkins; the United States Army had mobilized these men into a special force, focused and disciplined, ready to hurl
themselves at an enemy.

The two most important questions in science are "What can I know?"
and "How can I know it?"

Science and religion in fact part ways over the first question, what
each can know. Religion, and to some extent philosophy, believes it can
know, or at least address, the question, "Why?"

For most religions the answer to this question ultimately comes down
to the way God ordered it. Religion is inherently conservative; even one
proposing a new God only creates a new order.

The question "why" is too deep for science. Science instead believes it can only learn "how" something occurs.

The revolution of modern science and especially medical science began as science not only focused on this answer to "What can I know?" but more importantly, changed its method of inquiry, changed its answer to "How can I know it?"

This answer involves not simply academic pursuits; it affects how a society governs itself, its structure, how its citizens live. If a society does set Goethe's "Word . . . supremely high," if it believes that it *knows* the truth and that it need not question its beliefs, then that society is more likely to enforce rigid decrees, and less likely to change. If it leaves room for doubt about the truth, it is more likely to be free and open.

In the narrower context of science, the answer determines how individuals explore nature—how one does science. And the way one goes about answering a question, one's methodology, matters as much as the question itself. For the method of inquiry underlies knowledge and often determines what one discovers: how one pursues a question often dictates, or at least limits, the answer.

Indeed, methodology matters more than anything else. Methodology subsumes, for example, Thomas Kuhn's well-known theory of how science advances. Kuhn gave the word "paradigm" wide usage by arguing that at any given point in time, a particular paradigm, a kind of perceived truth, dominates the thinking in any science. Others have applied his concept to nonscientific fields as well.

According to Kuhn, the prevailing paradigm tends to freeze progress, indirectly by creating a mental obstacle to creative ideas and directly by, for example, blocking research funds from going to truly new ideas, especially if they conflict with the paradigm. He argues that nonetheless researchers eventually find what he calls "anomalies" that do not fit the paradigm. Each one erodes the foundation of the paradigm, and when enough accrue to undermine it, the paradigm collapses. Scientists then cast about for a new paradigm that explains both the old and new facts.

But the process—and progress—of science is more fluid than Kuhn's concept suggests. It moves more like an amoeba, with soft and ill-defined edges. More importantly, method matters. Kuhn's own theory recognizes that the propelling force behind the movement from one explanation to another comes from the methodology, from what we call the scientific method. But he takes as an axiom that those who ask questions constantly test existing hypotheses. In fact, with a methodology that probes and tests hypotheses—regardless of any paradigm—progress is inevitable. Without such a methodology, progress becomes merely coincendental.

Yet the scientific method has not always been used by those who inquire into nature. Through most of known history, investigators trying to penetrate the natural world, penetrate what we call science, relied upon the mind alone, reason alone. These investigators believed that they could know a thing if their knowledge followed logically from what they considered a sound premise. In turn they based their premises chiefly on observation.

This commitment to logic coupled with man's ambition to see the entire world in a comprehensive and cohesive way actually imposed blinders on science in general and on medicine in particular. The chief enemy of progress, ironically, became pure reason. And for the bulk of two and a half millennia—twenty-five hundred years—the actual treatment of patients by physicians made almost no progress at all.

One cannot blame religion or superstition for this lack of progress. In the West, beginning at least five hundred years before the birth of Christ, medicine was largely secular. While Hippocratic healers—the various Hippocratic texts were written by different people—did run temples and accept pluralistic explanations for disease, they pushed for material explanations.

Hippocrates himself was born in approximately 460 B.C. *On the Sacred Disease,* one of the more famous Hippocratic texts and one often attributed to him directly, even mocked theories that attributed epilepsy to the intervention of gods. He and his followers advocated precise observation, then theorizing. As the texts stated, "For a theory is a composite memory of things apprehended with sense perception." "But conclusions which are merely verbal cannot bear fruit." "I approve of theorizing also if it lays its foundation in incident, and deduces its conclusion in accordance with phenomena."

But if such an approach sounds like that of a modern investigator, a modern scientist, it lacked two singularly important elements.

First, Hippocrates and his associates merely observed nature. They did not probe it.

This failure to probe nature was to some extent understandable. To dissect a human body then was inconceivable. But the authors of the Hippocratic texts did not test their conclusions and theories. A theory must make a prediction to be useful or scientific—ultimately it must say, *If this, then that*—and testing that prediction is the single most important element of modern methodology. Once that prediction is tested, it must advance another one for testing. It can never stand still.

Those who wrote the Hippocratic texts, however, observed passively and reasoned actively. Their careful observations noted mucus discharges, menstrual bleeding, watery evacuations in dysentery, and they very likely observed blood left to stand, which over time separates into several layers, one nearly clear, one of somewhat yellowy serum, one of darker blood. Based on these observations, they hypothesized that there were four kinds of bodily fluids, or "humours": blood, phlegm, bile, and black bile. (This terminology survives today in the phrase "humoral immunity," which refers to elements of the immune system, such as antibodies, that circulate in the blood.)

This hypothesis made sense, comported with observations, and could explain many symptoms. It explained, for example, that coughs were caused by the flow of phlegm to the chest. Observations of people coughing up phlegm certainly supported this conclusion.

In a far broader sense, the hypothesis also conformed to the ways in which the Greeks saw nature: they observed four seasons, four aspects of the environment—cold, hot, wet, and dry—and four elements—earth, air, fire, and water.

Medicine waited six hundred years for the next major advance, for Galen, but Galen did not break from these teachings; he systematized them, perfected them. Galen claimed, "I have done as much for medicine as Trajan did for the Roman Empire when he built the bridges and roads through Italy. It is I, and I alone, who have revealed the true path of medicine. It must be admitted that Hippocrates already staked out this path. . . . He prepared the way, but I have made it possible."

Galen did not simply observe passively. He dissected animals and, although he did not perform autopsies on humans, served as a physician to gladiators whose wounds allowed him to see deep beneath the skin. Thus his anatomic knowledge went far beyond that of any known predecessor. But he remained chiefly a theoretician, a logician; he imposed order on the Hippocratic body of work, reconciling conflicts, reasoning so clearly that, if one accepted his premises, his conclusions seemed inevitable. He made the humoral theory perfectly logical, and even elegant. As historian Vivian Nutton notes, he raised the theory to a truly conceptual level, separating the humours from direct correlation with bodily fluids and making them invisible entities "recognizable only by logic."

Galen's works were translated into Arabic and underlay both Western and Islamic medicine for nearly fifteen hundred years before facing any significant challenge. Like the Hippocratic writers, Galen believed that illness was essentially the result of an imbalance in the body. He also thought that balance could be restored by intervention; a physician thus could treat a disease successfully. If there was a poison in the body, then the poison could be removed by evacuation. Sweating, urinating, defecating, and vomiting were all ways that could restore balance. Such beliefs led physicians to recommend violent laxatives and other purgatives, as well as mustard plasters and other prescriptions that punished the body, that blistered it and theoretically restored balance. And of all the practices of medicine over the centuries, one of the the the most enduring—yet least understandable to us today—was a perfectly logical extension of Hippocratic and Galenic thought, and recommended by both.

This practice was bleeding patients. Bleeding was among the most common therapies employed to treat all manner of disorders.

Deep into the nineteenth century, Hippocrates and most of those who followed him also believed that natural processes must not be interfered with. The various kinds of purging were meant to augment and accelerate natural processes, not resist them. Since pus, for example, was routinely seen in all kinds of wounds, pus was seen as a necessary part of healing. Until the late 1800s, physicians routinely would do nothing to avoid the generation of pus, and were reluctant even to drain it. Instead they referred to "laudable pus."

Similarly, Hippocrates scorned surgery as intrusive, as interfering with nature's course; further, he saw it as a purely mechanical skill, beneath the calling of physicians who dealt in a far more intellectual realm. This intellectual arrogance would subsume the attitude of Western physicians for more than two thousand years.

This is not to say that for two thousand years the Hippocratic texts and Galen offered the only theoretical constructs to explain health and disease. Many ideas and theories were advanced about how the body worked, how illness developed. And a rival school of thought gradually developed within the Hippocratic-Galenic tradition that valued experience and empiricism and challenged the purely theoretical.

It is impossible to summarize all these theories in a few sentences, yet nearly all of them did share certain concepts: that health was a state of equilibrium and balance, and that illness resulted either from an internal imbalance within the body, or from external environmental influences such as an atmospheric miasma, or some combination of both.

But in the early 1500s three men began to challenge at least the methods of medicine. Paracelsus declared he would investigate nature "not by following that which those of old taught, but by our own observation of nature, confirmed by . . . experiment and by reasoning thereon."

Vesalius dissected human corpses and concluded that Galen's findings had come from animals and were deeply flawed. His *De humani corporis fabrica*, likely illustrated by a student of Titian, became a cornerstone of the Renaissance.

Fracastorius, an astronomer, mathematician, botanist, and poet, meanwhile hypothesized that diseases had specific causes and that contagion "passes from one thing to another and is originally caused by infection of the imperceptible particle." One medical historian called his body of work "a peak maybe unequalled by anyone between Hippocrates and Pasteur."

The contemporaries of these three men included Martin Luther and Copernicus, men who changed the world. In medicine the new ideas of Paracelsus, Vesalius, and Fracastorius did not change the world. In the actual practice of medicine they changed nothing at all.

But the approach they called for did create ripples while the scholasticism of the Middle Ages that stultified nearly all fields of inquiry was beginning to decay. In 1605 Francis Bacon in *Novum Organum* attacked the purely deductive reasoning of logic, calling "Aristotle . . . a mere bondservant to his logic, thereby rendering it contentious and well nigh useless." He also complained, "The logic now in use serves rather to fix and give stability to the errors which have their foundation in commonly received notions than to help the search after truth. So it does more harm than good."

In 1628 Harvey traced the circulation of the blood, arguably perhaps the single greatest achievement of medicine—and certainly the greatest achievement until the late 1800s. And Europe was in intellectual ferment. Half a century later Newton revolutionized physics and mathematics. Newton's contemporary John Locke, trained as a physician, emphasized the pursuit of knowledge through experience. In 1753 James Lind conducted a pioneering controlled experiment among British sailors and demonstrated that scurvy could be prevented by eating limes—ever since, the British have been called "limeys." David Hume, after this demonstration and following Locke, led a movement of "empiricism." His contemporary John Hunter made a brilliant scientific study of surgery, elevating it from a barber's craft. Hunter also performed model scientific experiments, including some on himself—as when he infected himself with pus from a gonorrheal case to prove a hypothesis.

Then in 1798 Edward Jenner, a student of Hunter's—Hunter had told him "Don't think. Try."—published his work. As a young medical student Jenner had heard a milkmaid say, "I cannot take the smallpox because I have had cowpox." The cowpox virus resembles smallpox so closely that exposure to cowpox gives immunity to smallpox. But cowpox itself only rarely develops into a serious disease. (The virus that causes cowpox is called "vaccinia," taking its name from vaccination.)

Jenner's work with cowpox was a landmark, but not because he was the first to immunize people against smallpox. In China, India, and Persia, different techniques had long since been developed to expose children to smallpox and make them immune, and in Europe at least as early as the 1500s laypeople—not physicians—took material from a pustule of those with a mild case of smallpox and scratched it into the skin of those who had not yet caught the disease. Most people infected this way developed mild cases and became immune. In 1721 in Massachusetts, Cotton Mather took the advice of an African slave, tried this technique, and staved off a lethal epidemic. But "variolation" could kill. Vaccinating with cowpox was far safer than variolation.

From a scientific standpoint, however, Jenner's most important contribution was his rigorous methodology. Of his finding he said, "I placed it upon a rock where I knew it would be immoveable before I invited the public to take a look at it."

But ideas die hard. Even as Jenner was conducting his experiments, despite the vast increase in knowledge of the body derived from Harvey and Hunter, medical practice had barely changed. And many, if not most, physicians who thought deeply about medicine still saw it in terms of logic and observation alone.

In Philadelphia, twenty-two hundred years after Hippocrates and sixteen hundred years after Galen, Benjamin Rush, a pioneer in his views on mental illness, a signer of the Declaration of Independence, and America's most prominent physician, still applied logic and observation alone to build "a more simple and consistent system of medicine than the world had yet seen."

In 1796 he advanced a hypothesis as logical and elegant, he believed, as Newtonian physics. Observing that all fevers were associated with flushed skin, he concluded that this was caused by distended capillaries and reasoned that the proximate cause of fever must be abnormal "convulsive action" in these vessels. He took this a step further and concluded that *all* fevers resulted from disturbance of capillaries, and, since the capillaries were part of the circulatory system, he concluded that a hypertension of the entire circulatory system was involved. Rush proposed to reduce this convulsive action by "depletion," i.e., venesection—bleeding. It made perfect sense.

He was one of the most aggressive of the advocates of "heroic medicine." The heroism, of course, was found in the patient. In the early 1800s praise for his theories was heard throughout Europe, and one London physician said Rush united "in an almost unprecedented degree, sagacity and judgment."

A reminder of the medical establishment's acceptance of bleeding exists today in the name of the British journal *The Lancet,* one of the leading medical journals in the world. A lancet was the instrument physicians used to cut into a patient's vein.

But if the first failing of medicine, a failing that endured virtually unchallenged for two millennia and then only gradually eroded over the next three centuries, was that it did not probe nature through experiments, that it simply observed and reasoned from observation to a conclusion, that failing was—finally—about to be corrected.

What can I know? How can I know it?
If reason alone could solve mathematical problems, if Newton could think his way through physics, then why could not man reason out the

ways in which the body worked? Why did reason alone fail so utterly in medicine?

One explanation is that Hippocratic and Galenic theory did offer a system of therapeutics that seemed to produce the desired effect. They seemed to work. So the Hippocratic-Galenic model lasted so long not only because of its logical consistency, but because its therapies seemed to have effect.

Indeed, bleeding—today called "phlebotomy"—can actually help in some rare diseases, such as polycythemia, a rare genetic disorder that causes people to make too much blood, or hemachromatosis, when the blood carries too much iron. And in far more common cases of acute pulmonary edema, when the lungs fill with fluid, it could relieve immediate symptoms and is still sometimes tried. For example, in congestive heart failure excess fluid in the lungs can make victims extremely uncomfortable and, ultimately, kill them if the heart cannot pump the fluid out. When people suffering from these conditions were bled, they may well have been helped. This reinforced theory.

Even when physicians observed that bleeding weakened the patient, that weakening could still seem positive. If a patient was flushed with a fever, it followed logically that if bleeding alleviated those symptoms— making the patient pale—it was a good thing. If it made the patient pale it worked.

Finally, a euphoric feeling sometimes accompanies blood loss. This too reinforced theory. So bleeding both made logical sense in the Hippocratic and Galenic systems and sometimes gave physicians and patients positive reinforcement.

Other therapies also did what they were designed to do—in a sense. As late as the nineteenth century—until well after the Civil War in the United States—most physicians and patients still saw the body only as an interdependent whole, still saw a specific symptom as a result of an imbalance or disequilibrium in the entire body, still saw illness chiefly as something within and generated by the body itself. As the historian Charles Rosenberg has pointed out, even smallpox, despite its known clinical course and the fact that vaccination prevented it, was still seen as a manifestation of a systemic ill. And medical traditions outside the Hippocratic-Galenic model—from the "subluxations" of chiropractic to the "yin and yang" of

Chinese medicine—have also tended to see disease as a result of imbalance within the body.

Physicians and patients wanted therapies to augment and accelerate, not block, the natural course of disease, the natural healing process. The state of the body could be altered by prescribing such toxic substances as mercury, arsenic, antimony, and iodine. Therapies designed to blister the body did so. Therapies designed to produce sweating or vomiting did so. One doctor, for example, when confronted with a case of pleurisy, gave camphor and recorded that the case was "suddenly relieved by profuse perspiration." His intervention, he believed, had cured.

Yet a patient's improvement, of course, does not prove that a therapy works. For example, the 1889 edition of the *Merck Manual of Medical Information* recommended one hundred treatments for bronchitis, each one with its fervent believers, yet the current editor of the manual recognizes that "none of them worked." The manual also recommended, among other things, champagne, strychnine, and nitrogylcerin for seasickness.

And when a therapy clearly did not work, the intricacies—and intimacies—of the doctor-patient relationship also came into play, injecting emotion into the equation. One truth has not changed from the time of Hippocrates until today: when faced with desperate patients, doctors often do not have the heart—or, more accurately, they have too much heart—to do nothing. And so a doctor, as desperate as the patient, may try anything, including things he or she knows will not work as long as they will not harm. At the least, the patient will get some solace.

One cancer specialist concedes, "I do virtually the same thing myself. If I'm treating a teary, desperate patient, I will try low-dose alpha interferon, even though I do not believe it has ever cured a single person. It doesn't have side effects, and it gives the patient hope."

Cancer provides other examples as well. No truly scientific evidence shows that echinacea has any effect on cancer, yet it is widely prescribed in Germany today for terminal cancer patients. Japanese physicians routinely prescribe placebos in treatment. Steven Rosenberg, a National Cancer Institute scientist who was the first person to stimulate the immune system to cure cancer and who led the team that performed the first human gene therapy experiments, points out that for years chemotherapy was recommended to virtually all victims of pancreatic cancer even though not a single chemotherapy regimen had ever been shown to prolong their lives for one day. (At this writing, investigators have just demonstrated that gemcitabine can extend median life expectancy by one to two months, but it is highly toxic.)

Another explanation for the failure of logic and observation alone to advance medicine is that unlike, say, physics, which uses a form of logic—mathematics—as its natural language, biology does not lend itself to logic. Leo Szilard, a prominent physicist, made this point when he complained that after switching from physics to biology he never had a peaceful bath again. As a physicist he would soak in the warmth of a bathtub and contemplate a problem, turn it in his mind, reason his way through it. But once he became a biologist, he constantly had to climb out of the bathtub to look up a fact.

In fact, biology is chaos. Biological systems are the product not of logic but of evolution, an inelegant process. Life does not choose the logically best design to meet a new situation. It adapts what already exists. Much of the human genome includes genes which are "conserved"; i.e., which are essentially the same as those in much simpler species. Evolution has built upon what already exists.

The result, unlike the clean straight lines of logic, is often irregular, messy. An analogy might be building an energy efficient farmhouse. If one starts from scratch, logic would impel the use of certain building materials, the design of windows and doors with kilowatt hours in mind, perhaps the inclusion of solar panels on the roof, and so on. But if one wants to make an eighteenth-century farmhouse energy efficient, one adapts it as well as possible. One proceeds logically, doing things that make good sense given what one starts with, given the existing farmhouse. One seals and caulks and insulates and puts in a new furnace or heat pump. The old farmhouse will be—maybe—the best one could do given where one started, but it will be irregular; in window size, in ceiling height, in building materials, it will bear little resemblance to a new farmhouse designed from scratch for maximum energy efficiency.

For logic to be of use in biology, one has to apply it from a given starting point, using the then-extant rules of the game. Hence Szilard had to climb out of the bathtub to look up a fact.

Ultimately, then, logic and observation failed to penetrate the workings of the body not because of the power of the Hippocratic hypothesis, the Hippocratic paradigm. Logic and observation failed because neither one tested the hypothesis rigorously.

Once investigators began to apply something akin to the modern scientific method, the old hypothesis collapsed.

By 1800 enormous advances had been made in other sciences, beginning centuries earlier with a revolution in the use of quantitative measurement. Bacon and Descartes, although opposites in their views of the usefulness of pure logic, had both provided a philosophical framework for new ways of seeing the natural world. Newton had in a way bridged their differences, advancing mathematics through logic while relying upon experiment and observation for confirmation. Joseph Priestley, Henry Cavendish, and Antoine-Laurent Lavoisier created modern chemistry and penetrated the natural world. Particularly important for biology was Lavoisier's decoding of the chemistry of combustion and use of those insights to uncover the chemical processes of respiration, of breathing.

Still, all these advances notwithstanding, in 1800 Hippocrates and Galen would have recognized and largely agreed with most medical practice. In 1800 medicine remained what one historian called "the withered arm of science."

In the nineteenth century that finally began to change—and with extraordinary rapidity. Perhaps the greatest break came with the French Revolution, when the new French government established what came to be called "the Paris clinical school." One leader of the movement was Xavier Bichat, who dissected organs, found them composed of discrete types of material often found in layers, and called them "tissues"; another was René Laennec, inventor of the stethoscope.

Meanwhile, medicine began to make use of other objective measurements and mathematics. This too was new. Hippocratic writings had stated that the physician's senses mattered far more than any objective measurement, so despite medicine's use of logic, physicians had always avoided applying mathematics to the study of the body or disease. In the 1820s, two hundred years *after* the discovery of thermometers, French clinicians began using them. Clinicians also began taking advantage of methods discovered in the 1700s to measure other bodily functions precisely.

By then in Paris Pierre Louis had taken an even more significant step.

In the hospitals, where hundreds of charity cases awaited help, using the most basic mathematical analysis—nothing more than arithmetic—he correlated the different treatments patients received for the same disease with the results. For the first time in history, a physician was creating a reliable and systematic database. Physicians could have done this earlier. To do so required neither microscopes nor technological prowess; it required only taking careful notes.

Yet the real point at which modern medicine diverged from the classic was in the studies of pathological anatomy by Louis and others. Louis not only correlated treatments with results to reach a conclusion about a treatment's efficacy (he rejected bleeding patients as a useless therapy), he and others also used autopsies to correlate the condition of organs with symptoms. He and others dissected organs, compared diseased organs to healthy ones, learned their functions in intimate detail.

What he found was astounding, and compelling, and helped lead to a new conception of disease as something with an identity of its own, an objective existence. In the 1600s Thomas Sydenham had begun classifying diseases, but Sydenham and most of his followers continued to see disease as a result of imbalances, consistent with Hippocrates and Galen. Now a new "nosology," a new classification and listing of disease, began to evolve.

Disease began to be seen as something that invaded solid parts of the body, as an independent entity, instead of being a derangement of the blood. This was a fundamental first step in what would become a revolution.

Louis's influence and that of what became known as "the numerical system" could not be overstated. These advances—the stethoscope, laryngoscope, opthalmoscope, the measurements of temperature and blood pressure, the study of parts of the body—all created distance between the doctor and the patient, as well as between patient and disease; they objectified humanity. Even though no less a personage than Michel Foucault condemned this Parisian movement as the first to turn the human body into an object, these steps had to come to make progress in medicine.

But the movement was condemned by contemporaries also. Complained one typical critic, "The practice of medicine according to this view is entirely empirical, is shorn of all rational induction, and takes a position among the lower grades of experimental observations and fragmentary facts."

Criticism notwithstanding, the numerical system began winning convert after convert. In England in the 1840s and 1850s, John Snow began applying mathematics in a new way: as an epidemiologist. He had made meticulous observations of the patterns of a cholera outbreak, noting who got sick and who did not, where the sick lived and how they lived, where the healthy lived and how they lived. He tracked the disease down to a contaminated well in London. He concluded that contaminated water caused the disease. It was brilliant detective work, brilliant epidemiology. William Budd borrowed Snow's methodology and promptly applied it to the study of typhoid.

Snow and Budd needed no scientific knowledge, no laboratory findings, to reach their conclusions. And they did so in the 1850s, before the development of the germ theory of disease. Like Louis's study that proved that bleeding was worse than useless in nearly all circumstances, their work could have been conducted a century earlier or ten centuries earlier. But their work reflected a new way of looking at the world, a new way of seeking explanations, a new methodology, a new use of mathematics as an analytical tool.*

*The effort to correlate treatments and results has not yet triumphed. A "new" movement called "evidence-based medicine" has emerged recently, which continues to try to determine the best treatments and communicate them to physicians. No good physician today would discard the value of statistics, of evidence accumulated systematically in careful studies. But individual doctors, convinced either by anecdotal evidence from their own personal experience or by tradition, still criticize the use of statistics and probabilities to determine treatments and accept conclusions only reluctantly. Despite convincing studies, for example, it took years before cancer surgeons stopped doing radical mastectomies for all breast cancers.

A related issue involves the methodology in "clinical studies"—i.e., studies using people. To stay with cancer as an example, Vince DeVita, former director of the National Cancer Institute; Samuel Hellman, a leading oncologist; and Steven Rosenberg, chief of the Surgery Branch of the National Cancer Institute coauthor a standard reference for physicians on cancer treatments. DeVita and Rosenberg believe that carefully controlled randomized studies—experiments in which random chance determines the treatment given a patient—are necessary to find out what treatment works best. Yet Hellman has argued in the *New England Journal of Medicine* that randomized trials are unethical. He believes that physicians must always use their best judgment to determine treatment and cannot rely on chance, even when the effectiveness of a treatment is unknown, even to answer a question about what treatment works best, even when the patient has given fully informed consent.

.   .   .

At the same time, medicine was advancing by borrowing from other sciences. Insights from physics allowed investigators to trace electrical impulses through nerve fibers. Chemists were breaking down the cell into its components. And when investigators began using a magnificent new tool—the microscope equipped with new achromatic lenses, which came into use in the 1830s—an even wider universe began to open.

In this universe Germans took the lead, partly because fewer French than Germans chose to use microscopes and partly because French physicians in the middle of the nineteenth century were generally less aggressive in experimenting, in creating controlled conditions to probe and even manipulate nature. (It was no coincidence that the French giants Pasteur and Claude Bernard, who did conduct experiments, were not on the faculty of any medical school. Echoing Hunter's advice to Jenner, Bernard, a physiologist, told one American student, "Why think? Exhaustively experiment, then think.")

In Germany, meanwhile, Rudolf Virchow—both he and Bernard received their medical degrees in 1843—was creating the field of cellular pathology, the idea that disease began at the cellular level. And in Germany great laboratories were being established around brilliant scientists who, more than elsewhere, did actively probe nature with experiments. Jacob Henle, the first scientist to formulate the modern germ theory, echoed Francis Bacon when he said, "Nature answers only when she is questioned."

And in France, Pasteur was writing, "I am on the edge of mysteries and the veil is getting thinner and thinner."

Never had there been a time so exciting in medicine. A universe was opening.

Still, with the exception of the findings on cholera and typhoid—and even these won only slow acceptance—little of this new scientific knowledge could be translated into curing or preventing disease. And much that was being discovered was not understood. In 1868, for example, a Swiss investigator isolated deoxyribonucleic acid, DNA, from a cell's nucleus, but he had no idea of its function. Not until three-quarters of a century later, at the conclusion of some research directly related to the 1918 influenza pandemic, did anyone even speculate, much less demonstrate, that DNA carried genetic information.

So the advances of science actually, and ironically, led to "therapeutic nihilism." Physicians became disenchanted with traditional treatments, but they had nothing with which to replace them. In response to the findings of Louis and others, in 1835 Harvard's Jacob Bigelow had argued in a major address that in "the unbiased opinion of most medical men of sound judgment and long experience . . . the amount of death and disaster in the world would be less, if all disease were left to itself."

His address had impact. It also expressed the chaos into which medicine was being thrown and the frustration of its practitioners. Physicians were abandoning the approaches of just a few years earlier and, less certain of the usefulness of a therapy, were becoming far less interventionist. In Philadelphia in the early 1800s Rush had called for wholesale bloodletting and was widely applauded. In 1862 in Philadelphia a study found that, out of 9,502 cases, physicians had cut a vein "in one instance only."

Laymen as well were losing faith in and becoming reluctant to submit to the tortures of heroic medicine. And since the new knowledge developing in traditional medicine had not yet developed new therapies, rival ideas of disease and treatment began to emerge. Some of these theories were pseudoscience, and some owed as little to science as did a religious sect.

This chaos was by no means limited to America. Typical was Samuel Hahnemann, who developed homeopathy in Germany, publishing his ideas in 1810, just before German science began to emerge as the dominant force on the Continent. But nowhere did individuals feel freer to question authority than in America. And nowhere was the chaos greater.

Samuel Thomson, founder of a movement bearing his name that spread widely before the Civil War, argued that medicine was simple enough to be comprehended by everyone, so anyone could act as a physician. "May the time soon come when men and women will become their own priests, physicians, and lawyers—when self-government, equal rights and moral philosophy will take the place of all popular crafts of every description," argued his movement's publication. His system used "botanic" therapeutics, and he charged, "False theory and hypothesis constitute nearly the whole art of physic."

Thomsonism was the most popular layman's medical movement but hardly the only one. Dozens of what can only be called sects arose across the countryside. A Thomsonian rhyme summed up the attitude: "The nest of college-birs are three, / *Law, Physic and Divinity;* / And while these three remain combined, / They keep the world oppressed and blind / . . . Now is the time to be set free, / From priests' and Doctors' slavery."

As these ideas spread, as traditional physicians failed to demonstrate the ability to cure anyone, as democratic emotions and anti-elitism swept the nation with Andrew Jackson, American medicine became as wild and democratic as the frontier. In the 1700s Britain had relaxed licensing standards for physicians. Now several state legislatures did away with the licensing of physicians entirely. Why should there be any licensing requirements? Did physicians know anything? Could they *heal* anyone? Wrote one commentator in 1846, "There is not a greater aristocratic monopoly in existence, than this of regular medicine—neither is there a greater humbug." In England the title "Professor" was reserved for those who held university chairs, and, even after John Hunter brought science to surgery, surgeons often went by "Mister." In America the titles "Professor" and "Doctor" went to anyone who claimed them. As late as 1900, forty-one states licensed pharmacists, thirty-five licensed dentists, and only thirty-four licensed physicians. A typical medical journal article in 1858 asked, "To What Cause Are We to Attribute the Diminished Respectability of the Medical Profession in the Esteem of the American Public?"

By the Civil War, American medicine had begun to inch forward, but only inch. The brightest lights involved surgery. The development of anesthesia, first demonstrated in 1846 at Massachusetts General Hospital, helped dramatically, and, just as Galen's experience with gladiators taught him much anatomy, American surgeons learned enough from the war to put them a step ahead of Europeans.

In the case of infectious and other disease, however, physicians continued to attack the body with mustard plasters that blistered the body, along with arsenic, mercury, and other poisons. Too many physicians continued their adherence to grand philosophical systems, and the Civil War showed how little the French influence had yet penetrated American medicine. European medical schools taught the use of thermometers, stethoscopes, and ophthalmoscopes, but Americans rarely used them and the largest Union army had only half a dozen thermometers. Americans still relieved pain by applying opiate powders on a wound, instead of injecting opium with syringes. And when Union Surgeon General William Hammond banned some of the violent purgatives, he was both court-martialed and condemned by the American Medical Association.

After the Civil War, America continued to churn out prophets of new, simple, complete, and self-contained systems of healing, two of which, chiropractic and Christian Science, survive today. (Evidence does suggest that spinal manipulation can relieve musculoskeletal conditions, but no evidence supports chiropractic claims that disease is caused by misalignment of vertebrae.)

Medicine had discovered drugs—such as quinine, digitalis, and opium—that provided benefits, but, as one historian has shown, they were routinely prescribed indiscriminately, for their overall effect on the body, not for a specific purpose; even quinine was prescribed generally, not to treat malaria. Hence Oliver Wendell Holmes, the physician father of the Supreme Court justice, was not much overstating when he declared, "I firmly believe that if the whole materia medica, as now used, could be sunk to the bottom of the sea, it would be all the better for mankind—and all the worse for the fishes."

There was something else about America. It was such a practical place. If it was a nation bursting with energy, it had no patience for dalliance or daydreaming or the waste of time. In 1832, Louis had told one of his most promising protégés—an American—to spend several years in research before beginning a medical practice. The student's father was also a physician, James Jackson, a founder of Massachusetts General Hospital, who scornfully rejected Louis's suggestion and protested to Louis that "in this country his course would have been so singular, as in a measure to separate him from other men. We are a business doing people. . . . There is a vast deal to be done and he who will not be doing must be set down as a drone."

In America the very fact that science was undermining therapeutics made institutions uninterested in supporting it. Physics, chemistry, and the practical arts of engineering thrived. The number of engineers particularly was exploding—from 7,000 to 226,000 from the late nineteenth century to just after World War I—and they were accomplishing extraordinary things. Engineers transformed steel production from an art into a science, developed the telegraph, laid a cable connecting America to Europe, built railroads crossing the continent and skyscrapers that climbed upward, developed the telephone—with automobiles and airplanes not far behind. The world was being transformed. Whatever was being learned in the laboratory about biology was building basic knowledge, but with the exception of anesthesia, laboratory research had only proven actual medical practice all but useless while providing nothing with which to replace it.

Still, by the 1870s, European medical schools required and gave rigorous scientific training and were generally subsidized by the state. In contrast, most American medical schools were owned by a faculty whose profits and salaries—even when they did not own the school—were paid by student fees, so the schools often had no admission standards other than the ability to pay tuition. No medical school in America allowed medical students to routinely either perform autopsies or see patients, and medical education often consisted of nothing more than two four-month terms of lectures. Few medical schools had any association with a university, and fewer still had ties to a hospital. In 1870 even at Harvard a medical student could fail four of nine courses and still get an M.D.

In the United States, a few isolated individuals did research—outstanding research—but it was unsupported by any institution. S. Weir Mitchell, America's leading experimental physiologist, once wrote that he dreaded anything "removing from me the time or power to search for new truths that lie about me so thick." Yet in the 1870s, after he had already developed an international reputation, after he had begun experiments with snake venom that would lead directly to a basic understanding of the immune system and the development of antitoxins, he was denied positions teaching physiology at both the University of Pennsylvania and Jefferson Medical College; neither had any interest in research, nor a laboratory for either teaching or research purposes. In 1871 Harvard did create the first laboratory of experimental medicine at any American university, but that laboratory was relegated to an attic and paid for by the professor's father. Also in 1871 Harvard's professor of pathologic anatomy confessed he did not know how to use a microscope.

But Charles Eliot, a Brahmin with a birth defect that deformed one side of his face—he never allowed a photograph to show that side—had become Harvard president in 1869. In his first report as president, he declared, "The whole system of medical education in this country needs thorough reformation. The ignorance and general incompetency of the average graduate of the American medical Schools, at the time when he receives the degree which turns him loose upon the community, is something horrible to contemplate."

Soon after this declaration, a newly minted Harvard physician killed three successive patients because he did not know the lethal dose of morphine. Even with the leverage of this scandal, Eliot could push through only modest reforms over a resistant faculty. Professor of Surgery Henry Bigelow, the most powerful faculty member, protested to the Harvard Board of Overseers, "[Eliot] actually proposes to have written examinations for the degree of doctor of medicine. I had to tell him that he knew nothing about the quality of the Harvard medical students. More than half of them can barely write. Of course they can't pass written examinations. . . . No medical school has thought it proper to risk large existing classes and large receipts by introducing more rigorous standards."

Many American physicians were in fact enthralled by the laboratory advances being made in Europe. But they had to go to Europe to learn them. Upon their return they could do little or nothing with their knowledge. Not a single institution in the United States supported any medical research whatsoever.

As one American who had studied in Europe wrote, "I was often asked in Germany how it is that no scientific work in medicine is done in this country, how it is that many good men who do well in Germany and show evident talent there are never heard of and never do any good work when they come back here. The answer is that there is no opportunity for, no appreciation of, no demand for that kind of work here. . . . The condition of medical education here is simply horrible."

In 1873, Johns Hopkins died, leaving behind a trust of $3.5 million to found a university and hospital. It was to that time the greatest gift ever to a university. Princeton's library collection was then an embarrassment of only a few books—and the library was open only one hour a week. Columbia was little better: its library opened for two hours each afternoon, but freshmen could not enter without a special permission slip. Only 10 percent of Harvard's professors had a Ph.D.

The trustees of Hopkins's estate were Quakers who moved deliberately but also decisively. Against the advice of Harvard president Charles Eliot, Yale president James Burril Angell, and Cornell president Andrew D. White, they decided to model the Johns Hopkins University after the greatest German universities, places thick with men consumed with creating new knowledge, not simply teaching what was believed.

The trustees made this decision precisely because there was no such university in America, and precisely because they recognized the need after doing the equivalent of market research. A board member later explained, "There was a strong demand, among the young men of this country, for opportunities to study beyond the ordinary courses of a college or a scientific school. . . . The strongest evidence of this demand was the increased attendance of American students upon lectures of German universities." The trustees decided that quality would sell. They intended to hire only eminent professors and provide opportunities for advanced study.

Their plan was in many ways an entirely American ambition: to create a revolution from nothing. For it made little sense to locate the new institution in Baltimore, a squalid industrial and port city. Unlike Philadelphia, Boston, or New York, it had no tradition of philanthropy, no social elite ready to lead, and certainly no intellectual tradition. Even the architecture of Baltimore seemed exceptionally dreary, long lines of row houses, each with three steps, crowding against the street and yet virtually no street life—the people of Baltimore seemed to live inward, in backyards and courtyards.

In fact, there was no base whatsoever upon which to build . . . except the money, another American trait.

The trustees hired as president Daniel Coit Gilman, who left the presidency of the newly organized University of California after disputes with state legislators. Earlier he had helped create and had led the Sheffield Scientific School at Yale, which was distinct from Yale itself. Indeed, it was created partly because of Yale's reluctance to embrace science as part of its basic curriculum.

At the Hopkins, Gilman immediately recruited an internationally respected—and connected—faculty, which gave it instant credibility. In Europe, people like Huxley saw the Hopkins as combining the explosive energy and openness of America with the grit of science; the potential could shake the world.

To honor the Hopkins upon its beginnings, to honor this vision, to proselytize upon this new faith, Thomas Huxley came to America.

The Johns Hopkins would have rigor. It would have such rigor as no school in America had ever known.

The Hopkins opened in 1876. Its medical school would not open until 1893, but it succeeded so brilliantly and quickly that, by the outbreak of World War I, American medical science had caught up to Europe and was about to surpass it.

Influenza is a viral disease. When it kills, it usually does so in one of two ways: either quickly and directly with a violent viral pneumonia so damaging that it has been compared to burning the lungs; or more slowly and indirectly by stripping the body of defenses, allowing bacteria to invade the lungs and cause a more common and slower-killing bacterial pneumonia.

By World War I, those trained directly or indirectly by the Hopkins already did lead the world in investigating pneumonia, a disease referred to as "the captain of the men of death." They could in some instances prevent it and cure it.

And their story begins with one man.

CHAPTER TWO

NOTHING ABOUT the boyhood or youth of William Henry Welch suggested his future.

So it is apt that the best biography of him begins not with his childhood but with an extraordinary eightieth-birthday celebration in 1930. Friends, colleagues, and admirers gathered for the event not only in Baltimore, where he lived, but in Boston, in New York, in Washington; in Chicago, Cincinnati, and Los Angeles; in Paris, London, Geneva, Tokyo, and Peking. Telegraph and radio linked the celebrations, and their starting times were staggered to allow as much overlap as time zones made possible. The many halls were thick with scientists in many fields, including Nobel laureates, and President Herbert Hoover's tribute to Welch at the Washington event was broadcast live over American radio networks.

The tribute was to a man who had become arguably the single most influential scientist in the world. He had served as president of the National Academy of Sciences, president of the American Association for the Advancement of Science, president of the American Medical Association, and president or dominant figure of literally dozens of other scientific groups. At a time when no government funds went to research, as both chairman of the Executive Committee of the Carnegie Institution of Washington and president—for thirty-two years—of the Board of Scientific Directors of the Rockefeller Institute for Medical Research (now

Rockefeller University), he had also directed the flow of money from the two greatest philanthropic organizations in the country.

And yet Welch had been no great pioneer even in his own field of medical research—no Louis Pasteur, no Robert Koch, no Paul Ehrlich, no Theobald Smith. He had generated no brilliant insights, made no magnificent discoveries, asked no deep and original questions, and left no significant legacy in the laboratory or in scientific papers. He did little work—a reasonable judge might say he did no work—so profound as to merit even membership in, much less the presidency of, the National Academy of Sciences.

Nonetheless, these hundreds of the world's leading scientists had measured him as coldly and objectively as they measured everything and found him worthy. They had gathered to celebrate his life, if not for his science then for what he had done for science.

In his lifetime the world had changed radically, from horse and buggy to radio, airplanes, even the first television. Coca-Cola had been invented and rapidly spread across the country before 1900, by the 1920s Woolworth's had over fifteen hundred stores, and a technocratic makeover of America had accompanied the Progressive Age, culminating in 1930 in a White House conference on children that proclaimed the superiority of experts to parents in child raising, because "it is beyond the capacity of an individual parent to train her child to fit into the intricate, interwoven, and interdependent social and economic system we have developed."

Welch had of course played no role in those changes. But he had played a large and direct role in an equivalent makeover of medicine and especially American medicine.

He had served first as a kind of avatar, his own experience embodying and epitomizing that of many in his generation. Yet he was no simple symbol or representative. Like an Escher drawing, his life both represented that of others and simultaneously defined the lives of those who followed him, and those who followed them, and those who followed them, down to the present.

For if he did no revolutionary science, he lived a revolutionary life. He was personality and theater; he was impresario, creator, builder. Like an actor on a live stage, his life was a performance given once, leaving its impact upon his audience, and only through them echoing in time and place. He led the movement that created the greatest scientific medical enterprise, and possibly the greatest enterprise in any of the sciences, in the world. His legacy was not objectively measurable, but it was nonetheless real. It lay in his ability to stir other men's souls.

Welch was born in 1850 in Norfolk, Connecticut, a small town in the northern part of the state that remains even today a hilly and wooded retreat. His grandfather, great-uncle, father, and four uncles were physicians. His father also served a term in Congress and in 1857 addressed the graduates of Yale Medical School. In that speech he demonstrated a significant grasp of the latest medical developments, including a technique that would not be mentioned at Harvard until 1868 and the striking new "cell theory with its results in physiology and pathology," a reference to the work of Rudolf Virchow, who had then published only in German-language journals. He also declared, "All positive knowledge obtained . . . has resulted from the accurate observation of facts."

Yet if it seemed foreordained that Welch would become a physician, this was not the case. Years later he told the great surgeon Harvey Cushing, a protégé, that in his youth medicine had filled him with repugnance.

Perhaps part of that repugnance came from his circumstances. Welch's mother died when he was six months old. His sister, three years older, was sent away, and his father was distant both emotionally and physically. Throughout Welch's life he would be closer to his sister than to any other living soul; over the years their correspondence revealed what intimacies he was willing to share.

His childhood was marked by what would become a pattern throughout his life: loneliness masked by social activity. At first he sought to fit in. He was not isolated. Neighbors included an uncle and cousins his age with whom he played routinely, but he longed for greater intimacy and begged his cousins to call him "brother." They refused. Elsewhere, too, he sought to fit in, to belong. At the age of fifteen, submitting to evangelical fervor, he formally committed himself to God.

He attended Yale where he found no conflict between his religious commitment and science. While the college had begun teaching such practical arts as engineering, it kept a measured distance from the scientific ferment of these years immediately following the Civil War, purposely setting itself up as a conservative, Congregationalist counterbalance to the Unitarian influence at Harvard. But if Welch's intellectual interests developed only after college, his personality had already formed. Three attributes in particular stood out. Their combination would prove powerful indeed.

His intelligence did shine through, and he graduated third in his class. But the impression left on others came not from his brilliance but from his personality. He had the unusual ability to simultaneously involve himself passionately in something yet retain perspective. One student described him as "the only one who kept cool" during heated discussions, and he would carry this trait through the rest of his life.

There was something about him that made others want him to think well of them. Hazing of freshmen was brutal at the time, so brutal that a classmate was advised to keep a pistol in his room to prevent sophomores from abusing him. Yet Welch was left entirely alone. Skull and Bones, perhaps the single most secret society in the United States, which marks its members powerfully with the embrace of the establishment, inducted him, and he would remain deeply attached to Bones his entire life. Perhaps that satisfied his desire to belong. At any rate, his earlier desperation to fit in was replaced by a self-sufficiency. His roommate on parting left him an extraordinary note: "I ought to try to express my great indebtedness for the kindness which you always manifested toward me, the pure example you set me, . . . I feel now more deeply the truth of what I often said to others if not to you—that I was utterly unworthy of such a chum as yourself. I often pitied you, to think that you had to room with me, your inferior in ability, dignity and every noble and good quality."

It is the kind of note that a biographer might interpret as homoerotic. Perhaps it was. At least one other man would later devote himself to Welch with what could only be called ardor. Yet for the rest of Welch's life he also seemed somehow, in some indefinable way, to generate similar if less intense sentiments in others. He did so without effort. He charmed without effort. He inspired without effort. And he did so without his reciprocating any personal connection, much less attachment. A later age would call this "charisma."

His class rank entitled him to give an oration at commencement. In an undergraduate essay entitled "The Decay of Faith," Welch had decried mechanistic science, which viewed the world as a machine "unguided by a God of justice." Now, in 1870, a decade after Darwin published *Origin of Species,* in his oration Welch attempted to reconcile science and religion.

He found it a difficult task. Science is at all times potentially revolutionary; any new answer to a seemingly mundane question about "how" something occurs may uncover chains of causation that throw all preceding order into disarray and that threaten religious beliefs as well. Welch personally was experiencing the pains that many in the last half of the nineteenth century experienced for the first time as adults as science threatened to supplant the natural order, God's order, with an order defined by mankind, an order that promised no one knew what, an order that, as Milton wrote in *Paradise Lost*, "Frighted the reign of Chaos and old night."

Taking a step backward from what his father had said a dozen years before, Welch rejected the personal God of Emerson and the Unitarians, reiterated the importance of revealed truth in Scripture, argued that revelation need not submit to reason, and spoke of that which "man could never discover by the light of his own mind."

Welch would ultimately devote his life to discovering all the world with his own mind, and to spurring others to do the same. But not yet.

He had studied classics and he had hoped to teach Greek at Yale. Yale did not, however, offer him a position, and he became a tutor at a new private school. That school closed, Yale still offered him nothing, and, with no immediate prospects for employment, with his family importuning him to become a physician, he returned to Norfolk and apprenticed to his father.

It was an old-fashioned practice. Nothing his father did reflected his knowledge of the newest medical concepts. Like most American physicians, he ignored objective measurements such as temperature and blood pressure, and he even mixed prescriptions without measuring dosages, often relying on taste. This apprenticeship was not a happy time for Welch. In his own later accounts of his training, he passed over it as if it had never occurred. But sometime during it his views of medicine changed.

At some point he decided that if he was going to become a physician, he would do so in his own way. Routinely those preparing for medicine apprenticed for six months or a year, and then attended medical school. He had served his apprenticeship. But in the next step he took he marked out a new course. Welch returned to school all right, but he did not attend medical school. He learned chemistry.

Not only did no medical school in the United States require entering students to have either any scientific knowledge or a college degree, neither did any American medical school emphasize science. Far from it. In 1871, a senior professor at the Harvard Medical School argued, "In an age of science, like the present, there is more danger that the average medical student will be drawn from what is practical, useful, and even essential by the well-meant enthusiasm of the votaries of the applicable sciences, than that he will suffer from the want of knowledge of these. . . . [We] should not encourage the medical student to while away his time in the labyrinths of Chemistry and Physiology."

Welch had a different view. Chemistry seemed to him a window into the body. By then Carl Ludwig, later Welch's mentor, and several other leading German scientists had met in Berlin and determined to "constitute physiology on a chemico-physical foundation and give it equal scientific rank with physics."

It was highly unlikely that Welch knew of that determination, but his instincts were the same. In 1872 he entered Yale's Sheffield Scientific School to study chemistry. He considered the facilities there "excellent . . . certainly better than in any medical school, where chemistry as far as I can learn is very much slighted."

After half a year of grounding, he began medical school at the College of Physicians and Surgeons in New York City, which was not yet connected to Columbia University. (He disdained Yale's medical school; fifty years later he was asked to give a speech on Yale's early contributions to medicine and replied that there hadn't been any.) It was a typical good American medical school, with no requirements for admission and no grades in any course. As elsewhere, faculty salaries came directly from student fees, so faculty wanted to maximize the number of students. Instruction came almost entirely through lectures; the school offered no laboratory work of any kind. This, too, was typical. In no American school did students use a microscope. In fact, Welch's work in one course won him the great prize of a microscope; he cherished it but did not know how to use it, and no professor offered to instruct him. Instead he enviously watched them work, commenting, "I can only admire without understanding how to use its apparently complicated mechanism."

But unlike in many other schools, students at the College of Physicians and Surgeons could examine cadavers. Pathological anatomy—

using autopsies to decipher what was happening within organs—
enthralled Welch. New York City had three medical schools. He took the
course in pathological anatomy at all three.

Then he completed his school's single requirement for an M.D. He
passed a final examination. Welch called it "the easiest examination I ever
entered since leaving boarding school."

Shortly before Welch took this test, Yale finally offered him the position
he had so earnestly sought earlier—professor of Greek. He declined it.

To his father he wrote, "I have chosen my profession, am becoming
more and more interested in it, and do not feel at all inclined to relinquish it for anything else."

He was interested indeed.

He was also beginning to be recognized. Francis Delafield, one of his professors, had studied pathological anatomy in Paris with Pierre Louis and,
like Louis, kept detailed records of hundreds of autopsies. Delafield's was
the best work in America, the most precise, the most scientific. Delafield
now brought Welch into his fold and allowed him the extraordinary privilege of entering his own autopsy findings into Delafield's sacred notes.

Yet huge gaps in Welch's knowledge remained. He still did not know
how to use his microscope. Delafield, an expert in microscopic technique
who had made his own microtome (a device for cutting exquisitely thin
slices of tissue), would sit for hours with one eye glued to the lens, smoking a pipe, while Welch watched impotently. But Delafield did let Welch
perform a huge number of autopsies for someone in his junior position.
From each one he tried to learn.

That knowledge did not satisfy him. His best professors had studied
in Paris, Vienna, and Berlin. Although Welch still intended to practice
clinical medicine—not a single physician in the United States then made
a living doing research—he borrowed from family and friends and, having
run through all that his American professors could teach him, on April
19, 1876, a few months before Huxley spoke at the inauguration of the
Johns Hopkins University, Welch sailed for Europe to continue his scientific education. Simon Flexner, Welch's protégé and a brilliant scientist in
his own right, declared this trip "a voyage of exploration that was in its
results perhaps the most important ever taken by an American doctor."

■   ■   ■

He was hardly alone in seeking more knowledge in Germany, where the best science was then being done. One historian has estimated that between 1870 and 1914, fifteen thousand American doctors studied in Germany or Austria, along with thousands more from England, France, Japan, Turkey, Italy, and Russia.

The overwhelming majority of these physicians were interested solely in treating patients. In Vienna professors established a virtual assembly line to teach short courses on specific aspects of clinical medicine to foreign doctors, especially Americans. These Americans took the courses partly out of desire to learn and partly to gain an edge over competitors at home.

Welch himself expected to have to practice medicine to make a living, and he recognized how helpful to such a career studying in Germany could be. He assured his sister and brother-in-law as well as his father, all of whom were helping support him financially, "The prestige and knowledge which I should acquire by a year's study in Germany would decidedly increase my chance of success. The young doctors who are doing well in New York are in a large majority those who have studied abroad."

But his real interest lay with the tiny minority of Americans who went to Germany to explore a new universe. He wanted to learn laboratory science. In America he had already acquired a reputation as knowing far more than his colleagues. In Germany he was refused acceptance into two laboratories because he knew so little. This inspired rather than depressed him. Soon he found a place to start and excitedly wrote home, "I feel as if I were only just initiated into the great science of medicine. My previous experiences compared with the present are like the difference between reading of a fair country and seeing it with one's own eyes. To live in the atmosphere of these scientific workshops and laboratories, to come into contact with the men who have formed and are forming the science of today, to have the opportunity of doing a little original investigation myself are all advantages, which, if they do not prove fruitful in later life, will always be to me a source of pleasure and profit."

Of Leipzig's university, he said, "If you could visit the handsome and thoroughly equipped physiological, anatomical, pathological and chemical laboratories and see professors whose fame is already world-wide, with their corps of assistants and students hard at work, you would realize how by concentration of labor and devotion to study Germany has outstripped other countries in the science of medicine."

He focused on learning how to learn and stayed constantly alert to technique, to anything offering another window into the new world, anything that allowed him to see more clearly and deeply. "The chief value" of his work with one scientist was "in teaching me certain important methods of handling fresh tissues, especially in isolating particular elements." Of another scientist whom he disliked, he said, "What is of greater importance, I have acquired a knowledge of methods of preparing and mounting specimens so that I can carry on investigations hereafter."

By now he was attracting attention from his mentors, who included some of the leading scientists in the world, but they left a more distinct impression upon him. One was Carl Ludwig, whom he called "my ideal of a scientific man, accepting nothing upon authority, but putting every scientific theory to the severest test. . . . I hope I have learned from Professor Ludwig's precept and practice that most important lesson for every man of science, not to be satisfied with loose thinking and half-proofs, not to speculate and theorize but to observe closely and carefully."

Julius Cohnheim, another mentor, taught him a new kind of curiosity: "Cohnheim's interest centers on the explanation of the fact. It is not enough for him to know that congestion of the kidney follows heart disease. . . . He is constantly inquiring why does it occur under these circumstances. . . . He is almost the founder and certainly the chief representative of the so-called experimental or physiological school of pathology."

Welch began to analyze everything, including his most deeply held beliefs. Five years earlier he had condemned the concept of a world ruled other than by a God of justice. Now he told his father that he embraced Darwin: "That there is anything irreligious about the doctrine of evolution I cannot see. . . . In the end our preconceived beliefs must change and adapt themselves. The facts of science never will change."

He also analyzed the means by which German science had achieved such stature. Its three most important elements, he decided, were the thorough preparation required of students by German medical schools, the schools' independent financing, and the support of research by the government and universities.

In 1877, a year after the Johns Hopkins University opened, its president, Daniel Gilman, laid plans to assemble the greatest medical school faculty in America, one to rival any in Europe. The decision to launch a national—indeed international—search was itself revolutionary. With the exception of the University of Michigan, located in tiny Ann Arbor, every medical school in the United States filled its faculty exclusively from the ranks of local physicians. To perform the search Gilman chose the perfect man: Dr. John Shaw Billings.

Billings lay behind America's first great contribution to scientific medicine: a library. This library grew out of the detailed medical history of the Civil War ordered by the army surgeon general. The army also created a medical "museum," which was actually a library of specimens.

Both the museum and the history were remarkable. In 1998 scientists at the Armed Forces Institute of Pathology, a direct descendant of this museum, used specimens preserved in 1918 to determine the genetic makeup of the 1918 influenza virus. And the medical history was extraordinarily precise and useful. Even Virchow said he was "constantly astonished at the wealth of experience therein found. The greatest exactness in detail, careful statistics even in the smallest matters, and a scholarly statement embracing all sides of medical experience are here united."

Billings did not write that history, but it did inspire him to create a medical library of comparable quality. He built what one medical historian judged "probably the greatest and most useful medical library in the world." By 1876 it already held eighty thousand volumes; ultimately it grew into today's National Library of Medicine.

But he did more than collect books and articles. Knowledge is useless unless accessible. To disseminate knowledge, Billings developed a cataloging system far superior to any in Europe, and he began publishing the *Index Medicus,* a monthly bibliography of new medical books and articles appearing in the Americas, Europe, Japan. No comparable bibliography existed anywhere else in the world.

And no one else in the world had a better sense of what was going on in all the world's laboratories than Billings.

He traveled to Europe to meet possible candidates for the Hopkins faculty, including established scientists of international renown. But he also sought out young men, the next generation of leaders. He had heard of Welch, heard of his potential, heard that he had exposed himself not to one or two of the great scientists but to many, heard that he seemed to know everyone in Germany, including—even before they emerged as arguably the two greatest medical scientists of the nineteenth or early twentieth century—Robert Koch and Paul Ehrlich. (In fact, when Koch, then unknown, first made his dramatic demonstration of the life cycle of anthrax, Welch was in the same laboratory.)

Billings met with Welch in an ancient Leipzig beer hall, a hall that itself belonged to myth. On the wall were murals depicting the sixteenth-century meeting of Faust and the Devil, for the meeting had supposedly occurred in that very room. Billings and Welch talked passionately of science deep into the night, while the murals endowed their words with conspiratorial irony. Billings spoke of the plans for the Hopkins: unheard-of admission standards for students, labs that filled great buildings, the most modern hospital in the world, and of course a brilliant faculty. They talked also about life, about each other's goals. Welch knew perfectly well he was being interviewed. In response, he opened his soul.

After the dinner Billings told Francis King, president of the yet-to-be-built Johns Hopkins Hospital, that Welch "should be one of the first men to be secured, when the time came."

That time would not come for a while. The Hopkins had begun as a graduate school only, without even any undergraduate students, although it quickly expanded to include a college. Further expansion abruptly became problematic since its endowment was chiefly in Baltimore & Ohio Railroad stock. The country had been wallowing in depression for four years when the B&O and the Pennsylvania Railroad cut wages 10 percent, sparking violent strikes by railroad workers in Maryland that soon spread to Pittsburgh, Chicago, St. Louis, and farther west. B&O stock collapsed, and the plans to open the medical school had to be put off. There were no new faculty posts at the Hopkins to fill.

So in 1877 Welch returned to New York desperate for "some opportunity" in science "and at the same time making a modest livelihood." Failing to find one, he returned to Europe. In 1878 he was back in New York.

At no time in history had medicine been advancing so rapidly. The thousands who flocked to Europe were proof of American physicians' intense interest in those advances. Yet in the United States neither Welch nor anyone else could support himself by either joining in that great march or teaching what had been learned.

Welch proposed to a former mentor at the College of Physicians and Surgeons that he teach a laboratory course. The school had no laboratory and wanted none. No medical school in the United States used a laboratory for instruction. The school rejected his suggestion but did offer to let Welch lecture—without salary—in pathology.

Welch turned to Bellevue, a medical school with a lesser reputation. It let him offer his course and provided three rooms for it, equipped only with empty kitchen tables. There were no microscopes, no glassware, no incubators, no instruments. Facing the empty rooms, discouraged, he wrote, "I cannot make much of a success out of the affair at present. I seem to be thrown entirely upon my own resources for equipping the laboratory and do not think that I can accomplish much."

He was also worried. His entire compensation would come from student fees, and the three-month course was not required. He confided to his sister, "I sometimes feel rather blue when I look ahead and see that I am not going to be able to realize my aspirations in life. . . . There is no opportunity in this country, and it seems unlikely there ever will be. . . . I can teach microscopy and pathology, perhaps get some practice and make a living after a while, but that is all patchwork and the drudgery of life and what hundreds do."

He was wrong.

In fact he would catalyze the creation of an entire generation of scientists who would transform American medicine, scientists who would confront influenza in 1918, scientists whose findings from that epidemic still echo today.

CHAPTER THREE

WELCH'S COURSE quickly became extraordinarily popular. Soon students from all three of New York City's medical schools were lining up for it, attracted as Welch had been to this new science, to the microscope, to experimentation. And Welch did not simply teach; he inspired. His comments always seemed so solid, well grounded, well reasoned. A colleague observed, "He would leak knowledge." And the excitement! Each time a student fixed a specimen on a slide and looked through a microscope, an entire universe opened to him! To some, discovering that universe, entering into it, beginning to manipulate it, was akin to creating it; they must have felt almost godlike.

The College of Physicians and Surgeons had to offer a laboratory course to compete. It beseeched Welch to teach it. He declined out of loyalty to Bellevue but recommended the hiring of T. Mitchell Prudden, an American he had known—and considered a rival for the Hopkins job—in Europe. It was the first of what would be uncounted job offers that he engineered. Meanwhile one of his students recalled "his serious, eager look, his smiling face, his interest in young men which bound them to him. He was always ready to drop any work in which he was engaged and answer even trivial questions on any subject—in fact he was never without an answer for his knowledge was encyclopedic. I felt instinctively that he was wasted at Bellevue, and was destined to have a larger circle of hearers."

But despite the throngs of motivated students taking the two courses, neither Prudden nor Welch prospered. Two years went by, then three, then four. To cobble together a living, Welch did autopsies at a state hospital, served as an assistant to a prominent physician, and tutored medical students before their final exams. As he passed his thirtieth birthday he was doing no real science. He was making a reputation and it was clear if he chose to concentrate on practice he could become wealthy. Little medical research was being done in America—although the little that was done was significant—but even that little he had no part of. In Europe science was marching from advance to advance, breakthrough to breakthrough. The most important of these was the germ theory of disease.

Proving and elaborating upon the germ theory would ultimately open the way to confronting all infectious disease. It would also create the conceptual framework and technical tools that Welch and others later used to fight influenza.

Simply put, the germ theory said that minute living organisms invaded the body, multiplied, and caused disease, and that a specific germ caused a specific disease.

There was need for a new theory of disease. As the nineteenth century progressed, as autopsy findings were correlated with symptoms reported during life, as organs from animals and cadavers were put under a microscope, as normal organs were compared to diseased ones, as diseases became more defined, localized, and specific, scientists finally discarded the ideas of systemic illness and the humours of Hippocrates and Galen and began looking for better explanations.

Three theories stood as rivals to the germ theory.

The first involved "miasma." Several variations of this concept existed, but they basically argued that many diseases were caused by some kind of putrefaction in the atmosphere, or by some climactic influence, or by noxious fumes from decaying organic materials. (In China the wind was originally regarded as a demon that caused illness.) Miasmas seemed a particularly good explanation of epidemics, and the unhealthiness of swamp regions seemed to support the theory. In 1885, when Welch considered the germ theory as proven, the New York City Board of Health warned that "laying of all telegraph wires under ground in one season . . .

would prove highly detrimental to the health of the city . . . through the exposure to the atmosphere of so much subsoil, saturated, as most of it is, with noxious gases. . . . Harlem Flats [had] a sufficient supply of rotting filth to generate fetid gases adequate to the poisoning of half the population." As late as the 1930s one prominent and highly regarded British epidemiologist continued to advocate the miasma theory, and after the 1918 influenza pandemic, climatic conditions were scrutinized in a search for correlations.

The "filth" theory of disease was almost a corollary of the miasma theory. It also suited Victorian mores perfectly. Fear of "swamp gas"—often a euphemism for the smells of fecal matter—and installation of indoor toilets were all part of the Victorian drive to improve sanitation and simultaneously to separate the human body from anything Victorians found distasteful. And filth often is associated with disease: lice carry typhus; contaminated water spreads typhoid and cholera; rats through their fleas spread plague.

Both the miasma and filth theories had sophisticated adherents, including public health officials and some extremely gifted scientists, but the most scientific rival of the germ theory explained disease in terms purely of chemistry. It saw disease as a chemical process. This theory had much to recommend it.

Not only had scientists used chemistry as a lens that brought much of biology into focus, but some chemical reactions seemed to mimic the actions of disease. For example, advocates of the chemical theory of disease argued that fire was a chemical process and a single match could set off a chain reaction that ignited an entire forest or city. They hypothesized that chemicals they called "zymes" acted like a match. A zyme started a series of chemical reactions in the body that could launch the equivalent of fermentation—infection. (The chemical theory of disease, without the name, has in fact largely been validated. Scientists have clearly demonstrated that chemicals, radiation, and environmental factors can cause disease, although usually only through long-term or massive exposure and not, as the zymote theory hypothesized, by suddenly igniting a cascade of reactions.)

Ultimately this theory evolved to suggest that zymes could reproduce in the body; thus they acted as both catalysts and living organisms. In fact, this more sophisticated version of the zymote theory essentially describes what is today called a virus.

Yet these theories left many scientists unsatisfied. Disease often seemed to germinate, grow, and spread. Did there not then have to be a point of origin, a seed? Jacob Henle in his 1840 essay "On Miasmata and Contagia" first formulated the modern germ theory; he also offered evidence for the theory and laid out criteria that, if met, would prove it.

Then, in 1860, Pasteur proved that living organisms, not a chemical chain reaction, caused fermentation, winning converts to the germ theory. The most important early convert was Joseph Lister, who immediately applied these findings to surgery, instituting antiseptic conditions in the operating room and slashing the percentage of patients who died from infections after surgery.

But the work of Robert Koch was most compelling. Koch himself was compelling. The son of an engineer, brilliant enough to teach himself to read at age five, he studied under Henle, was offered research posts, but became a clinician to support his family. He did not, however, stop investigating nature. Working alone, he conducted a series of experiments that met the most rigid tests and discovered the complete life cycle of the anthrax bacillus, showing that it formed spores that could lie dormant in the soil for years. In 1876 he walked into the laboratory of Ferdinand Cohn, one of Welch's mentors, and presented his findings. They brought him instant fame.

He subsequently laid down what came to be known as "Koch's postulates," although Henle had earlier proposed much the same thing. The postulates state that before a microorganism can be said to cause a given disease, first, investigators had to find the germ in every case of the disease; second, they had to isolate the germ in pure culture; third, they had to inoculate a susceptible animal with the germ and the animal then had to get the disease; and, fourth, the germ had to be isolated from the test animal. Koch's postulates became a standard almost immediately. (Meeting the standard is not simple; finding a test animal that suffered the same symptoms as humans when infected with a human pathogen, for example, is not always possible.)

In 1882 Koch's discovery of the tubercle bacillus, the cause of tuberculosis, shook the scientific world and further confirmed the germ theory.

Tuberculosis was a killer. Laymen called it "consumption," and that name spoke to the awfulness of the disease. It consumed people. Like cancer, it attacked the young as well as the old, sucked the life out of them, turned them into cachectic shells, and then killed them.

It would be difficult to overstate the importance of Koch's discovery to the believers in bacteriology. In New York, one of Welch's friends came running into his bedroom with a newspaper account of the discovery. Welch jumped out of bed and together they rushed to tell another friend. Almost immediately afterward, Welch felt the excitement directly. He demonstrated Koch's discovery to his class, copying Koch's method, his class watching steam rise from the plate while he stained sputum from a consumption patient with carbol-fuchsin, the stain binding to the bacillus so that it became visible on a slide. Here was the newest and greatest of discoveries! Students looked at the slide through the microscope, saw what Koch had seen, and were electrified, many recalling the moment vividly years later. One of those students was Hermann Biggs, who became a giant in his own right; at that moment he decided to spend his life in bacteriology.

But for Welch, reproducing Koch's finding must have been bittersweet. He knew the Germans, knew nearly all of these men adventuring into the unknowns of science. Yet here he was only keeping track of their work, doing none himself.

Then, in 1883, Koch achieved the first great triumph of science over disease. Earlier in the nineteenth century, two cholera epidemics had devastated Europe and the United States. As a new epidemic in Egypt threatened the borders of Europe, France dispatched investigators in this new field of bacteriology to track down the cause of the disease. Germany dispatched Koch.

Before this, medicine's great successes had come about almost serendipitously, beginning with an observation. With smallpox Jenner started out by taking seriously the experiences of country folk inoculating themselves. But not here. In this case the target had been fixed in advance. Both the French and Koch rationally designed an approach, then turned the general tools of the laboratory and bacteriology to a particular target.

The French failed. Louis Thuillier, the youngest member of the expedition, died of cholera. Despite the bitter and nationalistic rivalry between Pasteur and Koch, Koch returned with the body to France and served as pallbearer at Thuillier's funeral, dropping into the grave a laurel wreath "such as are given to the brave."

Koch then returned to Egypt, isolated the cholera bacillus, and followed it to India to explore his findings in greater depth. John Snow's earlier epidemiological study in London had proved only to some that contaminated water caused the disease. Now, in conjunction with Koch's evidence, the germ theory seemed proven in cholera—and by implication the germ theory itself seemed proven.

Most leading physicians around the world, including in the United States, agreed with a prominent American public health expert who declared in 1885: "What was theory has become fact."

But a minority, both in the United States and Europe, still resisted the germ theory, believing that Pasteur, Koch, and others had proven that germs existed but not that germs *caused* disease—or at least that they were the sole cause of disease.*

The most notable critic was Max von Pettenkofer, who had made real and major scientific contributions. He insisted that Koch's bacteria were only one of many factors in the causation of cholera. His dispute with Koch became increasingly bitter and passionate. With a touch of both Barnum and a tightrope walker about him, Pettenkofer, determined to prove himself right, prepared test tubes thick with lethal cholera bacteria. Then he and several of his students drank them down. Amazingly, although two students developed minor cases of cholera, all survived. Pettenkofer claimed victory, and vindication.

It was a costly claim. In 1892 cholera contaminated the water supply of Hamburg and Altona, a smaller adjacent city. Altona filtered the water, and its citizens escaped the disease; Hamburg did not filter the water, and there 8,606 people died of cholera. Pettenkofer became not only a mocked but a reviled figure. He later committed suicide.

There was still no cure for cholera, but now science had demonstrated—

---

*The critics made some valid points. Clearly the attacking organism does not entirely determine whether someone gets sick. The same organism can attack two people, kill one, and not cause any symptoms in the other. An individual's genes, immune system, environment, and even such factors as stress all affect susceptibility.

As late as 1911 the head of the school training French army doctors in public health said that germs alone were "powerless to create an epidemic." But that particular view was by then an idiosyncratic, not simply minority, opinion.

the dead in Hamburg were the final evidence—that protecting the water supply and testing for the bacteria would prevent the disease. After that only an isolated and discredited group of recalcitrants continued to reject the germ theory.

By then Welch had arrived at the Hopkins. It had not been an easy journey to Baltimore.

When the offer finally came in 1884, Welch had become comfortable in New York, and wealth was his for the asking. Virtually every student who had ever passed through his course had the utmost respect for him, and by now many were physicians. He had already made a reputation; that and his charm entered him into society as much as he desired.

His closest friend was his preparatory school roommate Frederick Dennis, wealthy son of a railroad magnate and also a physician who had studied in Germany. At every opportunity Dennis had advanced Welch's career, extolling his talents to editors of scientific journals, using his society connections to help him in New York, occasionally even subsidizing him indirectly. Indeed, Dennis behaved more like a lover trying to win affection than a friend, even a close friend.

But Dennis had always demanded a kind of fealty. Welch had heretofore been willing to give it. Now Dennis demanded that Welch stay in New York. When Welch did not immediately agree, Dennis orchestrated an elaborate campaign to keep him there. He convinced Welch's father to advise him to stay, he convinced Andrew Carnegie to donate $50,000 for a laboratory at Bellevue, and he convinced Bellevue itself to pledge another $45,000; that would match any laboratory in Baltimore. And not only Dennis urged Welch to stay. A prominent attorney whose son had studied under Welch warned him that going to Baltimore would be "the mistake of your life. It is not in a century that a man of your age has acquired the reputation which you have gained." Even the president of the United States Trust Company sent a message that "however bright the prospect is in Baltimore it is darkness compared with the career" before him in New York.

The pressure was not without effect. Dennis did get Welch to set conditions that, if met, would cause him to stay. For Welch had his own doubts. Some related to his own fitness. He had done almost no real science in the years since returning from Germany. He had only talked for years about how his need to make a living prevented him from conducting original research.

The Hopkins expected more than talk. It had been open for eight years and, tiny as it was, had earned an international reputation. Welch confessed to his stepmother, "Such great things are expected of the faculty at the Johns Hopkins in the way of achievement and of reform of medical education in this country that I feel oppressed by the weight of responsibility. A reputation there will not be so cheaply earned as at Bellevue."

Yet precisely for that reason the Hopkins offered, he wrote, "undoubtedly the best opportunity in this country." Declining would reveal him as a hypocrite and a coward. Meanwhile in New York, the conditions he had set were not met, although Dennis considered them to have been.

Welch accepted the Hopkins offer.

Dennis was furious. His friendship with Welch had been, at least on Dennis's side, of great emotional depth and intensity. Now Dennis felt betrayed.

Welch confided to his stepmother, "I grieve that a life-long friendship should thus come to an end, but . . . [i]t looks almost as if Dr. Dennis thought he had a lien upon my whole future life. When he appealed to what he had done for me I told him that was a subject which I would in no way discuss with him."

Later Dennis sent Welch a letter formally breaking off their friendship, a letter written with enough intensity that in the letter itself he asked Welch to burn it after reading.

For Welch too the breaking off of the friendship was intense. He would not have another. Over much of the next half century, Welch's closest collaborator would be his protégé Simon Flexner. Together they would achieve enormous things. And yet Flexner too was kept distant. Flexner himself wrote that after Welch's estrangement from Dennis, "Never again would he allow any person, woman or colleague, close. . . . The bachelor scientist moved on a high plane of loneliness that may have held the secret of some of his power."

For the rest of his life Welch would remain alone. More than just alone, he would never dig in, never entrench himself, never root.

He never married. Despite working with others in ways that so often bind people together as comrades, with the single possible exception of the great and strange surgeon William Halsted—and that exception only a rumored possibility*—he had no known intimate relationship, sexual or otherwise, with either man or woman. Although he would live in Baltimore for half a century, he would never own a home there nor even have his own apartment; despite accumulating considerable wealth, he would live as a boarder, taking two rooms in the home of the same landlady, then moving with his landlady when she moved, and allowing his landlady's daughter to inherit him as a boarder. He would take nearly every dinner in one of his gentlemen's clubs, retreating to a world of men, cigars, and the conversations of an evening for the rest of his life. And he would, observed a young colleague, "deliberately break off relationships which seemed to threaten too strong an attachment."

But if he lived on the surface of ordinary life, his life was not ordinary. He was free, not just alone but free, free of entanglements of people, free of encumbrances of property, utterly free.

He was free to do extraordinary things.

At the Hopkins—it became simply "Hopkins" gradually, over several decades—Welch was expected to create an institution that would alter American medicine forever. When he accepted this charge in 1884, he was thirty-four years old.

The Hopkins went about achieving its goal both directly and indirectly. It served as home, however temporary, to much of the first generation of men and women who were beginning the transformation of American medical science. And its example forced other institutions to follow its path—or disappear.

In the process Welch gradually accumulated enormous personal power, a power built slowly, as a collector builds a collection. His first step was to return to Germany. Already he had worked under Cohn, to whom Koch had brought his anthrax studies, Carl Ludwig, and Cohnheim,

---

*Halsted had known Welch well in New York; both of them were trying to apply science to medicine. But Halsted began studying cocaine and became addicted. His life collapsed and he moved to Baltimore to be close to Welch. Once Halsted ended his addiction, Welch gave him a chance at the Hopkins, where he linked surgery to physiological research and became the most influential surgeon in the country and arguably the world. Halsted did marry, but he was eccentric and erratic and became addicted to morphine. It was unclear if Welch knew of this addiction.

three of the leading scientists in the world, and had met the young Paul Ehrlich, his hands multicolored and dripping with dyes, whose insights combined with his knowledge of chemistry would allow him to make some of the greatest theoretical contributions to medicine of all.

Now Welch visited nearly every prominent investigator in Germany. He had rank now, for he happily reported that the Hopkins "already has a German reputation while our New York medical schools are not even known by name." He could entertain with stories, recite a Shakespeare sonnet, or bring to bear an enormous and growing breadth of scientific knowledge. Even those scientists so competitive as to be nearly paranoid opened their laboratories and their private speculations to him. His combination of breadth and intelligence allowed him to see into the depths of their work as well as its broadest implications.

He also learned bacteriology from two Koch protégés. One gave a "class" whose students were scientists from around the world, many of whom had already made names for themselves. In this group too he shined; his colleagues gave him the honor of offering the first toast of appreciation to their teacher at a farewell banquet. And Welch learned the most from Koch himself, the greatest name in science, who accepted him into his famous course—given only once—for scientists who would teach others bacteriology.

Then, back in Baltimore, years before its hospital or medical school actually opened, even without patients and without students, the Hopkins began to precipitate change. For although the Hopkins medical hospital did not open until 1889, and the medical school until 1893, its laboratory opened almost immediately. That alone was enough.

In just its first year, twenty-six investigators not on the Hopkins faculty used the laboratories. Welch's young assistant William Councilman—who later remade Harvard's medical school in the Hopkins's image—kept them supplied with organs by riding his tricycle to other hospitals, retrieving the organs, and carrying them back in buckets suspended from the handlebars. Many of these guests or graduate students were or became world-class investigators, including Walter Reed, James Carroll, and Jesse Lazear, three of the four doctors who defeated yellow fever. Within a few more years, fifty physicians would be doing graduate work at the same time.

And the Hopkins began assembling a faculty. Its institutional vision combined with Welch himself allowed it to recruit an extraordinary one. Typical was Franklin Mall.

Mall had gotten his medical degree from the University of Michigan in 1883 at age twenty-one, gone to Germany and worked with Carl Ludwig, done some graduate work at the Hopkins, and had already made a mark. He expected—required—the highest conceivable standards, and not just from his students. Victor Vaughan, dean of the Michigan medical school and second only to Welch in his influence on American medical education, considered the school's chemistry lab the best in America and comparable to the best in the world. Mall dismissed it as "a small chemical lab" and called his Michigan education equal to that of a good high school.

When Welch offered Mall a job, Mall was at the University of Chicago where he was planning the expenditure of $4 million, an enormous sum— John D. Rockefeller was the major donor to Chicago—to do what Welch was attempting, to build a great institution. Mall responded to Welch's offer by proposing instead that Welch leave the Hopkins for Chicago at a significant increase in salary.

By contrast, the Hopkins was desperate for resources but Welch rejected Mall's proposal and replied, "I can think of but one motive which might influence you to come here with us and that is the desire to live here and a belief in our ideals and our future. . . . They will not appeal to the great mass of the public, not even to the medical public, for a considerable time. What we shall consider success, the mass of doctors will not consider a success."

Mall considered the alternatives. At Chicago he had already, as he told Welch, "formulated the biological dept, got its outfit for $25,000 and have practically planned its building which will cost $200,000," all of it funded, with more to come from Rockefeller. At the Hopkins there was a medical school faculty and, by now, a hospital, but no money yet with which to even open the school. (Its medical school finally opened only when a group of women, many of whom had also recently founded Bryn Mawr College, offered a $500,000 endowment provided that the medical school would accept women. The faculty and trustees reluctantly agreed.) But there was Welch.

Mall wired him, "Shall cast my lot with Hopkins. . . . I consider you the greatest attraction. You make the opportunities."

. . .

Yet it was not Welch's laboratory investigations that attracted, that made opportunities. For, unknown to Gilman and Billings, who hired him, and even to Welch himself, he had a failing.

Welch knew the methods of science, all right, could grasp immediately the significance of an experimental result, could see and execute the design of further experiments to confirm a finding or probe more deeply. But he had had those abilities during his six years in New York, when he did no science. He had told himself and others that the demands of making a living had precluded research.

Yet he had no family to support and others did magnificent science under far greater burdens. No scientist had faced more adverse conditions than George Sternberg, an autodidact whom Welch called "the real pioneer of modern bacteriologic work in this country . . . [who] mastered the technique and literature by sheer persistence and native ability."

In 1878, as Welch met Billings in the same beer hall where legend had Faust meeting the Devil, Sternberg was an army medical officer in combat with the Nez Perce Indians. From there he traveled by stagecoach for four hundred and fifty miles—enduring day after day after day of the stink of sweat, of bone-shattering bumps that shot up the spine, of choking on the dust—only to reach a train, then by train for another twenty-five hundred miles of steaming discomfort, jostling elbows, and inedible food. He endured all this to attend a meeting of the American Public Health Association. While Welch was bemoaning his lack of facilities in New York, Sternberg was building a laboratory largely at his own expense at a frontier army post. In 1881 he became the first to isolate the pneumococcus, a few weeks before Pasteur and Koch. (None of the three recognized the bacteria's full importance.) Sternberg also first observed that white blood cells engulfed bacteria, a key to understanding the immune system. He failed to follow up on these observations, but many of his other achievements were remarkable, especially his pioneering work taking photographs through microscopes and his careful experiments that determined both the temperature at which various kinds of bacteria died and the power of different disinfectants to kill them. That information allowed the creation of antiseptic conditions in both laboratory and public health work. Sternberg began that work too in a frontier post.

Meanwhile, in New York City Welch was swearing that if only he were free of economic worries his own research would flower.

In Baltimore his work did not flower. For there, even with talented young investigators helping him, his failing began to demonstrate itself.

His failing was this: in science as in the rest of his life, he lived upon the surface and did not root. His attention never settled upon one important or profound question.

The research he did was first-rate. But it was only first-rate—thorough, rounded, and even irrefutable, but not deep enough or provocative enough or profound enough to set himself or others down new paths, to show the world in a new way, to make sense out of great mysteries. His most important discoveries would be the bacteria now called *Bacillus welchii,* the cause of gas gangrene, and the finding that staphylococci live in layers of the skin, which meant that a surgeon had to disinfect not only the skin surface during an operation but layers beneath it. These were not unimportant findings, and, even in the absence of any single more brilliant success, if they had represented a tiny piece of a large body of comparable work, they might have added up to enough to rank Welch as a giant.

Instead they would be the only truly significant results of his research. In the context of an entire lifetime, especially at a time when an entire universe lay naked to exploration, this work did not amount to much.

The greatest challenge of science, its art, lies in asking an important question and framing it in a way that allows it to be broken into manageable pieces, into experiments that can be conducted that ultimately lead to answers. To do this requires a certain kind of genius, one that probes vertically and sees horizontally.

Horizontal vision allows someone to assimilate and weave together seemingly unconnected bits of information. It allows an investigator to see what others do not see, and to make leaps of connectivity and creativity. Probing vertically, going deeper and deeper into something, creates new information. Sometimes what one finds will shine brilliantly enough to illuminate the whole world.

At least one question connects the vertical and the horizontal. That question is "So what?" Like a word on a Scrabble board, this question can connect with and prompt movement in many directions. It can eliminate a piece of information as unimportant or, at least to the investigator asking the question, irrelevant. It can push an investigator to probe more deeply to understand a piece of information. It can also force an investigator to step back and see how to fit a finding into a broader context. To see questions in these ways requires a *wonder,* a deep wonder focused by discipline, like a lens focusing the sun's rays on a spot of paper until it bursts into flame. It requires a kind of conjury.

Einstein reportedly once said that his own major scientific talent was his ability to look at an enormous number of experiments and journal articles, select the very few that were both correct and important, ignore the rest, and build a theory on the right ones. In that assessment of his own abilities, Einstein was very likely overly modest. But part of his genius was an instinct for what mattered and the ability to pursue it vertically and connect it horizontally.

Welch had a vital and wide curiosity, but he did not have this deeper wonder. The large aroused him. But he could not see the large in the small. No question ever aroused a great passion in him, no question ever became a compulsion, no question ever forced him to pursue it until it was either exhausted or led him to new questions. Instead he examined a problem, then moved on.

In his first years at the Hopkins he would constantly refer to his work, refer to his need to return to the laboratory. Later he abandoned the pretense and ceased even attempting to do research. Yet he never fully accepted his choice; to the end of his life he would sometimes express the wish that he had devoted himself to the laboratory.

Nonetheless, despite this lack of scientific achievement, Welch did not live one of those lives that began with great promise and ended in bitterness and disappointment. Despite his minimal production in the laboratory, people like Mall were drawn to him. As a prominent scientist said, "Everyone agrees that Welch himself was the great attraction at the Pathological. . . . [H]is example, his intelligence, and his comprehensive knowledge formed the keystone of the arch of scientific medicine in America."

For William Welch's real genius lay in two areas.

First, he had not only knowledge but judgment. He had an extraordinary ability to hear someone describe his or her experiments, or read a paper, and immediately define the crucial points still obscure, the crucial series of experiments needed to clarify them. It was as if, although he could not himself conjure, he knew the techniques of conjuring and could teach others conjury.

He had an equally extraordinary ability to judge people, to identify those with the promise to do what he had not done. He largely chose the medical school faculty, and he chose brilliantly. All were young when appointed. Welch was thirty-four; William Osler, a Canadian and arguably the most famous clinical physician of the modern era, forty; William Halsted, a surgeon who changed the way surgeons thought, thirty-seven; Howard Kelly, a gynecologist and pioneer in radiation therapy, thirty-one; J. J. Abel, a chemist and pharmacologist who would discover adrenaline and help revolutionize pharmacopoeia, thirty-six; W. H. Howell, a physiologist, thirty-three; and Mall, thirty-one. (Howell, Abel, and Mall had been graduate students at the Hopkins.)

Second, Welch inspired. He inspired unconsciously, simply by being himself. In the early days of the school, Welch was heavy but not yet fat, short, with bright blue eyes that flashed above a dark beard called an "imperial"—a mustache and pointed goatee. He dressed conservatively but well in dark clothes and often carried a derby hat in his hand. Despite his bulk, his hands and feet were conspicuously small and made him appear almost delicate. But his most singular quality was not physical. He seemed so centered and comfortable with himself that he gave comfort to those around him. He exuded confidence without arrogance, smugness, or pomposity. In his disputes—and he had many with those outsiders who resisted changes—he never raised his voice, never seemed to feel, according to a man who watched him for decades, "the exuberant joy of putting an opponent down."

Everything about him was positive. His intelligence and the depth and breadth of his knowledge stimulated his teaching as well. He walked into the classroom without notes or preparation, often not knowing what subject he was to lecture on, and in an instant began discoursing lucidly and logically in ways that provoked thought and excitement. He was paternal without being paternalistic. Physicians sent him pathology samples for analysis and paid a hefty fee. His assistants did the work; he wrote up the results and gave them the money. He loved to eat and hosted lavish dinners at his club, the Maryland Club, often inviting junior colleagues or graduate students; one of them called these dinners among his "rosiest memories" because of Welch's conversation, his ability to make students feel "the richness of the world"—the world of art and literature as well as science.

The total effect, said Simon Flexner, "made for an atmosphere of achievement . . . The desire to be like Welch, the desire to win his approval, these were the principal incentives of the eager young men who crowded his lab."

Finally, a certain mystery clung to Welch. Although this was not part of his genius it explained part of his impact. For all his cordiality he remained distant. The cordiality itself was a barrier others could not penetrate. He paid little, and decreasing, attention to students until they did something significant enough to get his attention. He seemed casual, even sloppy. He would get so animated in conversation that his cigar ash would routinely drop onto his coat, where it would lie unnoticed. He was never on time. His desk would be piled with months of unanswered correspondence. Younger colleagues gave him a nickname, a nickname that spread from the Hopkins to younger scientists everywhere. They called him, never to his face, "Popsy."

It was a comfortable, paternal, and warm nickname. But if he gave comfort, he took comfort from no one. Although he helped all whom he deemed worthy, although he surrounded himself with people, he neither encouraged nor allowed anyone to confide personal troubles to him. And he confided in no one. Mall once wrote his sister that he longed for a real friendship with Welch, not just an acquaintanceship. Even Mall would not get it. Welch took vacations alone in Atlantic City, where he enjoyed its tackiness.

The students had a chant: "Nobody knows where Popsy eats / Nobody knows where Popsy sleeps / Nobody knows whom Popsy keeps / But Popsy."

The Hopkins medical school sat on the city's outskirts atop a hill, miles from the main campus of the university and downtown. The main building, the Pathological Laboratory, was ugly and squat, two stories of stone, with six tall windows on each floor, and square chimneys towering above the building itself. Inside, an amphitheater for autopsies hollowed out the building, and students on the top floor could peer down over railings; a long narrow room lined each floor, a pathology laboratory on the first floor, a bacteriology laboratory on the second.

Even without the school, once the hospital opened in 1889, with sixteen buildings on fourteen acres, a small community began to develop. People breakfasted together and lunched together every day, and often met in the evening. Every Monday night a slightly more formal group of thirty to forty people gathered, including faculty, students who already had an M.D. or Ph.D., and clinicians. They would discuss current research or cases, and comments routinely generated new questions. Senior faculty sometimes dined in evening clothes at the "high table" in a bay window overlooking the grounds. The younger men played poker together, entertained each other, and went to the "Church" together—Hanselmann's restaurant and bar, at Wolfe and Monument, where they drank beer. A Harvard professor compared the Hopkins to a monastery. Harvey Cushing said, "In the history of medicine there was never anything quite like it." And they did have a mission.

Elias Canetti, a Nobel laureate in literature, observed in his book *Crowds and Power* that large movements were often generated by what he called "crowd crystals, . . . the small, rigid groups of men, strictly delimited and of great constancy, which serve to precipitate crowds. Their structure is such that they can be comprehended and taken in at a glance. Their unity is more important than their size. Their role must be familiar; people must know what they are there for. . . . The crowd crystal is *constant*. . . . Its members are trained in both action and faith. . . . The clarity, isolation, and constancy of the crystal form an uncanny contrast with the excited flux of the surrounding crowd."

In the same way that precipitates fall out of solution and coalesce around a crystal, individuals with extraordinary abilities and a shared vision had now coalesced about Welch at the Hopkins. Together, with a handful of others around the country, they intended to precipitate a revolution.

CHAPTER FOUR

AMERICAN MEDICAL EDUCATION needed a revolution. When the Hopkins medical school did at last open in 1893, most American medical schools had still not established any affiliation with either a teaching hospital or a university, most faculty salaries were still paid by student fees, and students still often graduated without ever touching a patient. Nor did Welch exaggerate when he said that, other than the Hopkins, no American "medical school requires for admission knowledge approaching that necessary for entrance into the freshman class of a respectable college. . . . [S]ome require no evidence of preliminary education whatever."

By contrast, the Hopkins itself, not student fees, paid faculty salaries, and it required medical students to have not only a college degree but fluency in French and German and a background of science courses. Indeed, these requirements were so rigorous that Welch and Osler worried that the Hopkins would attract no students.

But students did come. They came flocking. Motivated and self-selected, they flocked to a school where students did not simply listen to lectures and take notes. They trooped through hospital rooms and examined patients, made diagnoses, heard the crepitant rales of a diseased lung, felt the alien and inhuman marble texture of a tumor. They performed autopsies, conducted laboratory experiments, and they explored: they explored organs with scalpels, nerves and muscles with electric currents, the invisible with microscopes.

Those at the Hopkins were hardly alone in seeking reform. The need had been recognized for decades. Leaders at a few other medical schools—especially Vaughan at Michigan, William Pepper Jr. at the University of Pennsylvania, William Councilman (Welch's assistant until 1892) at Harvard, others at Northwestern, at New York's College of Physicians and Surgeons, at Tulane—were advancing the same values that Welch and the Hopkins were, and they were doing so with equal urgency. The American Medical Association had pushed reform since its inception, and individual physicians sought better training as well; the thousands who studied in Europe proved that.

But relatively little change had occurred in the bulk of medical schools, and even at Harvard, Penn, and elsewhere, change had often come only after violent infighting, with continual rear-guard actions fought by reluctant faculty. William Pepper had made Penn good enough that the Hopkins raided its faculty, yet after sixteen years of fighting he spoke not of achievement but of "long and painful controversy."

Even where change had occurred, a gap between the Hopkins and elsewhere still remained. Harvey Cushing trained at Harvard and came to Baltimore as Halsted's assistant. Nothing in Boston had prepared him for the difference. He found the Hopkins "strange. . . . The talk was of pathology and bacteriology of which I knew so little that much of my time the first few months was passed alone at night in the room devoted to surgical pathology looking at specimens with a German textbook at hand."

The Hopkins did not limit its influence to medicine. Half a century after it opened, of 1,000 men starred in the 1926 edition of *American Men of Science,* 243 had Hopkins degrees; second was Harvard with 190. Even Harvard's Charles Eliot conceded that the Harvard Graduate School "started feebly" and "did not thrive, until the example of Johns Hopkins. . . . And what was true of Harvard was true of every other university in the land."

But in medicine the Hopkins made its chief mark. As early as 1900 Welch noted that at the Harvard-run Boston City Hospital "they have only Hopkins men there, and want no others." By 1913 a European acknowledged that research in the United States in his field rivaled that done in any European country and gave credit "to one man—Franklin P. Mall at the Johns Hopkins University." Of the first four American Nobel laureates in physiology or medicine, the Hopkins had trained three, while the fourth had received his highest degree in Europe.

In patient care its impact was similar. As with all medical schools, most of its graduates became practicing physicians. And within thirty-five years after opening, more than 10 percent of *all* Hopkins graduates had become full professors, with many younger graduates on track to do so. Many of these men transformed entire medical schools at other universities—people like Councilman and Cushing at Harvard, William MacCallum at Columbia, Eugene Opie at Washington University, Milton Winternitz at Yale, George Whipple (a Nobel laureate) at Rochester.

Howard Kelly, for all his strangeness—a fundamentalist who preached to prostitutes on street corners of whom one student said, "The only interest he manifested in my classmates was whether they were saved"—revolutionized gynecology and pioneered radiation therapy. And no individual had more impact on patient care than William Halsted, who introduced rubber gloves into surgery, who insisted upon preparation and thought prior to every step. He took such care that William Mayo once joked that his patients were healed by the time he finished, but the Mayo brothers also stated that they owed him a tremendous debt. So did all of American surgery: of seventy-two surgeons who served as residents or assistant residents under him, fifty-three became professors.

In the meantime, Henry James described the Hopkins as a place where, despite "the immensities of pain" one thought of "fine poetry . . . and the high beauty of applied science. . . . Grim human alignments became, in their cool vistas, delicate symphonies in white. . . . Doctors ruled, for me, so gently, the whole still concert."

Behind this still concert lay Welch, the impresario. By the first decade of the twentieth century, Welch had become the glue that cemented together the entire American medical establishment. His own person became a central clearinghouse of scientific medicine. Indeed, he became *the* central clearinghouse. As founding editor of the *Journal of Experimental Medicine,* the first and most important American research journal, he read submissions that made him familiar with every promising new idea and young investigator in the country.

He became a national figure, first within the profession, then within science, then in the larger world, serving as president or chairman of nineteen different major scientific organizations, including the American Medical Association, the American Association for the Advancement of

Science, and the National Academy of Sciences. Stanford president Ray Wilbur neither flattered nor overstated when in 1911 he wrote him, "Not to turn to you for information in regard to the best men to fill vacancies in our medical school would be to violate all the best precedents of American medical education." Welch had, said one colleague, "the power to transform men's lives almost by the flick of a wrist."

But his use of power in placing people in positions—or for that matter using it for such things as defeating antivivisection legislation, which would have prevented using animals as experimental models and thus crippled medical research—was trivial in its impact compared to his application of power to two other areas.

One area involved completing the reform of all medical education. The example of the Hopkins had forced more and faster reforms at the best schools. But too many medical schools remained almost entirely unaffected by the Hopkins example. Those schools would learn a harsh lesson, and soon.

Welch's second interest involved starting and directing the flow of tens of millions of dollars into laboratory research.

In Europe governments, universities, and wealthy donors helped support medical research. In the United States, no government, institution, or philanthropist even began to approach a similar level of support. As the Hopkins medical school was opening, American theological schools enjoyed endowments of $18 million, while medical school endowments totaled $500,000. The difference in financial support as well as educational systems largely explained why Europeans had achieved the bulk of medical advances.

Those advances had been extraordinary, for medicine in the late nineteenth and early twentieth centuries was experiencing arguably its most golden age—including anytime since. The germ theory had opened the door to that progress. Finally investigators began using that door.

In 1880 Pasteur—who observed, "Chance favors the prepared mind"— was trying to prove he had isolated the cause of chicken cholera. He inoculated healthy chickens with the bacteria. They died. Then chance intervened. He had put aside a virulent culture for several days, then used it to inoculate more chickens. They lived. More significantly, those same chickens survived when exposed to other virulent cultures. Crediting Jenner for the idea, he tried to weaken, or "attenuate," his word, cultures and use them to immunize birds against lethal bacteria. He succeeded.

He began applying these techniques to other infections. With anthrax he was not the first to experiment with weakened cultures, but his work was both definitive and very public. While a gallery of newspapermen and officials watched, he inoculated cattle, then exposed them to anthrax; the inoculuated ones lived, while the controls died. Three years later 3.3 million sheep and 438,000 cattle were vaccinated against anthrax in France. He also saved the life of a boy bitten by a rabid dog by giving him gradually stronger injections of fluid containing the pathogen. The next year, 1886, an international fund-raising drive created the Pasteur Institute. Almost immediately the German goverment funded research institutes for Koch and a few other outstanding investigators, and research institutes were founded in Russia, Japan, and Britain.

Meanwhile, public health measures were containing cholera and typhoid, and in Germany, Richard Pfeiffer, Koch's greatest disciple, and Wilhelm Kolle immunized two human volunteers with heat-killed typhoid bacilli. In Britain Sir Almroth Wright advanced upon this work and developed a vaccine against typhoid.

All these advances *prevented* infectious disease. But no physician could yet *cure* a patient who was dying of one. That was about to change.

One of the deadliest of childhood diseases was diphtheria. Usually it killed by choking its victims to death—by generating a membrane that closed the breathing passages. In Spain the disease was called *el garrotillo,* "the strangler."

In 1884, German scientist Friedrich Loeffler isolated the diphtheria bacillus from throats of patients, grew it on a special medium (laboratories today still use "Loeffler's serum slope" to grow the bacteria from suspected cases), and began careful experiments in animals that took several years. His work suggested that the bacteria themselves did not kill; the danger came from a toxin, a poison, that the bacteria excreted.

In 1889 Pasteur's protégés Émile Roux and Alexandre Yersin grew broth thick with diphtheria bacteria and used compressed air to force the broth through a filter of unglazed porcelain. (The filter was designed by Charles Chamberland, a physicist working with Pasteur; though only a tool, the filter itself would prove to be immensely important.) No bacteria or solids could pass through the porcelain. Only liquid could. They then sterilized this liquid. It still killed. That proved that a soluble toxin did the killing.

Meanwhile, an American physiologist named Henry Sewall at the University of Michigan was studying snake venom, which chemically resembles many bacterial toxins. In 1887 he immunized pigeons against rattlesnake poison.

If pigeons could be immunized, humans likely could be too. As they had with cholera, French and German scientists raced each other, building upon Sewall's and each other's advances, studying both diphtheria and tetanus. In December 1890, Koch protégés Emil Behring, who would later win the Nobel Prize, and Shibasaburo Kitasato showed that serum—the fluid left after all solids are removed from blood—drawn from one animal made immune to tetanus could be injected into a different animal and protect it from disease.

The paper shook the scientific world. Work on diphtheria at a level of intensity heretofore unknown proceeded in laboratories. Over the Christmas holiday in 1891 in Berlin, the first attempt to cure a person of diphtheria was made. It succeeded.

Scientists had discovered a way not simply to prevent a disease. They had found a way to cure disease. *It was the first cure.*

Over the next few years work continued. In 1894, Émile Roux of the Pasteur Institute read his paper summarizing experiments with diphtheria antitoxin before the International Congress on Hygiene in Budapest.

Many of the greatest scientists in the world sat in the audience. As Roux finished, these men, each renowned in his own right, began to clap, then stood on their seats, their hands making thunderous sounds, their voices shouting applause in half a dozen languages, their hats thrown to the ceiling. Welch then reported American experiences confirming the work of both the French and Germans. And each delegate returned to his home with a bottle of this marvelous curative agent in his possession.

In the keynote speech at the next meeting of the Association of American Physicians, an association created to foster scientific medicine, Welch said, "The discovery of the healing serum is entirely the result of laboratory work. In no sense was the discovery an accidental one. Every step leading to it can be traced, and every step was taken with a definite purpose and to solve a definite problem. These studies and resulting discoveries mark an epoch in the history of medicine."

His comment was a declaration not of war but of victory. Scientific medicine had developed technologies that could both prevent and cure diseases that had previously killed in huge numbers, and killed gruesomely.

And if French and German scientists had found the antitoxin, Americans William Park, chief of the laboratory division of the New York City Health Department, and Anna Williams, his deputy and perhaps the leading female bacteriologist in this country—possibly anywhere—transformed it into something that every doctor in the developed world had easy access to. They were an odd couple: he with an original and creative mind but staid, even stolid, extremely precise and well organized; she, wild, risk taking, intensely curious, a woman who took new inventions apart to see how they worked. They complemented each other perfectly.

In 1894 they discovered a way to make a toxin five hundred times as potent as that used by Europeans. This lethality made a far more efficient stimulator of antitoxin and slashed the cost to one-tenth what it had been. Park then broke the production process into tasks that ordinary workers, not scientists, could perform and turned part of the laboratory into a virtual factory. It soon became by far the cheapest, most efficient, and reliable producer of the antitoxin in the world. Diphtheria-antitoxin production today is still based on their methods.

The lab distributed it free in New York and sold it elsewhere. Park used the money to subsidize basic research and make the city laboratories into arguably the best medical research institution in the country at the time. Its annual reports soon contained, according to one historian of medicine, "a body of research of which any Institute in the world would be proud."

And the antitoxin suddenly became available around the world. Diphtheria fatality rates quickly fell by almost two-thirds, and country doctors began to perform miracles. It was only the first miracle of what promised to be many.

■   ■   ■

As the use of this antitoxin was becoming widespread, Frederick Gates, an intellectually curious Baptist minister who had a gift for seeing opportunities to exploit and was an assistant to John D. Rockefeller, picked up a medical textbook written by William Osler called *The Principles and Practice of Medicine,* a textbook that would go through many editions and find a readership among both physicians and informed laymen. In it Osler traced the evolution of medical ideas, explored controversies, and, most significantly, admitted uncertainty and ignorance.

Gates had started working for Rockefeller as a philanthropic adviser, but nothing limited him to eleemosynary concerns. He organized several Rockefeller business ventures, pulling, for example, a $50 million profit out of the Mesabi iron range in Minnesota. Rockefeller himself used a homeopathic physician, and Gates had also read *The New Testament of Homeopathic Medicine,* written by Samuel Hahnemann, founder of the movement. Gates decided that Hahnemann "must have been, to speak charitably, little less than lunatic."

Osler's book impressed Gates in very different ways for it presented a paradox. First, it showed that medical science had immense promise. But it also showed that that promise was far from being realized. "It became clear to me that medicine could hardly hope to become a science," Gates explained, "until . . . qualified men could give themselves to uninterrupted study and investigation, on ample salary, entirely independent of practice. . . . Here was an opportunity, to me the greatest, which the world could afford, for Mr. Rockefeller to become a pioneer."

Meanwhile, John D. Rockefeller Jr. talked about the idea of funding medical research with two prominent physicians, L. Emmett Holt and Christian Herter, both former students of Welch. Both eagerly endorsed the idea.

On January 2, 1901, Rockefeller Sr.'s grandchild John Rockefeller McCormick, also the grandchild of Cyrus McCormick, died of scarlet fever in Chicago.

Later that year the Rockefeller Institute for Medical Research was incorporated. It would change everything.

Welch declined the offer to head the new institute but he assumed all the duties of launching it, chairing both the institute board itself and its board of scientific directors. That scientific board included Welch's old friend T. Mitchell Prudden, Holt, Herter, two other prominent scientists who had been students of Welch, and Harvard's Theobald Smith. Smith, one of the leading bacteriologists in the world, had been Welch's first choice for director but had declined because he had done most of his research on animal diseases—for example, developing a vaccine to prevent hog cholera—and thought it would be more politic to have a director who had investigated human disease.

So Welch offered the position to Simon Flexner, who had left the Hopkins to take a highly prestigious professorship at the University of Pennsylvania's medical school. (Flexner had rejected an offer of an $8,000 salary from Cornell to take the position at Penn at $5,000.) But his appointment had been contentious, and at the meeting where he was chosen one faculty member said that accepting the Jew as a professor did not involve accepting him as a man. Daily he fought with other faculty over both personal and substantive issues.

Flexner accepted Welch's offer, and a raise. But the launching of the institute remained firmly under Welch's control. In this, Flexner said, Welch "accepted no assistance, not even clerical. Every detail was attended to with his own hand, every letter handwritten."

The European research institutes were either dedicated to infectious disease or designed to allow freedom to individuals such as Pasteur, Koch, and Ehrlich. The Rockefeller Institute saw medicine itself as its field; from its earliest existence, scientists there studied infectious disease, but they also laid the groundwork in surgery for organ transplants, established links between viruses and cancer, and developed a method to store blood.

At first the institute gave modest grants to scientists elsewhere, but in 1903 it opened its own laboratory, in 1910 its own hospital. And Flexner began to come into his own.

There was a roughness about Simon Flexner, something left over from the streets, from his growing up the black sheep in an immigrant Jewish family in Louisville, Kentucky. Older and younger brothers were brilliant students, but he quit school in the sixth grade. Sullen and flirting with delinquency, he was fired even by an uncle from a menial job in a photography studio. Next he worked for a dry-goods dealer who defrauded people and fled the city. A druggist fired him. His father gave him a tour of the city jail to try to frighten him into obedience, then arranged a plumbing apprenticeship, but the plumber balked when Simon's old principal warned him "not to have anything to do with Simon Flexner."

At the age of nineteen Flexner got another job with a druggist, washing bottles. The shop had a microscope and the druggist forbade him to touch it. He ignored the order. Flexner hated any kind of tedium, and taking orders. What the microscope showed him was not at all tedious.

Abruptly his mind engaged. He was fascinated. He began making sudden impossible leaps. In a single year he finished a two-year program at the Louisville College of Pharmacy and won the gold medal for best student. He began working for his older brother Jacob, another druggist who also had a microscope; now Simon did not have sneak to use it. Simultaneously he went to a medical school—at night. Flexner later recalled, "I never made a physical examination. I never heard a heart or lung sound."

But he did get an M.D. His younger brother Abraham had graduated from the Hopkins, and Simon sent some of his microscopic observations to Welch. Soon Simon was studying at the Hopkins himself.

Welch took to him though they were opposites. Flexner was small and wiry, almost wizened, and no one ever called him charming. He had an edgy insecurity and said, "I have never been educated in any branch of learning. There are great gaps in my knowledge." To fill the gaps, he read. "He read," his brother Abraham said, "as he ate." He devoured books, read everything, read omnivorously, from English literature to Huxley and Darwin. He felt he had to learn. His insecurities never fully left him. He talked of "sleepless nights and days of acute fear . . . a maddening nervousness which prevented me from having a quiet moment."

Yet others recognized in him extraordinary possibilities. Welch arranged a fellowship for him in Germany, and four years later he became professor of pathology at the Hopkins. Often he went into the field: to a mining town to study meningitis, to the Philippines to study dysentery, to Hong Kong to study plague. Nobel laureate Peyton Rous later called Flexner's scientific papers "a museum in print, only they stir with life; for he experimented as well as described."

He never lost his street toughness but his sharp hard edges did become rounded. He married a woman who was herself extraordinary enough to captivate Bertrand Russell (sixty letters from him were in her papers) and whose sister was a founder of Bryn Mawr. The famed jurist Learned Hand became a close friend. And he left his mark on the Rockefeller Institute.

Emerson said that an institution is the lengthened shadow of one man, and the institute did reflect Simon Flexner. Raymond Fosdick, later president of the Rockefeller Foundation, talked of the "steely precision of his reason. His mind was like a searchlight that could be turned at will on any question that came before him." A Rockefeller researcher said he had "a logic far beyond that of most men, final as a knife."

But in place of the comfort and monastic purpose and intimacy that Welch gave the Hopkins, Flexner made Rockefeller sharp, edgy, cold. Once, when the usefulness ended of horses that had been immunized against a disease, then bled over and over to produce antiserum, he never considered turning them out to pasture; he considered only either selling them for slaughter "to manufacturers or they can be bled further, with the idea of sacrificing them"—bleeding them to death for a final harvest of serum. He could dismiss a person as easily, ridding the institute of what he termed "unoriginal" men as soon as he made that determination. The room most feared in the institute was Flexner's office. He could be brutal there, and several prominent scientists were afraid of him. Even at Flexner's memorial service, a Nobel laureate said, "Individuals were as nothing to Dr. Flexner compared with the welfare of the institute."

He sought attention for the institute from the press and credit from the scientific community. His own work created controversy. Shortly after the Rockefeller Institute was established, a meningitis epidemic struck the eastern United States. Desperate measures were used to fight the infection. Diphtheria antitoxin was tried, and some physicians even tried the ancient practice of bleeding patients. At the Hopkins, Cushing tried draining pus-filled fluid from the spinal canal.

At the Rockefeller Institute, the meningitis epidemic seemed a particular challenge. Rockefeller and Gates wanted results. Flexner wanted to produce them.

Ten years earlier William Park, who had perfected diphtheria antitoxin, had developed a serum against meningococci. In every laboratory test his serum had worked. But it had had no effect on people. Now two Germans developed a similar serum, but they injected it directly into the spinal column instead of into veins or muscle. Normally the mortality rate from the disease was 80 percent. In 102 patients they cut the mortality to 67 percent, suggestive but not a statistically significant improvement.

Still, Flexner's instincts told him it meant something. He repeated the German experiments. His patients died at a 75 percent rate. Instead of discarding the approach, however, he persisted; he began a long series of experiments, both in the laboratory, to improve the serum's potency, and physiologically, searching for the best way to administer it to monkeys. After three years of work, he settled upon the method: first, to insert a needle intrathecally—under a thin membrane lining the spinal cord—and withdraw 50 ccs of spinal fluid, and then to inject 30 ccs of serum. (Unless fluid was withdrawn first, the injection could increase pressure and cause paralysis.) It worked. In 712 people the mortality rate fell to 31.4 percent.

Physicians from Boston, San Francisco, Nashville—all confirmed the work, with one noting, "Remarkable results were obtained in the use of this serum by the country practitioners."

Not all accepted Flexner's role. Later, in a bacteriology textbook, Park implied that Flexner had contributed little to the development of the serum. Flexner responded with an angry visit to Park's lab; a shouting matching ensued. There would be further disputes between the two, public enough that newspapers reported on one.

Ultimately Flexner cut the death rate for patients infected by the meningococcus, the most common cause of bacterial meningitis, to 18 percent. According to a recent *New England Journal of Medicine* study, today with antibiotics patients at Massachusetts General Hospital, one of the best hospitals in the world, suffering from bacterial meningitis have a mortality rate of 25 percent.

He and the institute received massive amounts of publicity. He liked it and wanted more. So did Gates and Rockefeller. In the first decade of the institute especially, whenever someone there seemed on the edge of something exciting, Flexner hovered about. His constant attention seemed to demand results, and he routinely urged investigators to publish, writing, for example, "In view of the rapidity with which publications are appearing from Belgium and France, I advise the publication of your present results. Please see me about this promptly."

The pressure did not all come from Flexner. It simply flowed down through him. At a 1914 dinner Gates declared, "Who has not felt the throbbing desire to be useful to the whole wide world? The discoveries of this institute have already reached the depths of Africa with their healing ministrations. . . . You announce a discovery here. Before night your discovery will be flashed around the world. In 30 days it will be in every medical college on earth."

The result was a publicity machine. Highly respected investigators mocked the institute for, said one who himself spent time there, "frequent ballyhoo of unimportant stuff as the work of genius" because of "administrators and directors impelled by the desire for institutional advertising."

Yet Flexner also had a large vision. In his own work, he had what Welch lacked: the ability to ask a large question and frame it in ways that made answering it achievable. And when he judged an investigator original, an asset to the institute, he gave his full support. He did so with Nobel laureates Alexis Carrel and Karl Landsteiner, both of whose work was recognized early, but he also gave freedom and support to young investigators who had not yet made their mark. Peyton Rous, whose undergraduate and medical degrees both came from the Hopkins, would win the Nobel Prize for his discovery that a virus could cause cancer. He made that finding in 1911. The prize did not come until 1966. Initially the scientific community mocked him; it took that long for his work first to be confirmed, then appreciated. Yet Flexner always stood by him. Thomas Rivers, a Hopkins-trained scientist at Rockefeller who defined the difference between viruses and bacteria, recalled, "I am not saying Flexner wasn't tough or couldn't be mean—he could, believe me—but he also was tender with people."

Even in a formal report to the board of scientific directors, thinking of Rous perhaps, or perhaps Paul Lewis, an extraordinarily promising young scientist working directly with Flexner, Flexner said, "The ablest men are often the most diffident and self-deprecatory. They require in many cases to be reassured and made to believe in themselves." When another scientist Flexner had faith in wanted to switch fields, Flexner told him, "It will take two years for you to find your way. I won't expect anything from you until after that."

And finally Flexner believed in openness. He welcomed disagreement, expected friction and interaction, wanted the institute to become a living thing. The lunchroom was as important to Flexner as the laboratory. There colleagues working in different areas exchanged ideas. "Rous was a brilliant conversationalist, Jacques Loeb, Carrel," recalled Michael Heidelberger, then a junior investigator. Although Rous and Carrel won the Nobel Prize, Loeb may have been the most provocative. "These were really remarkable sessions sometimes. They were a great inspiration."

Each Friday especially mattered; investigators routinely presented their most recent work in a casual setting, and colleagues made comments, suggested experiments, added different contexts. It was a place of excitement, of near holiness, even though some men—Karl Landsteiner, for instance, another Nobel laureate—almost never made presentations. Flexner actively sought out individualists who did not fit in elsewhere, whether they be loners or prima donnas. The mix was what mattered. Flexner, Rous said, made the institute "an organism, not an establishment."

And Flexner's impact, like Welch's, was extending far beyond anything he did personally in the laboratory, or for that matter, in the Rockefeller Institute itself.

Even before the institute had exerted wide influence, American medical science was attaining world class. In 1908 the International Congress on Tuberculosis was held in Washington. Robert Koch came from Germany, great and imperious, prepared to pass judgment and issue decrees.

At a meeting of the section on pathology and bacteriology, which Welch headed, Park read a paper stating that "it is now absolutely established that quite a number of children have contracted fatal generalized tuberculosis from bacilli" in cow's milk. Koch insisted Park was wrong, that no evidence supported the idea that cattle gave tuberculosis to man. Theobald Smith then rose and supported Park. Arguments broke out all over the room. But the congress as a whole was convinced; a few days later, it passed a resolution calling for preventive measures against the spread of tuberculosis from cattle to man. Koch snapped, "Gentlemen, you may pass your resolutions, but posterity will decide!"

One delegate noted, "Dr. Koch isolated the tubercle bacillus; today, science isolated Dr. Koch."

Science is not democratic. Votes do not matter. Yet this vote marked the coming of age of American medicine. It was by no means due solely to the Hopkins. Neither Park nor Smith had trained or taught there. But the Hopkins and the Rockefeller Institute were about to fit two more pieces into place that would give American medicine a true claim to scientific leadership.

CHAPTER FIVE

THE MEN WHO CREATED the Rockefeller Institute always intended to have a small affiliated hospital built to investigate disease. No patient would pay for treatment and only those suffering from diseases being studied would be admitted. No other research institute in the world had such a facility. That much William Welch, Simon Flexner, Frederick Gates, and John D. Rockefeller Jr. did intend. But they did not plan to have what Rufus Cole, the hospital's first director, all but forced upon them.

Tall, mustached, and elegant, with an ancestor who arrived at Plymouth, Massachusetts, in 1633, Cole did not appear to be a forceful man, did not seem someone capable of confronting Flexner. But he always remained true to those things that he had thought out, and his thinking was powerful. Then he yielded only to evidence, not to personality, and advanced his own ideas calmly and with tenacity. His longtime colleague Thomas Rivers called him "a modest man, a rather timid man," who "would go out of his way to dodge" a confrontation. But, Rivers added, "He was considered the brightest man that ever graduated from Hopkins at the time he graduated. . . . If you get him mad, get him in a corner and kind of back him up, . . . [y]ou would find, generally to your sorrow, that the old boy wasn't afraid to fight."

Cole had wide interests and late in life wrote a two-volume, 1,294-page study of Oliver Cromwell, the Stuarts, and the English Civil War.

But at the institute lunch table he focused. Heidelberger recalled, "He would sit there and listen to whatever was going on, and then he'd ask a question. Sometimes the question seemed almost naive for a person who was supposed to know as much as he did, but the result always was to bring out things that hadn't been brought out before and to get much deeper down into the problem than one had before. Dr. Cole was really quite remarkable in that way."

His father and two uncles were doctors, and at the Hopkins his professor Lewellys Barker had established laboratories next to patient wards to study disease, not just conduct diagnostic tests. There Cole had done pioneering research. He came away from that experience with ideas that would influence the conduct of "clinical" research—research using patients instead of test tubes or animals—to this day.

Flexner saw the hospital as a testing ground for ideas generated by laboratory scientists. The scientists would control experimental therapies. The doctors treating the patients would do little more than play the role of a technician caring for a lab animal.

Cole had other ideas. He would not allow the hospital and its doctors to serve, said Rivers, as a "handmaiden. He and his boys were not going to test Noguchi's ideas, Meltzer's ideas, or Levens's ideas. Cole was adamant that people caring for patients do the research on them."

In a letter to the directors Cole explained that the clinicians should be full-fledged scientists conducting serious research: "One thing that has most seriously delayed the advancement of medicine has been the physical and intellectual barrier between the laboratory and the wards of many of our hospitals. Clinical laboratories most often exist merely to aid diagnosis. I would therefore urge that the hospital laboratory be developed as a true research laboratory, and that moreover [the doctors] of the hospital be permitted and urged to undertake experimental work."

This was no simple question of turf or bureaucratic power. Cole was setting an enormously important precedent. He was calling for—demanding—that physicians treating patients undertake rigorous research involving patients with disease. Precedents for this kind of work had been seen elsewhere, but not in the systematic way Cole envisioned.

Such studies not only threatened the power of the scientists doing purely laboratory research at the institute but, by implication, also changed the doctor-patient relationship. They were an admission that doctors did not know the answers and could not learn them without the patients' help. Since any rigorous study required a "control," this also meant that random chance, as opposed to the best judgment of the physician, might dictate what treatment a patient got.

Timid of nature or not, Cole would not yield. Flexner did. As a result, the Rockefeller Institute Hospital applied science directly to patient care, creating *the* model of clinical research—a model followed today by the greatest medical research facility in the world, the Clinical Center at the National Institutes of Health in Bethesda, Maryland. That model allowed investigators to learn. It also prepared them to act.

The Rockefeller Institute Hospital opened in 1910. By then the best of American medical science and education could compete with the best in the world. But an enormous gap existed in the United States between the best medical practice and the average, and an unbridgeable chasm separated the best from the worst.

In effect, there were outstanding generals, colonels, and majors, but they had no sergeants, corporals, or privates; they had no army to lead, at least not a reliable one. The gap between the best and the average had to be closed, and the worst had to be eliminated.

Physicians already practicing were unreachable. They had on their own either chosen to adopt scientific methods or not. Thousands had. Simon Flexner himself received his M.D. from a terrible medical school but had more than compensated, confirming Welch's observation: "The results were better than the system."

But the system of medical education still needed massive reform. Calls for reform had begun in the 1820s. Little had been accomplished outside a handful of elite schools.

Even among elite schools change came slowly. Not until 1901 did Harvard, followed soon by Penn and Columbia, join the Hopkins in requiring medical students to have a college degree. But even the best schools failed to follow the Hopkins's lead in recruiting quality faculty, instead choosing professors in clinical medicine from among local physicians. The official history of Penn's medical school conceded, "Inbreeding of a faculty could hardly go farther." Harvard's clinical professors were actually selected by a group of doctors who had no status at Harvard and met at the Tavern Club to make their decisions, which were usually based on seniority. Not until 1912 would Harvard select a clinical professor from outside this group.

Pressure did come from within the profession to improve. Not only those at the Hopkins, Michigan, Pennsylvania, Harvard, and other leading medical schools devoted themselves to reform. So did a large number of individual physicians and surgeons. In 1904 the American Medical Association finally formed a Council on Medical Education to organize the reform movement. The council began inspecting all 162 medical schools—more than half of all the medical schools in the world—in the United States and Canada.

Three years later the AMA council issued a blistering—but confidential—report. It concluded that at the better schools improvement was occurring, although, despite enormous effort by many reformers, not at a rapid enough pace. But the worst schools had barely changed at all. Faculty still owned most of them, most still had no connection to a university or hospital and no standards for admission, and tuition still funded faculty salaries. One school had graduated 105 "doctors" in 1905, none of whom had completed any laboratory work whatsoever; they had not dissected a single cadaver, nor had they seen a single patient. They would wait for a patient to enter their office for that experience.

The report had some effect. Within a year, fifty-seven medical schools were requiring at least one year of college of their applicants. But that still left two-thirds of the schools with lower or no requirements, and it did not address the content of the education itself.

Unable to confront its own membership again—in 1900 the AMA had only eight thousand members out of one hundred ten thousand doctors and feared antagonizing the profession—the AMA gave its report to the Carnegie Foundation, insisted that it remain confidential, and asked for help. In turn, the Carnegie Foundation commissioned Simon Flexner's brother Abraham to survey medical education. Although not a doctor, Flexner had been an undergraduate at the Hopkins—he said that even among undergraduates "research was the air we breathed"—and had already demonstrated both a ruthless, unforgiving judgment and a commitment to advancing model educational institutions. In his first job after college, he had taught in a Louisville high school—where he failed his entire class of fifteen students—and had experimented with new ways of teaching. Later he would create the Institute for Advanced Study at Princeton, and personally recruit Albert Einstein to it.

Abraham Flexner began his study by talking at length to Welch and Franklin Mall. Their views influenced him, to say the least. He stated, "The rest of my study of medical education was little more than an amplification of what I had learned during my initial visit to Baltimore."

In 1910, the same year the Rockefeller Institute Hospital opened, his report *Medical Education in the United States and Canada* appeared. It soon came to be known simply as "The Flexner Report."

According to it, few—very, very few—schools met his standards, or any reasonable standard. He dismissed many schools as "without redeeming features of any kind . . . general squalor . . . clinical poverty. . . . [O]ne encounters surgery taught without patient, instrument, model, or drawing; recitations in obstetrics without a manikin in sight—often without one in the building." At Temple, at Halifax University, at the Philadelphia College of Osteopathy, the dissecting rooms "defy description. The smell is intolerable, the cadavers now putrid." At North Carolina Medical College Flexner quoted a faculty member saying, "'It is idle to talk of real laboratory work for students so ignorant and clumsy. Many of them, gotten through advertising, would make better farmers.'"

Flexner concluded that more than 120 of the 150-plus medical schools in operation should be closed.

It was the Progressive Era. Life was becoming organized, rationalized, specialized. In every field "professionals" were emerging, routing the ideas of the Jacksonian period, when state legislatures deemed that licensing even physicians was antidemocratic. Frederick Taylor was creating the field of "scientific management" to increase efficiencies in factories, and Harvard Business School opened in 1908 to teach it. This rationalization of life included national advertising, which was now appearing, and retail chains, which were stretching across the continent; United Drug Stores the largest, had 6,843 locations.

But the Flexner report did not merely reflect the Progressive Era. Nor did it reflect the context in which one Marxist historian tried to place scientific medicine, calling it "a tool developed by members of the medical profession and the corporate class to . . . legitimize" capitalism and shift attention from social causes of disease. Noncapitalist societies, including Japan, Russia, and China, were adopting scientific medicine as well. The report reflected less the Progressive Era than science. Not surprisingly, progressives failed in a similar effort to standardize training of lawyers. Anyone could read a statute; only a trained specialist could isolate a pathogen from someone sick.

The Progressive Era was, however, also the muckraking era. Flexner's report raked muck and created a sensation. Fifteen thousand copies were printed. Newspapers headlined it and investigated local medical schools. Flexner received at least one death threat.

The impact was immediate. Armed now with the outcry Flexner had generated, the AMA's Council on Medical Education began rating schools as "Class A" and fully satisfactory; "Class B," which were "redeemable"; or "Class C," which were "needing complete reorganization." Schools owned and operated by faculty were automatically rated C.

Less than four years after Flexner's report was issued, thirty-one states denied licensing recognition to new graduates of Class C institutions, effectively killing the schools outright. Class B schools had to improve or merge. Medical schools at such universities as Nebraska, Colorado, Tufts, George Washington, and Georgetown kept a tenuous hold on AMA approval but survived. In Baltimore three Class B schools consolidated into the present University of Maryland medical school. In Atlanta, Emory absorbed two other schools. Medical schools at such institutions as Southern Methodist, Drake, Bowdoin, and Fordham simply collapsed.

By the late 1920s, before the economic pressure of the Depression, nearly one hundred medical schools had closed or merged. The number of medical students, despite a dramatic increase in the country's population, declined from twenty-eight thousand in 1904 to fewer than fourteen thousand in 1920; in 1930, despite a further increase in the country's population, the number of medical students was still 25 percent less than in 1904.

Later, Arthur Dean Bevan, leader of the AMA reform effort, insisted, "The AMA deserved practically all the credit for the reorganization of medical education in this country. . . . 80% of the Flexner report was taken from the work of the Council on Medical Education." Bevan was wrong.

The AMA wanted to avoid publicity, but only the leverage of the publicity— indeed, the scandal—Flexner generated could force change. Without the report, reform would have taken years, perhaps decades. And Flexner influenced the direction of change as well. He defined a model.

The model for the schools that survived was, of course, the Johns Hopkins.

Flexner's report had indirect impact as well. It greatly accelerated the flow, already begun, of philanthropic funds into medical schools. Between 1902 and 1934, nine major foundations poured $154 million into medicine, nearly half the total funds given away to all causes. And this understates the money generated, because the gifts often required the school to raise matching funds. This money saved some schools. Yale, for example, was rated a weak Class B school but it launched a fund-raising drive and increased its endowment from $300,000 to almost $3 million; its operating budget leaped from $43,000 to $225,000. The states also began pouring money into schools of state universities.

The largest single donor remained the Rockefeller Foundation. John D. Rockefeller himself continued to see a homeopathic physician.

Welch had turned the Hopkins model into a force. He and colleagues at Michigan, at Penn, at Harvard, and at a handful of other schools had in effect first formed an elite group of senior officers of an army; then, in an amazingly brief time, they had revolutionized American medicine, created and expanded the officer corps, and begun training their army, an army of scientists and scientifically grounded physicians.

On the eve of America's entry into World War I, Welch had one more goal. In 1884, when the Hopkins first offered Welch his position, he had urged the establishment of a separate school to study public health in a scientific manner. Public health was and is where the largest numbers of lives are saved, usually by understanding the epidemiology of a disease— its patterns, where and how it emerges and spreads—and attacking it at its weak points. This usually means prevention. Science had first contained smallpox, then cholera, then typhoid, then plague, then yellow fever, all through large-scale public health measures, everything from filtering water to testing and killing rats to vaccination. Public health measures lack the drama of pulling someone back from the edge of death, but they save lives by the millions.

Welch had put that goal aside while he focused on transforming American medicine, on making it science-based. Now he began to pursue that goal again, suggesting to the Rockefeller Foundation that it fund a school of public health.

There was competition to get this institution, and others tried to convince the foundation that though creating a school of public health made good sense, putting it in Baltimore did not. In 1916, Harvard president Charles Eliot wrote bluntly to the foundation—and simultaneously paid Welch a supreme compliment—when he dismissed the entire Hopkins medical school as "one man's work in a new and small university. . . . The more I consider the project of placing the Institute of Hygiene at Baltimore, the less suitable expedient I find it. . . . In comparison with either Boston or New York, it conspicuously lacks public spirit and beneficent community action. The personality and career of Dr. Welch are the sole argument for putting it in Baltimore—and he is almost 66 years old and will have no similar successor."

Nonetheless, that "sole argument" sufficed. The Johns Hopkins School of Hygiene and Public Health was scheduled to open October 1, 1918. Welch had resigned as a professor at the medical school to be its first dean.

The study of epidemic disease is, of course, a prime focus of public health.

Welch was sick the day of the scheduled opening, and getting sicker. He had recently returned from a trip to investigate a strange and deadly epidemic. His symptoms were identical to those of the victims of that epidemic, and he believed he too had the disease.

The army Welch had created was designed to attack, to seek out particular targets, if only targets of opportunity, and kill them. On October 1, 1918, the abilities of that army were about to be tested by the deadliest epidemic in human history.

■ Part II
THE SWARM

CHAPTER SIX

Haskell County, Kansas, lies west of Dodge City, where cattle drives up from Texas reached a railhead, and belongs geographically to and, in 1918, not far in time from, the truly Wild West. The landscape was and is flat and treeless, and the county was, literally, of the earth. Sod houses built of earth were still common then, and even one of the county's few post offices was located in the dug-out sod home of the postmaster, who once a week collected the mail by riding his horse forty miles round-trip to the county seat in Santa Fe, a smattering of a few wooden buildings that was already well on its way to becoming the ghost town it would be in another ten years—today only its cemetery remains as a sign of its existence. But other towns nearby did have life. In Copeland, Stebbins Cash Store sold groceries, shoes, dry goods, dishes, hardware, implements, paints, and oils, while in Sublette, in the absence of a bank, S. E. Cave loaned money on real estate for 7.5 percent.

Here land, crops, and livestock were everything, and the smell of manure meant civilization. Farmers lived in close proximity to hogs and fowl, with cattle, pigs, and poultry everywhere. There were plenty of dogs too, and owners made sure to teach their dogs not to chase someone else's cattle; that could get them shot.

It was a land of extremes. It was dry enough that the bed of the Cimarron River often lay cracked and barren of water, dry enough that the front page of the local newspaper proclaimed in February 1918, "A

slow rain fell all day, measuring 27 one hundredths. It was well appreciated." Yet torrential rains sometimes brought floods, such as the one in
1914 that drowned ranchers and wiped out the first and largest permanent business in the area, a ranch that ran thirty thousand head of cattle.
In summer the sun bleached the prairie, parching it under a heat that
made light itself quiver. In winter unearthly gales swept unopposed
across the plains for hundreds of miles, driving the windchill past fifty
degrees below zero; then the country seemed as frozen and empty as the
Russian steppes. And storms, violent storms, from tornadoes to literally
blinding blizzards, plagued the region. But all these extremes of nature
came every season. Another extreme of nature came only once.

Epidemiological evidence suggests that a new influenza virus originated in Haskell County, Kansas, early in 1918. Evidence further suggests
that this virus traveled east across the state to a huge army base, and from
there to Europe. Later it began its sweep through North America, through
Europe, through South America, through Asia and Africa, through isolated islands in the Pacific, through all the wide world. In its wake followed
a keening sound that rose from the throats of mourners like the wind.
The evidence comes from Dr. Loring Miner.

Loring Miner was an unusual man. A graduate of the oldest university in
the West, Ohio University in Athens, Ohio, a classicist enamored of ancient
Greece, he had come in 1885 to this region. Despite a background so
unlike those of his fellow frontiersmen, he had taken to the country and
done well.

Miner was a big man in many ways: physically large, with angular
features and a handlebar mustache, gruff, someone who didn't suffer
fools—especially when he drank, which was often. A certain rebellious-
ness was part of his bigness as well. He hadn't seen the inside of a church
in years. Periodically he reread the classics in Greek but he ate peas with
his knife. And in thirty years on that prairie he had built a small empire
apart from medicine. In the Odd Fellows he was a past noble grand, he
had chaired the county Democratic Party, had been county coroner, was
county health officer. He owned a drugstore and grocery and expected
his patients to buy from him, and he married into the family of the
largest landowners in western Kansas. Even in Haskell there was a social
order, and now, during the war, his wife used her social standing as head

of the county Red Cross Woman's Work Committee. When she asked for something few said no to her, and most women in the county did Red Cross work—real work, hard work, almost as hard as farmwork.

But Miner also personified Welch's comment that the results of medical education were better than the system. Although an isolated country doctor who began practicing before the establishment of the germ theory of disease, he had quickly accepted it, kept up with the astounding advances in his profession, built a laboratory in his office, learned how to use the new antitoxins for diphtheria and tetanus. By 1918 one of his sons had also become a doctor with a fully scientific education, and was already in the navy. He prided himself on his own scientific knowledge and puzzled over problems. His patients said they'd rather have him drunk than someone else sober.

His practice ranged over hundreds of square miles. Perhaps that was what Miner liked about it, the great expanse, the extremes, the lonely wind that could turn as violent as a gunshot, the hours spent making his way to a patient, sometimes in a horse and buggy, sometimes by car, sometimes by train—conductors would hold the train for him, and in winter stationmasters would violate the rules and let him wait inside the office by the stove.

But in late January and early February 1918, Miner had other concerns. One patient presented with what seemed common symptoms, although with unusual intensity—violent headache and body aches, high fever, nonproductive cough. Then another. And another. In Satanta, in Sublette, in Santa Fe, in Jean, in Copeland, on isolated farms.

Miner had seen influenza often. He diagnosed the disease as influenza. But he had never seen influenza like this. This was violent, rapid in its progress through the body, and sometimes lethal. This influenza killed. Soon dozens of his patients—the strongest, the healthiest, the most robust people in the county—were being struck down as suddenly as if they had been shot.

Miner turned all his energies to this disease. He drew blood, urine, and sputum samples, and used the laboratory skills his son had helped him improve. He searched all his medical texts and journals. He called his few colleagues in that part of the state. He contacted the U.S. Public Health Service, which offered him neither assistance nor advice. Meanwhile he likely did what little he could, trying diphtheria antitoxin with no effect, perhaps even trying tetanus antitoxin—anything that might stimulate the body's immune system against disease.

The local paper, the *Santa Fe Monitor*, apparently worried about hurting morale in wartime, said little about deaths but on inside pages reported, "Mrs. Eva Van Alstine is sick with pneumonia. Her little son Roy is now able to get up. . . . Ralph Lindeman is still quite sick. . . . Goldie Wolgehagen is working at the Beeman store during her sister Eva's sickness. . . . Homer Moody has been reported quite sick. . . . Mertin, the young son of Ernest Elliot, is sick with pneumonia. . . . We are pleased to report that Pete Hesser's children are recovering nicely. . . . Mrs J. S. Cox is some better but is very weak yet. . . . Ralph McConnell has been quite sick this week."

By now the disease overwhelmed Miner with patients. He pushed everything else aside, slept sometimes in his buggy while the horse made its own way home—one advantage over the automobile—through frozen nights. Perhaps he wondered if he was being confronted with the Plague of Athens, a mysterious disease that devastated the city during the Peloponnesian Wars, killing possibly one-third the population.

Then the disease disappeared. By mid-March the schools reopened with healthy children. Men and women returned to work. And the war regained its hold on people's thoughts.

The disease still, however, troubled Miner deeply. It also frightened him, not only for his own people but for the people beyond. Influenza was neither a "reportable" disease—not a disease that the law required physicians to report—nor a disease that any state or federal public health agency tracked.

Yet Miner considered his experience so unusual, and this eruption of the disease so dangerous, that he formally warned national public health officials about it.

Public Health Reports was a weekly journal published by the U.S. Public Health Service to alert health officials to outbreaks of all communicable diseases, not only in North America and Europe but anywhere in the world—in Saigon, Bombay, Madagascar, Quito. It tracked not just deadly diseases such as yellow fever and plague but far lesser threats; especially in the United States, it tracked mumps, chickenpox, and measles.

In the first six months of 1918, Miner's warning of "influenza of severe type" was the only reference in that journal to influenza anywhere in the world. Other medical journals that spring carried articles on influenza outbreaks, but they all occurred after Haskell's, and they were not issued as public health warnings. Haskell County remains the first outbreak in 1918 suggesting that a new influenza virus was adapting, violently, to man.

As it turned out, the death rate in Haskell as a percentage of the entire county's population was only a fraction of what the death rate for the United States would be later that year, when influenza struck in full force.

People suffering from influenza shed virus—expel viruses that can infect others—for usually no more than seven days after infection and often even less. After that, although they may continue to cough and sneeze, they will not spread the disease. As sparsely populated and isolated as Haskell was, the virus infecting the county might well have died there, might well have failed to spread to the outside world. That would be so except for one thing: this was wartime.

The same week that Homer Moody and a dozen others in Jean, Kansas, fell ill, a young soldier named Dean Nilson came home to Jean on leave from Camp Funston, located three hundred miles away within the vast Fort Riley military reservation. The *Santa Fe Monitor* noted, "Dean looks like soldier life agrees with him." After his leave, of course, he returned to the camp. Ernest Elliot left Sublette, in Haskell County, to visit his brother at Funston just as his child fell ill; by the time Elliot returned home, the child had pneumonia. Of nearby Copeland on February 21, the paper said, "Most everybody over the country is having lagrippe or pneumonia." On February 28 it reported that John Bottom just left Copeland for Funston: "We predict John will make an ideal soldier."

Camp Funston, the second-largest cantonment in the country, held on average fifty-six thousand green young troops. The camp was built at the confluence of the Smoky Hill and Republican Rivers, where they form the Kansas River. Like all the other training camps in the country, Funston had been thrown together in literally a few weeks in 1917. There the army prepared young men for war.

It was a typical camp, with typical tensions between army regulars and men who had until recently been civilians. When Major John Donnelly was stopped by military police for speeding, for example, he defended himself to the commanding general: "I have, on a few occasions, corrected (enlisted) personnel along the road parallel to that camp for failure to salute; cases that I could not conscientiously overlook, there being no excuse whatever for their failure to do so. This, like my attempted correction of this guard, may not have been taken in the proper spirit, resulting in a feeling of insubordinate revenge and animosity towards me by members of this organization."

There were also the usual clashes of egos, especially since Camp Funston and Fort Riley had different commanding officers. These clashes ended when Major General C. G. Ballou, who commanded the cantonment, sent a missive to Washington. He had developed what he described as a "training ground for specialists" at Smoky Hill Flat. In fact, Smoky Hill Flat was the best of three polo fields on the base. The commanding officer of Fort Riley, only a colonel, established the post dump beside it. The general requested and received authority "to exercise command over the entire reservation of Fort Riley," and the colonel was relieved of his command.

Funston was typical in another way. The winter of 1917–18 was one of record cold, and, as the army itself conceded, at Funston as elsewhere "barracks and tents were overcrowded and inadequately heated, and it was impossible to supply the men with sufficient warm clothing."

So army regulations—written for health reasons—detailing how much space each man should have were violated, and men were stacked in bunks with insufficient clothing and bedding and inadequate heating. That forced them to huddle ever more closely together around stoves.

Men inducted into the army from Haskell County trained at Funston. There was a small but constant flow of traffic between the two places.

On March 4 a private at Funston, a cook, reported ill with influenza at sick call. Within three weeks more than eleven hundred soldiers were sick enough to be admitted to the hospital, and thousands more—the precise number was not recorded—needed treatment at infirmaries scattered around the base. Pneumonia developed in 237 men, roughly 20 percent of those hospitalized, but only thirty-eight men died. While that was a higher death toll than one would normally expect from influenza, it was not so high as to draw attention, much less than the death rate in Haskell, and only a tiny fraction of the death rate to come.

All influenza viruses mutate constantly. The timing of the Funston explosion strongly suggests that the influenza outbreak there came from Haskell; if Haskell was the source, whoever carried it to Funston brought a mild version of the virus, but it was a version capable of mutating back to lethality.

Meanwhile Funston fed a constant stream of men to other American bases and to Europe, men whose business was killing. They would be more proficient at it than they could imagine.

CHAPTER SEVEN

N O ONE WILL EVER KNOW with absolute certainty whether the 1918–19 influenza pandemic actually did originate in Haskell County, Kansas. There are other theories of origin. (For a fuller discussion of them see pages 456 through 458.) But Frank Macfarlane Burnet, a Nobel laureate who lived through the pandemic and spent most of his scientific career studying influenza, later concluded that the evidence was "strongly suggestive" that the 1918 influenza pandemic began in the United States, and that its spread was "intimately related to war conditions and especially the arrival of American troops in France." Numerous other scientists agree with him. And the evidence does strongly suggest that Camp Funston experienced the first major outbreak of influenza in America; if so, the movement of men from an influenza-infested Haskell to Funston also strongly suggests Haskell as the site of origin.

Regardless of where it began, to understand what happened next one must first understand viruses and the concept of the mutant swarm.

Viruses are themselves an enigma that exist on the edges of life. They are not simply small bacteria. Bacteria consist of only one cell, but they are fully alive. Each has a metabolism, requires food, produces waste, and reproduces by division.

Viruses do not eat or burn oxygen for energy. They do not engage in any process that could be considered metabolic. They do not produce waste. They do not have sex. They make no side products, by accident or design. They do not even reproduce independently. They are less than a fully living organism but more than an inert collection of chemicals.

Several theories of their origin exist, and these theories are not mutually exclusive. Evidence exists to support all of them, and different viruses may have developed in different ways.

A minority view suggests that viruses originated independently as the most primitive molecules capable of replicating themselves. If this is so, more advanced life forms could have evolved from them.

More virologists think the opposite: that viruses began as more complex living cells and evolved—or, more accurately, devolved—into simpler organisms. This theory does seem to fit some organisms, such as the "rickettsia" family of pathogens. Rickettsia used to be considered viruses but are now thought of as halfway between bacteria and viruses; researchers believe they once possessed but lost activities necessary for independent life. The leprosy bacillus also seems to have moved from complexity— doing many things—toward simplicity—doing fewer. A third theory argues that viruses were once *part* of a cell, an organelle, but broke away and began to evolve independently.

Whatever the origin, a virus has only one function: to replicate itself. But unlike other life forms (if a virus is considered a life form), a virus does not even do that itself. It invades cells that have energy and then, like some alien puppet master, it subverts them, takes them over, forces them to make thousands, and in some cases hundreds of thousands, of new viruses. The power to do this lies in their genes.

In most life forms, genes are stretched out along the length of a filament-like molecule of DNA, deoxyribonucleic acid. But many viruses—including influenza, HIV, and the coronavirus that causes SARS (Severe Acute Respiratory Syndrome)—encode their genes in RNA, ribonucleic acid, an even simpler but less stable molecule.

Genes resemble software; just as a sequence of bits in a computer code tells the computer what to do—whether to run a word processing program, a computer game, or an Internet search, genes tell the cell what to do.

Computer code is a binary language: it has only two letters. The genetic code uses a language of four letters, each representing the chemicals adenine, guanine, cytosine, and thymine (in some cases uracil substitutes for thymine).

DNA and RNA are strings of these chemicals. In effect they are very long sequences of letters. Sometimes these letters do not form words or sentences that make any known sense: in fact, 97 percent of human DNA does not contain genes and is referred to as "nonsense" or "junk" DNA.

But when the letters spell out words and sentences that do make sense, then that sequence is by definition a gene.

When a gene in a cell is activated, it orders the cell to make particular proteins. Proteins can be used like bricks as building blocks of tissue. (The proteins that one eats generally do end up building tissue.) But proteins also play crucial roles in most chemical reactions within the body, as well as in carrying messages to start and stop different processes. Insulin, for example, is a hormone but also a protein; it helps regulate the metabolism and it particularly affects blood glucose levels.

When a virus successfully invades a cell, it inserts its own genes into the cell's genome, and the viral genes seize control from the cell's own genes. The cell's internal machinery then begins producing what the viral genes demand instead of what the cell needs for itself.

So the cell turns out hundreds of thousands of viral proteins, which bind together with copies of the viral genome to form new viruses. Then the new viruses escape. In this process the host cell almost always dies, usually when the new viral particles burst through the cell surface to invade other cells.

But if viruses perform only one task, they are not simple. Nor are they primitive. Highly evolved, elegant in their focus, more efficient at what they do than any fully living being, they have become nearly perfect infectious organisms. And the influenza virus is among the most perfect of these perfect organisms.

Louis Sullivan, the first great modern architect, declared that form follows function.

To understand viruses, or for that matter to understand biology, one must think as Sullivan did, in a language not of words, which simply name things, but in a language of three dimensions, a language of shape and form.

For in biology, especially at the cellular and molecular levels, nearly all activity depends ultimately upon form, upon physical structure—upon what is called "stereochemistry."

The language is written in an alphabet of pyramids, cones, spikes, mushrooms, blocks, hydras, umbrellas, spheres, ribbons twisted into every imaginable Escher-like fold, and in fact every shape imaginable. Each form is defined in exquisite and absolutely precise detail, and each carries a message.

Basically everything in the body—whether it belongs there or not—either carries a form on its surface, a marking, a piece that identifies it as a unique entity, or its entire form and being comprises that message. (In this last case, it is pure information, pure message, and it embodies perfectly Marshall McLuhan's observation that "the medium is the message.")

Reading the message, like reading braille, is an intimate act, an act of contact and sensitivity. Everything in the body communicates in this way, sending and receiving messages by contact.

This communication occurs in much the same way that a round peg fits into a round hole. When they fit together, when they match each other in size, the peg "binds" to the hole. Although the various shapes in the body are usually more complex than a round peg, the concept is the same.

Within the body, cells, proteins, viruses, and everything else constantly bump against one another and make physical contact. When one protuberance fits the other not at all, each moves on. Nothing happens.

But when one complements the other, the act becomes increasingly intimate; if they fit together well enough, they "bind." Sometimes they fit as loosely as the round peg in the round hole, in which case they may separate; sometimes they fit more snugly, like a skeleton key in a simple lock on a closet door; sometimes they fit with exquisite precision, like a variegated key in a far more secure lock.

Then events unfold. Things change. The body reacts. The results of this binding can be as dramatic, or destructive, as any act of sex or love or hate or violence.

There are three different types of influenza viruses: A, B, and C. Type C rarely causes disease in humans. Type B does cause disease, but not epidemics. Only influenza A viruses cause epidemics or pandemics, an epidemic being a local or national outbreak, a pandemic a worldwide one.

Influenza viruses did not originate in humans. Their natural home is in wild aquatic birds, and many more variants of influenza viruses exist in birds than in humans. But the disease is considerably different in birds and humans. In birds, the virus infects the gastrointestinal tract. Bird droppings contain large amounts of virus, and infectious virus can contaminate cold lakes and other water supplies.

Massive exposure to an avian virus can infect man directly, but an avian virus cannot go from person to person. It cannot, that is, unless it first changes, unless it first adapts to humans.

This happens rarely, but it does happen. The virus may also go through an intermediary mammal, especially swine, and jump from swine to man. Whenever a new variant of the influenza virus does adapt to humans, it will threaten to spread rapidly across the world. It will threaten a pandemic.

Pandemics often come in waves, and the cumulative "morbidity" rate—the number of people who get sick in all the waves combined—often exceeds 50 percent. One virologist considers influenza so infectious that he calls it "a special instance" among infectious diseases, "transmitted so effectively that it exhausts the supply of susceptible hosts."

Influenza and other viruses—not bacteria—combine to cause approximately 90 percent of all respiratory infections, including sore throats.*

Coronaviruses (the cause of the common cold as well as SARS), parainfluenza viruses, and many other viruses all cause symptoms akin to influenza, and all are often confused with it. As a result, sometimes people designate mild respiratory infections as "flu" and dismiss them.

But influenza is not simply a bad cold. It is a quite specific disease, with a distinct set of symptoms and epidemiological behavior. In humans the virus directly attacks only the respiratory system, and it becomes increasingly dangerous as it penetrates deeper into the lungs. Indirectly it affects many parts of the body, and even a mild infection can cause pain in muscles and joints, intense headache, and prostration. It may also lead to far more grave complications.

The overwhelming majority of influenza victims usually recover fully within ten days. Partly because of this, and partly because the disease is confused with the common cold, influenza is rarely viewed with concern.

*Nonetheless, people today often demand antibiotics from physicians and the physicians too often accommodate them. But antibiotics have no effect whatsoever on viruses. Administering them serves only to increase resistance to antibiotics by bacteria: bacteria that survive exposure to antibiotics become immune to them.

Yet even when outbreaks are not deadly as a whole, influenza strikes so many people that even the mildest viruses almost always kill. Currently in the United States, even without an epidemic or pandemic, the Centers for Disease Control estimates that influenza kills on average 36,000 people a year.

It is, however, not only an endemic disease, a disease that is always around. It also arrives in epidemic and pandemic form. And pandemics can be more lethal—sometimes much, much more lethal—than endemic disease.

Throughout known history there have been periodic pandemics of influenza, usually several a century. They erupt when a new influenza virus emerges. And the nature of the influenza virus makes it inevitable that new viruses emerge.

The virus itself is nothing more than a membrane—a sort of envelope—that contains the genome, the eight genes that define what the virus is. It is usually spherical (it can take other shapes), about 1/10,000 of a millimeter in diameter, and it looks something like a dandelion with a forest of two differently shaped protuberances—one roughly like a spike, the other roughly like a tree—jutting out from its surface.

These protuberances provide the virus with its actual mechanism of attack. That attack, and the defensive war the body wages, is typical of how shape and form determine outcomes.

The protuberances akin to spikes are hemagglutinin. When the virus collides with the cell, the hemagglutinin brushes against molecules of sialic acid that jut out from the surface of cells in the respiratory tract.

Hemagglutinin and sialic acid have shapes that fit snugly together, and the hemagglutinin *binds* to the sialic acid "receptor" like a hand going into a glove. As the virus sits against the cell membrane, more spikes of hemagglutinin bind to more sialic acid receptors; they work like grappling hooks thrown by pirates onto a vessel, lashing it fast. Once this binding holds the virus and cell fast, the virus has achieved its first task: "adsorption," adherence to the body of the target cell.

This step marks the beginning of the end for the cell, and the beginning of a successful invasion by the virus.

Soon a pit forms in the cell membrane beneath the virus, and the virus slips through the pit to enter entirely within the cell in a kind of bubble called a "vesicle." (If for some reason the influenza virus cannot penetrate the cell membrane, it can detach itself and then bind to another cell that it *can* penetrate. Few other viruses can do this.)

By entering the cell, as opposed to fusing with the cell on the cell membrane—which many other viruses do—the influenza virus hides from the immune system. The body's defenses cannot find it and kill it.

Inside this vesicle, this bubble, shape and form shift and create new possibilities as the hemagglutinin faces a more acidic environment. This acidity makes it cleave in two and refold itself into an entirely different shape. The refolding process somewhat resembles taking a sock off a foot, turning it inside out, and sticking a fist in it. The cell is now doomed.

The newly exposed part of the hemagglutinin interacts with the vesicle, and the membrane of the virus begins to dissolve. Virologists call this the "uncoating" of the virus and "fusion" with the cell. Soon the genes of the virus spill into the cell, then penetrate to the cell nucleus, insert themselves into the cell's genome, displace some of the cell's own genes, and begin issuing orders. The cell begins to produce viral proteins instead of its own. Within a few hours these proteins are packaged with new copies of the viral genes.

Meanwhile, the spikes of neuraminidase, the other protuberance that jutted out from the surface of the virus, are performing another function. Electron micrographs show neuraminidase to have a boxlike head extending from a thin stalk, and attached to the head are what look like four identical six-bladed propellers. The neuraminidase breaks up the sialic acid remaining on the cell surface. This destroys the acid's ability to bind to influenza viruses.

This is crucial. Otherwise, when new viruses burst from the cell they could be caught as if on fly paper; they might bind to and be trapped by sialic acid receptors on the dead cell's disintegrating membrane. The neuraminidase guarantees that new viruses can escape to invade other cells. Again, few other viruses do anything similar.

From the time an influenza virus first attaches to a cell to the time the cell bursts generally takes about ten hours, although it can take less time or, more rarely, longer. Then a swarm of between 100,000 and 1 million new influenza viruses escapes the exploded cell.

The word "swarm" fits in more ways than one.

. . .

Whenever an organism reproduces, its genes try to make exact copies of themselves. But sometimes mistakes—mutations—occur in this process.

This is true whether the genes belong to people, plants, or viruses. The more advanced the organism, however, the more mechanisms exist to prevent mutations. A person mutates at a much slower rate than bacteria, bacteria mutate at a much slower rate than a virus—and a DNA virus mutates at a much slower rate than an RNA virus.

DNA has a kind of built-in proofreading mechanism to cut down on copying mistakes. RNA has no proofreading mechanism whatsoever, no way to protect against mutation. So viruses that use RNA to carry their genetic information mutate much faster—from 10,000 to 1 million times faster—than any DNA virus.

Different RNA viruses mutate at different rates as well. A few mutate so rapidly that virologists consider them not so much a population of copies of the same virus as what they call a "quasi species" or a "mutant swarm."

These mutant swarms contain trillions and trillions of closely related but different viruses. Even the viruses produced from a single cell will include many different versions of themselves, and the swarm as a whole will routinely contain almost every possible permutation of its genetic code.

Most of these mutations interfere with the functioning of the virus and will either destroy the virus outright or destroy its ability to infect. But other mutations, sometimes in a single base, a single letter, in its genetic code will allow the virus to adapt rapidly to a new situation. It is this adaptability that explains why these quasi species, these mutant swarms, can move rapidly back and forth between different environments and also develop extraordinarily rapid drug resistance. As one investigator has observed, the rapid mutation "confers a certain randomness to the disease processes that accompany RNA [viral] infections."

Influenza is an RNA virus. So is HIV and the coronavirus. And of all RNA viruses, influenza and HIV are among those that mutate the fastest. The influenza virus mutates so fast that 99 percent of the 100,000 to 1 million new viruses that burst out of a cell in the reproduction process are too defective to infect another cell and reproduce again. But that still leaves between 1,000 and 10,000 viruses that *can* infect another cell.

Both influenza and HIV fit the concept of a quasi species, of a mutant swarm. In both, a drug-resistant mutation can emerge within days. And the influenza virus reproduces rapidly—far faster than HIV. Therefore it adapts rapidly as well, often too rapidly for the immune system to respond.

CHAPTER EIGHT

A N INFECTION is an act of violence; it is an invasion, a rape, and the body reacts violently. John Hunter, the great physiologist of the eighteenth century, defined life as the ability to resist putrefaction, resist infection. Even if one disagrees with that definition, resisting putrefaction certainly does define the ability to live.

The body's defender is its immune system, an extraordinarily complex, intricate, and interwoven combination of various kinds of white blood cells, antibodies, enzymes, toxins, and other proteins. The key to the immune system is its ability to distinguish what belongs in the body, "self," from what does not belong, "nonself." This ability depends, again, upon reading the language of shape and form.

The components of the immune system—white blood cells, enzymes, antibodies, and other elements—circulate throughout the body, penetrating everywhere. When they collide with other cells or proteins or organisms, they interact with and read physical markings and structures just as the influenza virus does when it searches for, finds, and latches on to a cell.

Anything carrying a "self" marking, the immune system leaves alone. (It does, that is, when the system works properly. "Autoimmune diseases" such as lupus or multiple sclerosis develop when the immune system attacks its own body.) But if the immune system feels a "nonself" marking—either foreign invaders or the body's own cells that have become diseased—it responds. In fact, it attacks.

The physical markings that the immune system feels and reads and then binds to are called "antigens." The word refers to, very simply, anything that stimulates the immune system to respond.

Some elements of the immune system, such as so-called natural killer cells, will attack anything that bears any nonself-marking, any foreign antigen. This is referred to as "innate" or "nonspecific" immunity, and it serves as a first line of defense that counterattacks within hours of infection.

But the bulk of the immune system is far more targeted, far more focused, far more specific. Antibodies, for example, carry thousands of receptors on their surface to recognize and bind to a target antigen. Each one of those thousands of receptors is identical. So antibodies bearing these receptors will recognize and bind *only* to, for example, a virus bearing that antigen. They will not bind to any other invading organism.

One link between the nonspecific and specific immune response is a particular and rare kind of white blood cell called a dendritic cell. Dendritic cells attack bacteria and viruses indiscriminately, engulf them, then "process" their antigens and "present" those antigens—in effect they chop up an invading microorganism into pieces and display the antigens like a trophy flag.

The dendritic cells then travel to the spleen or the lymph nodes, where large numbers of other white blood cells concentrate. There these other white blood cells learn to recognize the antigen as a foreign invader and begin the process of producing huge numbers of antibodies and killer white cells that will attack the target antigen and anything attached to the antigen.

The recognition of a foreign antigen also sets off a parallel chain of events as the body releases enzymes. Some of these affect the entire body, for example, raising its temperature and causing fever. Others directly attack and kill the target. Still others serve as chemical messengers, summoning white blood cells to areas of invasion or dilating capillaries so killer cells can exit the bloodstream at the point of attack. Swelling, redness, and fever are all side effects of the release of these chemicals.

All this together is called the "immune response," and once the immune system is mobilized it is formidable indeed. But all this takes time. The delay can allow infections to gain a foothold in the body, even to advance in raging cadres that can kill.

In the days before antibiotics, an infection launched a race to the death between the pathogen and the immune system. Sometimes a victim would become desperately ill; then, suddenly and almost miraculously, the fever would break and the victim would recover. This "resolution by crisis" occurred when the immune system barely won the race, when it counterattacked massively and successfully.

But once the body survives an infection, it gains an advantage. For the immune system epitomizes the saying that that which does not kill you makes you stronger.

After it defeats an infection, specialized white cells (called "memory T cells") and antibodies that bind to the antigen remain in the body. If any invader carrying the same antigen attacks again, the immune system responds far more quickly than the first time. When the immune system can respond so quickly that a new infection will not even cause symptoms, people become immune to the disease.

Vaccinations expose people to an antigen and mobilize the immune system to respond to that disease. In modern medicine some vaccines contain only the antigen, some contain whole killed pathogens, and some contain living but weakened ones. They all alert the immune system and allow the body to mount an immediate response if anything bearing that antigen invades the body.

The same process occurs in the body naturally with the influenza virus. After people recover from the disease, their immune systems will very quickly target the antigens on the virus that infected them.

But influenza has a way to evade the immune system.

The chief antigens of the influenza virus are the hemagglutinin and neuraminidase protruding from its surface. But of all the parts of the influenza virus that mutate, the hemagglutinin and neuraminidase mutate the fastest. This makes it impossible for the immune system to keep pace.

By no means do the antigens of all viruses, even all RNA viruses, mutate rapidly. Measles is an RNA virus and mutates at roughly the same rate as influenza. Yet measles antigens do not change. Other parts of the virus do, but the antigens remain constant. (The most likely reason is that the part of the measles virus that the immune system recognizes as an antigen plays an integral role in the function of the virus itself. If it changes shape, the virus cannot survive.) So a single exposure to measles usually gives lifetime immunity.

Hemagglutinin and neuraminidase, however, can shift into different forms and still function. The result: their mutations allow them to evade the immune system but do not destroy the virus. In fact, they mutate so rapidly that even during a single epidemic both the hemagglutinin and neuraminidase often change.

Sometimes the mutations cause changes so minor that the immune system can still recognize them, bind to them, and easily overcome a second infection from the same virus.

But sometimes mutations change the shape of the hemagglutinin or neuraminidase enough that the immune system can't read them. The antibodies that bound perfectly to the old shapes do not fit well to the new one.

This phenomenon happens so often it has a name: "antigen drift."

When antigen drift occurs, the virus can gain a foothold even in people whose immune system has loaded itself with antibodies that bind to the older shapes. Obviously, the greater the change, the less efficiently the immune system can respond.

One way to conceptualize antigen drift is to think of a football player wearing a uniform with white pants, a green shirt, and a white helmet with a green *V* emblazoned on it. The immune system can recognize this uniform instantly and attack it. If the uniform changes slightly—if, for example, a green stripe is added to the white pants while everything else remains the same—the immune system will continue to recognize the virus with little difficulty. But if the uniform goes from green shirt and white pants to white shirt with green pants, the immune system may not recognize the virus so easily.

Antigen drift can create epidemics. One study found nineteen discrete, identifiable epidemics in the United States in a thirty-three-year period—more than one every other year. Each one caused between ten thousand and forty thousand "excess deaths" in the United States alone—an excess over and above the death toll usually caused by the disease. As a result influenza kills more people in the United States than any other infectious disease, including AIDS.

Public health experts monitor this drift and each year adjust the flu vaccine to try to keep pace. But they will never be able to match up perfectly, because even if they predict the direction of mutation, the fact that influenza viruses exist as mutating swarms means some will always be different enough to evade both the vaccine and the immune system.

But as serious as antigen drift can be, as lethal an influenza as that phenomenon can create, it does not cause great pandemics. It does not create firestorms of influenza that spread worldwide such as those in 1889–90, in 1918–19, in 1957, and in 1968.

Pandemics generally develop only when a radical change in the hemagglutinin, or the neuraminidase, or both, occurs. When an entirely new gene coding for one or both replaces the old one, the shape of the new antigen bears little resemblance to the old one.

This is called "antigen shift."

To use the football-uniform analogy again, antigen shift is the equivalent of the virus changing from a green shirt and white pants to an orange shirt and black pants.

When antigen shift occurs, the immune system cannot recognize the antigen at all. Few people in the world will have antibodies that can protect them against this new virus, so the virus can spread through a population at an explosive rate.

Hemagglutinin occurs in fifteen known basic shapes, neuraminidase in nine, and they occur in different combinations with subtypes. Virologists use these antigens to identify what particular virus they are discussing or investigating. "H1N1," for example, is the name given the 1918 virus, currently found in swine. An "H3N2" virus is circulating among people today.

Antigen shift occurs when a virus that normally infects birds attacks humans directly or indirectly. In Hong Kong in 1997 an influenza virus identified as "H5N1" spread directly from chickens to people, infecting eighteen and killing six.

Birds and humans have different sialic-acid receptors, so a virus that binds to a bird's sialic-acid receptor will not normally bind to—and thus infect—a human cell. In Hong Kong what most likely happened was that the eighteen people who got sick were subjected to massive exposure to the virus. The swarm of these viruses, the quasi species, likely contained a mutation that could bind to human receptors, and the massive exposure allowed that mutation to gain a foothold in the victims. Yet the virus did not adapt itself to humans; all those who got sick were infected directly from chickens.

But the virus can adapt to man. It can do so directly, with an entire animal virus jumping to humans and adapting with a simple mutation. It can also happen indirectly. For one final and unusual attribute of the influenza virus makes it particularly adept at moving from species to species.

The influenza virus not only mutates rapidly, but it also has a "segmented" genome. This means that its genes do not lie along a continuous strand of its nucleic acid, as do genes in most organisms, including most other viruses. Instead, influenza genes are carried in unconnected strands of RNA. Therefore, if two different influenza viruses infect the same cell, "reassortment" of their genes becomes very possible.

Reassortment mixes some of the segments of the genes of one virus with some from the other. It is like shuffling two different decks of cards together, then making up a new deck with cards from each one. This creates an entirely new hybrid virus, which increases the chances of a virus jumping from one species to another.

If the Hong Kong chicken influenza had infected someone who was simultaneously infected with a human influenza virus, the two viruses might easily have reassorted their genes. They might have formed a new virus that could pass easily from person to person. And the lethal virus might have adapted to humans.

The virus may also adapt indirectly, through an intermediary. Some virologists theorize that pigs provide a perfect "mixing bowl," because the sialic-acid receptors on their cells can bind to both bird and human viruses. Whenever an avian virus infects swine at the same time that a human virus does, reassortment of the two viruses can occur. And an entirely new virus can emerge that can infect man. In 1918 veterinarians noted outbreaks of influenza in pigs and other mammals, and pigs today still get influenza from a direct descendant of the 1918 virus. But it is not clear whether pigs caught the disease from man or man caught it from pigs.

And Dr. Peter Palese at Mount Sinai Medical Center in New York, one of the world's leading experts on influenza viruses, considers the mixing-bowl theory unnecessary to explain antigen shift: "It's equally likely that co-infection of avian and human virus in a human in one cell in the lung [gives] rise to the virus. . . . There's no reason why mixing couldn't occur in the lung, whether in pig or man. It's not absolute that there are no sialic acid receptors of those types in other species. It's not absolute that the avian receptor is really that different from the human, and, with one single amino acid change, the virus can go much better in another host."*

Antigen shift, this radical departure from existing antigens, led to major pandemics long before modern transportation allowed rapid movement of people. There is mixed opinion as to whether several pandemics in the fifteenth and sixteenth centuries were influenza although most medical historians believe that they were, largely because of the speed of their movement and the number of people who fell ill. In 1510 a pandemic of pulmonary disease came from Africa and "attacked at once and raged all over Europe not missing a family and scarce a person." In 1580 another pandemic started in Asia, then spread to Africa, Europe, and America. It was so fierce "that in the space of six weeks it afflicted almost all the nations of Europe, of whom hardly the twentieth person was free of the disease," and some Spanish cities were "nearly entirely depopulated by the disease."

There is no dispute, though, that other pandemics in the past were influenza. In 1688, the year of the Glorious Revolution, influenza struck England, Ireland, and Virginia. In these places "the people dyed . . . as in a plague." Five years later, influenza spread again across Europe: "all conditions of persons were attacked. . . . [T]hose who were very strong and hardy were taken in the same manner as the weak and spoiled, . . . the youngest as well as the oldest." In January 1699 in Massachusetts, Cotton Mather wrote, "The sickness extended to allmost all families. Few or none escaped, and many dyed especially in Boston, and some dyed in a strange or unusual manner, in some families all weer sick together, in some towns allmost all weer sick so that it was a time of disease."

At least three and possibly six pandemics struck Europe in the eighteenth century, and at least four struck in the nineteenth century. In 1847

---

*In 2001 Australian scientist Mark Gibbs advanced a theory that the influenza virus can also "recombine" its genes. Recombination means taking part of one gene and combining it with part of another gene. It is like cutting all the cards of two decks in pieces, taping the pieces together randomly, then assembling the first fifty-two for a new deck. Recombination has been demonstrated, but most virologists are skeptical of Gibbs's hypothesis.

and 1848 in London, more people died from influenza than died of cholera during the great cholera epidemic of 1832. And in 1889 and 1890, a great and violent worldwide pandemic—although nothing that even approached 1918 in violence—struck again. In the twentieth century, three pandemics struck. Each was caused by an antigen shift, by radical changes in either the hemagglutinin or the neuraminidase antigens, or both, or by changes in some other gene or genes.

Influenza pandemics generally infect from 15 to 40 percent of a population; any influenza virus infecting that many people and killing a significant percentage would be beyond a nightmare. In recent years public health authorities have at least twice identified a new virus infecting humans but successfully prevented it from adapting to man. To prevent the 1997 Hong Kong virus, which killed six of eighteen people infected, from adapting to people, public health authorities had every single chicken then in Hong Kong, 1.2 million of them, slaughtered. (The action did not wipe out this H5N1 virus. It survives in chickens and in 2003 it infected two more people, killing one. A vaccine for this particular virus has been developed, although it has not been stockpiled.)

An even greater slaughter of animals occurred in the spring of 2003 when a new H7N7 virus appeared in poultry farms in the Netherlands, Belgium, and Germany. This virus infected eighty-two people and killed one, and it also infected pigs. So public health authorities killed nearly thirty million poultry and some swine.

This costly and dreadful slaughter was done to prevent what happened in 1918. It was done to stop either of these influenza viruses from adapting to, and killing, man.

One more thing makes influenza unusual. When a new influenza virus emerges, it is highly competitive, even cannibalistic. It usually drives older types into extinction. This happens because infection stimulates the body's immune system to generate all its defenses against all influenza viruses to which the body has ever been exposed. When older viruses attempt to infect someone, they cannot gain a foothold. They cease replicating. They die out. So, unlike practically every other known virus, only one type—one swarm or quasi species—of influenza virus dominates at any given time. This itself helps prepare the way for a new pandemic, since the more time passes the fewer people's immune systems will recognize other antigens.

Not all pandemics are lethal. Antigen shift guarantees that the new virus will infect huge numbers of people, but it does not guarantee that it will kill large numbers. The twentieth century saw three pandemics.

The most recent new virus attacked in 1968, when the H3N2 "Hong Kong flu" spread worldwide with high morbidity but very low mortality—that is, it made many sick, but killed few. The "Asian flu," an H2N2 virus, came in 1957; while nothing like 1918, this was still a violent pandemic. Then of course there was the H1N1 virus of 1918, the virus that created its own killing fields.

■ Part III
THE TINDERBOX

CHAPTER NINE

I N THE SPRING OF 1918 death was no stranger to the world. Indeed, by then the bodies of more than five million soldiers had already been fed into what was called "the sausage factory" by generals whose stupidity was matched only by their brutality.

German generals, for example, had decided to bleed France into submission by matching it death for death at Verdun, believing that Germany's greater population would leave it victorious. The French later replied with their own massive offensive, believing that their *élan vital* would triumph.

Only slaughter triumphed. Finally one French regiment refused orders to make a suicidal charge. The mutiny spread to fifty-four divisions, stopped only by mass arrests, the conviction of twenty-three thousand men for mutiny, with four hundred sentenced to death and fifty-five actually executed.

Yet nothing expressed the brutality of this war as did a sanitation report on the planned eradication of rats in the trenches to prevent the spread of disease. A major noted, "Certain unexpected problems are involved in the rat problem. . . . The rat serves one useful function—he consumes the corpses on No Man's Land, a job which the rat alone is willing to undertake. For this reason it has been found desirable to control rather than eliminate the rat population."

All of Europe was weary of the war. Only in the United States

Anglophiles and Francophiles, most of them concentrated on the East Coast and many of them holding positions of power or influence, were not weary. Only in the United States Anglophiles and Francophiles still regarded war as glorious. And they put intense pressure on President Woodrow Wilson to enter the war.

The war had begun in 1914. Wilson had withstood this pressure. A German submarine had sunk the *Lusitania* in 1915 and he had not gone to war despite outrage in the press, instead winning a German commitment to limit submarine warfare. He had resisted other justifications for war. He could fairly campaign for reelection in 1916 on the slogan "He Kept Us Out of War." And he warned, "If you elect my opponent, you elect a war."

On election night he went to bed believing he had lost, but woke up reelected by one of the narrowest margins in history.

Then Germany took a great gamble. On January 31, 1917, giving only twenty-four hours' notice, it announced unrestricted submarine warfare against neutral and merchant vessels. It believed that it could starve Britain and France into submission before the United States—if the United States did at last declare war—could help. The action utterly outraged the nation.

Still Wilson did not go to war.

Then came the Zimmermann note: captured documents revealed that the German foreign minister had proposed to Mexico that it join Germany in war against the United States and reconquer parts of New Mexico, Texas, and Arizona.

Wilson's critics sputtered in fury at his pusillanimity. In a famous essay, pacifist and socialist Randolph Bourne, who later died in the influenza epidemic, lamented, "The war sentiment, begun so gradually but so perseveringly by the preparedness advocates who come from the ranks of big business, caught hold of one after another of the intellectual groups. With the aid of [Theodore] Roosevelt, the murmurs became a monotonous chant, and finally a chorus so mighty that to be out of it was at first to be disreputable and finally almost obscene. And slowly a strident rant was worked up against Germany."

On April 2, three weeks after the disclosure of the note, after his cabinet unanimously called for war, Wilson finally delivered his war message to Congress. Two days later he explained to a friend, "It was necessary for me by very slow stages and with the most genuine purpose to avoid war to lead the country on to a single way of thinking."

And so the United States entered the war filled with a sense of selfless mission, believing glory still possible, and still keeping itself separate from what it regarded as the corrupt Old World. It fought alongside Britain, France, Italy, and Russia not as an "ally" but as an "Associated Power."

Anyone who believed that Wilson's reluctant embrace of war meant that he would not prosecute it aggressively knew nothing of him. He was one of those rare men who believed almost to the point of mental illness in his own righteousness.

Wilson believed in fact that his will and spirit were informed by the spirit and hope of a people and even of God. He talked of his "sympathetic connection which I am sure that I have with" all American citizens and said, "I am sure that my heart speaks the same thing that they wish their hearts to speak." "I will not cry 'peace' so long as there is sin and wrong in the world," he went on. "America was born to exemplify that devotion to the elements of righteousness which are derived from the revelations of Holy Scripture."

He is probably the only American president to have held to this belief with quite such conviction, with no sign of self-doubt. It is a trait more associated with crusaders than politicians.

To Wilson this war was a crusade, and he intended to wage total war. Perhaps knowing himself even more than the country, he predicted, "Once lead this people into war, and they'll forget there ever was such a thing as tolerance. To fight you must be brutal and ruthless, and the spirit of ruthless brutality will enter into the very fibre of our national life, infecting Congress, the courts, the policeman on the beat, the man in the street."

America had never been and would never be so informed by the will of its chief executive, not during the Civil War with the suspension of habeas corpus, not during Korea and the McCarthy period, not even during World War II. He would turn the nation into a weapon, an explosive device.

As an unintended consequence, the nation became a tinderbox for epidemic disease as well.

∎   ∎   ∎

Wilson declared, "It isn't an army we must shape and train for war, it is a nation."

To train the nation, Wilson used an iron fist minus any velvet glove. He did have some legitimate reasons for concern, reasons to justify a hard line.

For reasons entirely unrelated to the war, America was a rumbling chaos of change and movement, its very nature and identity shifting. In 1870 the United States numbered only forty million souls, 72 percent of whom lived in small towns or on farms. By the time America entered the war, the population had increased to roughly 105 million. Between 1900 and 1915 alone, fifteen million immigrants flooded the United States; most came from Eastern and Southern Europe, with new languages and religions, along with darker complexions. And the first census after the war would also be the first one to find more people living in urban areas than rural.

The single largest ethnic group in the United States was German-American and a large German-language press had been sympathetic to Germany. Would German-Americans fight against Germany? The Irish Republican Army had launched an uprising against British rule on Easter, 1916. Would Irish-Americans fight to help Britain? The Midwest was isolationist. Would it send soldiers across an ocean when the United States had not been attacked? Populists opposed war, and Wilson's own secretary of state, William Jennings Bryan, three times the Democratic nominee for president, had resigned from the cabinet in 1915 after Wilson responded too aggressively for him to Germany's torpedoing the *Lusitania*. Socialists and radical unionists were strong in factories, in mining communities in the Rockies, in the Northwest. Would they, drafted or not, defend capitalism?

The hard line was designed to intimidate those reluctant to support the war into doing so, and to crush or eliminate those who would not. Even before entering the war, Wilson had warned Congress, "There are citizens of the United States, I blush to admit, . . . who have poured the poison of disloyalty into the very arteries of our national life. . . . Such creatures of passion, disloyalty, and anarchy must be crushed out."

He intended to do so.

His fire informed virtually everything that happened in the country, including fashion: to save cloth, a war material—everything was a war material—designers narrowed lapels and eliminated or shrank pockets. And his fury particularly informed every act of the United States government. During the Civil War Lincoln had suspended the writ of habeas corpus, imprisoning hundreds of people. But those imprisoned presented a real threat of armed rebellion. He left unchecked extraordinarily harsh criticism. Wilson believed he had not gone far enough and told his cousin, "Thank God for Abraham Lincoln. I won't make the mistakes that he made."

The government compelled conformity, controlled speech in ways, frightening ways, not known in America before or since. Soon after the declaration of war, Wilson pushed the Espionage Act through a cooperative Congress, which balked only at legalizing outright press censorship—despite Wilson's calling it "an imperative necessity."

The bill gave Postmaster General Albert Sidney Burleson the right to refuse to deliver any periodical he deemed unpatriotic or critical of the administration. And, before television and radio, most of the political discourse in the country went through the mails. A southerner, a narrow man and a hater, nominally a populist but closer to the Pitchfork Ben Tillman wing of the party than to that of William Jennings Bryan, Burleson soon had the post office stop delivery of virtually all publications and any foreign-language publication that hinted at less-than-enthusiastic support of the war.

Attorney General Thomas Gregory called for still more power. Gregory was a progressive largely responsible for Wilson's nominating Louis Brandeis to the Supreme Court, a liberal and the court's first Jew. Now, observing that America was "a country governed by public opinion," Gregory intended to help Wilson rule opinion and, through opinion, the country. He demanded that the Librarian of Congress report the names of those who had asked for certain books and also explained that the government needed to monitor "the individual casual or impulsive disloyal utterances." To do the latter, Gregory pushed for a law broad enough to punish statements made "from good motives or . . . [if] traitorous motives weren't provable."

The administration got such a law. In 1798, Federalist President John Adams and his party, under pressure of undeclared war with France, passed the Sedition Act, which made it unlawful to "print, utter, or publish . . . any false, scandalous, or malicious writing" against the government. But that law inflamed controversy, contributed to Adams's reelection defeat, and led to the only impeachment of a Supreme Court justice in history, when Samuel Chase both helped get grand jury indictments of critics and then sentenced these same critics to maximum terms.

Wilson's administration went further, yet engendered little opposition. The new Sedition Act made it punishable by twenty years in jail to "utter, print, write or publish any disloyal, profane, scurrilous, or abusive language about the government of the United States." One could go to jail for cursing the government, or criticizing it, even if what one said was true. Oliver Wendell Holmes wrote the Supreme Court opinion that found the act constitutional—after the war ended, upholding lengthy prison terms for the defendants—arguing that the First Amendment did not protect speech if "the words used . . . create a clear and present danger."

To enforce that law, the head of what became the Federal Bureau of Investigation agreed to make a volunteer group called the American Protective League an adjunct to the Justice Department, and authorized them to carry badges identifying them as "Secret Service." Within a few months the APL would have ninety thousand members. Within a year, two hundred thousand APL members were operating in a thousand communities.

In Chicago a "flying squad" of league members and police trailed, harassed, and beat members of the International Workers of the World. In Arizona, league members and vigilantes locked twelve hundred IWW members and their "collaborators" into boxcars and left them on a siding in the desert across the state line in New Mexico. In Rockford, Illinois, the army asked the league for help in gaining confessions from twenty-one black soldiers accused of assaulting white women. Throughout the country, the league's American Vigilance Patrol targeted "seditious street oratory," sometimes calling upon the police to arrest speakers for disorderly conduct, sometimes acting more . . . directly. And everywhere the league spied on neighbors, investigated "slackers" and "food hoarders," demanded to know why people didn't buy—or didn't buy more—Liberty Bonds.

States outlawed the teaching of German, while an Iowa politician warned that "ninety percent of all the men and women who teach the German language are traitors." Conversations in German on the street or over the telephone became suspicious. Sauerkraut was renamed "Liberty cabbage." The *Cleveland Plain Dealer* stated, "What the nation demands is that treason, whether thinly veiled or quite unmasked, be stamped out." Every day the *Providence Journal* carried a banner warning, "Every German or Austrian in the United States unless known by years of association should be treated as a spy." The Illinois Bar Association declared that lawyers who defended draft resisters were "unpatriotic" and "unprofessional." Columbia University president Nicholas Murray Butler, a national leader of the Republican Party, fired faculty critical of the government and observed, "What had been tolerable became intolerable now. What had been wrongheadedness was now sedition. What had been folly was now treason."

Thousands of government posters and advertisements urged people to report to the Justice Department anyone "who spreads pessimistic stories, divulges—or seeks—confidential military information, cries for peace, or belittles our effort to win the war." Wilson himself began speaking of the "sinister intrigue" in America carried on "high and low" by "agents and dupes."

Even Wilson's enemies, even the supposedly internationalist Communists, distrusted foreigners. Two Communist parties initially emerged in the United States, one with a membership of native-born Americans, one 90 percent immigrants.

Judge Learned Hand, one of Simon Flexner's closest friends, later observed, "That community is already in the process of dissolution where each man begins to eye his neighbor as a possible enemy, where nonconformity with the accepted creed, political as well as religious, becomes a mark of disaffection; where denunciation, without specification or backing, takes the place of evidence; where orthodoxy chokes freedom of dissent."

But American society hardly seemed to be dissolving. In fact it was crystallizing around a single focal point; it was more intent upon a goal than it had ever been, or might possibly ever be again.

Wilson's hard line threatened dissenters with imprisonment. The federal government also took control over much of national life. The War Industries Board allocated raw materials to factories, guaranteed profits, and controlled production and prices of war materials, and, with the National War Labor Board, it set wages as well. The Railroad Administration virtually nationalized the American railroad industry. The Fuel Administration controlled fuel distribution (and to save fuel it also instituted daylight savings time). The Food Admininstration—under Herbert Hoover— oversaw agricultural production, pricing, and distribution. And the government inserted itself in the psyche of America by allowing only its own voice to be heard, by both threatening dissenters with prison and shouting down everyone else.

Prior to the war Major Douglas MacArthur had written a long proposal advocating outright censorship if the nation did fight. Journalist Arthur Bullard, who was close to Wilson confidant Colonel Edward House, argued for another approach. Congress's rejection of censorship settled the argument in Bullard's favor.

Bullard had written from Europe about the war for *Outlook, Century,* and *Harper's Weekly.* He pointed out that Britain was censoring the press and had misled the British people, undermining trust in the government and support for the war. He urged using facts only. But he had no particular affection for truth per se, only for effectiveness: "Truth and falsehood are arbitrary terms. . . . There is nothing in experience to tell us that one is always preferable to the other. . . . There are lifeless truths and vital lies. . . . The force of an idea lies in its inspirational value. It matters very little if it is true or false."

Then, probably at the request of House, Walter Lippmann wrote Wilson a memo on creating a publicity bureau on April 12, 1917, a week after America declared war. One outgrowth of the Progressive Era, of the emergence of experts in many fields, was the conviction that an elite knew best. Typically, Lippmann later called society "too big, too complex" for the average person to comprehend, since most citizens were "mentally children or barbarians. . . . Self-determination [is] only one of the many interests of a human personality." Lippmann urged that self-rule be subordinated to "order," "rights," and "prosperity."

The day after receiving the memo, Wilson issued Executive Order 2594, creating the Committee on Public Information—the CPI—and named George Creel its head.

Creel was passionate, intense, handsome, and wild. (Once, years after the war and well into middle age, he literally climbed onto a chandelier in a ballroom and swung from it.) He intended to create "one white-hot mass . . . with fraternity, devotion, courage, and deathless determination."

To do so, Creel used tens of thousands of press releases and feature stories that were routinely run unedited by newspapers. And those same publications instituted a self-censorship. Editors would print nothing that they thought might hurt morale. Creel also created a force of "Four Minute Men"—their number ultimately exceeded one hundred thousand—who gave brief speeches before the start of meetings, movies, vaudeville shows, and entertainment of all kinds. Bourne sadly observed, "[A]ll this intellectual cohesion—herd-instinct—which seemed abroad so hysterical and so servile comes to us here in highly rational terms."

Creel began intending to report only facts, if carefully selected ones, and conducting only a positive campaign, avoiding the use of fear as a tool. But this soon changed. The new attitude was embodied in a declaration by one of Creel's writers that, "Inscribed in our banner even above the legend Truth is the noblest of all mottoes—'We Serve.'" They served a cause. One poster designed to sell Liberty Bonds warned, "I am Public Opinion. All men fear me! . . . [I]f you have the money to buy and do not buy, I will make this No Man's Land for you!" Another CPI poster asked, "Have you met this Kaiserite? . . . You find him in hotel lobbies, smoking compartments, clubs, offices, even homes. . . . He is a scandal-monger of the most dangerous type. He repeats all the rumors, criticism, and lies he hears about our country's part in the war. He's very plausible. . . . People like that . . . through their vanity or curiosity or *treason* they are helping German propagandists sow the seeds of discontent. . . ."

Creel demanded "100% Americanism" and planned for "every printed bullet [to] reach its mark." Simultaneously, he told the Four Minute Men that fear was "an important element to be bred in the civilian population. It is difficult to unite a people by talking only on the highest ethical plane. To fight for an ideal, perhaps, must be coupled with thoughts of self-preservation."

"Liberty Sings"—weekly community events—spread from Philadelphia across the country. Children's choruses, barbershop quartets, church choirs—all performed patriotic songs while the audiences sang along. At each gathering a Four Minute Man began the ceremonies with a speech.

Songs that might hurt morale were prohibited. Raymond Fosdick, a student of Wilson's at Princeton and board member (and later president) of the Rockefeller Foundation, headed the Commission on Training Camp

Activities. This commission banned such songs as "I Wonder Who's Kissing Her Now" and "venomous parodies" such as "Who Paid the Rent for Mrs. Rip Van Winkle While Mr. Rip Van Winkle Was Away?" along with "questionable jokes and other jokes, which while apparently harmless, have a hidden sting—which leave the poison of discontent and worry and anxiety in the minds of the soldiers and cause them to fret about home. . . . [T]he songs and jokes were the culmination of letter writing propaganda instigated by the Huns in which they told lying tales to the men of alleged conditions of suffering at home."

And Wilson gave no quarter. To open a Liberty Loan drive, Wilson demanded, "Force! Force to the utmost! Force without stint or limit! the righteous and triumphant Force which shall make Right the law of the world, and cast every selfish dominion down in the dust."

That force would ultimately, if indirectly, intensify the attack of influenza and undermine the social fabric. A softer path that Wilson also tried to lead the nation down would mitigate—but only somewhat—the damage.

The softer path meant the American Red Cross.

If the American Protective League mobilized citizens, nearly all of them men, to spy upon and attack anyone who criticized the war, the American Red Cross mobilized citizens, nearly all of them women, in more productive ways. The International Red Cross had been founded in 1863 with its focus on war, on the decent treatment of prisoners as set forth in the first Geneva Convention. In 1881 Clara Barton founded the American Red Cross, and the next year the United States accepted the guidelines of the convention. By World War I, all the combatants were members of the International Red Cross. But each national unit was fully independent.

The American Red Cross was a quasi-public institution whose titular president was (and is) the president of the United States. Officially chartered by Congress to serve the nation in times of emergency, the American Red Cross grew even closer to the government during the war. The chairman of its Central Committee was Wilson's presidential predecessor William Howard Taft, and Wilson had appointed its entire "War Council," the real ruling body of the organization.

As soon as the United States entered World War I, the American Red

Cross declared that it would "exert itself in any way which . . . might aid our allies. . . . The organization seeks in this great world emergency to do nothing more and nothing less than to coordinate the generosity and the effort of our people toward achieving a supreme aim."

There was no more patriotic organization. It had full responsibility for supplying nurses, tens of thousands of them, to the military. It organized fifty base hospitals in France. It equipped several railroad cars as specialized laboratories in case of disease outbreaks—but reserving them for use only by the military, not by civilians—and stationed them "so that one may be delivered at any point [in the country] within 24 hours." (The Rockefeller Institute also outfitted railroad cars as state-of-the-art laboratories and placed them around the country.) It cared for civilians injured or made homeless after several explosions in munitions factories.

But its most important role had nothing to do with medicine or disasters. Its most important function was to bind the nation together, for Wilson used it to reach into every community in the country. Nor did the Red Cross waste the opportunity to increase its presence in American life.

It had already made a reputation in several disasters: the Johnstown flood in 1889, when a dam broke and water smashed down upon the Pennsylvania city like a hammer, killing twenty-five hundred people; the San Francisco earthquake in 1906; major floods on the Ohio and Mississippi Rivers in 1912. It had also served American troops in the Spanish-American War and during the insurrection in the Philippines that followed.

Still, the American Red Cross began the Great War with only 107 local chapters. It finished with 3,864 chapters.

It reached into the largest cities and into the smallest villages. It made clear that to participate in Red Cross activities was to join the great crusade for civilization, and especially for American civilization. And it used subtlety and social pressure to all but compel participation. It identified the most prominent and influential man in a city, a person whom others could refuse only with difficulty, and asked him to chair the local Red Cross chapter; it appealed to him, told him how important he was to the war effort, how needed he was. Almost invariably he agreed. And it asked the leading hostess, the leader of "society" in cities—in Philadelphia, Mrs. J. Willis Martin, who started the nation's first garden club and whose family and husband's family were as established as any on the Main

Line—or whatever passed for "society" in small towns—in Haskell County, Mrs. Loring Miner, whose father was the largest landowner in southwest Kansas—to chair a woman's auxiliary.

In 1918 the Red Cross counted thirty million Americans—out of a total population of 105 million—as active supporters. Eight million Americans, nearly 8 percent of the entire population, served as production workers in local chapters. (The Red Cross had more volunteers in World War I than in World War II despite a 30 percent increase in the nation's population.) Women made up nearly all this enormous volunteer workforce, and they might as well have worked in factories. Each chapter received a production quota, and each chapter produced that quota. They produced millions of sweaters, millions of blankets, millions of socks. They made furniture. They did everything requested of them, and they did it well. When the Federal Food Administration said that pits from peaches, prunes, dates, plums, apricots, olives, and cherries were needed to make carbon for gas masks, newspapers reported, "Confectioners and restaurants in various cities have begun to serve nuts and fruit at cost in order to turn in the pits and shells, a patriotic service. . . . Every American man, woman or child who has a relative or friend in the army should consider it a matter of personal obligation to provide enough carbon making material for his gas mask." And so Red Cross chapters throughout the country collected thousands of tons of fruit pits—so many they were told, finally, to stop.

As William Maxwell, a novelist and *New Yorker* editor who grew up in Lincoln, Illinois, recalled, "[M]other would go down to roll bandages for the soldiers. She put something like a dish towel on her head with a red cross on the front and wore white, and in school we saved prune pits which were supposed to be turned into gas masks so that the town was aware of the war effort. . . . At all events there was an active sense of taking part in the war."

The war was absorbing all of the nation. The draft, originally limited to men aged twenty-one to thirty, was soon extended to men aged eighteen to forty-five. Even with the expanded base, the government declared that all men in that age group would be called within a year. *All* men, the government said.

The army would require as well at least one hundred thousand officers. The Student Army Training Corps was to provide many of that number: it would admit "men by voluntary induction, . . . placing them on active duty immediately."

In May 1918 Secretary of War Newton Baker wrote the presidents of all institutions "of Collegiate Grade," from Harvard in Cambridge, Massachusetts, to the North Pacific College of Dentistry in Portland, Oregon. He did not ask for cooperation, much less permission. He simply stated, "Military instruction under officers and non-commissioned officers of the Army will be provided in every institution of college grade which enroll 100 or more male students. . . . All students over the age of 18 will be encouraged to enlist. . . . The commanding officer . . . [will] enforce military discipline."

In August 1918 an underling followed Baker's letter with a memo to college administrators, stating that the war would likely necessitate "the mobilization of all physically-fit registrants under 21, within 10 months from this date. . . . The student, by voluntary induction, becomes a soldier in the United States Army, uniformed, subject to military discipline and with the pay of a private . . . on full active duty." Upon being activated, nearly all would be sent to the front. Twenty-year-olds would get only three months' training before activation, with younger men getting only a few months more. "In view of the comparatively short time during which most of the student-soldiers will remain in college and the exacting military duties awaiting them, academic instruction must necessarily be modified along the lines of direct military value."

Therefore the teaching of academic courses was to end, to be replaced by military training. Military officers were to take virtual command of each college in the country. High schools were "urged to intensify their instruction so that young men 17 and 18 years old may be qualified to enter college as quickly as possible."

The full engagement of the nation had begun the instant Wilson had chosen war. Initially the American Expeditionary Force in Europe was just that, a small force numbering little more than a skirmish line. But the American army was massing. And the forging of all the nation into a weapon was approaching completion.

That process would jam millions of young men into extraordinarily tight quarters in barracks built for far fewer. It would bring millions of workers into factories and cities where there was no housing, where men and women not only shared rooms but beds, where they not only shared beds but shared beds in shifts, where one shift of workers came home— if their room could be called a home—and climbed into a bed just vacated by others leaving to go to work, where they breathed the same air, drank from the same cups, used the same knives and forks.

That process also meant that through both intimidation and voluntary cooperation, despite a stated disregard for truth, the government controlled the flow of information.

The full engagement of the nation would thus provide the great sausage machine with more than one way to grind a body up. It would grind away with the icy neutrality that technology and nature share, and it would not limit itself to the usual cannon fodder.

CHAPTER TEN

WHILE AMERICA still remained neutral William Welch, then president of the National Academy of Sciences, and his colleagues watched as their European counterparts tried to perfect killing devices.

Technology has always mattered in war, but this was the first truly scientific war, the first war that matched engineers and their abilities to build not just artillery but submarines and airplanes and tanks, the first war that matched laboratories of chemists and physiologists devising or trying to counteract the most lethal poison gas. Technology, like nature, always exhibits the ice of neutrality however heated its effect. Some even saw the war itself as a magnificent laboratory in which to test and improve not just the hard sciences but theories of crowd behavior, of scientific management of the means of production, of what was thought of as the new science of public relations.

The National Academy had itself been created during the Civil War to advise the government on science, but it did not direct or coordinate scientific research on war technologies. No American institution did. In 1915 astronomer George Hale began urging Welch and others in the NAS to take the lead in creating such an institution. He convinced them, and in April 1916 Welch wrote Wilson, "The Academy now considers it to be its plain duty, in case of war or preparation for war, to volunteer its assistance and secure the enlistment of its members for any services we can offer."

Wilson had been a graduate student at the Hopkins when Welch had first arrived there and immediately invited him, Hale, and a few others to the White House. There they proposed to establish a National Research Council to direct all war-related scientific work. But they needed the president to formally request its creation. Wilson immediately agreed although he insisted the move remain confidential.

He wanted confidentiality because any preparation for war set off debate, and Wilson was about to use all the political capital he cared to in order to create the Council of National Defense, which was to lay plans for what would become, after the country entered the war, the virtual government takeover of the production and distribution of economic resources. The council's membership was comprised of six cabinet secretaries, including the secretaries of war and the navy, and seven men outside the government. (Ironically, considering Wilson's intense Christianity, three of the seven were Jews: Samuel Gompers, head of the American Federation of Labor; Bernard Baruch, the financier; and Julius Rosenwald, head of Sears. Almost simultaneously, Wilson appointed Brandeis to the Supreme Court. All this marked the first significant representation of Jews in government.)

But Wilson's silent approval was enough. Welch, Hale, and the others formed their new organization, bringing in respected scientists in several fields, scientists who asked other colleagues to conduct specific pieces of research, research that fitted in with other pieces, research that together had potential applications. And medicine, too, had become a weapon of war.

By then a kind of organizational chart had developed in American scientific medicine. This chart of course did not exist in any formal sense, but it was real.

At the top sat Welch, fully the impresario, capable of changing the lives of those upon whom his glance lingered, capable as well of directing great sums of money to an institution with a nod. Only he held such power in American science, and no one else has held such power since.

On the rung below him were a handful of contemporaries, men who had fought beside him to change medicine in the United States and who had well-deserved reputations. Perhaps Victor Vaughan ranked second to him as a builder of institutions; he had created a solid one at Michigan and been the single most important voice outside the Hopkins demanding reform of medical education. In surgery the brothers Charles and William Mayo were giants and immensely important allies in forcing change. In the laboratory Theobald Smith inspired. In public health Hermann Biggs had made the New York City Department of Health probably the best municipal health department in the world, and he had just taken over the state health department, while in Providence, Rhode Island, Charles Chapin had applied the most rigorous science to public health questions and reached conclusions that were revolutionizing public health practices. And in the U.S. Army, Surgeon General William Gorgas also had developed an international reputation, continuing and expanding upon George Sternberg's tradition.

Both the National Research Council and the Council of National Defense had medical committees that were controlled by Welch himself, Gorgas, Vaughan, and the Mayo brothers, all five of whom had already served as president of the American Medical Association. But conspicuous by his absence was Rupert Blue, then the civilian surgeon general and head of the U.S. Public Health Service (USPHS). Welch and his colleagues so doubted his abilities and judgment that they not only blocked him from serving on the committees but would not allow him even to name his own representative to them. Instead they picked a USPHS scientist they trusted. It was not a good sign that the head of the public health service was so little regarded.

From the beginning of their planning, these men focused on the biggest killer in war—not combat, but epidemic disease. Throughout the wars in history more soldiers had often died of disease than in battle or of their wounds. And epidemic disease had routinely spread from armies to civilian populations.

This was true not just in ancient times or in the American Civil War, in which two men died from disease for every battle-related death (counting both sides, one hundred eighty-five thousand troops died in combat or of their wounds, while three hundred seventy-three thousand died of disease). More soldiers had died of disease than combat even in the wars fought since scientists had adopted the germ theory and modern public health measures. In the Boer War that raged from 1899 to 1902 between Britain and the white settlers of South Africa, ten British troops died of disease for each combat-related death. (The British also put nearly a quarter of the Boer population in concentration camps, where 26,370 women and children died.) In the Spanish-American War in 1898, six American soldiers died of disease—nearly all of them from typhoid—for every one killed in battle or who died of his wounds.

The Spanish-American War deaths especially were entirely unnecessary. The army had expanded in a matter of months from twenty-eight thousand to two hundred seventy-five thousand, and Congress had appropriated $50 million for the military, but not a penny went to the army medical department; as a result, a camp of sixty thousand soldiers at Chickamauga had not a single microscope. Nor was army surgeon general Sternberg given any authority. Military engineers and line officers directly rejected his angry protests about a dangerously unsanitary camp design and water supply. Their stubbornness killed roughly five thousand American young men.

Other diseases could be equally dangerous. When even normally mild diseases such as whooping cough, chickenpox, and mumps invade a "virgin" human population, a population not previously exposed to them, they often kill in large numbers—and young adults are especially vulnerable. In the Franco-Prussian War in 1871, for example, measles killed 40 percent of those who fell ill during the siege of Paris, and a measles epidemic erupted in the U.S. Army in 1911, killing 5 percent of all the men who caught the disease.

Those facts were of deep concern to Welch, Vaughan, Gorgas, and the others. They committed themselves to ensuring that the best medical science be available to the military. Welch, sixty-seven years old, short, obese, and out of breath, put a uniform on, devoted much time to army business, and took a desk in Gorgas's personal office that he used whenever in Washington. Vaughan, sixty-five years old and equally obese at 275 pounds, put a uniform on and became head of the army's Division of Communicable Disease. Flexner at age fifty-four put a uniform on. Gorgas had them all commissioned majors, the highest rank then allowed (regulations were changed and they all later became colonels).

They thought not only about caring for soldiers wounded in combat. They thought not only about finding a source for digitalis, which was imported from Germany (Boy Scouts gathered foxglove in Oregon and tests found it produced a suitable drug), or surgical needles (these too were all imported, so they set up a U.S. factory to produce them), or discovering the most efficient way to disinfect huge amounts of laundry (they asked Chapin to look into this).

They thought about epidemic disease.

The single man who had the chief responsibility for the performance of military medicine was Surgeon General of the Army William Crawford Gorgas. The army gave him little authority with which to work—not much more than Sternberg had had. But he was a man able to accomplish much in the face of not only benign neglect but outright opposition from those above him.

Naturally optimistic and cheerful, devout, son of a Confederate officer who became president of the University of Alabama, Gorgas took up medicine ironically in pursuit of another aim: a military career. After he failed to get an appointment to West Point, it seemed his only way into the army, and he took it despite his father's bitter opposition. He soon became entirely comfortable in medicine and preferred to be addressed as "Doctor" rather than by rank, even as he rose to "General." He loved learning and set aside a fixed amount of minutes each day for reading, rotating his attention among fiction, science, and classical literature.

Gorgas had a distinct softness around his eyes that made him appear gentle, and he treated virtually everyone with whom he came into contact with dignity. His appearance and manner belied, however, his intensity, determination, focus, and occasional ferocity. In the midst of crisis or obstacles his public equanimity made him a center of calm, the kind that calmed and gave confidence to others. But in private, after encountering obtuseness if not outright stupidity in his superiors, he slammed drawers, hurled inkwells, and stormed out of his office muttering threats to quit.

Like Sternberg, he spent much of his early career at frontier posts in the West, although he also took Welch's course at Bellevue. Unlike Sternberg, he did not personally do any significant laboratory research. But he was every bit as tenacious, every bit as disciplined.

Two experiences epitomized both his abilities and his determination to do his job. The first came in Havana after the Spanish-American War. He did not belong to Walter Reed's team investigating yellow fever. Their work in fact did not convince him that the mosquito carried the disease. Nonetheless he was given the task of killing mosquitoes in Havana. He succeeded in this task—despite doubting its usefulness—so well that in

1902 yellow fever deaths there fell to zero. *Zero.* And malaria deaths fell by 75 percent. (The results convinced him that the mosquito hypothesis was correct.) An even more significant triumph came when he later took charge of clearing yellow fever from the construction sites along the Panama Canal. In this case his superiors rejected the mosquito hypothesis, gave him the barest minimum of resources, and tried to undermine his authority, his effort, and him personally, at one point demanding that he be replaced. He persisted—and succeeded—partly through his intelligence and insight into the problems disease presented, partly through his ability to maneuver bureaucratically. In the process he also earned a reputation as an international expert on public health and sanitation.

He became surgeon general of the army in 1914 and immediately began massaging congressmen and senators for money and authority to prepare in case the country went to war. He wanted no repeat of Sternberg's Spanish-American experience. Believing his work done, in 1917 he submitted his resignation to join a Rockefeller-sponsored international health project. When the United States entered the war, he withdrew his resignation.

Then sixty-three years old, white-haired, with a handlebar mustache, and thin—as a boy he had been almost fragile, and he remained thin despite an appetite for food that rivaled Welch's—he took as his first task surrounding himself with the best possible people, while simultaenously trying to inject his and their influence into army planning. His War Department seniors did not consult his department on the sites for its several dozen new cantonments, but army engineers did pay close attention to the medical department in the actual design of the training camps. They too wanted no repeat of the mistakes that had killed thousands of soldiers in 1898.

But only in one other area did the army medical department receive even a hearing from War Department leadership. That was its massive campaign against venereal disease, a campaign supported strongly by a political union of progressives, many of whom believed in perfecting secular society, and from Christian moralists. (The same political odd couple would soon unite to enact Prohibition.) Gorgas's office recognized "to what extremes the sexual moralist can go. How unpractical, how intolerant, how extravagant, even how unreasoning, if not scientifically dishonest, he can be." But it also knew that one-third of all workdays lost to illness in the army were caused by venereal disease. That loss the military would not tolerate.

The medical corps told enlisted men to masturbate instead of using prostitutes. It produced posters with such slogans as, "A Soldier who gets a dose is a traitor." It examined enlisted men twice a month for venereal disease, required any men infected to identify the person with whom or the building in which they had had sex, docked the pay of soldiers or sailors sick with venereal disease, and also made them subject to court-martial. With support from the most senior political leadership, the military by law prohibited prostitution and the sale of alcohol within five miles of any base—and the military had seventy bases with ten thousand or more soldiers or sailors scattered around the country. The health boards of twenty-seven states passed regulations allowing detention of people suffering venereal infection "until they are no longer a danger to the community." Eighty red-light districts were shut down. Even New Orleans had to close down its legendary Storyville, where prostitution was legal, where Buddy Bolden, Jelly Roll Morton, Louis Armstrong, and others had invented jazz in the whorehouses. And New Orleans mayor Martin Behrman was no reformer; he headed a political machine so tight it was called simply "the Ring."

But if Gorgas had the power to act decisively on venereal disease, if engineers listened to his sanitary experts in designing water supplies, the army paid him little heed on anything else. On no subject where he had only science behind him, science without political weight, could he get even a hearing from army superiors. Even when an American researcher developed an antitoxin for gangrene, Gorgas could not convince them to fund testing at the front. So Welch arranged for the Rockefeller Institute to pay the expenses of a team of investigators to go to Europe, and for the British army to test the antitoxin in British hospitals. (It worked, although not perfectly.)

In many ways, then, Gorgas, Welch, Vaughan, and their colleagues operated as a team independent of the army. But they could not operate independently in regard to epidemic disease, and they could not operate either independently or alone as camps filled with hundreds of thousands—in fact, millions—of young men.

When the war began there were one hundred forty thousand physicians in the United States. Only 776 of them were serving in the army or navy.

The military needed tens of thousands of physicians, and it needed them immediately. It would make no exceptions for scientists. Most would volunteer anyway. Most wanted to participate in this great crusade.

Welch and Vaughan joined the military, despite their being one hundred pounds overweight and past the regular army's mandatory retirement age, and they were not alone. Flexner joined at age fifty-four. Flexner's protégé Paul Lewis at Penn, Milton Rosenau at Harvard, and Eugene Opie at Washington University joined. All around the country laboratory scientists were joining.

And to avoid losing scientists piecemeal either as volunteers or to the draft, Flexner suggested to Welch that the entire Rockefeller Institute be incorporated into the army. Welch carried the idea to Gorgas, and Gorgas's deputy wired Flexner, "[U]nit will be arranged as you desire." And so the Rockefeller Institute became Army Auxiliary Laboratory Number One. There would be no auxiliary laboratory number two. Men in uniforms marched down laboratory and hospital corridors. An army adjutant commanded the technicians and janitors, maintained army discipline among them, and drilled them on parade on York Avenue. Lunch became "mess." A mobile hospital unit on wheels with buildings, wards, labs, laundry, and kitchen was rolled into the front yard of the institute from Sixty-fourth to Sixty-sixth Streets to treat soldiers with intractable wounds. Sergeants saluted scientists who—except for two Canadians who became privates—received officer rank.

This was no mere cosmetic change to allow life to go on as usual.* At Rockefeller the fiber of the work was rewoven. Nearly all research shifted to something war-related, or to instruction. Alexis Carrel, a Nobel laureate in 1912 who pioneered the surgical reattachment of limbs and organ transplantation as well as tissue culture—he kept part of a chicken heart alive for thirty-two years—taught surgical techniques to hundreds of newly militarized physicians. Others taught bacteriology. A biochemist studied poison gas. Another chemist explored ways to get more acetone from starch, which could be used both in making explosives and to stiffen the fabric that covered airplane wings. Peyton Rous, who had already

---

*During the Vietnam War many physician-scientists joined the Public Health Service to avoid the draft. But their work did go on as usual. They were assigned to the National Institutes of Health, which enjoyed some of its most productive years in history because of the influx of talent.

done the work that would later—decades later—win him a Nobel Prize, redirected his work to preserving blood; he developed a method still in use that led to the first blood banks being established at the front in 1917.

The war also consumed the supply of practicing physicians. Gorgas, Welch, and Vaughan had already laid plans for this. In December 1916 they had, through the Council of National Defense, asked state medical associations to secretly grade physicians. Roughly half of all practicing physicians were judged incompetent to serve. So when America did enter the war, the military first examined every male graduate of medical school in 1914, 1915, and 1916, seeking, as Vaughan said, the "best from these classes." This would supply approximately ten thousand doctors. Many of the best medical schools also sent much of their faculty to France, where the schools functioned as intact units, staffing and unofficially lending their names to entire military hospitals.

Yet these moves could not begin to satisfy the need. By the time the Armistice was signed thirty-eight thousand physicians would be serving in the military, at least half of all those under age forty-five considered fit for service.

The military, and especially the army, did not stop there. In April 1917 the army had fifty-eight dentists; in November 1918 it had 5,654. And the military needed nurses.

There were too few nurses. Nursing had, like medicine, changed radically in the late nineteenth century. It too had become scientific. But changes in nursing involved factors that went beyond the purely scientific; they involved status, power, and the role of women.

Nursing was one of the few fields that gave women opportunity and status, and that they controlled. While Welch and his colleagues were revolutionizing American medicine, Jane Delano, Lavinia Dock—both of whom were students in Bellevue's nursing program while Welch was exposing medical students there to new realities—and others were doing the same to nursing. But they fought not with an entrenched Old Guard in their own profession so much as with physicians. (Sometimes physicians, threatened by intelligent and educated nurses, waged a virtual guerrilla war; in some hospitals physicians replaced labels on drug bottles with numbers so nurses could not question a prescription.)

In 1912, before becoming surgeon general, Gorgas had anticipated that if war ever came, the army would need vast numbers of nurses, many more than would likely be available. He believed, however, that not all of them would have to be fully trained. He wanted to create a corps of "practical nurses," who lacked the education and training of "graduate nurses."

Others were also advancing this idea, but they were all men. The women who ran nursing would have none of it. Jane Delano had taught nursing and had headed the Army Nurse Corps. Proud and intelligent as well as tough, driven, and authoritarian, she had then just left the army to establish the Red Cross nursing program, and the Red Cross had all responsibility for supplying nurses to the army, evaluating, recruiting, and often assigning them.

She rejected Gorgas's plan, telling her colleagues it "seriously threatened" the status of professional nursing and warning, "Our Nursing Service would be of no avail with these groups of women unrelated to us, organized by physicians, taught by physicians, serving under their guidance." She told the Red Cross bluntly that "if this plan were put through I should at once sever my connection with the Red Cross . . . [and] every member of the State and Local Committee would go out with me."*

The Red Cross and the army surrendered to her. No training of nursing aides commenced. When the United States entered the war it had 98,162 "graduate nurses," women whose training probably exceeded that of many—if not most—doctors trained before 1910. The war sucked up nurses as it sucked up everything else. In May 1918 roughly sixteen thousand nurses were serving in the military. Gorgas believed that the army alone needed fifty thousand.

After Gorgas again pleaded with the Red Cross "to carry out the plans already formulated," after learning confidential information about the desperation in combat hospitals, Delano reversed herself, supported Gorgas, and tried to convince her colleagues of the need for "practical" nurses.

Her professional colleagues rebuffed them both. They refused to participate in organizing any large training program of such aides, and

---

*It would seem nurses needed their status protected. In the summer of 1918, the Treasury Department informed the secretary of war that army nurses taken captive, unlike soldiers, were not entitled to pay while they were prisoners of war. Outrage later forced a reversal of this policy.

agreed only to establish an Army Nursing School. By October 1918 this new nursing school had produced not a single fully trained nurse.

The triumph of the nursing profession at large over the Red Cross and the United States Army, an army at war, was extraordinary. That the victors were women made it more extraordinary. Ironically, this triumph reflected as well a triumph of George Creel's Committee on Public Information over the truth, for Creel's propaganda machine had prevented the public from learning just how profound the need for nurses was.

In the meantime the military's appetite for doctors and nurses only grew. Four million American men were under arms with more coming, and Gorgas was planning for three hundred thousand hospital beds. The number of trained medical staff he had simply could not handle that load. So the military suctioned more and more nurses and physicians into cantonments, aboard ships, into France, until it had extracted nearly all the best young physicians. Medical care for civilians deteriorated rapidly. The doctors who remained in civilian life were largely either incompetent young ones or those over forty-five years of age, the vast majority of whom had been trained in the old ways of medicine. The shortage of nurses would prove even more serious. Indeed, it would prove deadly, especially in civil society.

All this added kindling to the tinderbox. Still more kindling would come.

CHAPTER ELEVEN

WILSON HAD DEMANDED that "the spirit of ruthless brutality . . . enter into the very fibre of national life." To carry out that charge Creel had wanted to create "one white-hot mass," a mass driven by "deathless determination." He was doing so. This was truly total war, and that totality truly included the medical profession.

Creel's spirit even injected itself into *Military Surgeon,* a journal published by the army for its physicians, which said, "Every single activity of this country is directed towards one single object, the winning of the war; nothing else counts now, and nothing will count ever if we don't win it. No organization of any kind should be countenanced that has not this object in immediate view and is likely to help in the most efficient way. . . . Thus the medical sciences are applied to war, the arts are applied in perfecting camouflage, in reviving the spirits of our soldiers by entertainment, etc."

This medical journal, this journal for physicians whose goal was to save life, also declared, "The consideration of human life often becomes quite secondary. . . . The medical officer has become more absorbed in the general than the particular, and the life and limb of the individual, while of great importance, are secondary to measures pro bono publico." And this same journal expressed its opinion of what constituted pro bono publico when it quoted approvingly advice from Major Donald McRae, a combat veteran who said, "If any enemy wounded are found (in the trench) they should be bayonetted, if sufficient prisoners [for inter-rogation] have been taken."

Gorgas did not share the views of the journal's editors. When the investi-gator funded by Rockefeller found his gangrene antitoxin effective, he wanted to publish his results—which could help the Germans. Both Gor-gas and Secretary of War Newton Baker agreed that he should do so, and he did. Welch told Flexner, "I was very glad that both the Secretary and Surgeon General without any hesitation took this position."

But Gorgas had more important things to do than police the editors of *Military Surgeon*. He was focusing upon his mission, and he was pursu-ing it with the obsessiveness of a missionary. For Gorgas had a nightmare.

The U.S. Army had exploded from a few tens of thousands of soldiers before the war to millions in a few months. Huge cantonments, each holding roughly fifty thousand men, were thrown together in a matter of weeks. Hundreds of thousands of men occupied them before the camps were completed. They were jammed into those barracks that were fin-ished, barracks designed for far less than their number, while tens of thousands of young soldiers lived through the first winter in tents. Hos-pitals were the last buildings to be constructed.

These circumstances not only brought huge numbers of men into this most intimate proximity but exposed farm boys to city boys from hun-dreds of miles away, each of them with entirely different disease immuni-ties and vulnerabilities. Never before in American history—and possibly never before in any country's history—had so many men been brought together in such a way. Even at the front in Europe, even with the impor-tation there of labor from China, India, and Africa, the concentration and throwing together of men with different vulnerabilities may not have been as explosive a mix as that in American training camps.

Gorgas's nightmare was of an epidemic sweeping through those camps. Given the way troops moved from camp to camp, if an outbreak of infectious disease erupted in one, it would be extraordinarily difficult to isolate that camp and keep the disease from spreading to others. Thou-sands, possibly tens of thousands, could die. Such an epidemic might spread to the civilian population as well. Gorgas intended to do all within his power to prevent his nightmare from becoming real.

．　　　．　　　．

By 1917 medical science was far from helpless in the face of disease. It stood in fact on the banks of the river Styx. If it was able to wade into those waters and pull only a few people back from that crossing, in its laboratories lay the promise of much more.

True, science had so far developed only a single one of the "magic bullets" envisaged by Paul Ehrlich. He and a colleague had tried nine hundred different chemical compounds to cure syphilis before retesting the 606th one. It was an arsenic compound; this time they made it work, curing syphilis without poisoning the patient. Named Salversan, it was often called just "606."

But science had achieved considerable success in manipulating the immune system and in public health. Vaccines prevented a dozen diseases that devastated livestock, including anthrax and hog cholera. Investigators had also gone far beyond the first success against smallpox and were now developing vaccines to prevent a host of diseases as well as antitoxins and serums to cure them. Science had triumphed over diphtheria. Sanitary and public health measures were containing typhoid, cholera, yellow fever, and bubonic plague, and vaccines against typhoid, cholera, and plague also appeared. Antitoxin for snake bites went into production. An antiserum for dysentery was found. A tetanus antitoxin brought magical results—before its widespread use, in 1903 in the United States 102 people died out of every 1,000 treated for tetanus; ten years later universal use of the antitoxin lowered the death rate to 0 per 1,000 treated. Meningitis had been checked, if not conquered, largely by Flexner's antiserum. In 1917 an antitoxin for gangrene was developed; although it was not nearly as effective as other antitoxins, scientists could improve it as they had improved others, over time. The possibilities of manipulating the immune system to defeat infectious disease seemed to hold enormous promise.*

At the management level Gorgas was taking action too. He saw to it

---

*When antibiotics first appeared in the late 1930s and 1940s, they performed like magic, and much of this research was abandoned; in the early 1960s, public health officials were declaring victory over infectious disease. Now, with dozens of strains of bacteria developing resistance to drugs, with viruses gaining resistance even faster, with such diseases as tuberculosis, once considered conquered, making comebacks, investigators have returned to searching for ways to stimulate the immune system against everything from infections to cancer.

that many of the new army doctors assigned to the cantonments were trained at the Rockefeller Institute by some of the best scientists in the world. He began stockpiling huge quantities of vaccines, antitoxins, and sera. He did not rely for these products on drug manufacturers; they were unreliable and often useless. In 1917 in fact New York State health commissioner Hermann Biggs tested commercial products for several diseases and found them so poor that he banned all sales from all drug manufacturers in New York State. So Gorgas assigned production to people he could rely upon. The Army Medical School would make enough typhoid vaccine for five million men. The Rockefeller Institute would produce sera for pneumonia, dysentery, and meningitis. The Hygienic Laboratory in Washington, which ultimately grew into the National Institutes of Health, would prepare smallpox vaccine and antitoxins for diphtheria and tetanus.

He also transformed several railroad cars into the most modern laboratory facilities—the equipping of these cars was paid for not by the government but by the Rockefeller Institute and the American Red Cross—and stationed these rolling laboratories at strategic points around the country, ready, as Flexner told Gorgas's deputy for scientific matters, Colonel Frederick Russell, to "be sent to any one of the camps at which pneumonia or other epidemic disease prevails."

Also, even before construction began on the cantonments, Gorgas created a special unit for "the prevention of infectious disease." He assigned the very best men to it. Welch, who had already toured British and French camps and was alert to possible weak points, headed this unit, and its five other members were Flexner, Vaughan, Russell, Biggs, and Rhode Island's Charles Chapin. Each of them had international renown. They laid out precise procedures for the army to follow to minimize the chances of an epidemic.

Meanwhile, as troops were pouring into the camps in 1917, Rockefeller Institute colleagues Rufus Cole, Oswald Avery, and others who had turned their focus to pneumonia issued a specific warning: "Although pneumonia occurs chiefly in endemic form, small and even large epidemics are not unknown. It was the most serious disease which threatened the construction of the Panama Canal"—more so even than yellow fever, as Gorgas well knew—"and its prevalence in regions where large numbers of susceptible workers are brought together renders it of great importance. . . . Pneumonia [seems] especially likely to attack raw recruits. The experience among the small number of troops in the Mexican border, where pneumonia occurred in epidemic form [in 1916], should be a warning of what is likely to happen in our national army when large numbers of susceptible men are brought together during the winter months."

Gorgas's army superiors ignored the advice. As a result, the army soon suffered a taste of epidemic disease. It would be a test run, for both a virus and medicine.

The winter of 1917–18 was the coldest on record east of the Rocky Mountains, barracks were jam-packed, and hundreds of thousands of men were still living in tents. Camp hospitals and other medical facilities had not yet been finished. An army report conceded the failure to provide warm clothing or even heat. But most dangerous was the overcrowding.

Flexner warned that the situation "was as if the men had pooled their diseases, each picking up the ones he had not had, . . . greatly assisted by the faulty laying out of the camps, poor administration, and lack of adequate laboratory facilities." Vaughan protested impotently and later called army procedures "insane. . . . How many lives were sacrificed I can not estimate. . . . The dangers in mobilization steps followed were pointed out to the proper authorities before there was any assembly, but the answer was: 'The purpose of mobilization is to convert civilians into trained soldiers as quickly as possible and not to make a demonstration in preventive medicine.'"

In that bitterly cold winter, measles came to the army's barracks, and it came in epidemic form. Usually, of course, measles infects children and causes only fever, rash, cough, runny nose, and discomfort. But like many other children's diseases—especially viral diseases—when measles strikes adults, it often strikes hard. (Early in the twenty-first century, measles is still causing one million deaths a year worldwide.)

This outbreak racked its victims with high fever, extreme sensitivity to light, and violent coughs. Complications included severe diarrhea, meningitis, encephalitis (inflammation of the brain), violent ear infections, and convulsions.

As infected soldiers moved from camp to camp, the virus moved with them, rolling through camps like a bowling ball knocking down pins.

Vaughan reported, "Not a troop train came into Camp Wheeler [near Macon, Georgia] in the fall of 1917 without bringing from one to six cases of measles already in the eruptive stage. These men . . . distributed its seeds at the encampment and on the train. No power on earth could stop the spread of measles under these conditions."

Camp Travis outside San Antonio held 30,067 men. By Christmas, 4,571 men had come down with the disease. Funston had an average troop strength of over fifty-six thousand; three thousand were sick enough to require hospitalization. At Greenleaf in South Carolina, Devens in Massachusetts, the numbers were comparable. The 25,260 troops at Camp Cody in New Mexico were free of measles until soon after the arrival of men from Funston. Then measles began roaring through Cody, too.

And some young men began to die.

Investigators could develop neither a vaccine to prevent measles nor a serum to cure it, but most deaths were coming chiefly from secondary infections, from bacteria invading the lungs after the virus had weakened their defenses. And investigators at Rockefeller and elsewhere struggled to find a way to control these bacterial infections. They made some progress.

Meanwhile the army issued orders forbidding men from crowding around stoves, and officers entered barracks and tents to enforce it. But especially for the tens of thousands who lived in tents in the record cold, it was impossible to keep men from crowding around stoves.

Of all the complications of measles, the most deadly by far was pneumonia. In the six months from September 1917 to March 1918, before the influenza epidemic struck, pneumonia struck down 30,784 soldiers on American soil. It killed 5,741 of them. Nearly all these pneumonia cases developed as complications of measles. At Camp Shelby, 46.5 percent of all deaths—*all* deaths from all diseases, all car wrecks, all work accidents, all training mishaps combined—were a result of pneumonia following measles. At Camp Bowie, 227 soldiers died from disease in November and December 1917; 212 of them died of pneumonia after measles. The average death rate from pneumonia in twenty-nine cantonments was twelve times that of civilian men of the same age.

In 1918 the Republican-controlled Senate held hearings on the Wilson administration's mistakes in mobilizing the military. Republicans had despised Wilson since 1912, when he reached the White House despite winning only 41 percent of the vote. (Former Republican president and then third-party candidate Teddy Roosevelt and incumbent Republican president William Howard Taft split the GOP vote, and Socialist Eugene Debs also won 6 percent.) Mobilization failures seemed a perfect opportunity to embarrass him. And there was personal bitterness in the attacks: Congressman Augustus Peabody Gardner, son-in-law of Senate Majority Leader Henry Cabot Lodge, had resigned from Congress and enlisted, only to die of pneumonia in camp.

Gorgas was summoned to explain the measles fiasco. His testimony and his report on the epidemic to the chief of staff made front-page news. Like his mentor Sternberg during the typhoid debacle twenty years earlier, he lacerated his War Department colleagues and superiors for rushing troops to cantonments under living conditions that failed to meet minimum public health standards, for overcrowding, for exposing recruits to measles who had no immunity, for using untrained "country boys" to care for desperately sick men in poorly equipped hospitals and sometimes without hospitals at all. And he stated that the War Department seemed to consider the Medical Department of the army unimportant. "I was never in their confidence, no," he said in response to one senator's question.

He had hoped his testimony would force the army to give him more power to protect troops. Perhaps it did; the army initiated courts-martial at three cantonments. But his testimony also isolated him. He confided to his sister that, in the War Department, "All my friends seem to have deserted me and everybody is giving me a kick as I pass by."

Meanwhile, Welch visited one of the worst-hit camps, a camp where measles itself had left but where victims with complications still lingered. He told Gorgas that the mortality rate for troops developing pneumonia after measles "is stated to be 30% but more now in hospital will die. A good statistician needed in hospital—registrar not competent." To give the men in the hospital a better chance to survive, he continued, "Have Colonel Russell send directions for Avery's medicine for pneumococcus type work."

He was referring to the Rockefeller Institute's Oswald Avery, one of the Canadians there who had been inducted into the army as only a private. Private or not, he soon would be, if he was not already, the world's leading investigator of pneumonia. And conclusions Avery would reach would have import far—very, very far—beyond that subject. His findings would create a scientific revolution that would change the direction of all genetic research and create modern molecular biology. But that would come later.

Osler called pneumonia "the captain of the men of death." Pneumonia was the leading cause of death around the world, greater than tuberculosis, greater than cancer, greater than heart disease, greater than plague.

And, like measles, when influenza kills, it usually kills through pneumonia.

CHAPTER TWELVE

MEDICAL DICTIONARIES define pneumonia as "an inflammation of the lungs with consolidation." This definition omits mention of an infection, but in practice pneumonia is almost always caused by some kind of microorganism invading the lung, followed by an infusion of the body's infection-fighting weapons. The resulting inflamed mix of cells, enzymes, cell debris, fluid, and the equivalent of scar tissue thickens and leads to the consolidation; then the lung, normally soft and spongy, becomes firm, solid, inelastic. The disease kills usually when either the consolidation becomes so widespread that the lungs cannot transfer enough oxygen into the bloodstream, or the pathogen enters the bloodstream and carries the infection throughout the body.

Pneumonia maintained its position as the leading cause of death in the United States until 1936. It and influenza are so closely linked that modern international health statistics, including those compiled by the United States Centers for Disease Control, routinely classify them as a single cause of death. Even now, early in the twenty-first century, with antibiotics, antiviral drugs, oxygen, and intensive-care units, influenza and pneumonia combined routinely rank as the fifth or sixth—it varies year to year, usually depending on the severity of the influenza season—leading cause of death in the United States and the leading cause of death from infectious disease.

Influenza causes pneumonia either directly, by a massive viral invasion of the lungs, or indirectly—and more commonly—by destroying certain parts of the body's defenses and allowing so-called secondary invaders, bacteria, to infest the lungs virtually unopposed. There is also evidence that the influenza virus makes it easier for some bacteria to invade the lung not only by generally wiping out defense mechanisms but by specifically facilitating some bacteria's ability to attach to lung tissue.

Although many bacteria, viruses, and fungi can invade the lung, the single most common cause of pneumonia is the pneumococcus, a bacterium that can be either a primary or secondary invader. (It causes approximately 95 percent of lobar pneumonias, involving one or more entire lobes, although a far lesser percentage of bronchopneumonias.) George Sternberg, while working in a makeshift laboratory on an army post in 1881, first isolated this bacterium from his own saliva, inoculated rabbits with it, and learned that it killed. He did not recognize the disease as pneumonia. Neither did Pasteur, who discovered the same organism later but published first, so scientific etiquette gives him priority in the discovery. Three years later a third investigator demonstrated that this bacterium frequently colonized the lungs and caused pneumonia, hence its name.

Under the microscope the pneumococcus looks like a typical streptococcus, a medium-size elliptical or round bacterium usually linked with others in a chain, although the pneumococcus usually is linked only to one other bacterium—and is sometimes called a diplococcus—like two pearls side by side. When exposed to sunlight it dies within ninety minutes, but it survives in moist sputum in a dark room for ten days. It can be found occasionally on dust particles. In virulent form, it can be highly infectious—in fact it can itself cause epidemics.

As early as 1892 scientists tried to make a serum to treat it. They failed. In the next decades, while investigators were making enormous advances against other diseases, they made almost no progress against pneumonia. This was not through lack of trying. Whenever researchers made any progress against diphtheria, plague, typhoid, meningitis, tetanus, snake bite, and other killers, they immediately applied the same methods against pneumonia. Still nothing even hinted at success.

Investigators were working at the very outermost edge of science. Gradually they improved their ability to produce a serum that protected an animal, but not people. And they struggled to understand how this serum worked, advancing hypotheses that might eventually lead to therapies. Sir Almroth Wright, who was knighted for developing a typhoid vaccine, speculated that the immune system coated invading organisms with what he called "opsonins," which made it far easier for white blood cells to devour the invader. His insight was correct, but he was wrong in the conclusions he drew from this insight.

Nowhere was pneumonia more severe than among workers in South Africa's gold and diamond mines. Epidemic conditions were virtually constant and outbreaks routinely killed 40 percent of the men who got sick. In 1914 South African mine owners asked Wright to devise a vaccine against pneumonia. He claimed success. In fact he not only failed, his vaccinations could kill. This and other errors earned Wright the mocking nickname "Sir Almost Right" from competing investigators.

But by then two German scientists had found a clue to the problem in treating or preventing pneumonia. In 1910 they distinguished between what they called "typical" pneumococci and "atypical" pneumococci. They and others tried to develop this clue.

Yet as the Great War began so little progress had been made against pneumonia that Osler himself still recommended venesection—bleeding: "We employ it nowadays much more than we did a few years ago, but more often late in the disease than early. To bleed at the very onset in robust, healthy individuals in whom the disease sets in with great intensity and high fever is, I believe, a good practice."

Osler did not claim that bleeding cured pneumonia, only that it might relieve certain symptoms. He was wrong. The 1916 edition of his textbook also stated, "Pneumonia is a self-limited disease, which can neither be aborted nor cut short by any known means at our command."

Americans were about to challenge that conclusion.

When Rufus Cole came to the Rockefeller Institute to head its hospital, he decided to focus most of his own energies and those of the team he put together on pneumonia. It was an obvious choice, since it was the biggest killer.

To cure or prevent pneumonia required, as with all other infectious diseases at the time, manipulating the body's own defenses, the immune system.

In the diseases scientists could defeat, the antigen—the molecules on the surfaces of invading organisms that stimulated the immune system to respond, the target the immune response aimed at—did not change. In diphtheria the dangerous part was not even the bacteria itself but a toxin the bacteria produced.

The toxin was not alive, did not evolve, and had a fixed form, and the production of antitoxin had become routine. Horses were injected with gradually increasing doses of virulent bacteria. The bacteria made the toxin. In turn, the horse's immune system generated antibodies that bound to and neutralized the toxin. The horse was then bled, solids removed from the blood until only the serum remained, and this was then purified into the antitoxin that had become so common and lifesaving.

An identical process produced tetanus antitoxin, Flexner's serum against meningitis, and several other sera or antitoxins. Scientists were vaccinating the horse against a disease, then extracting the horse antibodies and injecting them into people. This borrowing of immune-system defenses from an outside source is called "passive immunity."

When vaccines are used to stimulate people's own immune systems directly, so that they develop their own defenses against bacteria or viruses, it is called "active immunity."

But in all the diseases treated successfully so far, the antigens, the target the immune system aimed at, remained constant. The target stayed still; it did not move. And so the target was easy to hit.

The pneumococcus was different. The discovery of "typical" and "atypical" pneumococci had opened a door, and investigators were now finding many types of the bacteria. Different types had different antigens. Sometimes also the same type was virulent, sometimes not, but why one killed and another caused mild or no disease was not yet a question anyone was designing experiments to answer. That lay out there for the future, a sort of undertow pulling at the data. The focus was far more immediate: finding a curative serum, a preventative vaccine, or both.

By 1912 Cole at Rockefeller had developed a serum that had measurable if not dramatic curative power against a single type of pneumococcus. He happened to read a paper by Avery on an entirely different subject—secondary infections in victims of tuberculosis. Although narrow and hardly a classic, the paper still made a deep impression on Cole. It was solid, thorough, tight, and yet was deeply analytical, showing an awareness of the potential implications of the conclusions and possible new directions for research. It also demonstrated Avery's knowledge of chemistry and ability to carry out a fully scientific laboratory investigation of illness in patients. Cole wrote Avery a note offering him a job at the institute. Avery did not reply. Cole sent a second note. Still he received no reply. Finally Cole visited Avery and raised the salary offer. Later he realized Avery rarely read his mail. It was typical of Avery; his focus was always on his experiments. Now he accepted. Soon after the Great War started, but before America's entry into it, Avery also began working on pneumonia.

Pneumonia was Cole's passion. For Avery it would become an obsession.

Oswald Avery was a short thin fragile man, a tiny man really who weighed at most 110 pounds. With his large head and intense eyes, he looked like someone who would have been laughed at as an "egghead," if that word had been in use then, and bullied in a schoolyard as a boy. If that was the case, it appeared to have left no scars; he seemed friendly, cheerful, even outgoing.

Born in Montreal, he grew up in New York City the son of a Baptist minister who preached at a church in the city. He had a good many talents. At Colgate University he tied for first prize in an oratory contest with classmate Harry Emerson Fosdick, who became among the most prominent preachers of the early twentieth century (Fosdick's brother Raymond ultimately headed the Rockefeller Foundation; John Rockefeller Sr. built Riverside Church for Harry). Avery also played cornet well enough to have performed in concert with the National Conservatory of Music—a concert conducted by Antonín Dvořák—and he often drew ink caricatures and painted landscapes.

Yet for all his outward friendliness and sociability, Avery spoke himself of what he called "the true inwardness of research."

René Dubos, an Avery protégé, recalled, "To a few of us who saw him in every day life, however, there was often revealed another aspect of his personality, . . . a more haunting quality, . . . a melancholy figure whistling gently to himself the lonely tune of the shepherd song in *Tristan and Isolde*. An acute need for privacy, even if it had to be bought at the cost of loneliness, conditioned much of Avery's behavior."

If the phone rang Avery would talk animatedly, as if happy to hear from the caller, but when he hung up, Dubos recalled, "It was as if a mask dropped, his smile replaced with a tired and almost tortured expression, the telephone pushed away on the desk as a symbol of protest against the encroaching world."

Like Welch, he never married, nor was he known to have had an emotional or intimate relationship with anyone of either sex. Like Welch, he could be charming and the center of attention; he did comic impersonations so well that one colleague called him "a natural born comedian." Yet he resented any kind of intrusion upon himself, resented even attempts by others to entertain him.

Everything else about him was the opposite of Welch. Welch read widely, had curiosity about everything, traveled throughout Europe, China, and Japan, and seemed to embrace the universe. Welch often sought relaxation in elaborate dinners and almost daily retreated to his club. And Welch as a very young man was recognized as marked for great things.

Avery was none of those things. He was certainly not considered a brilliant young investigator. When Cole hired him, he was almost forty years old. By forty Welch was moving in the highest circles of science internationally. By forty those of Avery's contemporaries who would leave any significant scientific legacy had already made names for themselves. Yet Avery, like much younger investigators at Rockefeller, was essentially on probation and had made no particular mark. Indeed, he had made no mark—but not from want of ambition, nor from lack of work.

While Welch constantly socialized and traveled, Avery had almost no personal life. He fled from one. He almost never entertained and rarely went out to dinner. Although he was close to and felt responsible for his younger brother and an orphaned cousin, his life, his world, was his research. All else was extraneous. Once the editor of a scientific journal asked him to write a memorial piece about Nobel laureate Karl Landsteiner, with whom he had worked closely at Rockefeller. In it Avery said nothing whatsoever about Landsteiner's personal life. The editor asked him to insert some personal details. Avery refused, stating that personal information would help the reader understand nothing that mattered, neither Landsteiner's achievements nor his thought processes.

(Landsteiner likely would have approved Avery's treatment. When he was notified he'd won the Nobel Prize, he continued working in his laboratory all day, got home so late that his wife was asleep, and did not wake her to give her the news.)

The research mattered, Avery was saying, not the life. And the life of research, like that of any art, lay within. As Einstein once said, "One of the strongest motives that lead persons to art or science is a flight from the everyday life. . . . With this negative motive goes a positive one. Man seeks to form for himself, in whatever manner is suitable for him, a simplified and lucid image of the world, and so to overcome the world of experience by striving to replace it to some extent by this image. This is what the painter does, and the poet, the speculative philosopher, the natural scientist, each in his own way. Into this image and its formation, he places the center of gravity of his emotional life, in order to attain the peace and serenity that he cannot find within the narrow confines of swirling personal experience."

With the possible exception of his love for music, Avery seemed to have no existence outside the laboratory. For years he shared the same apartment with Alphonse Dochez, another bachelor scientist who worked closely with him at Rockefeller, and a shifting cast of more temporary scientist-roommates who left when they got married or changed jobs. Avery's roommates lived normal lives, going out, going away for a weekend. When they came home, there would be Avery, ready to begin a lengthy conversation that lasted deep into the night about an experimental problem or result.

But if Avery had little personal life, he did have ambition. His desire to make a mark after so long in the wilderness led him to publish two papers soon after he arrived at Rockefeller. In the first, based on only a few experiments, he and Dochez formulated "a sweeping metabolic theory of virulence and immunity." In the second, Avery again reached well beyond his experimental evidence for a conclusion.

Both were quickly proved wrong. Humiliated, he was determined never to suffer such embarrassment again. He became extraordinarily careful, extraordinarily cautious and conservative, in anything he published or even said outside his own laboratory. He did not stop speculating— privately—about the boldest and most far-reaching interpretations of an experiment, but from then on he published only the most rigorously tested and conservative conclusions. From then on, Avery would only— in public—inch his way forward. An inch at a time, he would ultimately cover an enormous and startling distance.

•   •   •

When one inches along progress comes slowly, but it can still be decisive. Cole and Avery worked together precisely the way Cole had hoped for when he organized the Rockefeller hospital. More importantly, the work produced results.

In the laboratory Avery and Dochez took the lead. They worked in simple laboratories with simple equipment. Each room had a single deep porcelain sink and several worktables, each with a gas outlet for a Bunsen burner and drawers underneath. The tabletop space was filled with racks of test tubes, simple mason jars, petri dishes—droppers for various dyes and chemicals, and tin cans holding pipettes and platinum loops. On the same tabletop investigators performed nearly all their work: inoculating, bleeding, and dissecting animals. Also on the tabletop was a cage for the occasional animal kept as a pet. In the middle of the room were incubators, vacuum pumps, and centrifuges.

First they replicated earlier experiments, partly to familiarize themselves with techniques. They exposed rabbits and mice to gradually increasing dosages of pneumococci. Soon the animals developed antibodies to the bacteria. They drew blood from them, allowed solids to settle out, siphoned off the serum, added chemicals to precipitate remaining solids, then purified the serum by passing it through several filters. Others had done the equivalent. They succeeded in curing mice with the serum. Others had done that, too. But the mice were not people.

In a way, they weren't really mice either. Scientists had to keep as many factors constant as possible, limit variables, to make it easier to understand precisely what caused an experimental result. So mice were inbred until all mice in a given strain had virtually identical genes, except for sex differences. (Male mice were and are generally not used in experiments because they sometimes attack each other; the death or injury of a single mouse for any reason can distort experimental results and ruin weeks of work.) These mice were fully alive but also model systems, with as much of the complexity, diversity, and spontaneity of life eliminated as possible; they were bred to be as close to a test tube as a living thing can be.*

---

*The same genetic lines of laboratory mice used by Avery are still in use today; the mice have been inbred since at least 1909 to be a useful tool. As one scientist at the National Cancer Institute says, "I can cure cancer in a mouse one hundred percent of the time. If you can't do that, you may as well hang it up."

But if scientists were curing mice, no one anywhere had made any progress in curing people. Experiment after experiment had failed. Elsewhere other investigators trying similar approaches quit, convinced by their failures that their theories were wrong or that their techniques were not good enough to yield results—or they simply grew impatient and moved on to easier problems.

Avery did not move on. He saw snatches of evidence suggesting he was right. He persisted, experimenting repeatedly, trying to learn from each failure. He and Dochez grew hundreds of cultures of pneumococci, changing the strains, learning more and more about its metabolism, changing the composition of the media in which the bacteria grew. (Soon Avery became one of the best in the world at figuring out what medium would most effectively grow different bacteria.) His background in both chemistry and immunology began paying off, and they used every piece of information as a wedge, pounding it into the problem, cracking or prying open other secrets, improving techniques, and, finally, gradually inching past the work that others had done.

They and others identified three fairly uniform and common strains of pneumococci, which they called simply Type I, Type II, and Type III. Other pneumococci were designated as Type IV, a catchall for dozens of other strains (ninety have been identified) that appeared less often. The first three types gave them a far more specific target for an antiserum, which they made. When they exposed different cultures of pneumococci to the serum they discovered that the antibodies in the serum would bind only to its matching culture and not to any other. The binding was even visible in a test tube without a microscope; the bacteria and antibodies clumped together. The process was called "agglutination" and was a test for specificity.

But many things that work in vitro, in the narrow universe of a test tube, fail in vivo, in the nearly infinite complexity of life. Now they went through the cycle of testing in rabbits and mice again, testing different strains of the bacteria in animals for killing potential, testing how well they generated antibodies, how well the antibodies bound to them. They tried injecting massive dosages of killed bacteria, thinking it might spark a large immune response, then using the serum generated by that technique. They tried mixing small doses of living bacteria and massive doses of dead ones. They tried live bacteria. In mice they ultimately achieved spectacular cure rates.

At the same time, Avery's understanding of the bacteria deepened. It deepened enough that he forced scientists to change their thinking about the immune system.

One of the most puzzling aspects of pneumococci was that some were virulent and lethal, some were not. Avery thought he had a clue to the answer to this question. He and Dochez focused on the fact that some pneumococci—but only some—were surrounded by a capsule made of polysaccharides, a sugar, like the hard shell of sugar surrounding the soft insides of M&M candy. Avery's very first paper on the pneumococcus, in 1917, dealt with these "specific soluble substances." He would pursue this subject for more than a quarter of a century. As he tried to unravel this puzzle, he began calling the pneumococcus, this killing bacterium, the "sugar-coated microbe." His pursuit would yield a momentous discovery and a deep understanding of life itself.

Meanwhile, with the rest of the Western world already at war, Cole, Avery, Dochez, and their colleagues were ready to test their immune serum in people.

CHAPTER THIRTEEN

E VEN WHEN COLE first tried the new serum on patients it showed promise. He and Avery immediately devoted themselves to refining their procedures in the laboratory, in the methods of infecting horses and producing serum, in the way they administered it. Finally they began a careful series of trials with a finished product. They found that giving large dosages of serum—half a liter—intravenously cut the death rate of Type I pneumonias by more than half, from 23 percent to 10 percent.

It was not a cure. Pneumonias caused by other types of pneumococci did not yield so easily. And, as Avery and Cole stated, "Protection in man is inferior to protection in mice."

But of all pneumonias, those caused by Type I pneumococci were the single most common. Cutting the death rate by more than half in the single most common pneumonia was progress, real progress, enough progress that in 1917 the institute published a ninety-page monograph by Cole, Avery, Dochez, and Henry Chickering, another young Rockefeller scientist, entitled "Acute Lobar Pneumonia Prevention and Serum Treatment."

It was a landmark work, for the first time explaining step-by-step a way to prepare and use a serum that could cure pneumonia. And it very much anticipated outbreaks of the disease in army cantonments, noting, "Pneumonia bids fair in the present war to lead all diseases as a cause of death."

In October 1917, Gorgas told army hospital commanders that, "in view of the probability that pneumonia will be one of the most important diseases amongst the troops," they must send even more doctors to the Rockefeller Institute to learn how to prepare and administer this serum. Avery, still a private, was already diverting time from his research to teach bacteriology to officers who would be working in cantonments. Now he and his colleagues also taught this serum therapy. His students, rather than call him "Private," addressed him respectfully as "Professor"—a nickname already occasionally given him. His colleagues shortened it to "Fess," which stuck with him for the rest of his life.

Simultaneously Cole, Avery, and Dochez were developing a vaccine to prevent pneumonia caused by Types I, II, and III pneumococci. After proving it worked in animals, they and six other Rockefeller researchers turned themselves into guinea pigs, testing its safety in humans by giving each other massive doses. All of them had negative reactions to the vaccine itself; three had severe reactions. They decided that the vaccine was too dangerous to administer in those dosages but planned another experiment with lower doses administered once a week for four weeks, which gave recipients time to gradually build up immunity.

This vaccine came too late for any large-scale impact on the measles epidemic, but at Camp Gordon outside Atlanta, a vaccine against the strain of pneumococcus causing most of the pneumonias there was tested on one hundred men with measles, with fifty men vaccinated and fifty used as controls. Only two of those vaccinated developed this pneumonia, compared to fourteen unvaccinated men.

Meanwhile, Cole wrote Colonel Frederick Russell, who during his own scientific career in the army had significantly improved typhoid vaccine, about "the progress we have already made in the matter of prophylactic vaccination against pneumonia." But, Cole added, "The manufacture of large amounts of vaccine will be a big matter, much more difficult than the manufacture of typhoid vaccine. . . . I have been getting an organization together so that the large amounts of media necessary could be prepared, and so the vaccine could be made on a large scale."

Cole's organization was ready for a large test in March 1918, just as influenza was first surfacing among soldiers in Kansas. The vaccine was given to twelve thousand troops at Camp Upton on Long Island—that used up all the vaccine available—while nineteen thousand troops served as controls, receiving no vaccine. Over the next three months, not a single vaccinated soldier developed pneumonia caused by any of the types of pneumococci vaccinated against. The controls suffered 101 cases. This result was not absolutely conclusive. But it was more than suggestive. And it was a far better result than was being achieved anywhere else in the world. The Pasteur Institute was also testing a pneumonia vaccine, but without success.

If Avery and Cole could develop a serum or vaccine with real effectiveness against the captain of death . . . If they could do that, it would be the greatest triumph medical science had yet known.

Both the prospect of finally being able to defeat pneumonia and its appearance in the army camps only intensified Gorgas's determination to find a way to limit its killing. He asked Welch to create and chair a special board on the disease. Gorgas wanted the board run, literally, out of his own office; Welch's desk was in Gorgas's personal office.

Welch demurred and called Flexner. Both men agreed that the best man in the country, and probably in the world, to chair the board was Rufus Cole. The next day Flexner and Cole got on a train to Washington to meet Gorgas and Welch at the Cosmos Club. There they picked the members of the pneumonia board, a board to be supported by all the knowledge and resources of Gorgas, Welch, Flexner, and the institutions they represented.

They chose well. Each person selected would later be elected to membership in the National Academy of Sciences, arguably the most exclusive scientific organization in the world.

Avery would of course lead the actual laboratory investigations and stay in New York. Most of the others would work in the field. Lieutenant Thomas Rivers, a Hopkins graduate and Welch protégé, would become one of the world's leading virologists and succeed Cole as head of the Rockefeller Institute Hospital. Lieutenant Francis Blake, another Rockefeller researcher, would become dean of the Yale Medical School. Captain Eugene Opie, regarded as one of the most brilliant of Welch's pathology students, was already dean of the Washington University Medical School when he joined the army. Collaborating with them, although not actual board members, were future Nobel laureates Karl Landsteiner at Rockefeller and George Whipple at the Hopkins. Years later another Rockefeller scientist recalled, "It was really a privilege to be on the pneumonia team."

On a routine basis—if such urgency could be routine—Cole traveled to Washington to discuss the latest findings with Welch and senior army medical officers in Gorgas's office. Cole, Welch, Victor Vaughan, and Russell had also been conducting a series of the most rigorous inspection tours of cantonments, checking on everything from the quality of the camp's surgeons, bacteriologists, and epidemiologists right down to the way camp kitchens washed dishes. Any recommendations they made were immediately ordered to be carried out. But they did not simply dictate; many of the camp hospitals and laboratories were run by men they respected, and they listened to ideas as well.

Late that spring, Cole reported to the American Medical Association one of his conclusions about measles: that it "seems to render the respiratory mucous membrane especially susceptible to secondary infection." He also believed that these secondary infections, like measles itself, "occur chiefly in epidemic form. . . . Every new case of the infection adds not only to the extent but also to the intensity of the epidemic."

On June 4, 1918, Cole, Welch, and several other members of the pneumonia board appeared in Gorgas's office once more, this time with Hermann Biggs, New York State health commissoner; Milton Rosenau, a prominent Harvard scientist who was then a navy lieutenant commander; and L. Emmett Holt, one of those instrumental in the founding of the Rockefeller Institute. This time the discussion was wide-ranging, focusing on how to minimize the possibility of something worse than the measles epidemic. They were all worried about Gorgas's nightmare.

They were not particularly worried about influenza, although they were tracking outbreaks of the disease. For the moment those outbreaks were mild, not nearly as dangerous as the measles epidemic had been. They well knew that when influenza kills, it kills through pneumonia, but Gorgas had already asked the Rockefeller Institute to gear up its production and study of pneumonia serum and vaccine, and both the institute and the Army Medical School had launched major efforts to do so.

Then the conversation turned from the laboratory to epidemiological issues. The inspection tours of the camps had convinced Welch, Cole, Vaughan, and Russell that cross-infections had caused many of the measles-related pneumonia deaths. To prevent such a problem from recurring, Cole suggested creating contagious-disease wards with specially trained staffs, something the best civilian hospitals had. Welch pointed out that the British had isolation hospitals with entirely separate organizations and rigid discipline. Another possible solution to cross-infection involved using cubicles in hospitals—creating a warren of partitions around hospital beds.

They also discussed overcrowding in hospitals and isolation of troops. Since 1916 the Canadian army had segregated all troops arriving in Britain for twenty-eight days, to prevent their infecting any trained troops ready to go to the front. Welch advised establishing similar "detention camps for new recruits where men are kept for 10–14 days."

They all recognized the difficulty of convincing the army to do this, or of convincing the army to end the even more serious problem of overcrowding in barracks.

Still, another army medical officer injected one piece of good news. He said that the problem of overcrowding in the hospitals themselves had been eliminated. Every hospital in the army had at least one hundred empty beds as of May 15, with a total of twenty-three thousand beds empty. Every single epidemiological statistic the army collected showed improved overall health. He insisted that facilities and training were adequate.

Time would tell.

Man might be defined as "modern" largely to the extent that he attempts to control, as opposed to adjust himself to, nature. In this relationship with nature, modern humanity has generally been the aggressor and a daring one at that, altering the flow of rivers, building upon geological faults, and, today, even engineering the genes of existing species. Nature has generally been languid in its response, although contentious once aroused and occasionally displaying a flair for violence.

By 1918 humankind was fully modern, and fully scientific, but too busy fighting itself to aggress against nature. Nature, however, chooses its own moments. It chose this moment to aggress against man, and it did not do so prodding languidly. For the first time, modern humanity, a humanity practicing the modern scientific method, would confront nature in its fullest rage.

■ Part IV
IT BEGINS

CHAPTER FOURTEEN

IT IS IMPOSSIBLE to prove that someone from Haskell County, Kansas, carried the influenza virus to Camp Funston. But the circumstantial evidence is strong. In the last week of February 1918, Dean Nilson, Ernest Elliot, John Bottom, and probably several others unnamed by the local paper traveled from Haskell, where "severe influenza" was raging, to Funston. They probably arrived between February 28 and March 2, and the camp hospital first began receiving soldiers with influenza on March 4. This timing precisely fits the incubation period of influenza. Within three weeks eleven hundred troops at Funston were sick enough to require hospitalization.

Only a trickle of people moved back and forth between Haskell and Funston, but a river of soldiers moved between Funston, other army bases, and France. Two weeks after the first case at Funston, on March 18, influenza surfaced at both Camps Forrest and Greenleaf in Georgia; 10 percent of the forces at both camps would report sick. Then, like falling dominoes, other camps erupted with influenza. In total, twenty-four of the thirty-six largest army camps experienced an influenza outbreak that spring. Thirty of the fifty largest cities in the country, most of them adjacent to military facilities, also suffered an April spike in "excess mortality" from influenza, although that did not become clear except in hindsight.

At first it seemed like nothing to worry about, nothing like the measles outbreak with its pneumonic complications. Only in Haskell had influenza been severe. The only thing at all worrisome was that the disease was moving.

As Macfarlane Burnet later said, "It is convenient to follow the story of influenza at this period mainly in regard to the army experiences in America and Europe."

After the pandemic, outstanding epidemiologists searched military and civilian health records in the United States for any signs of uncommon influenza activity prior to the Funston outbreak. They found none. (The warning published about Haskell misstated the date, incorrectly putting it after Funston.) In France there had been some localized flare-ups of influenza during the winter, but they did not seem to spread and behaved like endemic, not epidemic, disease.

The first unusual outbreaks in Europe occurred in Brest in early April, where American troops disembarked. In Brest itself a French naval command was suddenly crippled. And from Brest the disease did spread, and quickly, in concentric circles.

Still, although many got sick, these outbreaks were, like those in the United States, generally mild. Troops were temporarily debilitated, then recovered. For example, an epidemic erupted near Chaumont involving U.S. troops and civilians: of 172 marines guarding headquarters there, most fell ill and fifty-four required hospitalization—but all of them recovered.

The first appearance in the French army came April 10. Influenza struck Paris in late April, and at about the same time the disease reached Italy. In the British army the first cases occurred in mid-April, then the disease exploded. In May the British First Army alone suffered 36,473 hospital admissions and tens of thousands of less serious cases. In the Second Army, a British report noted, "At the end of May it appeared with great violence. . . . The numbers affected were very great. . . . A brigade of artillery had one-third of its strength taken ill within forty-eight hours, and in the brigade ammunition column only fifteen men were available for duty one day out of a strength of 145." The British Third Army suffered equally. In June troops returning from the Continent introduced the disease into England.

But again the complications were few and nearly all the troops recovered. The only serious concern—and it was serious indeed—was that the disease would undermine the troops' ability to fight.

That seemed the case in the German army. German troops in the field suffered sharp outbreaks beginning in late April. By then German commander Erich von Ludendorff had also begun his last great offensive—Germany's last real chance to win the war.

The German offensive made great initial gains. From near the front lines Harvey Cushing, Halsted's protégé, recorded the German advance in his diary: "They have broken clean through. . . ." "The general situation is far from reassuring. . . . 11 P.M. The flow of men from the retreating Front keeps up." "Haig's most disquieting Order to the Army . . . ends as follows: 'With our backs to the wall, and believing in the justice of our cause, each one of us must fight to the end. The safety of our homes and the freedom of mankind depend alike upon the conduct of every one of us at this moment.'"

But then Cushing noted, "The expected third phase of the great German offensive gets put off from day to day." "When the next offensive will come off no one knows. It probably won't be long postponed. I gather that the epidemic of grippe which hit us rather hard in Flanders also hit the Boche worse, and this may have caused the delay."

Ludendorff himself blamed influenza for the loss of initiative and the ultimate failure of the offensive: "It was a grievous business having to listen every morning to the chiefs of staff's recital of the number of influenza cases, and their complaints about the weakness of their troops."

Influenza may have crippled his attack, stripped his forces of fighting men. Or Ludendorff may have simply seized upon it as an excuse. British, French, and American troops were all suffering from the disease themselves, and Ludendorff was not one to accept blame when he could place it elsewhere.

In the meantime, in Spain the virus picked up its name.

Spain actually had few cases before May, but the country was neutral during the war. That meant the government did not censor the press, and unlike French, German, and British newspapers—which printed nothing negative, nothing that might hurt morale—Spanish papers were filled with reports of the disease, especially when King Alphonse XIII fell seriously ill.

The disease soon became known as "Spanish influenza" or "Spanish flu," very likely because only Spanish newspapers were publishing accounts of the spread of the disease that were picked up in other countries.

It struck Portugal, then Greece. In June and July, death rates across England, Scotland, and Wales surged. In June, Germany suffered initial sporadic outbreaks, and then a full-fledged epidemic swept across all the country. Denmark and Norway began suffering in July, Holland and Sweden in August.

The earliest cases in Bombay erupted on a transport soon after its arrival May 29. First seven police sepoys who worked the docks were admitted to the police hospital; then men who worked at the government dockyard succumbed; the next day employees of the Bombay port fell ill, and two days later men who worked at a location that "abuts on the harbor between the government dockyard and Ballard Estate of the Port Trust." From there the disease spread along railroad lines, reaching Calcutta, Madras, and Rangoon after Bombay, while another transport brought it to Karachi.

Influenza reached Shanghai toward the end of May. Said one observer, "It swept over the whole country like a tidal wave." A reported half of Chungking lay ill. It jumped to New Zealand and then Australia in September; in Sydney it sickened 30 percent of the population.

But if it was spreading explosively, it continued to bear little resemblance to the violent disease that had killed in Haskell. Of 613 American troops admitted to the hospital during one outbreak in France, only one man died. In the French army, fewer than one hundred deaths resulted from forty thousand hospital admissions. In the British fleet, 10,313 sailors fell ill, temporarily crippling naval operations, but only four sailors died. Troops called it "three-day fever." In Algeria, Egypt, Tunisia, China, and India it was "everywhere of a mild form."

In fact, its mildness made some physicians wonder if this disease actually was influenza. One British army report noted that the symptoms "resembled influenza" but "its short duration and absence of complications" created doubt that it was influenza. Several different Italian doctors took a stronger position, arguing in separate medical journal articles that this "febrile disease now widely prevalent in Italy [is] not influenza." Three British doctors writing in the journal *The Lancet* agreed; they concluded that the epidemic could not actually be influenza, because the symptoms, though similar to those of influenza, were too mild, "of very short duration and so far absent of relapses or complications."

That issue of *The Lancet* was dated July 13, 1918.

· · ·

In March and April in the United States, when the disease began jumping from army camp to army camp and occasionally spreading to adjacent cities, Gorgas, Welch, Vaughan, and Cole showed little concern about it, nor did Avery commence any laboratory investigation. Measles was still lingering, and had caused many more deaths.

But as influenza surged across Europe, they began to attend to it. Despite the articles in medical journals about its generally benign nature, they had heard of some worrisome exceptions, some hints that perhaps this disease wasn't always so benign after all, that when the disease did strike hard, it was unusually violent—more violent than measles.

One army report noted "fulminating pneumonia, with wet hemor-rhagic lungs"—i.e., a rapidly escalating infection and lungs choked with blood—"fatal in from 24 to 48 hours." Such a quick death from pneumo-nia is extraordinary. And an autopsy of a Chicago civilian victim revealed lungs with similar symptoms, symptoms unusual enough to prompt the pathologist who performed the autopsy to send tissue samples to Dr. Ludwig Hektoen, a highly respected scientist who knew Welch, Flexner, and Gorgas well and who headed the John McCormick Memorial Insti-tute for Infectious Diseases. The pathologist asked Hektoen "to look at it as a new disease."

And in Louisville, Kentucky, a disturbing anomaly appeared in the in-fluenza statistics. There deaths were not so few, and—more surprisingly—40 percent of those who died were aged twenty to thirty-five, a statistically extraordinary occurrence.

In France in late May, at one small station of 1,018 French army recruits, 688 men were ill enough to be hospitalized and forty-nine died. When 5 percent of an entire population—especially of healthy young adults—dies in a few weeks, that is frightening.

By mid-June, Welch, Cole, Gorgas, and others were trying to gather as much information as possible about the progression of influenza in Europe. Cole could get nothing from official channels but did learn enough from such people as Hans Zinsser, a former (and future) Rocke-feller investigator in the army in France, to become concerned. In July, Cole asked Richard Pearce, a scientist at the National Research Council who was coordinating war-related medical research, to make "accurate information concerning the influenza prevailing in Europe" a priority, adding, "I have inquired several times in Washington at the Surgeon General's office"—referring to civilian Surgeon General Rupert Blue, head of the U.S. Public Health Service, not Gorgas—"but no one seems to have any definite information in regard to the matter." A few days later Cole showed more concern when he advised Pearce to put more resources into related research.

In response Pearce contacted several individual laboratory scientists, such as Paul Lewis in Philadelphia, as well as clinicians, pathologists, and epidemiologists, asking if they could begin new investigations. He would act as a clearinghouse for their findings.

Between June 1 and August 1, 200,825 British soldiers in France, out of two million, were hit hard enough that they could not report for duty even in the midst of desperate combat. Then the disease was gone. On August 10, the British command declared the epidemic over. In Britain itself on August 20, a medical journal stated that the influenza epidemic "has completely disappeared."

The *Weekly Bulletin* of the Medical Service of the American Expeditionary Force in France was less willing than the British to write off the influenza epidemic entirely. It did say in late July, "The epidemic is about at an end . . . and has been throughout of a benign type, though causing considerable noneffectiveness."

But it went on to note, "Many cases have been mistaken for meningitis. . . . Pneumonias have been more common sequelae in July than in April."

In the United States, influenza had neither swept through the country, as it had in Western Europe and parts of the Orient, nor had it completely died out.

Individual members of the army's pneumonia commission had dispersed to perform studies in several locations, and they still saw signs of it. At Fort Riley, which included Camp Funston, Captain Francis Blake, was trying to culture bacteria from the throats of both normal and sick troops. It was desultory work, far less exciting than what he was accustomed to, and he hated Kansas. He complained to his wife, "No letter from my beloved for two days, no cool days, no cool nights, no drinks, no movies, no dances, no club, no pretty women, no shower bath, no poker, no people, no fun, no joy, no nothing save heat and blistering sun and scorching winds and sweat and dust and thirst and long and stifling nights and working all hours and lonesomeness and general hell—that's Fort Riley Kansas." A few weeks later, he said it was so hot they kept their cultures of bacteria in an incubator so the heat wouldn't kill them. "Imagine going into an incubator to get cool," he wrote.

He also wrote, "Have been busy on the ward all day—some interesting cases. . . . But most of it influenza at present."

Influenza was about to become interesting.

For the virus had not disappeared. It had only gone underground, like a forest fire left burning in the roots, swarming and mutating, adapting, honing itself, watching and waiting, waiting to burst into flame.

CHAPTER FIFTEEN

THE 1918 INFLUENZA PANDEMIC, like many other influenza pandemics, came in waves. The first spring wave killed few, but the second wave would be lethal. Three hypotheses can explain this phenomenon.

One is that the mild and deadly diseases were caused by two entirely different viruses. This is highly unlikely. Many victims of the first wave demonstrated significant resistance to the second wave, which provides strong evidence that the deadly virus was a variant of the mild one.

The second possibility is that a mild virus caused the spring epidemic, and that in Europe it encountered a second influenza virus. The two viruses infected the same cells, "reassorted" their genes, and created a new and lethal virus. This could have occurred and might also explain the partial immunity some victims of the first wave acquired, but at least some scientific evidence directly contradicts this hypothesis, and most influenza experts today do not believe this happened.

The third explanation involves the adaptation of the virus to man.

In 1872 the French scientist C. J. Davaine was examining a specimen of blood swarming with anthrax. To determine the lethal dose he measured out various amounts of this blood and injected it into rabbits. He found it required ten drops to kill a rabbit within forty hours. He drew blood from this rabbit and infected a second rabbit, which also died. He repeated the process, infecting a third rabbit with blood from the second, and so on, passing the infection through five rabbits.

Each time he determined the minimum amount of blood necessary to kill. He discovered that the bacteria increased in virulence each time, and after going through five rabbits a lethal dose fell from 10 drops of blood to 1/100 of a drop. At the fifteenth passage, the lethal dose fell to 1/40,000 of a drop of blood. After twenty-five passages, the bacteria in the blood had become so virulent that less than 1/1,000,000 of a drop killed.

This virulence disappeared when the culture was stored. It was also specific to a species. Rats and birds survived large doses of the same blood that killed rabbits in infinitesimal amounts.

Davaine's series of experiments marked the first demonstration of a phenomenon that became known as "passage." This phenomenon reflects an organism's ability to adapt to its environment. When an organism of weak pathogenicity passes from living animal to living animal, it reproduces more proficiently, growing and spreading more efficiently. This often increases virulence.

In other words, it becomes a better and more efficient killer.

Changing the environment even in a test tube can have the same effect. As one investigator noted, a strain of bacteria he was working with turned deadly when the medium used to grow the organism changed from beef broth to veal broth.

But the phenomenon is complex. The increase in killing efficiency does not continue indefinitely. If a pathogen kills too efficiently, it will run out of hosts and destroy itself. Eventually its virulence stabilizes and even recedes. Especially when jumping species, it can become less dangerous instead of more dangerous. This happens with the Ebola virus, which does not normally infect humans. Initially Ebola has extremely high mortality rates, but after it goes through several generations of human passages, it becomes far milder and not particularly threatening.

So passage can also weaken a pathogen. When Pasteur was trying to weaken or, to use his word, "attenuate" the pathogen of swine erysipelas, he succeeded only by passing it through rabbits. As the bacteria adapted to rabbits, it lost some of its ability to grow in swine. He then inoculated pigs with the rabbit-bred bacteria, and their immune systems easily destroyed it. Since the antigens on the weak strain were the same as those on normal strains, the pigs' immune systems learned to recognize—and destroy—normal strains as well. They became immune to the disease. By 1894, veterinarians used Pasteur's vaccine to protect 100,000 pigs in France; in Hungary over 1 million pigs were vaccinated.

The influenza virus is no different in its behavior from any other pathogen, and it faces the same evolutionary pressures. When the 1918 virus jumped from animals to people and began to spread, it may have suffered a shock of its own as it adapted to a new species. Although it always retained hints of virulence, this shock may well have weakened it, making it relatively mild; then, as it became better and better at infecting its new host, it turned lethal.

Macfarlane Burnet won his Nobel Prize for work on the immune system, but he spent the bulk of his career investigating influenza, including its epidemiological history. He noted an occasion when passage turned a harmless influenza virus into a lethal one. A ship carrying people sick with influenza visited an isolated settlement in east Greenland. Two months after the ship's departure, a severe influenza epidemic erupted, with a 10 percent mortality rate; 10 percent of those with the disease died. Burnet was "reasonably certain that the epidemic was primarily virus influenza" and concluded that the virus passed through several generations—he estimated fifteen or twenty human passages—in mild form before it adapted to the new population and became virulent and lethal.

In his study of the 1918 pandemic, Burnet concluded that by late April 1918 "the essential character of the new strain seems to have been established." He continued, "We must suppose that the ancestral virus responsible for the spring epidemics in the United States passaged and mutated. . . . The process continued in France."

Lethality lay within the genetic possibilities of this virus; this particular mutant swarm always had the potential to be more pestilential than other influenza viruses. Passage was sharpening its ferocity. As it smoldered in the roots, adapting itself, becoming increasingly efficient at reproducing itself in humans, passage was forging a killing inferno.

On June 30, 1918, the British freighter *City of Exeter* docked at Philadelphia after a brief hold at a maritime quarantine station. She was laced with deadly disease, but Rupert Blue, the civilian surgeon general and head of the U.S. Public Health Service, had issued no instructions to the maritime service to hold influenza-ridden ships. So she was released.

Nonetheless, the condition of the crew was so frightening that the British consul had arranged in advance for the ship to be met at a wharf empty of anything except ambulances whose drivers wore surgical masks. Dozens of crew members "in a desperate condition" were taken immediately to Pennsylvania Hospital where, as a precaution against infectious disease, a ward was sealed off for them. Dr. Alfred Stengel, who had initially lost a competition for a prestigious professorship at the University of Pennsylvania to Simon Flexner but who did get it when Flexner left, had gone on to become president of the American College of Physicians. An expert on infectious diseases, he personally oversaw the sailors' care. Despite Stengel's old rivalry with Flexner, he even called in Flexner's protégé Paul Lewis for advice. Nonetheless, one after another, more crew members died.

They seemed to die of pneumonia, but it was a pneumonia accompanied, according to a Penn medical student, by strange symptoms, including bleeding from the nose. A report noted, "The opinion was reached that they had influenza."

In 1918 all infectious disease was frightening. Americans had already learned that "Spanish influenza" was serious enough that it had slowed the German offensive. Rumors now unsettled the city that these deaths too came from Spanish influenza. Those in control of the war's propaganda machine wanted nothing printed that could hurt morale. Two physicians stated flatly to newspapers that the men had not died of influenza. They were lying.

The disease did not spread. The brief quarantine had held the ship long enough that the crew members were no longer contagious when the ship docked. This particular virulent virus, finding no fresh fuel, had burned itself out. The city had dodged a bullet.

By now the virus had undergone numerous passages through humans. Even while medical journals were commenting on the mild nature of the disease, all over the world hints of a malevolent outbreak were appearing.

In London the week of July 8, 287 people died of influenzal pneumonia, and 126 died in Birmingham. A physician who performed several autopsies noted, "The lung lesions, complex or variable, struck one as being quite different in character to anything one had met with at all commonly in the thousands of autopsies one has performed during the last twenty years. It was not like the common broncho-pneumonia of ordinary years."

The U.S. Public Health Service's weekly *Public Health Reports* finally took notice, at last deeming the disease serious enough to warn the country's public health officials that "an outbreak of epidemic influenza . . . has been reported at Birmingham, England. The disease is stated to be spreading rapidly and to be present in other locations." And it warned of "fatal cases."

Earlier some physicians had insisted that the disease was not influenza because it was too mild. Now others also began to doubt that this disease was influenza—but this time because it seemed too deadly. Lack of oxygen was sometimes so severe that victims were becoming cyanotic—part or all of their bodies were turning blue, occasionally a very dark blue.

On August 3 a U.S. Navy intelligence officer received a telegram that he quickly stamped SECRET and CONFIDENTIAL. Noting that his source was "reliable," he reported, "I am confidentially advised . . . that the disease now epidemic throughout Switzerland is what is commonly known as the black plague, although it is designated as Spanish sickness and grip."

Many histories of the pandemic portray the eruption of deadly disease—the hammer blow of the second wave—as sudden and simultaneous in widely separated parts of the world, and therefore deeply puzzling. In fact the second wave developed gradually.

When water comes to a boil in a pot, first an isolated bubble releases from the bottom and rises to the surface. Then another. Then two or three simultaneously. Then half a dozen. But unless the heat is turned down, soon enough all the water within the pot is in motion, the surface a roiling violent chaos.

In 1918 each initial burst of lethality, isolated though it may have seemed, was much like a first bubble rising to the surface in a pot coming to boil. The flame may have ignited in Haskell and set off the first burst. The outbreak that killed 5 percent of *all* French recruits at one small base was another. Louisville was still another, as were the deaths on the *City of*

1. William Henry Welch, the single most powerful individual in the history of American medicine and one of the most knowledgeable. A wary colleague said he could "transform men's lives almost with the flick of a wrist." When Welch first observed autopsies of influenza victims, he worried, "This must be some new kind of infection or plague."

2. Welch and John D. Rockefeller Jr. (on the right) together created the Rockefeller Institute for Medical Research (now Rockefeller University), arguably the best scientific research institution in the world. Simon Flexner (on the left), a Welch protégé, was the institute's first head; he once said that no one could run an institution unless he had the capacity to be cruel.

3. Flexner brought the mortality rate for the most common bacterial meningitis down to 18 percent in 1910 without antibiotics. Today, with antibiotics, the mortality rate is 25 percent.

4. A dense jungle-like growth of epithelial cells covers a healthy mouse trachea.

5. Only seventy-two hours after infection the influenza virus transforms the same area into a barren and lifeless desert. White blood cells are patrolling the area, too late.

6. The virus swept first through military bases, where men were jammed together despite the objections of Welch and Army Surgeon General William Gorgas. This is an army emergency hospital, probably a ward for convalescents.

7. Army Surgeon General William Gorgas was determined that this would be the first war in which fewer American soldiers died of disease than from combat.

8. Rupert Blue, the civilian surgeon general and head of the U.S. Public Health Service, was a master bureaucrat but failed to heed warnings of, seek advance information about, or prepare for the epidemic.

9. Massachusetts was the first state to suffer huge numbers of civilian deaths. This is a hospital in Lawrence.

Preparing to Bury City's Influenza Victims

DIGGING TRENCH GRAVES FOR EPIDEMIC VICTIMS

10. In Philadelphia the number of dead quickly overwhelmed the city's ability to handle bodies. It was forced to bury people, without coffins, in mass graves and soon began using steam shovels to dig the graves.

11.

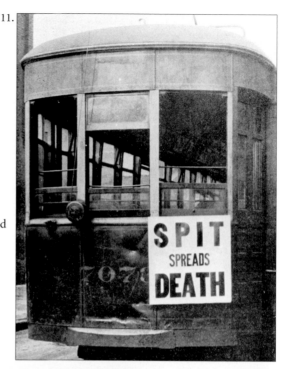

Posters and handouts spread warnings and advice. They also spread terror.

12.

13. The two messages in this photograph—the policeman's protective mask and patriotism—epitomized a conflict of interest in public officials.

14. All New York City workers wore masks. Note the absence of traffic on the street and pedestrians on the sidewalk. The same silent streets were seen everywhere. In Philadelphia a doctor said, "The life of the city had almost stopped."

15. Oswald T. Avery as a private, when the Rockefeller Institute became Army Auxiliary Laboratory Number One.

16. Avery in later life. Persistent and tenacious, he said, "Disappointment is my daily bread. I thrive on it." Welch asked him to find the cause of influenza. His work on influenza and pneumonia would ultimately lead him to one of the most important scientific discoveries of the twentieth century.

17. William Park, who made New York City's municipal laboratories a premier research institution. His rigorous scientific discipline, when teamed with the more creative temperament of Anna Williams [below], led to dramatic advances, including the development of a diphtheria antitoxin still in use. The National Academy of Sciences hoped they could develop a serum or vaccine for influenza.

18. Anna Wessel Williams was probably the leading female bacteriologist in the world. A lonely woman who never married, she told herself she would "rather [have] discontent than happiness through lack of knowledge," and wondered "if it would be worthwhile to make the effort to have friends and if so how I should go about it." From her earliest memories, she dreamed "about going places. Such wild dreams were seldom conceived by any other child."

19. The virus moved inexorably across the country. Here navy nurses and doctors await the onslaught.

20. Military commanders tried to protect healthy men; at Mare Island in San Francisco sheets were hung in barracks to screen men from each other's breathing.

21. In most cities all public meetings were banned, all public gathering places—churches, schools, theaters, and saloons—closed. Most churches simply canceled services but this one in California met outdoors, a technical violation of the closing order but a response to the congregation's need for prayer.

22. Rufus Cole, the Rockefeller Institute scientist who had led the successful effort to develop a pneumonia vaccine and treatment just before the outbreak of the epidemic. He also made the Rockefeller Institute Hospital a model for the way clinical research is conducted, including at the National Institutes for Health.

23.

Seattle, like many other places, became a masked city. Red Cross volunteers made tens of thousands of masks. All police wore them. Soldiers marched through the city's downtown wearing them.

24.

25.

26. More than one scientist called Paul A. Lewis "the brightest man I ever met." As a young investigator in 1908 he proved polio was caused by a virus and devised a vaccine that was 100 percent effective in protecting monkeys. It would be half a century before a polio vaccine could protect man. He too was one of the prime investigators searching for the cause of influenza, and a cure or preventative. Ultimately his ambition to investigate disease would cost him his life.

27. In the late 1920s Richard Shope, Lewis's protégé, unearthed a crucial clue in the search for the cause of influenza. While Lewis went to Brazilian jungles to investigate yellow fever, Shope continued his pursuit of influenza. He was the first to prove a virus caused the disease.

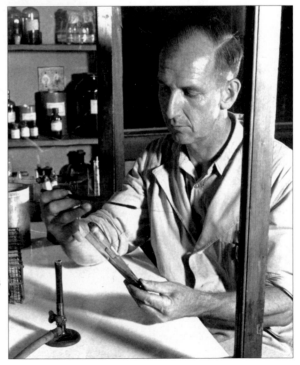

Exeter and the outbreak in Switzerland. All these were bursts of lethal disease, violent bubbles rising to the surface.

Epidemiological studies written relatively soon after the pandemic recognized this. One noted that army cantonments in the United States saw "a progressive increase in cases reported as influenza beginning with the week ending August 4, 1918, and of the influenzal pneumonia cases beginning with the week ending August 18. If this was really the beginning of the great epidemic wave we should expect that if these series of data were plotted out on a logarithmic scale the increase from week to week would plot out as a straight line following the usual logarithmic rise of an epidemic curve. . . . This condition is substantially fulfilled with the curve of rise plotting out on logarithmic paper as a practically straight line."

The report also found "definite outbreaks of increasing severity" occurring during the summer in both the United States and Europe, which "indistinguishably blend with the great Fall wave."

In early August the crew of a steamship proceeding from France to New York was hit so hard with influenza "that all of the seamen were prostrate on it and it had to put into Halifax," according to an epidemiologist in Gorgas's office, where it remained until enough crew members were well enough to proceed to New York.

On August 12 the Norwegian freighter *Bergensfjord* arrived in Brooklyn after burying four men at sea, dead of influenza. It carried two hundred people still sick with the disease; ambulances transported many of them to a hospital.

Royal Copeland, head of the New York City health department, and the port health officer jointly stated there was "not the slightest danger of an epidemic" because the disease seldom attacks "a well-nourished people." (Even had he been right, a study by his own health department had just concluded that 20 percent of city schoolchildren were malnourished.) He took no action whatsoever to prevent the spread of infection.

A navy bulletin warned of two steamships from Norway and one from Sweden arriving in New York City with influenza cases aboard on August 14 and 15. On August 18, New York papers described outbreaks on board the *Rochambeau* and *Nieuw Amsterdam;* men from both ships had been taken to St. Vincent's Hospital.

On August 20 even Copeland conceded that influenza, though mild and—he claimed—certainly not in epidemic form, was present in the city.

The lethal variant of the virus was finding its home in humans. Now, almost simultaneously, on three continents separated by thousands of miles of ocean—in Brest, in Freeport, Sierra Leone, and in Boston—the killing, rolling boil was about to begin.

Nearly 40 percent of the two million American troops who arrived in France—791,000 men—disembarked at Brest, a deepwater port capable of handling dozens of ships simultaneously. Troops from all over the world disembarked there. Brest had already seen a burst of influenza in the spring as had many other cities, albeit as in most of those other places that influenza had been mild. The first outbreak with high mortality occurred in July, in a replacement detachment of American troops from Camp Pike, Arkansas. They occupied an isolated camp and the outbreak initially seemed contained. It was not. By August 10, the same day the British army declared the influenza epidemic over, so many French sailors stationed at Brest were hospitalized with influenza and pneumonia that they overwhelmed the naval hospital there—forcing it to close. And the death rate among them began soaring.

The August 19 *New York Times* took note of another outbreak: "A considerable number of American negroes, who have gone to France on horse transports, have contracted Spanish influenza on shore and died in French hospitals of pneumonia."

Within another few weeks all the area around Brest was in flames. American troops continued pouring into and then out of the city, mixing with French troops also training in the vicinity. When soldiers of both armies left the vicinity, they dispersed the virus en masse.

Freetown, Sierra Leone, was a major coaling center on the West African coast, servicing ships traveling from Europe to South Africa and the Orient. On August 15 the HMS *Mantua* arrived there with two hundred crew suffering from influenza. Sweating black men loaded tons of coal into her, guided by several crew.

When the laborers returned to their homes, they carried more than their wages. Soon influenza spread through the force of men who coaled the ships. And this influenza was not mild. On August 24, two natives died of pneumonia while many others were still sick.

On August 27, the HMS *Africa* pulled into port. She too needed coal, but five hundred of the six hundred laborers of the Sierra Leone Coaling Company did not report to work that day. Her crew helped coal her, working side by side with African laborers. She carried a crew of 779. Within a few weeks, nearly six hundred were sick. And fifty-one were dead—7 percent of the entire crew died.

The transport HMS *Chepstow Castle*, carrying troops from New Zealand to the front, coaled at Freetown on August 26 and 27; within three weeks, out of her 1,150 men, influenza struck down nine hundred of them. The death toll on her was thirty-eight.

The *Tahiti* coaled at the same time; sixty-eight men aboard her died before she reached England, the same day as the *Chepstow Castle*. After docking, crew of the two ships suffered eight hundred more cases and 115 more deaths.

In Sierra Leone itself, officials soon after estimated that influenza killed 3 percent of the entire African population, nearly all of them dying within the next few weeks. More recent evidence suggests that the death toll was most likely considerably more than that, possibly double that figure—or higher.

Across the Atlantic, at Commonwealth Pier in Boston, the navy operated a "receiving ship." The name was a misnomer. It was actually a barracks where as many as seven thousand sailors in transit ate and slept in what the navy itself called "grossly overcrowded" quarters.

On August 27, two sailors reported to sick bay with influenza. On August 28, eight more sailors reported ill. On August 29, fifty-eight men were admitted.

As in Brest and Freetown and aboard ship, men began to die. Fifty of the men were quickly transferred to the Chelsea Naval Hospital, where Lieutenant Commander Milton Rosenau and his young assistant Lieutenant John J. Keegan, worked.

The sailors were in better than good hands. While Keegan would later become dean of the University of Nebraska Medical School, Rosenau was one of the giants of the day. Strong, solid, and thick-necked, he looked as intimidating and determined as a wrestler staring down an opponent. Yet he was uniformly polite and supportive, and people enjoyed working under him. A prime mover in creating the U.S. Public Health Service Hygienic Laboratory and later the president of the Society of American

Bacteriologists, he was best known for his textbook, *Preventive Medicine and Hygiene,* which was referred to as "The Bible" for both army and navy medical officers. Only a few weeks earlier, he had met with Welch, Gorgas, and Vaughan to discuss how to prevent or contain any new epidemic.*

Rosenau and Keegan immediately isolated the men and did everything possible to contain the disease, working backward from each victim to trace and isolate people with whom the patients had had contact. But the disease was too explosive. They turned their attention to bacteriological analysis, seeking the pathogen so they could prepare a vaccine or serum. Their findings did not satisfy them, and within a few weeks they began using human volunteers from the navy brig in the first experiments in the world to determine if a virus caused the disease.

Long before that any hopes of containing the disease had collapsed. On September 3 a civilian suffering from influenza was admitted to the Boston City Hospital. On September 4 students at the Navy Radio School at Harvard, in Cambridge across the Charles River from Boston proper, fell ill.

And then came Devens.

*Rosenau and Flexner had had a running but friendly competition for years. In 1911 Rosenau had shown that Flexner had made an important mistake. Two years later Rosenau won the American Medicine Gold Medal in 1913 for "proving" that stable flies transmitted poliomyelitis. Flexner proved that finding to be in error in 1915. Yet each respected the other, and they got along well. Shortly before the war, with Harvard still underfunding medical research, Flexner wrote him, "I am astonished and pained to learn that you have so small a budget for your lab," and promptly arranged for a Rockefeller grant to him. Their cooperation was routine, for example when Rosenau asked Flexner earlier in 1918, "Please send Chelsea Naval Hospital at once sufficient antimeningitis serum for 4 patients."

CHAPTER SIXTEEN

C AMP DEVENS sat on five thousand acres in rolling hills thirty-five miles northwest of Boston. It included fine farmland along the Nashua River, as well as what had been until recently heavily forested land cut down now to tree stumps. Like the other cantonments in the country it was thrown together with amazing speed, at the rate of 10.4 buildings a day. In August 1917 it opened with fifteen thousand men although the camp was incomplete—its sewage was still being discharged directly into the Nashua River.

Like most other camps, it had suffered from measles and pneumonia. The medical staff was first rate. An inspection of the Devens hospital had given it an excellent review down to its kitchen, noting, "The mess officer is well informed and alert."

In fact the Devens medical staff was so good that Frederick Russell was preparing to rely on it to launch several major new scientific investigations. One involved correlating the existence of streptococci in the mouths of healthy soldiers with streptococcal infections of the throat. Another sought an explanation for the far higher morbidity rates of pneumonia among blacks over whites. Still another involved measles. Late in the summer at Devens, Major Andrew Sellards had passed infectious material from a recent measles case through a porcelain filter to isolate the virus, had inoculated four monkeys with it, and on August 29 began inoculating a series of human volunteers.

The only problem at Devens was that it was built to hold a maximum of thirty-six thousand men. On September 6, Devens held just over forty-five thousand men. Still, the camp hospital could accommodate twelve hundred and it was caring for only eighty-four patients. With enough medical personnel to run several simultaneous research efforts, with a highly competent clinical staff, with a virtually empty hospital, Devens seemed ready for any emergency.

It wasn't.

A week before any reported illness in the harbor, Boston public health authorities worried: "A sudden and very significant increase reported the third week of August in the cases of pneumonia occurring in the army cantonment at Camp Devens in the district seems to justify a suspicion that an influenza epidemic may have started among the soldiers there."

While the eruption at Devens might still have come from the Navy Commonwealth Pier facility, it might also have developed independently. It might even have spread to Boston from Devens. At any rate, on September 1, four more soldiers at Devens were diagnosed with pneumonia and admitted to the hospital. In the next six days, twenty-two more new cases of pneumonia were diagnosed. None of these, however, were considered to be influenza.

On September 7, a soldier from D Company, Forty-second Infantry, was sent to the hospital. He ached to the extent that he screamed when he was touched, and he was delirious. He was diagnosed as having meningitis.

The next day a dozen more men from his company were hospitalized and suspected of having meningitis. It was a reasonable diagnosis. Symptoms did not resemble those of influenza, and a few months earlier the camp had suffered a minor epidemic of meningitis, and the doctors—lacking any false pride—had even called Rosenau for help. He had come himself, along with six bacteriologists; they had worked nearly around the clock for five days, identifying and quarantining 179 carriers of the disease. Rosenau had left the camp impressed with army medicine; even though he and his staff had done much of the work, he had advised navy superiors that the same effort would not have been possible in the navy.

Now, over the next few days, other organizations began reporting cases of influenza-like disease. The medical staff, good as it was, did not at first connect these various cases to each other or to the outbreak on Commonwealth Pier. They made no attempt to quarantine cases. In the first few days no records of influenza cases were even kept because they "were looked upon as being examples of the epidemic disease which attacked so many of the camps during the spring." In the overcrowded barracks and mess halls, the men mixed. A day went by. Two days. Then, suddenly, noted an army report, "Stated briefly, the influenza . . . occurred as an explosion."

It exploded indeed. In a single day, 1,543 Camp Devens soldiers reported ill with influenza. On September 22, 19.6 percent of the entire camp was on sick report, and almost 75 percent of those on sick report had been hospitalized. By then the pneumonias, and the deaths, had begun.

On September 24 alone, 342 men were diagnosed with pneumonia. Devens normally had twenty-five physicians. Now, as army and civilian medical staff poured into the camp, more than two hundred and fifty physicians were treating patients. The doctors, the nurses, the orderlies went to work at 5:30 A.M. and worked steadily until 9:30 P.M., slept, then went at it again. Yet on September 26 the medical staff was so overwhelmed, with doctors and nurses not only ill but dying, they decided to admit no more patients to the hospital, no matter how ill.

The Red Cross, itself by then overwhelmed by the spread of the disease to the civilian population, managed to find twelve more nurses to help and sent them. They were of little help. Eight of the twelve collapsed with influenza; two died.

For this was no ordinary pneumonia. Dr. Roy Grist, one of the army physicians at the hospital, wrote a colleague, "These men start with what appears to be an ordinary attack of LaGrippe or Influenza, and when brought to the Hosp. they very rapidly develop the most vicious type of Pneumonia that has ever been seen. Two hours after admission they have the Mahogany spots over the cheek bones, and a few hours later you can begin to see the Cyanosis extending from their ears and spreading all over the face, until it is hard to distinguish the coloured men from the white."

Blood carrying oxygen in arteries is bright red; without oxygen in veins it is blue. Cyanosis occurs when a victim turns blue because the lungs cannot transfer oxygen into the blood. In 1918 cyanosis was so extreme, turning some victims so dark—the entire body could take on color resembling that of the veins on one's wrists—it sparked rumors that the disease was not influenza at all, but the Black Death.

Grist continued, "It is only a matter of a few hours then until death comes. . . . It is horrible. One can stand it to see one, two or twenty men die, but to see these poor devils dropping like flies . . . We have been averaging about 100 deaths per day. . . . Pneumonia means in about all cases death. . . . We have lost an outrageous number of Nurses and Drs., and the little town of Ayer is a sight. It takes special trains to carry away the dead. For several days there were no coffins and the bodies piled up something fierce. . . . It beats any sight they ever had in France after a battle. An extra long barracks has been vacated for the use of the Morgue, and it would make any man sit up and take notice to walk down the long lines of dead soldiers all dressed and laid out in double rows. . . . Good By old Pal, God be with you till we meet again."

Welch, Cole, Victor Vaughan, and Fredrick Russell, all of them colonels now, had just finished a tour of southern army bases. It was not their first such tour, and as before, knowing that an army barracks offered explosive tinder, they had been inspecting camps to find and correct any practice that might allow an epidemic to gain a foothold. They also spent much time discussing pneumonia. After leaving Camp Macon in Georgia, they had retired for a few days of relaxation to Asheville, North Carolina, the most fashionable summer retreat in the South. The Vanderbilts had built one of the most elaborate estates in the country there, and not many miles away Welch's old colleague William Halsted had built a virtual castle in the mountains (today Halsted's home is a resort called the High Hamptons).

At the Grove Park Inn, one of the most elegant settings in the city, they listened to a concert. Welch lit a cigar. A bellboy promptly told him smoking was not allowed. He and Cole withdrew to the veranda and began talking. Another bellboy asked them to please be quiet during the concert. Welch left in disgust.

Meanwhile Russell wrote Flexner, "We are all well. Welch, Vaughan, and Cole, and I have had a very profitable trip and have begun to believe that immunity—" in this he was referring to efforts to manipulate the immune system—"is the most important thing in pneumonia, as in other infectious diseases. It makes a good working hypothesis and one we will try to follow up by working in the lab, wards, and in the field this fall and winter. Bonne chance."

The group returned to Washington on a Sunday morning relaxed and in good spirits. But their mood changed abruptly as they stepped off the train. An escort had been waiting for them and his anxiety quickly communicated itself. He was taking them to the surgeon general's office—immediately. Gorgas himself was in Europe. His deputy barely looked up as they opened the door: "You will proceed immediately to Devens. The Spanish influenza has struck that camp."

They arrived at Devens eight hours later in a cold and drizzling rain. The entire camp was in chaos, the hospital itself a battlefield. The war had come home indeed. As they entered the hospital, they watched a continuous line of men filing in from the barracks carrying their blankets or being themselves carried.

Vaughan recorded this sight: "hundreds of young stalwart men in the uniform of their country coming into the wards of the hospital in groups of ten or more. They are placed on the cots until every bed is full and yet others crowd in. The faces wear a bluish cast; a distressing cough brings up the blood-stained sputum."

Care was almost nonexistent. The base hospital, designed for twelve hundred, could accommodate at most—even with crowding "beyond what is deemed permissible," according to Welch—twenty-five hundred. It now held in excess of six thousand. All beds had long since been filled. Every corridor, every spare room, every porch was filled, crammed with cots occupied by the sick and dying. There was nothing antiseptic about the sight. And there were no nurses. When Welch arrived seventy out of two hundred nurses were already sick in bed themselves, with more falling ill each hour. Many of them would not recover. A stench filled the hospital as well. Bed linen and clothing were rank with urine and feces from men incapable of rising or cleaning themselves.

Blood was everywhere, on linens, clothes, pouring out of some men's nostrils and even ears while others coughed it up. Many of the soldiers, boys in their teens, men in their twenties—healthy, normally ruddy men—were turning blue. Their color would prove a deadly indicator.

The sight chilled even Welch and his colleagues. It was more chilling still to see corpses littering the hallways surrounding the morgue. Vaughan reported, "In the morning the dead bodies are stacked about the morgue like cord wood." As Cole recalled, "They were placed on the floor without any order or system, and we had to step amongst them to get into the room where an autopsy was going on."

In the autopsy room they saw the most chilling sights yet. On the table lay the corpse of a young man, not much more than a boy. When he was moved in the slightest degree fluid poured out of his nostrils. His chest was opened, his lungs removed, other organs examined carefully. It was immediately apparent this was no ordinary pneumonia. Several other autopsies yielded similar abnormalities.

Cole, Vaughan, Russell, the other members of this scientific team were puzzled, and felt an edge of fear. They turned to Welch.

He had studied with the greatest investigators in the world as a young man. He had inspired a generation of brilliant scientists in America. He had visited and seen diseases in China, the Philippines, and Japan that were unknown in the United States. He had read scientific journals in many languages for years, heard back-channel gossip from all the leading laboratories in the world. Surely he would be able to tell them something, have some idea.

He did not reassure. Cole stood beside him, thinking he had never seen Welch look nervous before, or excited in quite this way. In fact Cole was shaken: "It was not surprising that the rest of us were disturbed but it shocked me to find that the situation, momentarily at least was too much for Dr. Welch."

Then Welch said, "This must be some new kind of infection or plague."

Welch walked out of the autopsy room and made three phone calls, to Boston, New York, and Washington. In Boston he spoke to Burt Wolbach, a Harvard professor and chief pathologist at the the great Boston hospital the Brigham, and asked him to perform autopsies. Perhaps there was a clue to this strange disease there.

But Welch also knew that any treatment or prevention for this would have to come from the laboratory. From the Rockefeller Institute in New York he summoned Oswald Avery. Avery had been refused a commission in the Rockefeller army unit because he was Canadian, but on August 1 he had become an American citizen. By coincidence, the same day Welch called him, Avery was promoted from private to captain. More importantly, he had already begun the investigations that would ultimately revolutionize the biological sciences; influenza would confirm him in this work.

Later that day both Avery and Wolbach arrived and immediately began their respective tasks.

The third call Welch made was to Washington, to Charles Richard, the acting army surgeon general while Gorgas was at the front. Welch gave a detailed description of the disease and his expectations of its course at Devens and elsewhere. For this was going to spread. He urged that "immediate provision be made in every camp for the rapid expansion of hospital space."

Richard responded instantly, sending orders to all medical personnel to isolate and quarantine all cases and segregate soldiers from civilians outside the camps: "It is important that the influenza be kept out of the camps, as far as practicable. . . . Epidemics of the disease can often be prevented, but once established they cannot well be stopped." But he also conceded the difficulty: "There are few diseases as infectious as influenza. . . . It is probable that patients become foci of infection before the active symptoms. . . . No disease which the army surgeon is likely to see in this war will tax more severely his judgement and initiative."

He also warned both the army adjutant general and chief of staff, "New men will almost surely contract the disease. In transferring men from Camp Devens a virulent form of the disease will almost surely be conveyed to other stations. . . . During the epidemic new men should not be sent to Camp Devens, nor should men be sent away from that camp."

The next day, with reports already of outbreaks in other camps, Richard tried to impress upon the chief of staff the lethality of the disease, relating what Welch had told him: "The deaths at Camp Devens will probably exceed 500. . . . The experience at Camp Devens may be fairly expected to occur at other large cantonments. . . . With few exceptions they are densely populated, a condition which tends to increase the chance for 'contact' infection and the virulence and mortality of the disease. . . . It may be expected to travel westward and involve successively military stations in its course." And he urged that the transfer of personnel from one camp to another be all but eliminated except for the most "urgent military necessities."

Gorgas had fought his own war, to prevent epidemic disease from erupting in the camps. He had lost.

On August 27, the same day the first sailors at Commonwealth Pier fell ill, the steamer *Harold Walker* had departed Boston, bound for New Orleans. En route fifteen crew members had fallen ill; in New Orleans the ship unloaded its cargo and put three crewmen ashore. The three men died. By then the *Harold Walker* had proceeded to Mexico.

On September 4, physicians at the New Orleans naval hospital made the first diagnosis of influenza in any military personnel in the city; the sailor had arrived in New Orleans from the Northeast. That same date a second patient also reported ill with influenza; he was serving in New Orleans. Forty of the next forty-two patients who entered the hospital had influenza or pneumonia.

On September 7 three hundred sailors from Boston arrived at the Philadelphia Navy Yard. Many of them, mixing with hundreds of other sailors, were almost immediately transferred to the navy base in Puget Sound. Others had already gone from Boston to north of Chicago to the Great Lakes Naval Training Station, the largest facility of its kind in the world.

On September 8 at the Newport Naval Base in Rhode Island, more than one hundred sailors reported sick.

The virus was reaching south along the coast, jumping inland to the Midwest, spanning the nation to the Pacific.

Meanwhile, at the Chelsea Naval Hospital, Rosenau and his team of physicians were also overwhelmed—and well aware of the larger implications. Even before Avery arrived, he and Keegan had begun the first effort in the country, and possibly in the world, to create an immune serum that would work against this new mortal enemy. Simultaneously Keegan sent off a description of the disease to the *Journal of the American Medical Association,* warning that it "promises to spread rapidly across the entire country, attacking between 30 and 40 percent of the population, and running an acute course."

■   ■   ■

Keegan was incorrect only in that he limited his estimate to "the entire country." He should have said "the entire world."

This influenza virus, this "mutant swarm," this "quasi species," had always held within itself the potential to kill, and it had killed. Now, all over the world, the virus had gone through roughly the same number of passages through humans. All over the world, the virus was adapting to humans, achieving maximum efficiency. And all over the world, the virus was turning lethal.

Around the world from Boston, in Bombay, which like so many other cities had endured a mild epidemic in June, the lethal virus exploded almost simultaneously. There it quickly began killing at a rate more than double that of a serious epidemic of bubonic plague in 1900.

As the virus moved, two parallel struggles emerged.

One encompassed all of the nation. Within each city, within each factory, within each family, into each store, onto each farm, along the length of the track of the railroads, along the rivers and roads, deep into the bowels of mines and high along the ridges of the mountains, the virus would find its way. In the next weeks, the virus would test society as a whole and each element within it. Society would have to gather itself to meet this test, or collapse.

The other struggle lay within one tight community of scientists. They, men like Welch, Flexner, Cole, Avery, Lewis, Rosenau, had been drafted against their will into a race. They knew what was required. They knew the puzzle they needed to solve. They were not helpless. They had some tools with which to work. They knew the cost if they failed.

But they had very little time indeed.

■ Part V
EXPLOSION

CHAPTER SEVENTEEN

O N SEPTEMBER 7, three hundred sailors arrived from Boston at the Philadelphia Navy Yard. And what happened in Philadelphia from that point would prove—too often—to be a model for what would happen elsewhere.

Philadelphia was already typical in its war experiences. Every city was being flooded by people, and in Philadelphia shipbuilding alone had added tens of thousands of workers. In a few months a great marsh had been transformed into the Hog Island shipyard, the largest shipyard in the world, where thirty-five thousand workers toiled among furnaces and steel and machinery. Nearby the New York Shipbuilding yard worked eleven thousand five hundred men, and a dozen other shipyards each worked from three thousand to five thousand more. And the city was thick with other great industrial plants: several munitions factories each employed several thousands at a single location, the J. G. Brill Company turned out a streetcar an hour and employed four thousand, Midvale Steel had ten thousand workers, Baldwin Locomotive, twenty thousand.

Overcrowded before the war, with jobs sucking ever more workers into the city and the population swelling to 1.75 million, Philadelphia literally teemed with people. In 1918 a national publication for social workers judged living conditions in its slums, where most tenements still had outhouses servicing dozens of families, worse than on the Lower East Side of New York. Blacks endured even more squalid conditions and

Philadelphia had the largest African American population of any northern city, including New York or Chicago.

Housing was so scarce that Boy Scouts canvassed the area seeking rooms for newly arrived women with war jobs. Two, three, and four entire families would cram themselves into a single two- or three-room apartment, with children and teenagers sharing a bed. In rooming houses laborers shared not just rooms but beds, often sleeping in shifts just as they worked in shifts. In those same tenements, the city's own health department had conceded that during the winter of 1917–18 "the death rate . . . has gone up owing to the high cost of living and scarcity of coal."

The city offered the poor social services in the form of Philadelphia Hospital, known as "Blockley," a poorhouse, and an asylum. But it offered nothing else, not even an orphanage. The social elite and progressives ran whatever charitable activities that did exist. Even normal services such as schools were in short supply. Of the twenty largest cities in America, Philadelphia, the city of Benjamin Franklin and the University of Pennsylvania, spent less on education than all but one. In all of South Philadelphia, home to hundreds of thousands of Italians and Jews, there would be no high school until 1934.

All this made Philadelphia fertile ground for epidemic disease. So did a city government incapable of responding to a crisis. Muckraker Lincoln Steffens called Philadelphia "the worst-governed city in America." He may well have been right.

Even Tammany's use of power in New York was haphazard compared to that of the Philadelphia machine, which had returned to power in 1916 after a reformer's single term in office. Philadelphia's boss was Republican state senator Edwin Vare. He had bested and mocked people who considered themselves his betters, people who despised him, people with such names as Wharton, Biddle, and Wanamaker.

A short, thick-chested, and thick-bellied man—his nickname was "the little fellow"—Vare had his base in South Philadelphia. He had grown up there before the incursion of immigrants, on a pig farm in a then-rural area called "the Neck." He still lived there despite enormous wealth. The wealth came from politics.

All city workers kicked back a portion of their salary to Vare's machine. To make sure none ever missed a payment, city workers received their salary not where they worked or in City Hall—a classic and magnificent

Victorian building, with curved shoulders and windows reminiscent of weeping willow trees—but across the street from City Hall in Republican Party headquarters. The mayor himself kicked back $1,000 from his pay.

Vare was also the city's biggest contractor, and his biggest contract was for street cleaning, a contract he had held for almost twenty years. At a time when a family could live in comfort on $3,000 a year, in 1917 he had received over $5 million for the job. Not all of that money stayed in Vare's pockets, but even the part that left passed through them and paid a toll. Yet the streets were notoriously filthy, especially in South Philadelphia— where the need was greatest, where everything but raw sewage, and sometimes even that, ran through the gutters, and where the machine was strongest.

Ironically, the very lack of city services strengthened the machine since it provided what the city did not: food baskets to the poor, help with jobs and favors, and help with the police—the commissioner and many magistrates were in Vare's pocket. People paid for the favors with votes which, like a medieval alchemist, he transmuted into money.

The machine proved so lucrative that Edwin Vare and his brother William, a congressman, became philanthropists, giving so much to their church at Moyamensing Avenue and Morris Street that it was renamed the Abigail Vare Memorial Methodist Episcopal Church, after their mother. Not many churches are named after mere mortals, but this one was.

Yet nothing about the machine was saintly. On primary election day in 1917, several Vare workers blackjacked two leaders of an opposing faction, then beat to death a policeman who intervened. The incident outraged the city. Vare's chief lieutenant in 1918 was Mayor Thomas B. Smith. In his one term in office he would be indicted, although acquitted, on three entirely unrelated charges, including conspiracy to murder that policeman. That same election, however, gave Vare absolute control over both the Select and Common Councils, the city's legislature, and broad influence in the state legislature.

Director of the Philadelphia Department of Public Health and Charities was Dr. Wilmer Krusen, a political appointee who served at the mayor's pleasure and whose term automatically expired with the mayor's. Krusen, a decent man whose son would become a surgeon at the Mayo Clinic, was as good an appointment as the machine made. But he lacked background in, commitment to, or understanding of public health issues. And he was by nature someone who thought most problems disappeared on their own. He was not someone to rush into a thing.

He certainly would exert no pressure whatsoever on the machine to advance the public health. Although a gynecologist, he refused even to help the military in its massive national campaign against prostitution. Even New Orleans had succumbed to pressure to close Storyville, where prostitution was legal, but no pressure could make Philadelphia, where prostitution remained illegal, in any way hinder its flesh industry. So, according to a military report, the navy "actually took control of police affairs" outside its installations.

The city government was choking on corruption, with lines of authority split among Vare, precinct captains–turned–entrepreneurs, and the mayor. It did not wish to act, nor could it if it chose to.

Four days after the arrival of the sailors from Boston at the Navy Yard, nineteen sailors reported ill with symptoms of influenza.

Lieutenant Commander R. W. Plummer, a physician and chief health officer for the Philadelphia naval district, was well aware of the epidemic's rage on Commonwealth Pier and at Devens and its spread to the civilian population in Massachusetts. Determined to contain the outbreak, he ordered the immediate quarantine of the men's barracks and the meticulous disinfecting of everything the men had touched.

In fact, the virus had already escaped, and not only into the city. One day earlier 334 sailors had left Philadelphia for Puget Sound; many would arrive there desperately ill.

Plummer also immediately called in Paul Lewis.

Lewis had been expecting such a call.

He loved the laboratory more than he loved anyone or anything, and he had the full confidence of Welch, Theobald Smith, and Flexner. Lewis had won their confidence by his extraordinary performance as a young scientist under each of them in turn. He had already achieved much, and he held the promise of much more. He also knew his own worth, not in the sense that it made him smug but in that it gave him responsibility, making his promise at least as much burden as ambition. Only an offer to become the founding head of the new Henry Phipps Institute—Phipps had made millions at U.S. Steel with Andrew Carnegie, then, like

Carnegie, had become a prominent philanthropist—which was associated with the University of Pennsylvania, had lured him to Philadelphia from the Rockefeller Institute. He was modeling Phipps after the institute, although Phipps would focus much more narrowly on lung disease, particularly tuberculosis.

No one needed to tell Lewis the urgency of the situation. He knew the details of the British sailors who had died in early July, and he had very likely tried to culture bacteria from them and prepare a serum. Soon after learning that influenza had appeared in the Navy Yard, Lewis arrived there.

It was up to him to take charge of what would normally be the step-by-step, deliberate process of tracking down the pathogen and trying to develop a serum or vaccine. And there was no time for normal scientific procedures.

The next day eighty-seven sailors reported ill. By September 15, while Lewis and his assistants worked in labs at Penn and at the navy hospital, the virus had made six hundred sailors and marines sick enough to require hospitalization, and more men were reporting ill every few minutes. The navy hospital ran out of beds. The navy began sending ill sailors to the Pennsylvania Hospital at Eighth and Spruce.

On September 17, five doctors and fourteen nurses in that civilian hospital suddenly collapsed. None had exhibited any prior symptoms whatsoever. One moment they felt normal; the next, they were being carried in agony to hospital beds.

Navy personnel from Boston had been transferred elsewhere as well. As Philadelphia was erupting, so was the Great Lakes Naval Training Station, thirty-two miles above Chicago. Teddy Roosevelt had created the base in 1905, declaring that it would become the largest and best naval training station in the world. With forty-five thousand sailors it was the largest, and it had begun to generate a proud history. The "Seabees" naval construction battalions were born there, and during the war Lieutenant John Philip Sousa created fourteen regimental bands there; sometimes all fifteen hundred musicians played en masse on Ross Field, spectacle for tens of thousands who flocked to hear them. As the influenza virus swept through the base, there would be no massing of anyone, musicians or otherwise. At this base, influenza ripped through the barracks very much like an explosion.

Robert St. John had just been inducted into the navy there when he became one of the early victims. Given a cot in a drill hall where soon thousands of men—in that one hall—would lie unattended, he later recalled, "No one ever took our temperatures and I never even saw a doctor." He did make his first friend in the navy, a boy on the next cot who was too ill to reach for water. St. John himself barely had the strength to help him drink from his canteen. The next morning an orderly pulled the blanket over his friend's head, and two sailors put the body on a stretcher and carried it away. By then the medical department had already reported that "33 caskets to Naval Medical Supply Depot required." They would soon require far more than that.

One nurse at Great Lakes would later be haunted by nightmares. The wards had forty-two beds; boys lying on the floor on stretchers waited for the boy on the bed to die. Every morning the ambulances arrived and stretcher bearers carried sick sailors in and bodies out. She remembered that at the peak of the epidemic the nurses wrapped more than one living patient in winding sheets and put toe tags on the boys' left big toe. It saved time, and the nurses were utterly exhausted. The toe tags were shipping tags, listing the sailor's name, rank, and hometown. She remembered bodies "stacked in the morgue from floor to ceiling like cord wood." In her nightmares she wondered "what it would feel like to be that boy who was at the bottom of the cord wood in the morgue."

The epidemic was sweeping through the Philadelphia naval installations with comparable violence, as it had in Boston. Yet in Philadelphia, despite the news out of Boston, despite the Great Lakes situation, despite events at its own Navy Yard, Philadelphia public health director Wilmer Krusen had done absolutely nothing.

Not all the city's public health figures remained oblivious to the threat. The day after the first sailor fell ill, Dr. Howard Anders, a prominent public health expert who despised and had no faith in the Vare machine, wrote Navy Surgeon General William Braisted to ask would "the navy (federal) authorities directly come in, under this threat of influenza invasion, and insist upon safeguarding its men and collaterally the whole population of Philadelphia . . . ?" (Braisted declined.)

Krusen publicly denied that influenza posed any threat to the city. He seemed to believe that, for he made no contingency plans in case of emer-

gency, stockpiled no supplies, and compiled no lists of medical personnel who would be available in an emergency, even though 26 percent of Philadelphia's doctors and even a higher percentage of nurses were in the military. Indeed, despite building pressure from Lewis, from Anders, from physicians all over the city, from faculty at Penn and Thomas Jefferson Medical College—which refused to release six doctors who wanted to volunteer for military service just as the epidemic erupted—not until September 18, a full week after the disease appeared in the city, did Krusen even schedule a meeting with Plummer, Lewis, and several others.

In Krusen's fifth-floor office at City Hall they acquainted each other with the facts. In Massachusetts nearly one thousand had already died, with tens of thousands ill, and the Massachusetts governor had just issued a plea for doctors and nurses from neighboring regions. In Philadelphia hundreds of sailors were hospitalized. Few signs of disease had surfaced among civilians, but Lewis reported that as yet his research had not found an answer.

Even if Lewis succeeded in making a vaccine, it would take weeks to produce in sufficient quantities. Thus, only drastic action could prevent the spread of influenza throughout the city. Banning public meetings, closing businesses and schools, imposing an absolute quarantine on the Navy Yard and on civilian cases—all these things made sense. A recent precedent existed. Only three years earlier Krusen's predecessor—during the single term of the reform mayor—had imposed and enforced a strict quarantine when a polio epidemic had erupted, a disease Lewis knew more about than anyone in the world. Lewis certainly wanted a quarantine.

But Plummer was Lewis's commanding officer. He and Krusen wanted to wait. Both feared that taking any such steps might cause panic and interfere with the war effort. Keeping the public calm was their goal. Those polio restrictions had been imposed when the country wasn't fighting a war.

The meeting ended with nothing decided except to monitor developments. Krusen did promise to start a mass publicity campaign against coughing, spitting, and sneezing. Even that would take days to organize. And it would conflict with the downplaying of danger by Krusen and navy officials.

In Washington, Gorgas, who likely had heard from Lewis, was unsatisfied with these developments. By then influenza had erupted in two more cantonments, Camp Dix in New Jersey and Camp Meade in Maryland, that sandwiched the city. Lewis was in very close contact with the Philadelphia Tuberculosis Society, and Gorgas asked it to print and distribute twenty thousand large posters warning of influenza and stating a simple precaution that might help in at least a small way: "When obliged to cough or sneeze, always place a handkerchief, paper napkin, or fabric of some kind before the face."

Meanwhile the *Evening Bulletin* assured its readers that influenza posed no danger, was as old as history, and was usually accompanied by a great miasma, foul air, and plagues of insects, none of which were occurring in Philadelphia. Plummer assured reporters that he and Krusen would "confine this disease to its present limits, and in this we are sure to be successful. No fatalities have been recorded among Navy men. No concern whatever is felt by either the military and naval physicians or by the civil authorities."

The next day two sailors died of influenza. Krusen opened the Municipal Hospital for Contagious Diseases to the navy, and Plummer declared, "The disease has about reached its crest. We believe the situation is well in hand. From now on the disease will decrease."

Krusen insisted to reporters that the dead were not victims of an epidemic; he said that they had died of influenza but insisted it was only "old-fashioned influenza or grip." The next day fourteen sailors died. So did the first civilian, "an unidentified Italian" at Philadelphia General Hospital at South Thirty-fourth and Pine.

The following day more than twenty victims of the virus went to a morgue. One was Emma Snyder. She was a nurse who had cared for the first sailors to come to Pennsylvania Hospital. She was twenty-three years old.

Krusen's public face remained nothing but reassuring. He now conceded that there were "a few cases in the civilian population" and said that health inspectors were looking for cases among civilians "to nip the epidemic in the bud." But he did not say how.

On Saturday, September 21, the Board of Health made influenza a "reportable" disease, requiring physicians to notify health officials of any cases they treated. This would provide information about its movement. For the board to act on a Saturday was extraordinary in itself, but the board nonetheless assured the city that it was "fully convinced that the statement issued by Director Krusen that no epidemic of influenza prevails in the civil population at the present time is absolutely correct. Moreover, the Board feels strongly that if the general public will carefully and rigidly observe the recommendations [to] avoid contracting the influenza an epidemic can successfully be prevented."

The board's advice: stay warm, keep the feet dry and the bowels open—this last piece of advice a remnant of the Hippocratic tradition. The board also advised people to avoid crowds.

Seven days later, on September 28, a great Liberty Loan parade, designed to sell millions of dollars of war bonds, was scheduled. Weeks of organizing had gone into the event, and it was to be the greatest parade in Philadelphia history, with thousands marching in it and hundreds of thousands expected to watch it.

These were unusual times. The Great War made them so. One cannot look at the influenza pandemic without understanding the context. Wilson had realized his aims. The United States was waging total war.

Already two million U.S. troops were in France; it was expected that at least two million more would be needed. Every element of the nation, from farmers to elementary school teachers, was willingly or otherwise enlisted in the war. To Wilson, to Creel, to his entire administration, and for that matter to allies and enemies alike, the control of information mattered. Advertising was about to emerge as an industry; J. Walter Thompson—his advertising agency was already national, and his deputy became a senior Creel aide—was theorizing that it could engineer behavior; after the war the industry would claim the ability to "sway the ideas of whole populations," while Herbert Hoover said, "The world lives by phrases" and called public relations "an exact science."

Total war requires sacrifice and good morale makes sacrifices acceptable, and therefore possible. The sacrifices included inconveniences in daily life. To contribute to the war effort, citizens across the country endured the "meatless days" during the week, the one "wheatless meal" every day. All these sacrifices were of course voluntary, completely voluntary—although Hoover's Food Administration could effectively close businesses that did not "voluntarily" cooperate. And if someone chose to go for a drive in the country on a "gasless Sunday," when people were "voluntarily" refraining from driving, that someone was pulled over by hostile police.

The Wilson administration intended to make the nation cohere. Wilson informed the head of the Boy Scouts that selling bonds would give "every Scout a wonderful opportunity to do his share for the country under the slogan, 'Every Scout to Save a Soldier.'" Creel's one hundred fifty thousand Four Minute Men, those speakers who opened virtually every public gathering including movie and vaudeville shows, inspired giving. And when inspiration alone failed, other pressures could be exerted.

The preservation of morale itself became an aim. For if morale faltered, all else might as well. So free speech trembled. More than in the McCarthy period, more than during World War II itself, more than in the Civil War—when Lincoln was routinely vilified by opponents—free speech trembled indeed. The government had the two hundred thousand members of the American Protective League, who reported to the Justice Department's new internal security agency headed by J. Edgar Hoover and spied on neighbors and coworkers. Creel's organization advised citizens, "Call the bluff of anyone who says he has 'inside information.' Tell him that it's his patriotic duty to help you find the source of what he's saying. If you find a disloyal person in your search, give his name to the Department of Justice in Washington and tell them where to find him."

Socialists, German nationals, and especially the radical unionists in the International Workers of the World got far worse treatment. The *New York Times* declared, "The IWW agitators are in effect, and perhaps in fact, agents of Germany. The Federal authorities should make short work of these treasonable conspirators against the United States." The government did just that, raiding union halls, convicting nearly two hundred union men at mass trials in Illinois, California, and Oregon, and applying relentless pressure against all opponents; in Philadelphia on the same day that Krusen first discussed influenza with navy officials, five men who worked for the city's German-language paper *Tageblatt* were imprisoned.

What the government didn't do, vigilantes did. There were the twelve hundred IWW members locked in boxcars in Arizona and left on a siding in the desert. There was IWW member Frank Little, tied to a car and dragged through streets in Butte, Montana, until his kneecaps were scraped off, then hung by the neck from a railroad trestle. There was Robert Prager, born in Germany but who had tried to enlist in the navy, attacked by a crowd outside St. Louis, beaten, stripped, bound in an American flag, and lynched because he uttered a positive word about his country of origin. And, after that mob's leaders were acquitted, there was the juror's shout, "I guess nobody can say we aren't loyal now!" Meanwhile, a *Washington Post* editorial commented, "In spite of excesses such as lynching, it is a healthful and wholesome awakening in the interior of the country."

Socialist Eugene Debs, who in the 1912 presidential election had received nearly one million votes, was sentenced to ten years in prison for opposing the war, and in an unrelated trial Wisconsin congressman Victor Berger was sentenced to twenty years for doing the same. The House of Representatives thereupon expelled him and when his constituents reelected him anyway the House refused to seat him. All this was to protect the American way of life.

Few elites in America enjoyed more luxuries than did Philadelphia society, with its Biddles and Whartons. Yet the *Philadelphia Inquirer* reported approvingly that at "a dinner on the Main Line a dozen men were gathered at the table, and there was some criticism of the way the government was handling things. The host rose and said, 'Gentlemen, it is not my business to tell you what to say but there are four Secret Service agents here this evening.' It was a tactful way of putting a stop to conversation for which he did not care."

Meanwhile, Treasury Secretary William McAdoo believed that during the Civil War the government had made a "fundamental error" not selling bonds to average citizens: "Any great war must necessarily be a popular movement. It is a crusade; and, like all crusades, it sweeps along on a powerful stream of romanticism. [Lincoln's treasury secretary Salmon] Chase did not attempt to capitalize the emotions of the people. We went direct to the people, and that means to everybody—to businessmen, workmen, farmers, bankers, millionaires, schoolteachers, laborers. We capitalized on the profound impulse called patriotism. It is the quality of coherence that holds a nation together; it is one of the deepest and most powerful of human motives." He went still further and declared, "Every person who refuses to subscribe or who takes the attitude of let the other fellow do it, is a friend of Germany and I would like nothing better than to tell it to him to his face. A man who can't lend his govt $1.25 a week at the rate of 4% interest is not entitled to be an American citizen."

The Liberty Loan campaign would raise millions of dollars in Philadelphia alone. The city had a quota to meet. Central to meeting that quota was the parade scheduled for September 28.

Several doctors—practicing physicians, public health experts at medical schools, infectious disease experts—urged Krusen to cancel the parade. Howard Anders tried to generate public pressure to stop it, telling newspaper reporters the rally would spread influenza and kill. No newspaper quoted his warning—such a comment might after all hurt morale—so he demanded of at least one editor that the paper print his warning that the rally would bring together "a ready-made inflammable mass for a conflagration." The editor refused.

Influenza was a disease spread in crowds. "Avoid crowds" was the advice Krusen and the Philadelphia Board of Health gave. To prevent crowding the Philadelphia Rapid Transit Company had just limited the number of passengers in streetcars.

Army camps had already become so overwhelmed by influenza that on September 26 Provost Marshal Enoch Crowder canceled the next scheduled draft call. That same day, Massachusetts governor Samuel McCall formally pleaded for federal help and for doctors, nurses, and supplies from neighboring states.

If influenza was only beginning its assault on Philadelphia, it was already roaring full speed through the Navy Yard. Fourteen hundred sailors were now hospitalized with the disease. The Red Cross was converting the United Service Center at Twenty-second and Walnut into a five-hundred-bed hospital for the sole use of the navy. Krusen saw those reports and heard from those who wanted to cancel the parade, all right, but he did not seem to be listening. All he did was forbid the entertainment of soldiers or sailors by any organization or private party in the city. But military personnel could still visit stores, ride streetcars, go to vaudeville shows or moving picture houses.

In Philadelphia on September 27, the day before the parade, hospitals admitted two hundred more people—123 of them civilians—suffering from influenza.

Krusen felt intense and increasing pressure to cancel the parade, pressure coming from colleagues in medicine, from the news out of Massachusetts, from the fact that the army had canceled the draft. The decision whether to proceed or not was likely entirely his own. Had he sought guidance from the mayor, he would have found none. For a magistrate had just issued an arrest warrant for the mayor, who was now closeted with his lawyer, distracted and impossible to reach. Earlier, for the good of the city and the war effort, an uneasy truce had been forged between the Vare machine and the city's elite. Now Mrs. Edward Biddle, president of the Civic Club, married to a descendant of the founder of the Bank of the United States, resigned from a board the mayor had appointed her to, ending that truce, adding to the chaos in City Hall.

Krusen did hear some good news. Paul Lewis believed he was making progress in identifying the pathogen, the cause of influenza. If so, work on a serum and a vaccine could proceed rapidly. The press headlined this good news, although it did not report that Lewis, a careful scientist, was unsure of his findings.

Krusen declared that the Liberty Loan parade and associated rallies would proceed.

None of the anxiety of the moment was reported in any of the city's five daily papers, and if any reporter questioned either Krusen or the Board of Health about the wisdom of the parade's proceeding, no mention of it appeared in print.

On September 28, marchers in the greatest parade in the city's history proudly stepped forward. The paraders stretched at least two miles, two miles of bands, flags, Boy Scouts, women's auxiliaries, marines, sailors, and soldiers. Several hundred thousand people jammed the parade route, crushing against each other to get a better look, the ranks behind shouting encouragement over shoulders and past faces to the brave young men. It was a grand sight indeed.

Krusen had assured them they were in no danger.

The incubation period of influenza is twenty-four to seventy-two hours. Two days after the parade, Krusen issued a somber statement: "The epidemic is now present in the civilian population and is assuming the type found in naval stations and cantonments."

To understand the full meaning of that statement, one must understand precisely what was occurring in the army camps.

CHAPTER EIGHTEEN

DEVENS HAD BEEN STRUCK by surprise. The other cantonments and navy bases were not. Gorgas's office had issued immediate warnings of the disease, and medical staffs around the country took heed. Even so, the virus reached first and with most lethality into these military posts, invading the close cluster of young men in their barracks beds. Camp Grant was neither the worst hit, nor the least. Indeed, except for one particular and individual tragedy, it was quite typical.

The camp sprawled across rolling but mostly level country on the Rock River outside Rockford, Illinois. The soil there was rich and lush, and its first commandant had planted fifteen hundred acres on the base with sweet corn and "hog corn," hay, wheat and winter wheat, potatoes, and oats. Most recruits there came from northern Illinois and Wisconsin, farm boys with straw-colored hair and flush cheeks who knew how to raise the crops and produced them in plenty.

It was a remarkably orderly place, given the haste with which it had been built. It had neat rows of wooden barracks, and more rows and rows of large barrack-tents, eighteen men to each. All the roads were dirt and in the late summer dust filled the air, except when rain turned the roads to mud. The hospital was situated at one end of the camp and had two thousand beds, although the most patients it had cared for at one time was 852; several infirmaries were also scattered throughout the base.

In June 1918, Welch, Cole, Russell, and Richard Pearce of the National

Research Council—who rarely left Washington, usually being too busy coordinating research efforts—had inspected the camp and come away impressed. Welch judged Grant's chief medical officer, Lieutenant Colonel H. C. Michie, "capable and energetic," the hospital laboratory "excellent," the pathologist "a good man," while Joe Capps, a friend of Cole, was "of course an excellent chief of service" at the hospital itself. The veterinarian, who was responsible for several hundred horses and assorted livestock, had also impressed them favorably.

During that June visit they had all discussed pneumonia. Capps had started clinical experiments with a serum developed by Preston Kyes that differed from Cole's. Kyes was a promising University of Chicago investigator of whom Welch had said, "It is worth while for us to keep our eye on him." Capps and Cole exchanged information. Capps also spoke of seeing a disturbing trend toward a "different type of pneumonia . . . clinically more toxic and fatal . . . at autopsy often massive areas of consolidation . . . and also areas of hemorrhagic alveoli."

Then he demonstrated for them an innovation he had experimented with: the wearing of gauze masks by patients with respiratory disease. Welch called the mask "a great thing . . . an important contribution in prevention of spray infections." He encouraged Capps to write an article for the *Journal of the American Medical Association* and advised Pearce to conduct studies of the masks' effectiveness. Cole agreed: "This is a very important matter in connection with the prevention of pneumonia."

Welch also came away from that inspection, the last one of that tour, recommending two things. It confirmed in him his desire to have new arrivals at all camps assigned for three weeks to specially constructed detention camps; these men would eat, sleep, drill—and be quarantined—together to avoid any cross-infections with men already in camp. Second, he wanted Capps's use of masks extended to all camps.

Capps did write the *JAMA* article. He reported finding the masks so successful that after less than three weeks of experimenting he had abandoned testing and simply started using them as "a routine measure." He also made the more general point that "one of the most vital measures in checking contagion" is eliminating crowding. "Increasing the space between beds in barracks, placing the head of one soldier opposite the feet of his neighbor, stretching tent flags between beds, and suspending a curtain down the center of the mess table, are all of proved value."

To prevent a few arriving individuals from infecting an entire camp, he also repeated Welch's recommendation to isolate transferred troops. Grant had such a "depot brigade," a separate quarantine barracks for new recruits and transfers. Its stairways were built on the outside so guards could enforce the quarantine. But officers did not stay in the depot brigade; only enlisted men did.

Capps's article appeared in the August 10, 1918, issue of *JAMA*.

On August 8, Colonel Charles Hagadorn took command of Camp Grant. A short, brooding officer and a West Point graduate, still a bachelor at fifty-one years of age, he had devoted his life to the army and his men. He had also prepared for war all his life, studying it constantly and learning from experience as well as reading and analysis; one report "accredited [him] one of the most brilliant line experts of the regular army." He had fought the Spanish in Cuba, fought guerrillas in the Philippines, and chased Pancho Villa in Mexico just a year before. Sometimes he gave what seemed impulsive and even inexplicable orders, but they had a curve of reason behind them. He was determined to teach his soldiers to survive, and to kill. Not to die. He cared about his troops and liked being surrounded by them.

One problem that confronted him seemed to have little to do with war. The camp was over capacity. Only thirty thousand troops had been present when Welch had visited in June. Now the strength was in excess of forty thousand with no expectation of any decrease. Many men were forced into tents and winter—winter in northern Illinois, one year after a record cold—was only a few weeks away.

Army regulations defined how much space each soldier had in the barracks. These regulations had little to do with comfort and much to do with public health. In mid-September Hagadorn decided to ignore the army regulations on overcrowding and move even more men from tents into barracks. Already the nights were cold, and they would be more comfortable there.

But by then Gorgas's office had issued warnings about the epidemic and influenza had reached the Great Lakes Naval Training Station one hundred miles away. At Camp Grant, doctors watched for the first case. They even had an idea where it might occur. Dozens of officers had just arrived from Devens.

The camp senior medical staff confronted Hagadorn over his plan to increase crowding. Although no record exists of the meeting, these physicians were men whom Welch and Cole held in the highest regard, and in outstanding civilian careers they gave rather than took orders. The meeting had to have been contentious. For God's sake, they would have warned him, scattered cases of influenza had already appeared in Rockford.

But Hagadorn believed that disease could be controlled. In addition to his combat record, he had been chief of staff in the Canal Zone and had seen Gorgas control even tropical diseases there. Besides, he had tremendous confidence in his medical staff. He had more confidence in his doctors than they had in themselves, perhaps reminding them they had avoided even the measles epidemic that had plagued so many cantonments. On September 4 the camp's own epidemiologist had filed a report noting, "The epidemic diseases at this camp were at no time alarming. . . . Cases of Measles, Pneumonia, Scarlet fever, Diphtheria, Meningitis and the Smallpox occurred sporadically. None of these diseases ever assumed epidemic form."

And this was only influenza. Still, Hagadorn made a few concessions. On September 20 he issued several orders to protect the camp's health. To prevent the rise of dust, all roads would be oiled. And out of concern for influenza he agreed to a virtual quarantine: "Until further notice from these Headquarters, passes and permission to be absent from Camp . . . will not be granted to Officers or enlisted men, except from this office, and then only for the most urgent reasons."

But he issued one more order that day as well. It must have been particularly galling for Michie and Capps to see him use their authority to justify it: "There must as a military necessity be a crowding of troops. The Camp Surgeon under the circumstances authorizes a crowding in barracks . . . beyond the authorized capacity. . . . This will be carried out at once as buildings are newly occupied."

September 21, the day after Hagadorn issued his order, several men in the Infantry Central Officers Training School—the organization with officers from Devens—reported ill. They were immediately isolated in the base hospital.

It did little good. By midnight 108 men from the infantry school and the unit next to it were admitted to the hospital. There each patient had a gauze mask placed over his mouth and nose.

The two units were isolated from the rest of the camp, and men in the units were partly isolated from each other. Every bed had sheets hung around it, and twice a day each man was examined. All public gatherings—movies, YMCA functions, and the like—were canceled, and the men were ordered not "to mingle in any manner with men of other organizations at any time. . . . No visitors will be permitted in the area involved. . . . Any barracks from which several cases are reported will be quarantined; its occupants will not be permitted to mingle in any way with the occupants of other barracks in the same organization."

Guards enforced the orders strictly. But people infected with influenza can infect others before they feel any symptoms. It was already too late. Within forty-eight hours every organization in the camp was affected.

The next day hospital admissions rose to 194, the next 371, the next 492. Four days after the first officer reported sick, the first soldier died. The next day two more men died, and 711 soldiers were admitted to the hospital. In six days the hospital went from 610 occupied beds to 4,102 occupied, almost five times more patients than it had ever cared for.

There were too few ambulances to carry the sick to the hospital, so mules pulled ambulance carts until the mules, exhausted, stopped working. There were too few sheets for the beds, so the Red Cross ordered six thousand from Chicago. There were too few beds, so several thousand cots were crammed into every square inch of corridor, storage area, meeting room, office, and veranda.

It wasn't enough. Early on the medical detachment members had moved into tents so their own barracks could be transformed into a five-hundred-bed—or cot—hospital. Ten barracks scattered throughout the camp were also converted into hospitals. It still wasn't enough.

All training for war, for killing, ceased. Now men fought to stop the killing.

Healthy soldiers were consumed with attending, in one way or another, the sick. Three hundred and twenty men were sent to the hospital as general support staff, then 260 more were added. Another 250 men did nothing but stuff sacks with straw to make mattresses. Several hundred others unloaded a stream of railroad cars full of medical supplies. Hundreds more helped transport the sick or cleaned laundry—washing sheets, making masks—or prepared food. Meanwhile, barely in advance of a threatening thunderstorm, one hundred carpenters worked to enclose thirty-nine verandas with roofing paper to keep the rain off the hundreds of patients exposed to the elements. The gauze masks Capps was so proud of, the masks Welch had praised, were no longer being made; Capps ran out of material and personnel to make them.

The medical staff itself was collapsing from overwork—and disease. Five days into the epidemic five physicians, thirty-five nurses, and fifty orderlies were sick. That number would grow, and the medical staff would have its own death toll.

Seven days into the epidemic soldiers still capable of work converted nine more barracks into hospitals. There were shortages of aspirin, atropine, digitalis, glacial acetic acid (a disinfectant), paper bags, sputum cups, and thermometers—and thermometers that were available were being broken by men in delirium.

Forty more nurses arrived for the emergency, giving the hospital 383. It needed still more. All visitors to the base and especially to the hospital had already been prohibited "except under extraordinary circumstances." Now those extraordinary circumstances had become common, with visitors pouring in, Michie noted, "summoned by danger of death telegrams. . . ." Four hundred thirty-eight telegrams had been handled the day before.

That number was still climbing, and rapidly. To handle what soon became thousands of telegrams and phone calls each day, the Red Cross erected a large tent, floored, heated, wired for electricity, with its own telephone exchange and rows of chairs that resembled an auditorium where relatives waited to see desperately ill soldiers. More personnel were needed to escort these visitors to the sick. More personnel and more laundry facilities were needed just to wash the gown and mask that every visitor donned.

The hospital staff could not keep pace. Endless rows of men coughing, lying in bloodstained linen, surrounded by flies—orders were issued that "formalin should be added to each sputum cup to keep the flies away"—and the grotesque smells of vomit, urine, and feces made the relatives in some ways more desperate than the patients. They offered bribes to whoever seemed healthy—doctor, nurse, or orderly—to ensure care for their sons and lovers. Indeed, visitors begged them to accept bribes.

Michie responded sternly: "Devoting special personal care to any one patient whose condition is not critical is prohibited and the ward personnel is instructed to report any civilian or other person to the commanding officer who makes a special request that a certain patient be given special attention."

And there was something else, something still worse.

The same day that the first Camp Grant soldier died, 3,108 troops boarded a train leaving there for Camp Hancock outside Augusta, Georgia.

They left as a civilian health official several hundred miles away from Camp Grant demanded the quarantine of the entire camp, demanded that even escorts of the dead home be prohibited. They left with the memory of the trains carrying troops infected with measles, when Gorgas and Vaughan had protested uselessly that troops had "distributed its seeds at the encampment and on the train. No power on earth could stop the spread of measles under these conditions." They left after the provost general had had the foresight to cancel the next draft. And they left after Gorgas's office had urged that all movement of troops between infected and uninfected camps cease.

The army did order no "transfer of any influenza contacts" between camps or to bases under quarantine. But even that order came days later, at a time when each day's delay could cost literally thousands of lives. And the order also stated that "movements of officers and men not contacts will be effected promptly as ordered." Yet men could appear healthy while incubating influenza themselves, and they could also infect others before symptoms appeared.

The men leaving Grant on that train were jammed into the cars with little room to move about, layered and stacked as tightly as if on a submarine as they moved deliberately across 950 miles of the country. They would have been excited at first, for movement creates its own excitement, and then tedium would have set in, the minutes dragging out, the hours melding the passage into a self-contained world ten feet across and seven feet high, smelling of cigarette smoke and sweat, with hundreds of men in each car in far closer quarters than in any barracks, and with far less ventilation.

As the country rolled by men would have leaned out windows to suck in a wisp of air the way they sucked on cigarettes. And then one soldier would have broken into a coughing fit, another would have begun pouring out sweat, another would have suddenly had blood pouring out of his nose. Other men would have shrunk from them in fear, and then still others would have collapsed or erupted in fever or delirium or begun bleeding from their nose or possibly their ears. The train would have filled with panic. At stops for refueling and watering, men would have poured out of the train seeking any escape, mixed with workers and other civilians, obeyed reluctantly when officers ordered them back into the cars, into this rolling coffin.

When the train arrived, over seven hundred men—nearly one-quarter of all the troops on the train—were taken directly to the base hospital, quickly followed by hundreds more; in total, two thousand of the 3,108 troops would be hospitalized with influenza. After 143 deaths among them the statistics merged into those of other troops from Camp Hancock—Hancock, to which this shipment of virus was sent—and became impossible to track. But it is likely that the death toll approached, and possibly exceeded, 10 percent of all the troops on the train.

Hagadorn had become all but irrelevant to the running of the camp. Now he yielded on every point to the medical personnel, did everything they asked, made every resource available to them. Nothing seemed even to slow the disease.

On October 4, for the first time more than one hundred men at Camp Grant died in a single day. Nearly five thousand were ill, with hundreds more falling ill each day. And the graph of contagion still pointed nearly straight up.

Soon, in a single day, 1,810 soldiers would report ill. At some other army camps even more soldiers would collapse almost simultaneously; indeed, at Camp Custer outside Battle Creek, Michigan, twenty-eight hundred troops would report ill—in a *single* day.

Before the epidemic, Capps had begun testing Preston Kyes's pneumonia serum, prepared from chickens. Kyes had reasoned that since chickens were not susceptible to the pneumococcus, infecting them with highly virulent pneumococci might produce a very powerful serum. Capps had planned a series of "very carefully controlled" experiments.

But now, with nothing else to try, he administered the serum to all as it arrived—it was in short supply. It seemed to work. Two hundred and thirty-four men suffering from pneumonia received the serum; only 16.7 percent died, while more than half of those who did not receive it died. *But it was in short supply.*

Desperate efforts were being made to protect troops from the disease, or at least prevent complications. Germicidal solutions were sprayed into the mouths and noses of troops. Soldiers were ordered to use germicidal mouthwash and to gargle twice a day. Iodine in glycerine was tried in an attempt to disinfect mouths. Vaseline containing menthol was used in nasal passages, mouths washed with liquid albolene.

Despite every effort, the death toll kept rising. It rose so high that staff grew weary, weary of paperwork, weary even of identifying the dead. Michie was forced to issue orders warning, "The remains are labeled by placing an adhesive plaster bearing the name, rank, organization around the middle of the left forearm. It is the duty of the Ward Surgeon to see that this is done before the remains leave the ward. . . . A great deal of difficulty has been experienced in reading names on death certificates . . . Either have these certificates typewritten or . . . plainly printed. Any neglect on the part of responsible persons will be interpreted as a neglect of duty."

Michie also instructed all personnel, "The relatives and friends of persons dying at this hospital must not be sent to the base hospital morgue. . . . The handling of the effects of the deceased has grown into an enormous task."

Simultaneously, in that important fight to sustain the country's morale, the *Chicago Tribune* reported good news from Camp Grant. "Epidemic Broken!" blared the paper's headlines. "The small army of expert workers under the command of Lt. Col. H. C. Michie has battled the pneumonia epidemic to a standstill . . . deaths occurred among the pneumonia patients, but more than 100 fighting men pulled through the crisis of their illness . . . 175 patients have been released after winning their fight."

At that point Grant's death toll was 452. It showed no sign of slowing. Hoping to have some slight effect on it, hoping to prevent cross-infections, Michie and Capps reiterated their orders to place patients outside: "The crowding of patients in the wards must be reduced to the minimum. . . . The verandas must be used to the greatest advantage."

Perhaps that reminded Hagadorn of his earlier order authorizing overcrowding. Perhaps then too he got word of the hundreds of young men who had died on the train to Georgia, which, like the barracks overcrowding, he had ordered because of "military necessity." Perhaps these things caused him such personal pain that it explained why he abruptly ordered the withholding of the names of all soldiers who died from influenza. Perhaps somehow that allowed him to block the deaths from his mind.

A day later the death toll at the camp broke five hundred, with thousands more still desperately ill. "How far the pandemic will spread will apparently depend only upon the material which it can feed upon," wrote one army physician. "It is too early to foretell the end or to measure the damage which will be done before the pandemic disappears."

Many of the dead were more boys than men, eighteen years old, nineteen years old, twenty years old, twenty-one years old, boys filled with their lithe youth and sly smiles. Hagadorn, the bachelor, had made the army his home, his soldiers his family, the young men about him his life.

On October 8 Michie reported the latest death toll to Colonel Hagadorn in his headquarters office. The colonel heard the report, nodded, and, after an awkward moment, Michie rose to leave. Hagadorn told him to close the door.

Death was all about him, in the papers on his desk, in the reports he heard, literally in the air he breathed. It was an envelope sealing him in.

He picked up his phone and ordered his sergeant to leave the building and take with him all personnel in the headquarters and stand for inspection outside.

It was a bizarre order. The sergeant informed Captain Jisson and Lieutenant Rashel. They were puzzled but complied.

For half an hour they waited. The pistol shot, even from inside the building, came as a loud report.

Hagadorn was not listed as a casualty of the epidemic. Nor did his sacrifice stop it.

CHAPTER NINETEEN

TWO DAYS AFTER Philadelphia's Liberty Loan parade, Wilmer Krusen had issued that somber statement, that the epidemic in the civilian population "was assuming the type found in naval stations and cantonments."

Influenza was indeed exploding in the city. Within seventy-two hours after the parade, every single bed in each of the city's thirty-one hospitals was filled. And people began dying. Hospitals began refusing to accept patients—with nurses turning down $100 bribes—without a doctor's or a police order. Yet people queued up to get in. One woman remembered her neighbors going "to the closest hospital, the Pennsylvania Hospital at 5th and Lombard but when they got there there were lines and no doctors available and no medicine available. So they went home, those that were strong enough."

Medical care was making little difference anyway. Mary Tullidge, daughter of Dr. George Tullidge, died twenty-four hours after her first symptoms. Alice Wolowitz, a student nurse at Mount Sinai Hospital, began her shift in the morning, felt sick, and was dead twelve hours later.

On October 1, the third day after the parade, the epidemic killed more than one hundred people—117—in a single day. That number would double, triple, quadruple, quintuple, sextuple. Soon the daily death toll from influenza alone would exceed the city's average *weekly* death toll from all causes—all illnesses, all accidents, all criminal acts combined.

On October 3, only five days after Krusen had let the parade proceed, he banned all public meetings in the city—including, finally, further Liberty Loan gatherings—and closed all churches, schools, theaters. Even public funerals were prohibited. Only one public gathering place was allowed to remain open: the saloon, the key constituency of the Vare machine. The next day the state health commissioner closed them.

The first temporary facility to care for the sick was set up at Holmesburg, the city's poorhouse. It was called "Emergency Hospital #1"; the Board of Health knew more would follow. Its five hundred beds were filled in a day. Ultimately there would be twelve similar large hospitals run with city help, three of them located in converted Republican Clubs in South Philadelphia. It was where people had always gone for help.

In ten days—*ten days!*—the epidemic had exploded from a few hundred civilian cases and one or two deaths a day to hundreds of thousands ill and hundreds of deaths each day.

Federal, municipal, and state courts closed. Giant placards everywhere warned the public to avoid crowds and use handkerchiefs when sneezing or coughing. Other placards read "Spitting equals death." People who spat on the street were arrested—sixty in a single day. The newspapers reported the arrests—even while continuing to minimize the epidemic. Physicians were themselves dying, three one day, two another, four the next. The newspapers reported those deaths—on inside pages with other obituaries—even while continuing to minimize the epidemic. Health and city workers wore masks constantly.

What should I do? people wondered, with dread. *How long will it go on?* Each day people discovered that friends and neighbors who had been perfectly healthy a week—or a day—earlier were dead.

And city authorities and newspapers continued to minimize the danger. The *Public Ledger* claimed nonsensically that Krusen's order banning all public gatherings was not "a public health measure" and reiterated, "There is no cause for panic or alarm."

On October 5, doctors reported that 254 people died that day from the epidemic, and the papers quoted public health authorities as saying, "The peak of the influenza epidemic has been reached." When 289 Philadelphians died the next day, the papers said, "Believing that the peak of the epidemic has passed, health officials are confident."

In each of the next two days more than three hundred people died, and again Krusen announced, "These deaths mark the high water mark in the fatalities, and it is fair to assume that from this time until the epidemic is crushed the death rate will constantly be lowered."

The next day 428 people died, and the daily death toll would keep climbing for many days yet—approaching double even that figure.

Krusen said, "Don't get frightened or panic stricken over exaggerated reports."

But Krusen's reassurances no longer reassured.

One could not listen to Paul Lewis speak on any subject and not sense the depth of his knowledge and his ability to see into a problem, envision possible solutions and understand their ramifications. Other scientists in the city did not defer to him, but they looked to him.

He had been working on this problem for three weeks now. He hardly ever left his laboratory. Nor did his assistants, except for the ones who fell ill. Every scientist in Philadelphia was spending every waking minute in the laboratory as well.

The laboratory was his favorite place anyway, more even than home. Normally, everything in his work gave him peace; the laboratory gave him peace, including the mysteries that he embraced. He settled into them like a man casting off into an impenetrable ocean fog, a fog that made one feel both alone in and part of the world.

But this work did not give him peace. It wasn't the pressure exactly. It was that the pressure forced him off rhythm, forced him to abandon the scientific process. He developed a hypothesis and focused on it, but the shorthand process by which he arrived at it made him uncomfortable.

So did hearing the news of the deaths. The youth and vitality and promise of the dead horrified. The waste of their promise horrified. He worked harder.

Arthur Eissinger, president and "honor man" of Penn's class of 1918, died. Dudley Perkins, a Swarthmore football hero, died. Nearly two-thirds of the dead were under forty.

It was a common practice in 1918 for people to hang a piece of crepe on the door to mark a death in the house. There was crepe everywhere. "If it was a young person they'd put a white crepe at the door," recalled Anna Milani. "If it was a middle-aged person, they'd put a black crepe, and if it was an elderly one, they put a grey crepe at the door signifiying who died. We were children and we were excited to find out who died next and we were looking at the door, there was another crepe and another door."

There was always another door. "People were dying like flies," Clifford Adams said. "On Spring Garden Street, looked like every other house had crepe over the door. People was dead there."

Anna Lavin was at Mount Sinai Hospital: "My uncle died there. . . . My aunt died first. Their son was thirteen. . . . A lot of young people, just married, they were the first to die."

But the most terrifying aspect of the epidemic was the piling up of bodies. Undertakers, themselves sick, were overwhelmed. They had no place to put bodies. Gravediggers either were sick or refused to bury influenza victims. The director of the city jail offered to have prisoners dig graves, then rescinded the offer because he had no healthy guards to watch them. With no gravediggers bodies could not be buried. Undertakers' work areas were overflowing, they stacked caskets in halls, in their living quarters—many lived above their businesses.

Then undertakers ran short of coffins. The few coffins available suddenly became priceless. Michael Donohue's family operated a funeral home: "We had caskets stacked up outside the funeral home. We had to have guards kept on them because people were stealing the caskets. . . . You'd equate that to grave robbing."

There were soon no caskets left to steal. Louise Apuchase remembered most vividly the lack of coffins: "A neighbor boy about seven or eight died and they used to just pick you up and wrap you up in a sheet and put you in a patrol wagon. So the mother and father *screaming,* 'Let me get a macaroni box' [for a coffin]—macaroni, any kind of pasta, used to come in this box, about 20 pounds of macaroni fit in it—'please please let me put him in the macaroni box, don't take him away like that. . . .'"

Clifford Adams remembered "bodies stacked up . . . stacked up out to be buried. . . . They couldn't bury them." The bodies backed up more and more, backed up in the houses, were put outside on porches.

The city morgue had room for thirty-six bodies. Two hundred were stacked there. The stench was terrible; doors and windows were thrown open. No more bodies could fit. Bodies lay in homes where they died, as they died, often with bloody liquid seeping from the nostrils or mouths. Families covered the bodies in ice; even so the bodies began to putrefy and stink. Tenements had no porches; few had fire escapes. Families closed off rooms where a body lay, but a closed door could not close out the knowledge and the horror of what lay behind the door. In much of the city, a city more short of housing than New York, people had no room that could be closed off. Corpses were wrapped in sheets, pushed into corners, left there sometimes for days, the horror of it sinking in deeper each hour, people too sick to cook for themselves, too sick to clean themselves, too sick to move the corpse off the bed, lying alive on the same bed with the corpse. The dead lay there for days, while the living lived with them, were horrified by them, and, perhaps most horribly, became accustomed to them.

Symptoms were terrifying. Blood poured from noses, ears, eye sockets; some victims lay in agony; delirium took others away while living.

Routinely two people in a single family would die. Three deaths in a family were not uncommon. Sometimes a family suffered even more. David Sword lived at 2802 Jackson Street. On October 5 the sixth member of his family died of influenza, while the *North American* reported that three other family members in the hospital "may also die of the plague."

The plague. In the streets people had been whispering the word. The word slipped, somehow, once, by accident, into that newspaper. The "morale" issue, the self-censorship, the intent by editors to put every piece of news in the most positive possible context, all meant that no newspaper used that word again. Yet people did not need newspapers to speak of the Black Death. Some bodies were turning almost black. People had seen them, and they had lost faith in what they read anyway. One young medical student called in to treat hundreds of patients recalled, "The cyanosis reached an intensity that I have never seen since. Indeed the rumor got about that the Black Death had returned." The newspapers quoted Dr. Raymond Leopold, sounding reasonable: "There is abundant reason for such a rumor. . . . It is true that many bodies have assumed a dark hue and have given off a pronounced odor after death." But he gave his assurance, "There is no truth in the black plague assertion."

He was of course correct. But how many trusted the newspapers anymore? And even if the Black Death had not come, a plague had and, with it, so had terror.

The war had come home.

■   ■   ■

Long before Hagadorn's suicide, long before the marchers in Philadelphia began to parade down the city streets, influenza had seeded itself along the edges of the nation.

On September 4 it had reached New Orleans, with the three seamen—who soon died—carried to the hospital off the *Harold Walker* from Boston. On September 7 it had reached the Great Lakes Naval Training Station, with sailors transferred from Boston. In the next few days ports and naval facilities on the Atlantic and Gulf Coasts—in Newport, New London, Norfolk, Mobile, and Biloxi—also reported this new influenza. On September 17, 1918, "the extensive prevalence of an influenza-like disease" was reported in Petersburg, Virginia, outside Camp Lee. That same day, the several hundred sailors who had departed Philadelphia earlier for Puget Sound arrived; eleven men had to be carried from the ship on stretchers to a hospital, bringing the new virus to the Pacific.

The virus had spanned the country, establishing itself on the Atlantic, in the Gulf, on the Pacific, on the Great Lakes. It had not immediately erupted in epidemic form, but it had seeded itself. Then the seeds began to sprout into flowers of flame.

The virus followed rail and river into the interior of the continent, from New Orleans up the Mississippi River into the body of the nation, from Seattle to the East, from the Great Lakes training station to Chicago and from there along the railroad lines in many directions. From each original locus fingers reached out, unevenly, like sparks shooting out, often jumping over closer points to farther ones—from Boston to Newport, for example, and only then reaching backward to fill in Brockton and Providence and places in between.

On September 28, when the Liberty Loan paraders marched through Philadelphia streets, there were as yet only seven cases reported in Los Angeles, two in San Francisco. But the virus would get there soon enough.

In Philadelphia meanwhile fear came and stayed. Death could come from anyone, anytime. People moved away from others on the sidewalk, avoided conversation; if they did speak, they turned their faces away to avoid the other person's breathing. People became isolated, increasing the fear.

The impossibility of getting help compounded the isolation. Eight hundred fifty Philadelphia doctors and more nurses were away in the military. More than that number were sick. Philadelphia General Hospital had 126 nurses. Despite all precautions, despite wearing surgical masks and gowns, eight doctors and fifty-four nurses—43 percent of the staff—themselves required hospitalization. Ten nurses at this single hospital died. The Board of Health pleaded for help from retired nurses and doctors if they remembered "even a little" of their profession.

When a nurse or doctor or policeman did actually come, they wore their ghostly surgical masks, and people fled them. In every home where someone was ill, people wondered if the person would die. And someone was ill in every home.

Philadelphia had five medical schools. Each one dismissed its classes, and third- and fourth-year students manned emergency hospitals being set up in schools and empty buildings all over the city. The Philadelphia College of Pharmacy closed as well, sending its students out to help druggists.

Before University of Pennsylvania medical students went out to man the hospitals, they listened to a lecture from Alfred Stengel, the expert on infectious diseases who had treated the crew of the *City of Exeter* what seemed so long ago. Stengel reviewed dozens of ideas that had been advanced in medical journals. Gargles of various disinfectants. Drugs. Immune sera. Typhoid vaccine. Diphtheria antitoxin. But Stengel's message was simple: *This doesn't work. That doesn't work. Nothing worked.*

"His suggestion for treatment was negative," Isaac Starr, one of those Penn students, who became an internationally known cardiologist, recalled. "He had no confidence in any of the remedies that had been proposed."

Stengel was correct. Nothing they were yet doing worked. Starr went to Emergency Hospital #2 at Eighteenth and Cherry Streets. He did have help, if it could be called that, from an elderly physician who had not practiced in years and who brought Starr into touch with the worst of heroic medicine. Starr wouldn't forget that, the ancient arts of purging, of venesection, the ancient art of opening a patient's vein. But for the most part he and the other students elsewhere were on their own, with little help even from nurses, who were so desperately needed that in each of ten emergency hospitals supplied by the Red Cross only a single qualified nurse was available to oversee whatever women came as volunteers. And often the volunteers reported for their duty once and, from either fear or exhaustion, did not come again.

Starr had charge of an entire floor of an emergency hospital. He thought at first his patients had "what appeared to be a minor illness . . . with fever but little else. Unhappily the clinical features of many soon changed." Most striking again was the cyanosis, his patients sometimes turning almost black. "After gasping for several hours they became delirious and incontinent, and many died struggling to clear their airways of a blood-tinged froth that sometimes gushed from their nose and mouth."

Nearly one-quarter of all the patients in his hospital died *each day*. Starr would go home, and when he returned the next day, he would find that between one-quarter and one-fifth of the patients in the hospital had died, replaced by new ones.

Literally hundreds of thousands of people in Philadelphia were falling ill. Virtually all of them, along with their friends and relatives, were terrified that, no matter how mild the symptoms seemed at first, within them moved an alien force, a seething, spreading infection, a live thing with a will that was taking over their bodies—and could be killing them. And those who moved about them feared—feared both for the victims and for themselves.

The city was frozen with fear, frozen quite literally into stillness. Starr lived twelve miles from the hospital, in Chestnut Hill. The streets were silent on his drive home, silent. They were so silent he took to counting the cars he saw. One night he saw no cars at all. He thought, "The life of the city had almost stopped."

■ Part VI
THE PESTILENCE

CHAPTER TWENTY

THIS WAS INFLUENZA, only influenza.

This new influenza virus, like most new influenza viruses, spread rapidly and widely. As a modern epidemiologist already quoted has observed, *Influenza is a special instance among infectious diseases. This virus is transmitted so effectively that it exhausts the supply of susceptible hosts.* This meant that the virus sickened tens of millions of people in the United States—in many cities more than half of all families had at least one victim ill with influenza; in San Antonio the virus made more than half the entire population ill—and hundreds of millions across the world.

But this was influenza, only influenza. The overwhelming majority of victims got well. They endured, sometimes a mild attack and sometimes a severe one, and they recovered.

The virus passed through this vast majority in the same way influenza viruses usually did. Victims had an extremely unpleasant several days (the unpleasantness multiplied by terror that they would develop serious complications) and then recovered within ten days. The course of the disease in these millions actually convinced the medical profession that this was indeed only influenza.

But in a minority of cases, and not just in a tiny minority, the virus manifested itself in an influenza that did not follow normal patterns, that was unlike any influenza ever reported, that followed a course so different from the usual one for the disease that Welch himself had initially feared some new kind of infection or plague. If Welch feared it, those who suffered with the disease were terrified by it.

Generally in the Western world, the virus demonstrated extreme virulence or led to pneumonia in from 10 to 20 percent of all cases. In the United States, this translated into two to three million cases. In other parts of the world, chiefly in isolated areas where people had rarely been exposed to influenza viruses—in Eskimo settlements of Alaska, in jungle villages of Africa, in islands of the Pacific—the virus demonstrated extreme virulence in far more than 20 percent of cases. These numbers most likely translate into several hundred million severe cases around the world in a world with a population less than one-third that of today.

This was still influenza, only influenza. The most common symptoms then as now are well known. The mucosal membranes in the nose, pharynx, and throat become inflamed. The conjunctiva, the delicate membrane that lines the eyelids, becomes inflamed. Victims suffer headache, body aches, fever, often complete exhaustion, cough. As one leading clinician observed in 1918, the disease was "ushered in by two groups of symptoms: in the first place the constitutional reactions of an acute febrile disease—headache, general aching, chills, fever, malaise, prostration, anorexia, nausea or vomiting; and in the second place, symptoms referable to an intense congestion of the mucous membranes of the nose, pharynx, larynx, trachea, and upper respiratory tract in general, and of the conjunctivae." Another noted, "The disease began with absolute exhaustion and chill, fever, headache, conjunctivitis, pain in back and limbs, flushing of face. . . . Cough was often constant. Upper air passages were clogged." A third reported, "In nonfatal cases . . . the temperature ranged from 100 to 103F. Nonfatal cases usually recovered after an illness of about a week."

Then there were the cases in which the virus struck with violence.

To those who suffered a violent attack, there was often pain, terrific pain, and the pain could come almost anywhere. The disease also separated them, pushed them into a solitary and concentrated place.

In Philadelphia, Clifford Adams said, "I didn't think about anything. . . . I got to the point where I didn't care if I died or not. I just felt like that all my life was nothing but when I breathe."

Bill Sardo in Washington, D.C., recalled, "I wasn't expected to live, just like everybody else that had gotten it. . . . You were sick as a dog and you weren't in a coma but you were in a condition that at the height of the crisis you weren't thinking normally and you weren't reacting normally, you sort of had delusions."

In Lincoln, Illinois, William Maxwell felt "time was a blur as I was lying in that little upstairs room and I . . . had no sense of day or night, I felt sick and hollow inside and I knew from telephone calls my aunt had, I knew enough to be alarmed about my mother. . . . I heard her say, 'Will, oh no,' and then, 'if you want me to . . .' The tears ran down her face so she didn't need to tell me."

Josey Brown fell ill working as a nurse at the Great Lakes Naval Training Station and her "heart was racing so hard and pounding that it was going to jump out" of her chest and with terrible fevers she was "shaking so badly that the ice would rattle and would shake the chart attached to the end of the bed."

Harvey Cushing, Halsted's protégé who had already attained prominence himself but had yet to make his full reputation, served in France. On October 8, 1918, he wrote in his journal, "Something has happened to my hind legs and I wobble like a tabetic"—someone suffering from a long and wasting illness, like a person with AIDS who needs a cane—"and can't feel the floor when I unsteadily get up in the morning. . . . So this is the sequence of the grippe. We may perhaps thank it for helping us win the war if it really hit the German Army thus hard [during their offensive]." In his case what seemed to be the complications were largely neurological. On October 31, after spending three weeks in bed with headache, double vision, and numbness of both legs, he observed, "It's a curious business, unquestionably still progressing . . . with considerable muscular wasting. . . . I have a vague sense of familiarity with the sensation—as if I had met [it] somewhere in a dream." Four days later: "My hands now have caught up with my feet—so numb and clumsy that shaving's a danger and buttoning laborious. When the periphery is thus affected the brain too is benumbed and awkward."

Cushing would never fully recover.

And across the lines lay Rudolph Binding, a German officer, who described his illness as "something like typhoid, with ghastly symptoms of intestinal poisoning." For weeks he was "in the grip of the fever. Some days I am quite free; then again a weakness overcomes me so that I can barely drag myself in a cold perspiration onto my bed and blankets. Then pain, so that I don't care whether I am alive or dead."

Katherine Anne Porter was a reporter then, on the *Rocky Mountain News*. Her fiancé, a young officer, died. He caught the disease nursing her, and she, too, was expected to die. Her colleagues set her obituary in type. She lived. In *Pale Horse, Pale Rider* she described her movement toward death: "She lay on a narrow ledge over a pit she knew to be bottomless . . . and soft carefully shaped words like oblivion and eternity are curtains hung before nothing at all. . . . Her mind tottered and slithered again, broke from its foundation and spun like a cast wheel in a ditch. . . . She sank easily through deeps and deeps of darkness until she lay like a stone at the farthest bottom of life, knowing herself to be blind, deaf, speechless, no longer aware of the members of her own body, entirely withdrawn from all human concerns, yet alive with a peculiar lucidity and coherence; all notions of the mind, all ties of blood and the desires of the heart, dissolved and fell away from her, and there remained of her only a minute fiercely burning particle of being that knew itself alone, that relied upon nothing beyond itself for its strength; not susceptible to any appeal or inducement, being itself composed entirely of one single motive, the stubborn will to live. This fiery motionless particle set itself unaided to resist destruction, to survive and to be in its own madness of being, motiveless and planless beyond that one essential end."

Then, as she climbed back from that depth, "Pain returned, a terrible compelling pain running through her veins like heavy fire, the stench of corruption filled her nostrils, the sweetish sickening smell of rotting flesh and pus; she opened her eyes and saw pale light through a coarse white cloth over her face, knew that the smell of death was in her own body, and struggled to lift her hand."

These victims came with an extraordinary array of symptoms, symptoms either previously unknown entirely in influenza or experienced with previously unknown intensity. Initially, physicians, good physicians, intelligent physicians searching for a disease that fitted the clues before them—and influenza did not fit the clues—routinely misdiagnosed the disease.

Patients would writhe from agonizing pain in their joints. Doctors would diagnose dengue, also called "breakbone fever."

Patients would suffer extreme fever and chills, shuddering, shivering, then huddling under blankets. Doctors would diagnose malaria.

Dr. Henry Berg at New York City's Willard Parker Hospital—across the street from William Park's laboratory—worried that the patients' complaints of "a burning pain above the diaphragm" meant cholera. Noted another doctor, "Many had vomiting; some became tender over the abdomen indicating an intra-abdominal condition."

In Paris, while some physicians also diagnosed cholera or dysentery, others interpreted the intensity and location of headache pain as typhoid. Deep into the epidemic Parisian physicians still remained reluctant to diagnose influenza. In Spain public health officials also declared that the complications were due to "typhoid," which was "general throughout Spain."

But neither typhoid nor cholera, neither dengue nor yellow fever, neither plague nor tuberculosis, neither diphtheria nor dysentery, could account for other symptoms. No known disease could.

In *Proceedings of the Royal Society of Medicine,* a British physician noted "one thing I have never seen before—namely the occurrence of subcutaneous emphysema"—pockets of air accumulating just beneath the skin—"beginning in the neck and spreading sometimes over the whole body."

Those pockets of air leaking through ruptured lungs made patients crackle when they were rolled onto their sides. One navy nurse later compared the sound to a bowl of rice crispies, and the memory of that sound was so vivid to her that for the rest of her life she could not tolerate being around anyone who was eating rice crispies.

Extreme earaches were common. One physician observed that otitis media—inflammation of the middle ear marked by pain, fever, and dizziness—"developed with surprising rapidity, and rupture of the drum membrane was observed at times in a few hours after the onset of pain." Another wrote, "Otitis media reported in 41 cases. Otologists on duty day and night and did immediate paracentesis [insertion of a needle to remove fluid] on all bulging eardrums. . . ." Another: "Discharge of pus from the external ear was noted. At autopsy practically every case showed otitis media with perforation. . . . This destructive action on the drum seems to me to be similar to the destructive action on the tissues of the lung."

The headaches throbbed deep in the skull, victims feeling as if their heads would literally split open, as if a sledgehammer were driving a wedge not into the head but from inside the head out. The pain seemed to locate particularly behind the eye orbit and could be nearly unbearable when patients moved their eyes. There were areas of lost vision, areas where the normal frame of sight went black. Some paralysis of ocular muscles was frequently recorded, and German medical literature noted eye involvement with special frequency, sometimes in 25 percent of influenza cases.

The ability to smell was affected, sometimes for weeks. Rarer complications included acute—even fatal—renal failure. Reye's syndrome attacked the liver. An army summary later stated simply, "The symptoms were of exceeding variety as to severity and kind."

It was not only death but these symptoms that spread the terror.

This was influenza, only influenza. Yet to a layperson at home, to a wife caring for a husband, to a father caring for a child, to a brother caring for a sister, symptoms unlike anything they had seen terrified. And the symptoms terrified a Boy Scout delivering food to an incapacitated family; they terrified a policeman who entered an apartment to find a tenant dead or dying; they terrified a man who volunteered his car as an ambulance. The symptoms chilled laypeople, chilled them with winds of fear.

The world looked black. Cyanosis turned it black. Patients might have few other symptoms at first, but if nurses and doctors noted cyanosis they began to treat such patients as terminal, as the walking dead. If the cyanosis became extreme, death was certain. And cyanosis was common. One physician reported, "Intense cyanosis was a striking phenomenon. The lips, ears, nose, cheeks, tongue, conjunctivae, fingers, and sometimes the entire body partook of a dusky, leaden hue." And another: "Many patients exhibited upon admission a strikingly intense cyanosis, especially noticeable in the lips. This was not the dusky pallid blueness that one is accustomed to in a failing pneumonia, but rather [a] deep blueness." And a third: "In cases with bilateral lesions the cyanosis was marked, even to an indigo blue color. . . . The pallor was of particularly bad prognostic import."

Then there was the blood, blood pouring from the body. To see blood trickle, and in some cases spurt, from someone's nose, mouth, even from the ears or around the eyes, had to terrify. Terrifying as the bleeding was, it did not mean death, but even to physicians, even to those accustomed to thinking of the body as a machine and to trying to understand the disease process, symptoms like these previously unassociated with influenza had to be unsettling. For when the virus turned violent, blood was everywhere.*

In U.S. Army cantonments, from 5 percent to 15 percent of all men hospitalized suffered from epistaxis—bleeding from the nose—as with hemorrhagic viruses such as Ebola. There are many reports that blood sometimes spurted from the nose with enough power to travel several feet. Doctors had no explanation for these symptoms. They could only report them.

"15% suffered from epistaxis. . . ." "In about one-half the cases a foamy, blood-stained liquid ran from the nose and mouth when the head was lowered. . . ." "Epistaxis occurs in a considerable number of cases, in one person a pint of bright red blood gushing from the nostrils. . . ." "A striking feature in the early stages of these cases was a bleeding from some portion of the body. . . . Six cases vomited blood; one died from loss of blood from this cause."

What was this?

"One of the most striking of the complications was hemorrhage from mucous membranes, especially from the nose, stomach, and intestine. Bleeding from the ears and petechial hemorrhages in the skin also occurred."

One German investigator recorded "hemorrhages occurring in different parts of the interior of the eye" with great frequency. An American pathologist noted: "Fifty cases of subconjunctival hemorrhage [bleeding from the lining of the eye] were counted. Twelve had a true hemoptysis, bright red blood with no admixture of mucus. . . . Three cases had intestinal hemorrhage. . . ."

"Female patients had a hemorrhagic vaginal discharge which was at first considered to be coincident menstruation, but later was interpreted as hemorrhage from the uterine mucosa."

*Many mechanisms can cause bleeding in mucous membranes, and the precise way the influenza virus does this is unknown. Some viruses also attack platelets— which are necessary for clotting—directly or indirectly, and elements of the immune system may inadvertently attack platelets as well.

What was this?

Never did the virus cause only a single symptom. The chief diagnostician in the New York City Health Department summarized, "Cases with intense pain look and act like cases of dengue . . . hemorrhage from nose or bronchi. . . . Expectoration is usually profuse and may be bloodstained . . . paresis or paralysis of either cerebral or spinal origin . . . impairment of motion may be severe or mild, permanent or temporary . . . physical and mental depression. Intense and protracted prostration led to hysteria, melancholia, and insanity with suicidal intent."

The impact on the mental state of the victims would be one of the most widely noted sequelae.

During the course of the epidemic, 47 percent of all deaths in the United States, nearly half of all those who died from all causes combined—from cancer, from heart disease, from stroke, from tuberculosis, from accidents, from suicide, from murder, and from all other causes—resulted from influenza and its complications. And it killed enough to depress the average life expectancy in the United States by more than ten years.

Some of those who died from influenza and pneumonia would have died if no epidemic had occurred. Pneumonia was after all the leading cause of death. So the key figure is actually the "excess death" toll. Investigators today believe that in the United States the 1918–19 epidemic caused an excess death toll of about 675,000 people. The nation then had a population between 105 and 110 million, while it was approaching 300 million in 2006. So a comparable figure today would be approximately 1,750,000 deaths.

And there was something even beyond the gross numbers that gave the 1918 influenza pandemic terrifying immediacy, brought it into every home, brought it into homes with the most life.

Influenza almost always selects the weakest in a society to kill, the very young and the very old. It kills opportunistically, like a bully. It almost always allows the most vigorous, the most healthy, to escape, including young adults as a group. Pneumonia was even known as "the old man's friend" for killing particularly the elderly, and doing so in a relatively painless and peaceful fashion that even allowed time to say good-bye.

There was no such grace about influenza in 1918. It killed the young and strong. Studies worldwide all found the same thing. Young adults, the healthiest and strongest part of the population, were the most likely to die. Those with the most to live for—the robust, the fit, the hearty, the ones raising young sons and daughters—those were the ones who died.

In South African cities, those between the ages of twenty and forty accounted for 60 percent of the deaths. In Chicago the deaths among those aged twenty to forty almost quintupled deaths of those aged forty-one to sixty. A Swiss physician "saw no severe case in anyone over 50." In the "registration area" of the United States—those states and cities that kept reliable statistics—breaking the population into five-year increments, the single greatest number of deaths occurred in men and women aged twenty-five to twenty-nine, the second-greatest number in those aged thirty to thirty-four, the third-greatest in those aged twenty to twenty-four. And more people died in *each* of those five-year groups than the total deaths among *all* those over age sixty.

Graphs that correlate mortality rates and age in influenza outbreaks always—always, that is, except for 1918–19—start out with a peak representing infant deaths, then fall into a valley, then rise again, with a second peak representing people somewhere past sixty-five or so. With mortality on the vertical and age on the horizontal, a graph of the dead would like like a U.

But 1918 was different. Infants did die then in large numbers, and so did the elderly. But in 1918 the great spike came in the middle. In 1918 an age graph of the dead would look like a W.

It is a graph that tells a story of utter tragedy. Even at the front in France, Harvey Cushing recognized this tragedy and called the victims "doubly dead in that they died so young."

In the American military alone, influenza-related deaths totaled just over the number of Americans killed in combat in Vietnam. One in every sixty-seven soldiers in the army died of influenza and its complications, nearly all of them in a ten-week period beginning in mid-September.

But influenza of course did not kill only men in the military. In the United States it killed fifteen times as many civilians as military. And among young adults still another demographic stood out. Those most vulnerable of all to influenza, those most likely of the most likely to die, were pregnant women. As far back as the year 1557, observers connected influenza with miscarriage and the death of pregnant women. In thirteen studies of hospitalized pregnant women during the 1918 pandemic, the death rate ranged from 23 percent to 71 percent. Of the pregnant women who survived, 26 percent lost the child. And these women were the most likely group to already have other children, so an unknown but enormous number of children lost their mothers.

The most pregnant word in science is "interesting." It suggests something new, puzzling, and potentially significant. Welch had asked Burt Wolbach, the brilliant chief pathologist at the great Boston hospital known as "the Brigham," to investigate the Devens cases. Wolbach called it "the most interesting pathological experience I have ever had."

The epidemiology of this pandemic was *interesting*. The unusual symptoms were *interesting*. And the autopsies—and some symptoms revealed themselves only in autopsy—were *interesting*. The damage this virus caused and its epidemiology presented a deep mystery. An explanation would come—but not for decades.

In the meantime this influenza, for it was after all only influenza, left almost no internal organ untouched. Another distinguished pathologist noted that the brain showed "marked hyperemia"—blood flooding the brain, probably because of an out-of-control inflammatory response— adding, "the convolutions of the brain were flattened and the brain tissues were noticeably dry."

The virus inflamed or affected the pericardium—the sac of tissue and fluid that protects the heart—and the heart muscle itself, noted others. The heart was also often "relaxed and flabby, offering strong contrast to the firm, contracted left ventricle nearly always present in post-mortem in patients dying from lobar pneumonia."

The amount of damage to the kidneys varied but at least some damage "occurred in nearly every case." The liver was sometimes damaged. The adrenal glands suffered "necrotic areas, frank hemorrhage, and occasionally abscesses. . . . When not involved in the hemorrhagic process they usually showed considerable congestion."

Muscles along the rib cage were torn apart both by internal toxic processes and by the external stress of coughing, and in many other muscles pathologists noted "necrosis," or "waxy degeneration."

Even the testes showed "very striking changes . . . encountered in nearly every case. . . . It was difficult to understand why such severe toxic lesions of the muscle and the testis should occur. . . ."

And, finally, came the lungs.

Physicians had seen lungs in such condition. But those lungs had not come from pneumonia patients. Only one known disease—a particularly virulent form of bubonic plague called pneumonic plague, which kills approximately 90 percent of its victims—ripped the lungs apart in the way this disease did. So did weapons in war.

An army physician concluded, "The only comparable findings are those of pneumonic plague and those seen in acute death from toxic gas."

Seventy years after the pandemic, Edwin Kilbourne, a highly respected scientist who has spent much of his life studying influenza, confirmed this observation, stating that the condition of the lungs was "unusual in other viral respiratory infections and is reminiscent of lesions seen following inhalation of poison gas."

But the cause was not poison gas, and it was not pneumonic plague. It was only influenza.

CHAPTER TWENTY-ONE

IN 1918 IN PARTICULAR, influenza struck so suddenly that many victims could remember the precise instant they knew they were sick, so suddenly that throughout the world reports were common of people who toppled off horses, collapsed on the sidewalk.

Death itself could come so fast. Charles-Edward Winslow, a prominent epidemiologist and professor at Yale, noted, "We have had a number of cases where people were perfectly healthy and died within twelve hours." The *Journal of the American Medical Association* carried reports of death within hours: "One robust person showed the first symptom at 4:00 P.M. and died by 10:00 A.M." In *The Plague of the Spanish Lady: The Influenza Pandemic of 1918-1919*, writer Richard Collier recounted this: In Rio de Janeiro, a man asked medical student Ciro Viera Da Cunha, who was waiting for a streetcar, for information in a perfectly normal voice, then fell down, dead; in Cape Town, South Africa, Charles Lewis boarded a streetcar for a three-mile trip home when the conductor collapsed, dead. In the next three miles six people aboard the streetcar died, including the driver.

Lewis stepped off the streetcar and walked home.

It was the lungs that had attracted attention from pathologists first. Physicians and pathologists had many times seen lungs of those dead of pneumonia. Many of the deaths from influenzal pneumonia did look like these normal pneumonias. And the later in the epidemic a victim died, the higher was the percentage of autopsy findings that resembled normal pneumonia, bacterial pneumonia.

Those who died very quickly, a day or even less after the first symptoms, however, most likely died of an overwhelming and massive invasion of the virus itself. The virus destroyed enough cells in the lung to block the exchange of oxygen. This alone was unusual and puzzling. But the lungs of the men and women who died two days, three days, four days after the first symptom of influenza bore no resemblance to normal pneumonias at all. They were more unusual, more puzzling.

In April a Chicago pathologist had sent lung-tissue samples to the head of a research institute and asked him "to look over it as a new disease." British pathologists in France had commented on strange autopsy findings in the spring. Capps had mentioned unusual findings in the lungs to Welch, Cole, and other members of the inspection party in June. The lungs Welch himself had seen in the Devens autopsy room had made him fear that the disease was a new one.

The respiratory tract serves a single purpose: to transfer oxygen from the air into red blood cells. One can picture the entire system as an inverted oak tree. The trachea—the windpipe—carries air from the outside world into the lungs and is the equivalent of the tree trunk. This trunk then divides into two great branches, each called a "primary bronchus," which carry oxygen into the right and left lungs. Each primary bronchus subdivides into smaller and smaller bronchi, smaller branches, as they enter the lungs until they become "bronchioles." (Bronchi have cartilage, which helps give the lung a kind of architectural structure; bronchioles do not have cartilage.)

Each lung itself subdivides into lobes—the right lung has three, the left only two. The lobes subdivide into a total of nineteen smaller pockets. Within these pockets, sprouting like leaves from the smaller bronchi and the bronchioles, are clusters of tiny sacs called alveoli. They are much like tiny but porous balloons, and the average person has 300 million of them. The alveoli play a role comparable to that which leaves play in photosynthesis. In the alveoli, the actual transfer of oxygen into the blood takes place.

The right side of the heart pumps blood without oxygen into the lungs, where it passes into capillaries, the smallest blood vessels, so small that individual blood cells often move in single file. Capillaries surround the alveoli, and oxygen molecules slip through the membrane of the alveolar tissue and attach to the hemoglobin of the red blood cells as they circulate past them. After picking up oxygen, the blood returns to the left side of the heart, where it is pumped through arteries throughout the body. (The body's entire blood supply moves through the lungs each minute.)

In arteries, red blood cells carry oxygen and are bright red; in veins, such as those visible on one's wrist, the same cells without oxygen are bluish. When the lungs fail to oxygenate the blood, part of the body, and in some cases the entire body, can turn blue, causing cyanosis. Lack of oxygen, if extended for any length of time, damages and ultimately kills other organs in the body.

Healthy lung tissue is light, spongy, and porous, much lighter than water, and a good insulator of sound. A physician percussing the chest of a healthy patient will hear little. When normal lung tissue is manipulated, it "crepitates": as the air in the alevoli escapes, it makes a crackling noise similar to rubbing hairs together.

A congested lung sounds different from a healthy one: solid tissue conducts breathing sounds to the chest wall, so someone listening can hear "rales," crackling or wheezing sounds (although it can also sound either dull or hyperresonant). If the congestion is dense enough and widespread enough the lung is "consolidated."

In bronchopneumonia, bacteria—and many kinds of bacteria can do this—invade the alveoli themselves. Immune-system cells follow them there, and so do antibodies, fluid, and other proteins and enzymes. An infected alveolus becomes dense with this material, which prevents it from transferring oxygen to the blood. This "consolidation" appears in patches surrounding the bronchi, and the infection is usually fairly localized.

In lobar pneumonia, entire lobes become consolidated and transformed into a liverlike mass—hence the word "hepatization" to describe it. A hepatized lobe can turn various colors depending on the stage of disease; grey hepatization, for example, indicates that various kinds of white blood cells have poured into the lung to fight an infection. A diseased lung also includes the detritus of dissolved cells, along with various proteins such as fibrin and collagen that are part of the body's efforts to repair damage. (These repair efforts can cause their own problems.

"Fibrosis" occurs when too much fibrin interferes with the normal functioning of the lung.)

Roughly two-thirds of all bacterial pneumonias and an even higher percentage of lobar pneumonias are caused by a single group of bacteria, the various subtypes of the pneumococcus. (The pneumococcus is also the second leading cause of meningitis.) A virulent pneumococcus can spread through an entire lobe within a matter of hours. Even today, in 20 to 30 percent of the cases of lobar pneumonia, bacteria also spread through the blood to infect other areas of the body, and many victims still die. Some cyanosis is not unusual in lobar pneumonia, but most of the lung often still looks normal.

In 1918 pathologists did see at autopsy the normal devastation of the lungs caused by the usual lobar and bronchopneumonias. But the lungs from those who died quickly during the pandemic, the lungs that so confused even Welch, those lungs were different. Said one pathologist, "Physical signs were confusing. Typical consolidation was seldom found." And another: "The old classification by distribution of the lesions was inappropriate." And another: "Essentially toxic damage to alevolar walls and exudation of blood and fluid. Very little evidence of bacterial action could be found in some of these cases."

At a discussion reported in the *Journal of the American Medical Association,* several pathologists concurred, "The pathological picture was striking, and was unlike any type of pneumonia ordinarily seen in this country. . . . The lung lesions, complex and variable, struck one as being quite different in character to anything one had met with at all commonly in the thousands of autopsies one had performed during the last 20 years."

Normally when the lungs are removed they collapse like deflated balloons. Not now. Now they were full, but not of air. In bacterial pneumonias, normally the infection rages inside the alveoli, inside the tiny sacs. In 1918, while the alveoli were also sometimes invaded, the spaces between the alveoli were filled. This space, which makes up the bulk of the volume of the lung, was filled with the debris of destroyed cells and with every element of the immune system, from enzymes to white blood cells. And it was filled with blood.

One more observer concluded that "the acute death" he saw evidence of in the lungs "is a lesion which does not occur in other types of pulmonary infection. In influenza it is the lesion of characterization."

.   .   .

Victims' lungs were being ripped apart as a result of, in effect, collateral damage from the attack of the immune system on the virus. Since the respiratory tract must allow outside air to pass into the innermost recesses of the body, it is extremely well defended. The lungs became the battleground between the invaders and the immune system. Nothing was left standing on that battleground.

The immune system begins its defense far in advance of the lungs, with enzymes in saliva that destroy some pathogens (including HIV, which makes its home in most bodily fluids, but not in saliva, where enzymes kill it). Then it raises physical obstacles, such as nasal hairs that filter out large particles and sharp turns in the throat that force inhaled air to collide with the sides of breathing passageways.

Mucus lines these passageways and traps organisms and irritants. Underneath the layer of mucus lies a blanket of "epithelial cells," and from their surfaces extend "cilia," akin to tiny hairs which, like tiny oars, sweep upward continuously at from 1,000 to 1,500 beats a minute. This sweeping motion moves foreign organisms away from places they can lodge and launch an infection, and up to the larynx. If something does gain a foothold in the upper respiratory tract, the body first tries to flush it out with more fluid—hence the typical runny nose—and then expel it with coughs and sneezes.

These defenses are as physical as raising an arm to block a punch and do no damage to the lungs. Even if the body overreacts, this usually does no serious harm, although an increased volume of mucus blocks air passages and makes breathing more difficult. (In allergies these same symptoms occur because the immune system does overreact.)

There are more aggressive defenses. Macrophages and "natural killer" cells—two kinds of white blood cells that seek and destroy all foreign invaders, unlike other elements of the immune system that only attack a specific threat—patrol the entire respiratory tract and lungs. Cells in the respiratory tract secrete enzymes that attack bacteria and some viruses (including influenza) or block them from attaching to tissue beneath the mucus, and these secretions also bring more white cells and antibacterial enzymes into a counterattack; if a virus is the invader, white blood cells also secrete interferon, which can block viral infection.

All these defenses work so well that the lungs themselves, although directly exposed to outside air, are normally sterile.

But when the lungs do become infected, other defenses, lethal and violent defenses, come into play. For the immune system is at its core a killing machine. It targets infecting organisms, attacks with a complex arsenal of weapons—some of them savage weapons—and neutralizes or kills the invader.

The balance, however, between kill and overkill, response and overresponse, is a delicate one. The immune system can behave like a SWAT team that kills the hostage along with the hostage taker, or the army that destroys the village to save it.

In 1918 especially, this question of balance played a crucial role in the war between virus and immune system, and between life and death. The virus was often so efficient at invading the lungs that the immune system had to mount a massive response to it. What was killing young adults a few days after the first symptom was not the virus. The killer was the massive immune response itself.

The virus attaches itself normally to epithelial cells, which line the entire respiratory tract like insulation in a tube all the way to the alveoli. Within fifteen minutes after influenza viruses invade the body, their hemagglutinin spikes begin binding with the sialic-acid receptors on these cells. One after another these spikes attach to the receptors, each one a grappling hook binding the virus tighter and tighter to the cell. Generally about ten hours after the virus invades a cell, the cell bursts open, releasing between 1,000 and 10,000 viruses capable of infecting other cells. At even the lowest reproduction rate—1,000 times 1,000 times 1,000, and so on—one can easily understand how a victim could feel perfectly healthy one moment and collapse the next, just as the fifth or sixth generation of viruses matures and infects cells.

Meanwhile, the virus is also attacking the immune system directly, undermining the body's ability to protect itself; the virus inhibits the release of interferon, and interferon is usually the first weapon the body employs to fight viral infection. In 1918 the ability to inhibit the immune system was so obvious that researchers, even while overwhelmed by the pandemic, noticed that influenza victims had weakened immune responses to other stimuli; they used objective tests to prove it.

Even mild influenza viruses can utterly and entirely denude the upper respiratory tract of epithelial cells, leaving it bare, stripping the throat raw. (The repair process begins within a few days but takes weeks.)

Once an infection gains a foothold, the immune system responds initially with inflammation. The immune system can inflame at the site of an infection, causing the redness, heat, and swelling there, or it can inflame the entire body through fever, or both.

The actual process of inflammation involves the release by certain white blood cells of proteins called "cytokines." There are many kinds of white cells; several kinds attack invading organisms, while other "helper" cells manage attacks, and still others produce antibodies. There are even more kinds of cytokines. Some cytokines attack invaders directly, such as interferon, which attacks viruses. Some act as messengers carrying orders. Macrophages, for example, release "GM CSF," which stands for "granulocyte-macrophage colony-stimulating factor"; GM CSF stimulates the production in the bone marrow of more macrophages as well as granulocytes, another kind of white blood cell. Some cytokines also carry messages to parts of the body not normally considered belonging to the immune system; several cytokines can affect the hypothalamus, which acts like the body's thermostat. When these cytokines bind to receptors in the hypothalamus, body temperature goes up; the entire body becomes inflamed. (Fever is part of the immune response; some pathogens do not grow well at higher temperatures.) In influenza, fever routinely climbs to 103, and can go higher.

But cytokines themselves also have toxic effects. The typical symptoms of influenza outside the respiratory tract, the headache and body ache, are caused not by the virus but by cytokines. A side effect of cytokines' stimulating the bone marrow to make more white cells, for instance, is likely what aches in the bone.

Cytokines can cause more serious and permanent damage as well. "Tumor necrosis factor," to give one example, is a cytokine that gets its name from its ability to kill cancer cells—tumors exposed to TNF in the laboratory simply melt away; it also helps raise body temperature and stimulates antibody production. But TNF is extraordinarily lethal, and not just to diseased cells. It can destroy healthy ones as well. In fact, it can kill the entire body. TNF is a toxin and a major cause of toxic shock syndrome, and it is not the only toxic cytokine.

Routinely, the body fights off the influenza virus before it gains a solid foothold in the lungs themselves. But in 1918 the virus often succeeded in infecting epithelial cells not only in the upper respiratory tract but all the way down the respiratory tract into the innermost sanctuaries of the lungs, into the epithelial cells of the alveoli. This was viral pneumonia.

The immune system followed the virus into the lungs and there waged war. In this war the immune system held nothing back. It used all its weapons. And it killed. It killed particularly with "killer T cells," a white blood cell that targets the body's own cells when they are infected with a virus, and it killed with what is sometimes referred to as a "cytokine storm," a massive attack using every lethal weapon the body possesses.

The same capillaries that moved blood past the alveoli delivered this attack. The capillaries dilated, pouring out fluid, every kind of white blood cell, antibodies, other elements of the immune system, and cytokines into the lung. Then these cytokines and other enzymes virtually obliterated the capillaries. Even more fluid poured into the lung. The cells that line the alveoli were damaged, if they survived the virus itself. Pink glassy membranes, called hyaline membranes, formed on the insides of the alveoli. Once these membranes formed, "surfactant"—a slippery, soap-like protein that reduces surface tension and eases the transfer of oxygen into red blood cells—disappeared from the alveoli. More blood flooded the lungs. The body started producing fiberlike connective tissue. Areas of the lung became enmeshed in cell debris, fibrin, collagen, and other materials. Proteins and fluid filled the space between cells.

Macfarlane Burnet, the Nobel laureate, described what was happening inside the lungs: "acute inflammatory injection . . . very rapid necrosis of most of the epithelial lining of the bronchial tree down to and especially involving the smallest bronchioles. . . . Essentially toxic damage to alveolar walls and exudation of blood and fluid . . . [C]ontinued exudation of fluid in areas where blocking of smaller bronchi had occurred would produce eventually airless regions."

The immune system changes with age. Young adults have the strongest immune system in the population, most capable of mounting a massive immune response. Normally that makes them the healthiest element of the population. Under certain conditions, however, that very strength becomes a weakness.

In 1918 the immune systems of young adults mounted massive

responses to the virus. That immune response filled the lungs with fluid and debris, making it impossible for the exchange of oxygen to take place. The immune response killed.

The influenza outbreak in 1997 in Hong Kong, when a new virus jumped from chickens to humans, killed only six people and it did not adapt to man. More than a million chickens were slaughtered to prevent that from happening, and the outbreak has been much studied. In autopsies pathologists noticed extremely high cytokine levels, discovered even that the bone marrow, lymphoid tissue, spleen—all involved in the immune response—and other organs were themselves under attack from an immune system turned renegade. They believed that this proved "syndrome [was] not previously described with influenza." In fact, investigators in 1918 had seen the same thing.

This was still influenza, only influenza.

In the 1970s physicians began to recognize a pathological process in the lungs that could have many causes but, once the process began, looked the same and received the same treatment. They called it ARDS, which stands for Acute Respiratory Distress Syndrome. Almost anything that puts extreme stress on the lung can cause ARDS: near drowning, smoke inhalation, inhaling toxic fumes (or poison gas) . . . or influenzal viral pneumonia. Doctors today looking at pathology reports of lungs in 1918 would immediately designate the condition as ARDS.

One pulmonary expert describes ARDS as "a burn inside the lungs." It is a virtual scorching of lung tissue. When viral pneumonia causes the condition, the immune system toxins designed to destroy invaders are what, in effect, flame in the lung, scorching the tissue.

Whatever the causes of ARDS, even today there is no way of stopping the process of disintegration in the lung once it begins. The only care is supportive, keeping the victim alive until he or she can recover. This requires all the technology of modern intensive care units. Still, even with the best modern care, even with for example dramatically more efficient and effective administration of oxygen than in 1918, the mortality rate for ARDS patients in different studies ranges from 40 to 60 percent. Without intensive care—and hospitals have few beds in intensive-care units—the mortality rate would approach 100 percent.

(In 2003 a new coronavirus that causes SARS, "Severe Acute Respiratory Syndrome," appeared in China and quickly spread around the world. Coronaviruses cause an estimated 15 to 30 percent of all colds and, like the influenza virus, infect epithelial cells. When the coronavirus that causes SARS does kill, it often kills through ARDS, although since the virus replicates much more slowly than influenza, death from ARDS can come several weeks after the first symptoms.)

In ARDS, death can come from many causes. Organs outside the lungs fail because they get too little oxygen. The lungs can so fill with fluid that the right ventricle of the heart cannot empty it so the victim drowns. The strain of trying to pump blood out of the lung can cause heart failure. Or the victim can simply die from exhaustion: he or she must breathe so rapidly to get enough oxygen that muscles become exhausted. Breathing just stops.

ARDS by no means accounts for all the influenza deaths in 1918 and 1919, or even for a majority of them. It explains only those who died in a few days, and it explains why so many young healthy people died. Although influenza almost certainly killed some people in ways that had little to do with the lungs—for example, someone whose already weak heart could not stand the additional strain of fighting the disease— the overwhelming majority of non-ARDS deaths came from bacterial pneumonias.

The destruction of the epithelial cells eliminated the sweeping action that clears so much of the respiratory tract of bacteria, and the virus damaged or exhausted other parts of the immune system as well. That gave the normal bacterial flora of the mouth unimpeded entry into the lungs. Recent research also suggests that the neuraminidase on the influenza virus makes it easier for some bacteria to attach to lung tissue, creating a lethal synergy between the virus and these bacteria. And in the lungs, the bacteria began to grow.

Bacterial pneumonias developed a week, two weeks, three weeks after someone came down with influenza, including even a seemingly mild case of influenza. Often influenza victims seemed to recover, even returned to work, then suddenly collapsed again with bacterial pneumonia.

It is impossible to know what percentage of the dead were killed by a viral pneumonia and ARDS and how many died from bacterial pneumonias. Generally speaking, epidemiologists and historians who have written about this pandemic have assumed that the overwhelming majority of deaths came from secondary invaders, from bacterial pneumonias that can be fought with antibiotics.

The conclusion of the army's pneumonia commission, however, is chilling in terms of implications for today. This commission, comprised of half a dozen of the finest scientists in America, both conducted autopsies and reviewed pathology reports of others; it found signs of what would today be called ARDS in almost half the autopsies. A separate study limited to the pathology of the disease, conducted by Milton Winternitz, a Welch protégé and later dean of the Yale Medical School, reached the same conclusion.

That overstates the proportion of victims who died from ARDS—in effect from influenzal viral pneumonia—because the army study looked only at deaths among soldiers, men who were young and otherwise healthy, the group most likely to have been killed by their own immune systems. In the total population, viral pneumonias and ARDS would not account for as high a percentage of the deaths. Most deaths almost certainly did come from secondary bacterial infections, but probably not quite so many as has been assumed. That should, however, be small comfort for those who worry about the next influenza pandemic.

The 1957 pandemic was far milder than 1918, but even then 25 percent of the fatalities had viral pneumonia only; three-quarters of the deaths came from complications, generally bacterial pneumonia, even in that golden age of antibiotics. Since then bacterial resistance has become a major problem in medicine. Today the mortality rate for a bacterial pneumonia following influenza is still roughly 7 percent, and in some parts of the United States, 35 percent of pneumococcal infections are resistant to the antibiotic of choice. When *Staphylococcus aureus*, a bacterium that has become particularly troubling in hospitals because of its resistance to antibiotics, is the secondary invader, the death rate— today—rises to as high as 42 percent. That is higher than the general death rate from bacterial pneumonias in 1918.

■ Part VII
THE RACE

CHAPTER TWENTY-TWO

NATURE CHOSE to rage in 1918, and it chose the form of the influenza virus in which to do it. This meant that nature first crept upon the world in familiar, almost comic, form. It came in masquerade. Then it pulled down its mask and showed its fleshless bone.

Then, as the pathogen spread from cantonments to cities, as it spread within cities, as it moved from city to town to village to farmhouse, medical science began moving as well. It began its own race against the pathogen, moving more rapidly and with more purpose than it ever had.

Scientists did not presume to think that they would or could control this rage of nature. But they did not abandon their search for ways to control the damage of this rage. They still tried to save lives.

Worldwide their struggle, their race, commenced. In the United States that struggle would be fought by Welch, Gorgas, Cole, and their colleagues, as well as by the institutions they had built and the men and women they had trained. Neither these institutions nor these men and women had ever been tested like this. They had never imagined they would be tested like this. But any possibility of affecting the course of the disease lay in their hands.

To save lives they needed the answer to at least one of three questions. It was possible that even a single rough approximation of an answer would give them enough knowledge to intervene, to interrupt the disease at some critical juncture. But it was also possible they could learn detailed answers to all three questions and still remain helpless, utterly helpless.

First, they needed to understand the epidemiology of influenza, how it behaved and spread. Scientists had already learned to control cholera, typhoid, yellow fever, malaria, bubonic plague, and other diseases by understanding their epidemiology even before developing either a vaccine or cure.

Second, they needed to learn its pathology, what it did within the body, the precise course of the disease. That too might allow them to intervene in some way that saved lives.

Third, they needed to know what the pathogen was, what microorganism caused influenza. This could allow them to find a way to stimulate the immune system to prevent or cure the disease. It was also conceivable that even without knowing the precise cause, they could develop a serum or vaccine.

The easiest question to answer for influenza was its epidemiology. Although some respected investigators still believed in the miasma theory— they thought influenza spread too fast for person-to-person contact to account for it—most believed correctly it was an airborne pathogen. Breathing it in could cause the disease. They did not know the exact, precise details, that for example when the virus floats in the air it can infect someone else for anywhere from an hour to a day after it is exhaled (the lower the humidity, the longer the virus survives). But they did know that it was "a crowd disease," spread most easily in crowds.

They also had an accurate estimate that someone with influenza "sheds" the virus—can infect others—usually from the third to the sixth day after he or she is infected.

They also believed, correctly, that people could catch influenza not only by inhaling it but by hand-to-mouth or -nose contact. They rightly thought, for instance, that a sick person could cover his mouth with his hand when he coughed, then several hours later shake hands, and the second person could then rub his chin in thought or touch his nose or stick a piece of candy in his mouth and infect himself. Similarly, someone sick could cough into a hand, touch a hard surface such as a doorknob, and spread it to someone else who turns the doorknob and later brings a hand to face. (In fact, the virus can remain infectious on a hard surface for up to two days.)

Knowledge of influenza's epidemiology, then, was of little use. Only ruthless isolation and quarantine could affect its course. No scientist and no public health official had the political power to take such action. Some local authorities might take some action, but no national figure could. Even within the army Gorgas's urgent and desperate calls to end the transfer of troops were ignored.

Scientists were also learning too well about the pathology of the disease and its natural course. They were learning chiefly that they could do almost nothing to intervene in serious cases, in the cases that progressed to viral pneumonia and ARDS; even administering oxygen seemed to have no effect.

They believed they could, however, possibly save lives if they could prevent or treat the slower moving pneumonias caused by what they were fairly quickly suspecting to be secondary invaders. Some preventive measures involved only giving proper guidance, such as to rest in bed after influenza infection, or giving good care, which was becoming more and more impossible as the numbers of the sick rose, as nurses and doctors themselves succumbed.

But if they could find the pathogen . . . They had tools, they could manipulate the immune system, they could prevent and cure some pneumonias—including the most common pneumonias. The conquest of bacterial pneumonias seemed tantalizingly within the reach of science, tantalizingly at the very edge of scientists' reach—or just beyond it. If they could just find the pathogen . . .

All the energies of science rose to that challenge.

William Welch himself would not rise to it. From Camp Devens he had returned directly to Baltimore, neither stopping in New York City nor going on to report to the surgeon general's office in Washington. Others could perform that duty, and on the phone he had said what he had to say.

In the meantime Welch wasn't feeling very well. No doubt he tried to shrug off the discomfort. He had, after all, had an exceedingly difficult trip. Just before going to Devens he, Cole, and Vaughan had concluded their latest round of camp inspections and had just begun to relax for a few days in Asheville, North Carolina. He had even contemplated resigning his commission. Then they had been abruptly ordered to the surgeon general's office on a Sunday, gone straight on to Devens, and there discovered this terrible disease.

So he had every reason to be tired and out of sorts. Likely he told himself something akin to that. The rattling of the train would have disturbed him, exacerbating the first signs of a headache. Large a man as he was, he had difficulty getting comfortable on a train anyway.

But as the train moved south he felt worse and worse, perhaps suffering a sudden violent headache and an unproductive cough, cough in which nothing came up, and certainly with a fever. He would have looked at himself clinically, objectively, and made a correct diagnosis. He had influenza.

No record exists of his precise clinical course. All of Baltimore, all of the East Coast, was erupting in flames. The virus struck the Hopkins itself so hard that the university closed its hospital to all but its own staff and students. Three Hopkins medical students, three Hopkins nurses, and three Hopkins doctors would die.

Welch did not go to the hospital. Almost seventy years old, forty years older than those who were dying in the greatest numbers, having just left the horror at Devens and knowing the enormous strain on and therefore the likely poor care even at the Hopkins facility, he later said, "I could not have dreamed of going to a hospital at that time."

Instead, he went to bed immediately in his own rooms, and stayed there. He knew better than to push himself now: pushing oneself after infection with this disease could easily open the path for a secondary invader to kill. After ten days in bed at home, when he felt well enough to travel at all, to recuperate more he withdrew entirely to his beloved Hotel Dennis in Atlantic City, the odd tacky place that was his haven.

In the midst of the chaos that was everywhere, he returned to this familiar place that gave him comfort. What had he always liked about it? Perhaps the life that roared through it. Quiet resorts bored him: he described Mohonk, a mountain resort ninety miles above New York City, as "a kind of twin-lakes-resort with Miss Dares sitting in rockers on the broad piazza, . . . where it seems as if nine o'clock will never come so that one could go decently to bed . . . [C]olored neckties are not allowed." But Atlantic City! and "the most terrifying, miraculous, blood-curdling affair called the Flip-flap railroad . . . just built on a long pier out over the ocean . . . [Y]ou go down from a height of about 75 feet . . . with the head down and the feet up, so that you would drop out of the car, if it was not for the tremendous speed. As you go round the circle the effect is indescribable. . . . Crowds stand around and say they would not try it for $1000."

Yes, the life that roared through Atlantic City—the young men and women and their frolicking, the sensuality of sweat and surf and salt, the vibrancy and thrust of flesh about the ocean and boardwalk, all that— made one feel as if one were not merely observing but partaking. But now Atlantic City was quiet. It was October, off-season, the resorts quiet. And here, as everywhere, was influenza. Here, as everywhere, there was a shortage of doctors, a shortage of nurses, a shortage of hospitals, a short- age of coffins, its schools closed, its places of public amusement closed, its Flip-flap railroad closed.

He stayed in bed for several more weeks, recuperating. The disease, he told his nephew, "seems to have localized itself in my intestinal, rather than the respiratory tract, which is probably fortunate." He also insisted that his nephew, later a U.S. senator, make certain if any symptoms of influenza appeared at all in his family that the victim stay in bed "until the temperature has been normal for three days."

He had planned to attend a meeting on the disease at the Rockefeller Institute, but almost two weeks after arriving in Atlantic City, a month after first becoming ill, he canceled; he had not recovered enough to attend. He would play no further role in medical science for the course of the epidemic. He would not participate in the search for a solution. He had of course done no laboratory work in years, but he had often proved an extraordinarily useful conduit, knowing everyone and everything, a cross-pollinator recognizing how the work of one investigator might complement the work of another, and directly or indirectly putting the two in touch. Now he would not play even that role.

Coincidentally, both Flexner and Gorgas arrived in Europe on unre- lated business just as influenza erupted in America. The generation who had transformed American medicine had withdrawn from the race. If anything was to be done in the nature of a scientific breakthrough, their spiritual descendants would do the doing.

Welch had left Massachusetts with Burt Wolbach performing more autopsies, Milton Rosenau already beginning experiments on human vol- unteers, and Oswald Avery beginning bacteriological investigations. Other outstanding scientists had also already engaged this problem—William Park and Anna Williams in New York, Paul Lewis in Philadelphia, Preston

Kyes in Chicago, and others. If the country was lucky, very lucky indeed, one of them might find something soon enough to help.

For all the urgency, investigators could not allow themselves to be panicked into a disorderly approach. Disorder would lead nowhere. They began with what they knew and with what they could do.

They could kill pathogens outside the body. An assortment of chemicals could disinfect a room, or clothes, and they knew precisely the amount of chemicals needed and the duration of exposure necessary to fumigate a room. They knew how to disinfect instruments and materials. They knew how to grow bacteria, and how to stain bacteria to make them visible under microscopes. They knew that what Ehrlich called "magic bullets" existed that could kill infectious pathogens, and they even had started down the right pathways to find them.

Yet in the midst of crisis, with death everywhere, none of that knowledge was useful. Fumigation and disinfecting required too much labor to work on a mass scale, and finding a magic bullet required discovering more unknowns than was then possible. Investigators quickly recognized they would get no help from materia medica.

Medicine had, however, if not entirely mastered at least knew how to use one tool: the immune system itself.

Investigators understood the basic principles of the immune system. They knew how to manipulate those principles to prevent and cure some diseases. They knew how to grow and weaken or strengthen bacteria in the laboratory, and how to stimulate an immune response in an animal. They knew how to make vaccines, and they knew how to make antiserum.

They also understood the specificity of the immune system. Vaccines and antisera work only against the specific etiological agent, the specific pathogen or toxin causing the disease. Few investigators cared how elegant their experiments were as friends, families, and colleagues fell ill. But to have the best hope of protecting with a vaccine or curing with a serum, investigators needed to isolate the pathogen. They needed to answer a first question, the most important question—indeed, at this point the only question. What caused the disease?

Richard Pfeiffer believed he had found the answer to that question a quarter century earlier. One of Koch's most brilliant disciples, scientific director of the Institute for Infectious Disease in Berlin, and a general in the German army, he was sixty years old in 1918 and by then had become somewhat imperious. Over his career he had addressed some of the great questions of medicine, and he had made enormous contributions. By any standard he was a giant.

During and after the 1889–90 influenza pandemic—with the exception of 1918–19, the most severe influenza pandemic in the last three centuries—he had searched for the cause. Carefully, painstakingly, he had isolated tiny, slender, rod-shaped bacteria with rounded ends, although they sometimes appeared in somewhat different forms, from people suffering from influenza. He often found the bacteria the sole organism present, and he found it in "astonishing numbers."

This bacteria clearly had the ability to kill, although in animals the disease produced did not quite resemble human influenza. Thus, the evidence against it did not fulfill "Koch's postulates." But human pathogens often either do not sicken animals or cause different symptoms in them, and many pathogens are accepted as the cause of a disease without fully satisfying Koch's postulates.

Pfeiffer was confident that he had found the cause of influenza. He even named the bacteria *Bacillus influenzae*. (Today this bacteria is called *Hemophilus influenzae*.)

Among scientists the bacteria quickly became known as "Pfeiffer's bacillus," and, given his deserved reputation, few doubted the validity of his discovery.

Certainty creates strength. Certainty gives one something upon which to lean. Uncertainty creates weakness. Uncertainty makes one tentative if not fearful, and tentative steps, even when in the right direction, may not overcome significant obstacles.

To be a scientist requires not only intelligence and curiosity, but passion, patience, creativity, self-sufficiency, and courage. It is not the courage to venture into the unknown. It is the courage to accept—indeed, embrace—uncertainty. For as Claude Bernard, the great French physiologist of the nineteenth century, said, "Science teaches us to doubt."

A scientist must accept the fact that all his or her work, even beliefs, may break apart upon the sharp edge of a single laboratory finding. And just as Einstein refused to accept his own theory until his predictions were tested, one must seek out such findings. Ultimately a scientist has nothing to believe in but the process of inquiry. To move forcefully and aggressively even while uncertain requires a confidence and strength deeper than physical courage.

All real scientists exist on the frontier. Even the least ambitious among them deal with the unknown, if only one step beyond the known. The best among them move deep into a wilderness region where they know almost nothing, where the very tools and techniques needed to clear the wilderness, to bring order to it, do not exist. There they probe in a disciplined way. There a single step can take them through the looking glass into a world that seems entirely different, and if they are at least partly correct their probing acts like a crystal to precipitate an order out of chaos, to create form, structure, and direction. A single step can also take one off a cliff.

In the wilderness the scientist must create . . . *everything*. It is grunt work, tedious work that begins with figuring out what tools one needs and then making them. A shovel can dig up dirt but cannot penetrate rock. Would a pick then be best, or would dynamite be better—or would dynamite be too indiscriminately destructive? If the rock is impenetrable, if dynamite would destroy what one is looking for, is there another way of getting information about what the rock holds? There is a stream passing over the rock. Would analyzing the water after it passes over the rock reveal anything useful? How would one analyze it?

Ultimately, if the researcher succeeds, a flood of colleagues will pave roads over the path laid, and those roads will be orderly and straight, taking an investigator in minutes to a place the pioneer spent months or years looking for. And the perfect tool will be available for purchase, just as laboratory mice can now be ordered from supply houses.

Not all scientific investigators can deal comfortably with uncertainty, and those who can may not be creative enough to understand and design the experiments that will illuminate a subject—to know both where and how to look. Others may lack the confidence to persist. Experiments do not simply work. Regardless of design and preparation, experiments—especially at the beginning, when one proceeds by intelligent guesswork—rarely yield the results desired. An investigator must make them work. The less known, the more one has to manipulate and even force experiments to yield an answer.

Which raises another question: How does one know when one knows?

In turn this leads to more practical questions: How does one know when to continue to push an experiment? And how does one know when to abandon a clue as a false trail?

No one interested in any truth will torture the data itself, ever. But a scientist can—and should—torture an experiment to get data, to get a result, especially when investigating a new area. A scientist can—and should—seek any way to answer a question: if using mice and guinea pigs and rabbits does not provide a satisfactory answer, then trying dogs, pigs, cats, monkeys. And if one experiment shows a hint of a result, the slightest bump on a flat line of information, then a scientist designs the next experiment to focus on that bump, to create conditions more likely to get more bumps until they become either consistent and meaningful or demonstrate that the initial bump was mere random variation without meaning.

There are limits to such manipulation. Even under torture, nature will not lie, will not yield a consistent, reproducible result, unless it is true. But if tortured enough, nature will mislead; it will confess to something that is true only under special conditions—the conditions the investigator created in the laboratory. Its truth is then artificial, an experimental artifact.

One key to science is that work be *reproducible*. Someone in another laboratory doing the same experiment will get the same result. The result then is reliable enough that someone else can build upon it. The most damning condemnation is to dismiss a finding as "not reproducible." That can call into question not only ability but on occasion ethics.

If a reproducible finding comes from torturing nature, however, it is not useful. To be useful a result must not only be reproducible, it must be . . . perhaps one should call it *expandable*. One must be able to enlarge it, explore it, learn more from it, use it as a foundation to build structures upon.

These things become easy to discern in hindsight. But how does one know when to persist, when to continue to try to make an experiment work, when to make adjustments—and when finally to abandon a line of thought as mistaken or incapable of solution with present techniques?

How does one know when to do either?

The question is one of judgment. For the distinguishing element in science is not intelligence but judgment. Or perhaps it is simply luck.

George Sternberg did not pursue his discovery of the pneumococcus, and he did not pursue his discovery that white blood cells devoured bacteria. He did not because doing so would have deflected him from his unsuccessful pursuit of yellow fever. Given his abilities, had he focused on either of those other discoveries, his name would be well known instead of forgotten in the history of science.

Judgment is so difficult because a negative result does not mean that a hypothesis is wrong. Nor do ten negative results, nor do one hundred negative results. Ehrlich believed that magic bullets existed; chemical compounds could cure disease. His reasoning led him to try certain compounds against a certain infection. Ultimately he tried more than nine hundred chemical compounds. Each experiment began with hope. Each was performed meticulously. Each failed. Finally he found the compound that did work. The result was not only the first drug that could cure an infection; it confirmed a line of reasoning that led to thousands of investigators' following the same path.

How does one know when one knows? When one is on the edge one cannot know. One can only test.

Thomas Huxley advised, "Surely there is a time to submit to guidance and a time to take one's own way at all hazards."

Thomas Rivers was one of the young men from the Hopkins on the army's pneumonia commission. He would later—only a few years later—define the differences between viruses and bacteria, become one of the world's leading virologists, and succeed Cole as head of the Rockefeller Institute Hospital. He gave an example of the difficulty of knowing when one knows when he spoke of two Rockefeller colleagues, Albert Sabin and Peter Olitsky. As Rivers recalled, they "proved polio virus would grow only in nervous tissue. Elegant work, absolutely convincing. Everyone believed it."

Everyone believed it, that is, except John Enders. The virus Sabin and Olitsky were working with had been used in the laboratory so long that it had mutated. That particular virus *would* grow only in nervous tissue. Enders won a Nobel Prize for growing polio virus in other tissue, work that led directly to a polio vaccine. Sabin's career was hardly ruined by his error; he went on to develop the best polio vaccine. Olitsky did well, too. But had Enders pursued his intuition and been wrong, much of his own career would have been utterly wasted.

Richard Pfeiffer insisted he had discovered the cause, the etiological agent, of influenza. His confidence was so great he had even named it *Bacillus influenzae*. He had tremendous stature, half a rung below Pasteur, Koch, and Ehrlich. Surely his reputation stood higher than that of any American investigator before the war. Who would challenge him?

His reputation gave his finding tremendous weight. Around the world, many scientists believed it. Indeed, some accepted it as an axiom: without the bacteria there could be no influenza. "No influenza bacilli have been found in cases here," wrote one European investigator. Therefore the disease was, he concluded, "not influenza."

CHAPTER TWENTY-THREE

LABORATORIES EVERYWHERE had turned to influenza. Pasteur's protégé Émile Roux, one of those who had raced German competitors for a diphtheria antitoxin, directed the work at the Pasteur Institute. In Britain virtually everyone in Almroth Wright's laboratory worked on it, including Alexander Fleming, whose later discovery of penicillin he first applied to research on Pfeiffer's so-called influenza bacillus. In Germany, in Italy, even in revolution-torn Russia, desperate investigators searched for an answer.

But by the fall of 1918 these laboratories could function only on a far-reduced scale. Research had been cut back and focused on war, on poison gas or defending against it, on preventing infection of wounds, on ways to prevent diseases that incapacitated troops such as "trench fever," an infection related to typhus that was not serious in itself but had taken more troops out of the line than any other disease. Laboratory animals had become unavailable; armies consumed them for testing poison gas and similar purposes. The war had also sucked into itself technicians and young researchers.

Laboratories in both Europe and the United States were affected, but Europeans suffered far more, with their work limited by shortages not only of people but of everything from coal for heat to money for petri dishes. At least those resources Americans had. And if the United States still lagged behind Europe in the number of investigators, it no longer lagged in the quality of investigators. The Rockefeller Institute had already become arguably the best research institute in the world; out of a mere handful of scientists working there then, one man had already won the Nobel Prize and two would win it. In the most relevant area of work, in pneumonia, the Rockefeller Institute had a clear lead over the rest of the world. And Rockefeller scientists were hardly the only Americans doing world-class work.

For Welch, Michigan's Victor Vaughan, Harvard's Charles Eliot, Penn's William Pepper, and the handful of colleagues who had pushed so hard for change had succeeded. They had transformed American medical science. If that transformation had only just occurred, if it had only recently risen to the level of Europe, it also had the vitality that comes from recent conversion. And the nation at large was not so exhausted as Europe. It was not exhausted at all.

As influenza stretched its fingers across the country and began to crush out lives in its grip, virtually every serious medical scientist—and many simple physicians who considered themselves of scientific bent—began looking for a cure. They were determined to prove that science could indeed perform miracles.

Most of them, simply, were not good enough to address the problem with any hope of success. They tried anyway. Their attempt was heroic. It required not just scientific ability but physical courage. They moved among the dead and dying, reached swabs into mouths and nasal passages of the desperately ill, steeped themselves in blood in the autopsy room, dug deep into bodies, and struggled to grow from swabbings, blood, and tissue the pathogen that was killing more humans than any other in history.

A few of these investigators, possibly as few as a few dozen, were smart enough, creative enough, knowledgeable enough, skilled enough, and commanded enough resources that they were not on a fool's errand. They could confront this disease with at least the hope of success.

In Boston, Rosenau and Keegan continued to study the disease in the laboratory. The bulk of the army's pneumonia commission had been ordered to Camp Pike, Arkansas, where, even as Welch arrived at Devens, they began investigating "a new bronchopneumonia." The Rockefeller team whom Welch had brought to Devens headed back to New York, where they added Martha Wollstein, a respected bacteriologist also associated with the Rockefeller Institute, to the effort; she had studied the influenza bacillus since 1905. In Chicago at the Memorial Institute for Infectious Diseases, Ludwig Hektoen dove into the work. And at the Mayo Clinic, E. C. Rosenow did the same. The only civilian government research institution, the Public Health Service's Hygienic Laboratory and its director George McCoy joined in.

But of all those working on it in the United States, perhaps the most important were Oswald Avery at Rockefeller, William Park and Anna Williams at the New York City Department of Public Health, and Paul Lewis in Philadelphia.

Each of them brought a different style to the problem, a different method of doing science. For Park and Williams, the work would come as close to routine as something could be in the midst of such extreme crisis; their efforts would have no impact on their own lives in any personal sense, although they would help direct research on influenza down the path that ultimately yielded the right answer. For Avery the work would confirm him in a direction that he would follow for decades, decades first of enormous frustration but then of momentous discovery—in fact a discovery that opened the door to an entire universe even now just beginning to be explored. For Lewis, although he could not have known it, his work on influenza would mark a turning point in his own life, one that would lead to a great tragedy, for science, for his family, and for himself.

It was not a good time to confront a major new threat in the Bureau of Laboratories of the New York City Department of Public Health, the bureau Park ran and in which Williams worked. For they had a special problem: New York City politics.

On January 1, 1918, Tammany Hall reclaimed control of the city. Patronage came first. Hermann Biggs, the pioneer who had built the department, had left a year earlier to become state health commissoner; Biggs had been untouchable because he had treated a top Tammany leader who had protected the entire department during prior Tammany administrations. His successor was not untouchable. Mayor John Hylan replaced him two weeks after taking control. But most jobs in the Department of Health were not patronage positions, so to create vacancies Tammany began to smear the best municipal health department in the world. Soon Hylan demanded the firing of division chiefs and the removal of highly respected physicians on the advisory board.

Even the new Tammany-appointed health commissioner balked at that and resigned, leaving the department leaderless. The mayor was standing on the sidewalk outside City Hall when a crony introduced Royal Copeland to him, said he was a loyal Tammany man, and suggested the mayor name him the new health commissioner. But Copeland, dean of a homeopathic medical school, was not even an M.D.

Nonetheless the mayor agreed to appoint him. The three men then climbed the steps to his office, and Copeland was sworn in.

The best municipal public health department in the world was now run by a man with no belief in modern scientific medicine and whose ambitions were not in public health but in politics. If Tammany wanted vacancies to fill with loyalists, that is what he would give them. (Copeland once explained his loyalty to Tammany in simple terms: "Man is a social animal and cannot work without cooperation. Organization is a necessity and my organization is Tammany." A few years later Tammany would repay his loyalty by carrying him to the United States Senate.) So he continued the machine's efforts to disassemble the department. One of the best division heads was first threatened with criminal charges and when that failed he was hauled to a civil-service hearing on charges of "neglect of duty, inefficiency, and incompetency."

Park had run the department's laboratory division since 1893, had never involved himself in politics, and was himself untouchable. He continued to do excellent science in the midst of this turmoil; soon after Avery and Cole and others at Rockefeller developed their serum against Types I and II pneumococcus, Park developed a procedure for "typing" the pneumococcus so simple that any decent laboratory could perform it within thirty minutes, allowing nearly immediate use of the right serum for treatment.

But now he had to defend the department. He helped organize a defense, and the defense became national. Criticism rained down on Tammany from the city, the state, from Baltimore, Boston, Washington.

Welch and nearly every major figure in medicine attacked Tammany. Rupert Blue, the head of the U.S. Public Health Service, publicly called upon the mayor to desist.

Tammany backed off, and Copeland embarked on a public relations campaign to repair the damage to himself and his "organization," relying on patriotism to stifle criticism. By late summer the frenzy had died down, but what had been the best public health department in the world was demoralized. The internationally respected director of the Bureau of Public Health Education resigned. The deputy commissioner of health, in office twenty years, resigned, and the mayor replaced him with his personal physician.

On September 15, New York City's first influenza death occurred. By then the disease had long since begun leaking out of the army and navy bases into the civilian population of Massachusetts.

In two polio epidemics in the preceding decade, public health officials had all but closed down the city. But now Copeland did nothing. Three days later, as hospitals began filling with influenza cases, he made influenza and pneumonia reportable diseases, while simultaneously stating that "other bronchial diseases and not the so-called Spanish influenza are said to be responsible for the illness of the majority of persons who were reported to be ill with influenza. . . ."

A few days more and even Copeland could no longer deny reality. People could see disease all about them. Finally he imposed a quarantine on victims and warned, "The health department is prepared to compel patients who may be a menace to the community to go to hospitals." He also assured all concerned "that the disease is not getting away from the control of the health department but is decreasing."

Park knew better. As a student in Vienna in 1890 he had watched that influenza pandemic kill one of his professors and wrote, "We mourn for him and for ourselves." And for several months now he and others in his laboratory had followed the progress of the disease. He was well aware of the transformation of the *City of Exeter* into a floating morgue and of serious cases in July and August on ships arriving in New York harbor. Those cases did one good thing: they relieved the laboratory of political pressure and allowed him and it to concentrate on work.

In late August he and Anna Williams began devoting all their energies to the disease. In mid-September they were called to Camp Upton in Long Island. The disease had just reached there, and few deaths had occurred—yet—but already a single barracks, filled with soldiers from Massachusetts, had two thousand cases.

Park and Williams had collaborated now for a quarter of a century, and they complemented each other perfectly. He was a quiet brown-eyed man with a somewhat reserved, even aristocratic, bearing. He had a claim to the social elite; his father's ancestors arrived in America in 1630, his mother's in 1640. He also felt a calling. Three great-aunts had been missionaries and were buried in Ceylon, a cousin to whom he was very close became a minister, and Park himself had considered becoming a medical missionary.

He had a serious purpose and curiosity per se did not drive that purpose. His seeking of knowledge in the laboratory served his purpose only to the extent, as he saw it, that it served God's purpose. He donated his salary as professor of bacteriology at New York University to the laboratory, or at least into the hands of some of his professional workers who struggled on city salaries. He also involved himself directly with patients, often working the diphtheria wards at the city-run Willard Parker Hospital across the street from his laboratory. The hospital was a new, gleaming place, thirty-five iron bedsteads to each ward, with water closets and bathtubs of marble with porcelain lining, the polished hardwood floors washed every morning with a 1:1,000 solution of bichloride of mercury, the same solution in which patients themselves bathed at discharge and admission.

Methodical, somewhat stolid, he was a master bureaucrat in the best sense of the word; he had run the health department's Bureau of Laboratories for decades and had always looked for ways to make the system work. What drove him was the desire to bring laboratory research to patients. He was a pragmatist. Goethe observed that one searches where there is light. Some scientists try to create new light to shine on problems. Park was not one such; his forte was making exhaustive explorations with existing light.

It was his and Williams's work that had led to mass production of inexpensive diphtheria antitoxin. It was his work that had marked America's acceptance as a scientific equal of Europe, when that international conference had endorsed his views on tuberculosis over Koch's. His scientific papers were exact if not quite elegant, and he matched his precision with a deeply probing and careful mind.

It was that precision, and the missionary's sense of right and wrong, that had led to his public feud over meningitis serum a few years earlier with Simon Flexner and the Rockefeller Institute. In 1911 Park had created the Laboratory for Special Therapy and Investigation, at least in part to rival the Rockefeller Institute. He was a few years older now, but no mellower. He and Flexner remained "pretty acid" about each other, noted one scientist who knew them both well, with "no love lost between them," but despite their animosity both of them cooperated with the other whenever called upon, and neither held back information.

(This openness was a far cry from the atmosphere at some other laboratories, including the Pasteur Institute. Pasteur himself had once advised a protégé not to share information with outsiders, saying, "Keep your cadavers to yourself." When Anna Williams visited there, she was refused any information on a pneumonia antiserum until it was published, and also had to promise that after she left, she would say nothing about anything else she had seen until it was published. Even in publication Pasteur scientists did not tell everything. As Biggs wrote Park, "Marmorek has taught her how it's done—it is secret of course. In the usual way, he omitted the essential thing in his article.")

If Park was almost stolid, Anna Williams injected a certain wildness and creativity into the laboratory. She loved going up in airplanes with stunt fliers—a reckless act in pre–World War I airplanes—and loved sudden fast turns and out-of-control drops. She loved to drive and was always speeding; when traffic was stalled, she often simply pulled into the opposite side of the road and proceeded, and she had a string of traffic tickets to prove it. Once she took a mechanic's course and decided to take her Buick engine apart—but failed to put it back together. In her diary she wrote, "From my earliest memories, I was one of those who wanted to go places. When I couldn't go, I would have my dreams about going. And, such wild dreams were seldom conceived by any other child."

Despite—or more likely because of—her wildness, she had established herself as the premier woman medical scientist in America. Her achievement came at a price.

She was unhappy. She was also lonely. At the age of forty-five, she wrote, "I was told today that it was quite pathetic that I had no one particular friend." She and Park had worked together for decades but they maintained a careful distance. To her diary she confided, "There are degrees to everything, including friendship. . . . [T]here is no sentimentality about my friendships and little sentiment." Religion gave her no relief. She wanted too much from it. She told herself that Jesus knew that his anguish was momentary and that in exchange he was going to save the world. "This knowledge . . . if we were sure, oh! what would we not be willing to undergo." Of course she had no such knowledge. She could only recall "all the good things I have been taught . . . [and] act as if they were true."

Yet in the end, although jealous of those who lived a normal life, she still preferred "discontent rather than happiness through lack of knowledge." Instead she did content herself with the fact that "I have had thrills." Analyzing herself, she confided in her diary that what mattered to her more were "love of knowledge," "love of appreciation," "love of winning," "fear of ridicule," and "power to do, to think new things."

These were not Park's motives, but she and Park made a powerful combination. In science, at least, she had had thrills indeed.

She was fifty-five years old in 1918. Park was the same age. There were no thoughts of thrills on the long drive and rough roads from Manhattan to Camp Upton, even though Park indulged her and let her drive. At the camp the military doctors, knowing what was happening at Devens, begged for advice.

Park and Williams were experts on vaccine therapy. Even during the polio epidemics they had done excellent science, if only to prove the negative; Park had tried to develop but instead proved the ineffectiveness of several treatments. This time they felt hopeful; their work with streptococci and pneumococci, like that of the Rockefeller Institute's, was promising. But as yet Park and Williams had no advice to give; they could only swab the throats and nasal passages of the sick at Upton, return to their laboratory, and proceed from there.

They also got material from another source, which Williams never forgot. It was her first influenza autopsy; the body was that of, she later wrote, "a fine-looking youth from Texas" who shared her last name. She stood staring at his fine features wondering about him, wondering even if he was some distant relative, and noting, "Death occurring so quickly it left little or no marks of disease anywhere except for the lungs."

She could not have looked at his perfect form, perfect but for death, and not wondered just what the country was about to endure. The drive back to New York, the car filled with swabbings from mucosal membranes, sputum, and tissue samples of a mysterious and lethal disease, likely alternated between intense conversation and silence, conversation as they planned their experiments and silence knowing the silence of the laboratory that awaited them.

There was in fact nothing like Park's laboratory in the world. From outside on the street, Park could look up with pride on the six-story building, the floors of laboratories, knowing that his successes had built them. Entirely dedicated to diagnostic testing, production of sera and antitoxins, and medical research, his creation sat at the foot of East Sixteenth Street with the teeming wharfs of the East River just beyond.

Streetcars, horse-drawn carriages, and automobiles clattered past, and the smell of manure still mixed with that of gasoline and oil. There was all the sweat and ambition and failure and grit and money of New York City, all that made the city what it was and is.

Inside the building Park oversaw a virtual industry. More than two hundred workers reported to him, nearly half of them scientists or technicians in one laboratory or another, each one with lab tables laid out in horizontal rows, gas burners in virtually constant use on each table, glassware stacked on shelves above the tables as well as filling shelves along the walls, the rooms often hissing with steam and humidity from the autoclaves used to sterilize.

No other laboratory anywhere, not in any institute, not in any university, not sponsored by any government, not run by any pharmaceutical company, had the combination of scientific competence, epidemiological and public health expertise, and ability to carry out directed research— to focus all resources on one question and not be deflected from that search no matter how enticing or important a finding might be—intent on immediate practical results.

His laboratory could also function in extreme crisis. It had done so before: preventing outbreaks of cholera and typhoid, triumphing over diphtheria, helping in meningitis epidemics. It had done so not only in New York City but all over the country; when requested, Park had sent teams to fight outbreaks of disease elsewhere.

And one other ability made the department unique. If a solution was found, it could produce serum and vaccines in industrial quantities as quickly as—and of better quality than—any drug manufacturer in the world. Indeed, it had been so successful making antitoxins that drug makers and city physicians had combined to use all their political power to limit that production. But now Park could quickly gear back up. Because of the assignment to produce serum for the army, he had just quadrupled the number of horses he could infect and then bleed.

So it was not surprising that soon after Park returned from Camp Upton, he received a telegram from Richard Pearce, head of the National Research Council's section on medicine. Pearce was grabbing at any information he could get from the French, the British, even the Germans, and distributing it to investigators everywhere. He was also breaking the questions about influenza into pieces and asking each of a handful of investigators to focus on a single piece. From Park he wanted to know "the nature of the agent causing the so-called Spanish influenza . . . [and] pure cultures of the causative organism if obtainable. . . . Will your lab undertake the necessary bacteriological studies and make reports as quickly as possible to the undersigned?"

Park instantly wired back, "Will undertake work."

It was as if the laboratory had gone to war, and Park was confident of victory. As he reviewed every published and unpublished scrap of data on the disease from laboratories around the world, he was unimpressed and dismissed most of it with near contempt. Certain his lab could do better, believing that others' sloppiness at least partly contributed to their failure to understand the disease, he laid extraordinarily ambitious plans. In addition to finding the pathogen, in addition to finding a vaccine or serum or both, in addition to producing that drug in huge quantities, in addition to communicating to others the precise procedures to follow so they could produce it, he intended still more. He intended to make the most thorough study of any disease outbreak ever, selecting a large sample of people and, as many of them inevitably became ill, monitoring them through the most sophisticated possible laboratory and epidemiological means. The workload would be enormous, but he believed that his department could handle it.

But within days, almost within hours, the disease began to overwhelm the department. Park had already compensated for the loss of labor to the war by analyzing every system and maximizing efficiency (installing, for example, a vacuum pump that in fifteen minutes could fill three thousand tubes with individual vaccine doses), and even changing accounting methods. But now, as influenza struck first one janitor or technician or scientist at a time, then four at a time, then fifteen at a time, the laboratory reeled. Not so long before, when the Health Department had tracked a typhus outbreak to ground, four of his workers had died of typhus—most likely from laboratory infection. Now people in Park's own lab were again sick, some dying.

Influenza had humbled him, and quickly. He abandoned both his arrogance about the work of others and his own ambitious plans. Now he was trying to get just one thing right, the important thing. *What was the pathogen?*

Meanwhile, the world seemed to shift underfoot. To Park and Williams and to others in other laboratories racing to find an answer, it must have seemed as if they could see this great catastrophe approaching but had to remain frozen in place, all but incapable of doing anything to defeat or avoid it. It was almost as if one's foot were caught under rocks in a tidal pool while the tide came in—the water rising to the knees, to the waist, one sucking in a deep breath then doubling over to try to pry one's foot loose and straightening to feel the water at one's neck, the swell of a wave passing over one's head. . . .

New York City was panicking, terrified.

By now Copeland was enforcing strict quarantines on all cases. There were literally hundreds of thousands of people sick simultaneously, many of them desperately sick. The death toll ultimately reached thirty-three thousand for New York City alone, and that understated the number considerably since statisticians later arbitrarily stopped counting people as victims of the epidemic even though people were still dying of the disease at epidemic rates—still dying months later at rates higher than anywhere else in the country.

It was impossible to get a doctor, and perhaps more impossible to get a nurse. Reports came in that nurses were being held by force in the homes of patients too frightened and desperate to allow them to leave.

Nurses were literally being kidnapped. It did not seem possible to put more pressure on the laboratory. Yet more pressure came.

The pressure pushed Park to abandon more than his ambitious plans. He had always been meticulous, had never compromised, had built much of his scientific reputation on exposing the flawed work of others, always moving forward carefully, basing his own experiments upon well-established premises and with as few assumptions as possible. "On the basis of experimental facts," he had always said, "we are justified in . . ."

Now Park had no leisure for justification. If he was to have any impact on the course of the epidemic he would have to guess—and guess right. So those in his laboratory would, he reported, "study closely only the more dominant types that were demonstrated by our procedure. . . . We recognized that our methods . . . did not take into account . . . heretofore undescribed organisms that might have an etiologic relationship to these infections."

The laboratory had only two constants. One was an endless supply of samples, of swabbings, blood, sputum, and urine from live patients and organs from the dead. "We had plenty of material, I am sorry to say," Williams observed laconically.

And they had their routine. Only the need to keep to discipline saved the laboratory from utter chaos. There was nothing even faintly exciting about this work; it was pure tedium, and pure boredom. And yet every step involved contact with something that could kill, and every step involved passion. Technicians took sputum samples from patients in the hospital and immediately—they could not wait even an hour, or bacteria from the patient's mouth could penetrate into the sputum and contaminate it—began working with it. The steps began with "washing": placing each small lump of balled mucus in a bottle of sterile water, removing it and repeating the process five times, then breaking up the mucus, washing it more, passing a platinum loop—a thin circle of platinum, like something one uses to blow bubbles—through it to transfer it to a test tube, taking another loop and repeating the step half a dozen times. Each step took time, time while people died, but they had no choice. They needed each step, needed to dilute the bacteria to prevent too many colonies from growing in the same medium. Then they took more time, more steps, isolating each of these growths.

Everything mattered. The most tedious tasks mattered. Washing glassware mattered. Contaminated glassware could ruin an experiment, waste time, cost lives. In the course of this work, 220,488 test tubes, bottles, and flasks would be sterilized. Everything mattered, and yet no one knew who would report to work each day, who would not—and who would suddenly be carried across the street to the hospital—and if someone failed to come into work it was nearly impossible to keep track of such simple jobs as removing growing cultures from incubators.

There were dozens of ways to grow bacteria but often only one way to grow a particular kind. Some grow only without oxygen, others only with it in plentiful supply. Some require alkaline media, others acid. Some are extremely delicate, others stable.

Every step, every attempt to grow the pathogen, meant effort, and effort meant time. Every hour incubating a culture meant time. They did not have time.

Four days after accepting the task from Pearce, Park wired, "The only results so far that are of real importance have been obtained in two fatal cases, one a man coming from Brooklyn Navy Yard and one a doctor from the naval hospital in Boston. Both developed an acute septic pneumonia and died within a week of the onset of the first infection. In both cases the lungs showed a beginning pneumonia and in smears very abundant streptococci. . . . There were absolutely no influenza bacilli in either of the lungs."

The failure to find the "influenza bacillus" maddened Park. His best hope to produce a vaccine or serum would be to find a known pathogen, and the most likely suspect was the one Pfeiffer had named *Bacillus influenzae*. Pfeiffer had been and still was confident it caused the disease. Park would not hesitate to rule *B. influenzae* out if he did not find good evidence for it, but he had the utmost respect for Pfeiffer. Working in these desperate circumstances, he wanted to confirm rather than reject Pfeiffer's work. He wanted the answer to be Pfeiffer's bacillus. That would give them a chance, a chance to produce something that saved thousands of lives.

B. influenzae was a particularly difficult bacteria to isolate. It is tiny, even by the standards of bacteria, and usually occurs singly or in pairs rather than in large groups. It requires particular factors, including blood, in culture medium for it to grow. It grows only within a very narrow range of temperatures, and its colonies are minute, transparent, and without structure. (Most bacteria form distinctive colonies with a particular shape and color, distinctive enough that they can sometimes be identified just by looking at the colony in the same way that some ants can be identified by the form of their anthill.) *B. influenzae* grows only on the surface of the medium, since it depends heavily upon oxygen. It is also difficult to stain, hence difficult to see under the microscope. It is an easy target to miss unless one is specifically looking for it and unless one uses excellent technique.

While others in the lab searched for other organisms, Park asked Anna Williams to concentrate on finding Pfeiffer's. Anna Williams found it. She found it constantly. Ultimately, once she perfected her technique, she would find it in 80 percent of all samples from the Willard Parker Hospital, in every single sample from the Marine Hospital, in 98 percent of the samples from the Home for Children.

As much as Park wanted Williams to be right, he would not let his desire corrupt his science. He went a step further, to "the most delicate test of identity . . . agglutination."

"Agglutination" refers to a phenomenon in which antibodies in a test tube bind to the antigen of the bacterium and form clumps, often large enough to be visible to the naked eye.

Since the binding of antibodies to an antigen is *specific*, since the antibodies to the influenza bacillus will bind to only that bacterium and to no other, it is a precise confirmation of identity. The agglutination tests proved without doubt that Williams had found Pfeiffer's influenza bacillus.

Less than a week after first reporting his failure to find it, Park wired Pearce that *B. influenzae* "would seem to be the starting point of the disease." But he was well aware that his methods had been less than thorough, adding, "There is of course the possibility that some unknown filterable virus may be the starting point."

The report had consequences. Park's laboratory began the struggle to produce an antiserum and vaccine to Pfeiffer's bacillus. Soon they were culturing liters and liters of the bacteria, transporting it north, and injecting it into the horses on the Health Department's 175-acre farm sixty-five miles north of the city.

But the only way to know for certain that *B. influenzae* caused the disease was to follow Koch's postulates: isolate the pathogen, use it to re-create the disease in an experimental animal, and then re-isolate the pathogen from the animal. The bacillus did kill laboratory rats. But their symptoms did not resemble influenza.

The results, suggestive as they were, did not fully satisfy Koch's postulates. In this case the necessary experimental animal was man.

Human experiments had begun. In Boston, Rosenau and Keegan were already trying to give the disease to volunteers from a navy brig.

None of the volunteer subjects had yet gotten sick. One of the doctors conducting the study did. In fact he died of influenza. In a scientific sense, however, his death demonstrated nothing.

CHAPTER TWENTY-FOUR

WHILE PARK TRIED to produce an antiserum or vaccine against the disease in New York, Philadelphia was already approaching collapse. Its experience would soon be echoed in many cities around the country.

There Paul Lewis was searching for the answer as well. Few, including Park, were more likely to find it. The son of a physician, Lewis grew up in Milwaukee, went to the University of Wisconsin, and finished his medical training at Penn in 1904. Even before leaving medical school he knew he intended to spend his life in the laboratory, and he quickly acquired both a pedigree and a well-deserved reputation. He started as a junior investigator working on pneumonia under Welch, Osler, Biggs, and several others who comprised the Rockefeller Institute's Board of Scientific Advisers. Lewis impressed them all. Most impressed was Theobald Smith, one of the world's leading bacteriologists, for whom Lewis then worked in Boston. Later Smith recommended Lewis to Simon Flexner, saying that Harvard lacked the resources to allow Lewis to develop fully and that "[h]is heart lies in research."

From Smith there could come no higher compliment. Lewis deserved it. He seemed born for the laboratory. At least that was the only place where he was happy; he loved not only the work itself but the laboratory environment, loved disappearing into the laboratory and into thought. "Love" was not too strong a word; his passions lay in the lab. At Rockefeller, Lewis had started off pursuing his own ideas but when a polio epidemic erupted Flexner asked him to work with him on it. He agreed. It was a perfect match. Their polio work was a model combination of speed and good science. They not only proved that polio was a viral disease, still considered a landmark finding in virology, but they developed a vaccine that protected monkeys from polio 100 percent of the time. It would take nearly half a century to develop a polio vaccine for humans. In the course of this research Lewis became one of the leading experts in the world on viruses.

Flexner pronounced Lewis "one of the best men in the country, . . . a very gifted fellow." That may have been an understatement. Richard Shope worked closely with him in the 1920s, knew many of the world's best scientists (including Flexner, Welch, Park, Williams, and many Nobel laureates)—and himself became a member of the National Academy of Sciences. He called Lewis the smartest man he ever knew. Joseph Aronson, a prize-winning University of Pennsylvania scientist who had also done research at the Pasteur Institute, named his son after Lewis and, like Shope, said Lewis was the brightest man he had ever met.

When the war began, Pearce, the National Research Council official, told Lewis what he told only four or five other scientists in the country: to expect to be asked "for special service in connection with epidemic disease."

Lewis was ready. He received a navy commission and told Flexner he had "no onerous routine duties." His laboratory abilities were far more important. He was still cooperating with Cole and Avery on the development of pneumonia serum, and he was also, as he told Flexner, experimenting with dyes "as regards their capacity to inhibit the growth" of the bacteria that cause tuberculosis. The idea that dyes might kill bacteria was not original with him, but he was doing world-class work in the area and his instincts were right about its importance. Twenty years later a Nobel Prize would go to Gerhard Domagk for turning a dye into the first antibiotic, the first of the sulfa drugs.

But now the city did not need laboratory breakthroughs that deepened understanding. It needed instant successes. Lewis had reached his conclusions about polio with tremendous speed—roughly a year, and they had been both sound and pioneering conclusions. But now he had only weeks, even days. Now he was watching bodies literally pile up in the hospital morgue at the Navy Yard, in the morgues of civilian hospitals, in undertaking establishments, in homes.

He remembered Flexner's work on meningitis during an epidemic of that disease. Flexner had solved that problem and the success had made the reputation of the Rockefeller Institute. Knowing that Flexner had succeeded then made a solution to this seem possible. Perhaps Lewis could do the same.

He considered whether a filter-passing organism caused influenza. But to look for a virus Lewis would have to look in darkness. That was science, the best of science—at least to look into the gloaming was—but he was not now engaged only in science. Not right now. He was trying to save lives *now*.

He had to look where there was light.

First, light shone on a kind of blunt-force use of the immune system. Even if they could not find the pathogen, even if they could not follow normal procedures and infect horses with the pathogen and then prepare the blood from horses, there was one animal that was suffering from the disease that was scorching its way across the earth. That animal was man.

Most people who contracted the disease survived. Even most people who contracted pneumonia survived. It was quite possible that their blood and their serum held antibodies that would cure or prevent disease in others. Lewis and Flexner had had some success using this approach with polio in 1910. In Boston, Dr. W. R. Redden at the navy hospital also remembered, as he reported, "the experimental evidence presented by Flexner and Lewis with convalescent serum from poliomyelitis." Now Redden and a colleague drew blood from those who had survived an influenza attack, extracted the serum, and injected it into thirty-six pneumonia patients in a row, beginning October 1. This was not a scientific experiment with controls, and in a scientific sense the results proved nothing. But by the time they reported the results in the October 19 *JAMA,* thirty patients had recovered, five were still undergoing treatment, and only one had died.

Experiments began in Philadelphia using both the whole blood and serum of survivors of influenza as well. These too were not scientific experiments; they were desperate attempts to save lives. If there was any sign this procedure worked, the science could follow later.

Lewis let others conduct that blunt-force work. It took no truly special skills, and others could do it as well as he. He spent his time on four things. He did not do these things sequentially. He did them simultaneously, moving down different paths—setting up experiments to test each hypothesis—at the same time.

First, he tried to develop an influenza vaccine using the same methods he had used against polio. This was a more sophisticated version of the blunt-force approach of transfusing the blood or serum of influenza survivors. For he at least suspected a virus might cause influenza.

Second, he stayed in the laboratory following a shimmer of light. As Park had reasoned, so Lewis reasoned. Research could find bacteria. Pfeiffer had already pointed an accusing finger at one bacillus. Lewis and everyone in his laboratories were working hours and days without relief, taking only a few hours off for sleep, running procedure after procedure— agglutination, filtration, transferring culture growths, injecting laboratory animals. His team too searched for bacteria. They took more swabs from the throats and noses of the first victims, exposed the medium to it, and waited. They worked intensively, twenty-four hours a day in shifts, and then they waited, frustrated by the time it took bacteria to grow in the cultures, frustrated by the number of cultures that became contaminated, frustrated by everything that interfered with their progress.

In the first fifteen cases, Lewis found no *B. influenzae*. Ironically, the disease had exploded so quickly, spreading to hospital staff, that Lewis had little except sputum samples to work with: "The hospitals were so depleted [of staff] . . . I have had no autopsy material" except from four "badly decomposed" bodies, almost certainly too long dead to be of any use.

Then, like Park and Williams, Lewis adjusted his techniques and did begin to find the bacillus regularly. He gave this information to Krusen, the health commissioner. The *Inquirer* and other newspapers, desperate to say something positive, declared that he had found the cause of influenza and "armed the medical profession with absolute knowledge on which to base their campaign against the disease."

Lewis had no such absolute knowledge, nor did he believe he had it. True, he had isolated *B. influenzae*. But he had also isolated a pneumococcus and a hemolytic streptococcus. Some instinct pointed him another direction. He began third and fourth lines of inquiry. The third involved shifting his dye experiments from trying to kill tuberculosis bacteria to trying to kill pneumococci.

But death surrounded him, enveloped him. He turned his attention back to helping produce the only thing that might work *now*. After the emergency, if anything seemed to work he could always return to the laboratory and do careful, deliberate experimentation to understand it and prove its effectiveness.

So he chose as his targets the bacteria he and others had found. From the first instant he had seen the dying sailors, he had known he would have to begin work on it *now*. For even if he had guessed right, even if what he was doing could succeed, it would take time to succeed. So, in his laboratory and in other laboratories around the city, the investigators no longer investigated. They simply tried to produce. There was no certainty that anything they produced would work. There was only hope.

He started by preparing medium using beef peptone broth with blood added, and then growing cultures of the pathogens they had isolated from cases—*B. influenzae,* Types I and II of the pneumococcus, and hemolytic streptococcus. He personally prepared small batches of vaccine including these organisms and gave it to sixty people. Of those sixty, only three people developed pneumonia and none died. A control group had ten pneumonias and three deaths.

This seemed more than just promising. It was not proof. Many factors could explain the results, including random chance. But he could not wait for explanations.

His laboratory had no ability to produce the immense quantities of vaccine needed. It required an industrial operation. They needed vats to grow these things in, not petri dishes or laboratory flasks. They needed vats like those in a brewery.

He handed off this task to others in the city, including those who ran the municipal laboratory. It would take time to grow enough for tens of thousands of people.

The whole process, even in its most accelerated state, would take at least three weeks. And it would take time once they made the vaccine to administer it to thousands and thousands of people in a series of injections of increasing doses spaced several days apart. In all that time, the disease would be killing.

Meanwhile, Lewis began work on still a fifth line of inquiry, making a serum that could cure the disease. This work was trickier. They could make a vaccine with a shotgun approach, combining several organisms and protecting against all of them. (Today vaccines against diphtheria, pertussis—whooping cough—and tetanus are combined in a single shot; a single shot protecting against measles, mumps, and rubella is routinely given to children; and today's flu shots contain vaccines against several subtypes of influenza viruses, while the anti-pneumonia vaccine is a direct descendant of the work done at the Rockefeller Institute in 1917.

A serum had to aim at only one specific target; if it worked at all, it would work only against a single organism. To make a serum that worked, Lewis would have to pick a single target. If he had to aim at a single target, he had to choose the bacillus Pfeiffer had discovered, *B. influenzae*. It was still by far the most likely cause of the disease.

Developing a serum against this organism would likely be difficult. While Lewis was still at the Rockefeller Institute, Flexner himself had tried to do this in collaboration with Martha Wollstein. Wollstein—a fine scientist, although Flexner never treated her with the respect he gave to others—had experimented with *B. influenzae* almost continuously since 1906. But Flexner and she had made no progress whatsoever. They had not only failed to develop a serum that could help man; they had failed to cure any laboratory animals.

Lewis never understood precisely where Flexner had gone wrong in that attempt, although it certainly would have been the subject of many talks in the famous lunchroom where solutions to so many scientific problems were suggested. Now he had no opportunity to think deeply about the problem, think all the way through it, come up with a hypothesis with explanatory power, and test it.

Lewis could only hope that Flexner failed because his technique was faulty. That was quite possible. Flexner had sometimes been a little sloppy in the laboratory. He had once even conceded, "Technically, I am not well-trained in the sense of meticulous and complete accuracy."

So now Lewis hoped some technical error—perhaps in the preparation of the medium, perhaps in too rough a usage for the killed bacteria, perhaps somewhere else—accounted for Flexner's problems. It might have. For example, many years later a young graduate student entered a laboratory and saw a renowned Harvard professor at the sink washing glassware while his technician was perfoming a complex task at the workbench. The student asked him why the technician was not washing the glassware. "Because," the professor replied, "I always do the most important part of the experiment and in this experiment the most important thing is the cleanliness of the glassware."

Lewis turned all his attention in effect to washing the glassware, to the most mundane tasks, making certain there would no mistakes in the work itself, at the same time applying any knowledge about Pfeiffer's bacillus that had been learned since Flexner's failure.

Lewis knew full well that little of what he was doing was good science. It was all, or nearly all, based on informed guesswork. He only worked harder.

As he worked, the society about him teetered on the edge of collapse.

CHAPTER TWENTY-FIVE

W HEN WELCH had first seen autopsies of victims at Devens he had walked out of the morgue and made three calls: to a Harvard pathologist, asking him to conduct further autopsies; to Gorgas's office, warning of the coming of an epidemic; and to Oswald Avery at the Rockefeller Institute, asking him to get on the next train from New York. He hoped Avery could identify the pathogen killing the men at Devens.

Avery immediately left his own lab, walked the few blocks home for a change of clothes, then went to Pennsylvania Station, that magnificent and uplifting building. For the length of his train ride through the Connecticut countryside, through the teeming train stations of New Haven, Providence, and Boston, up to Devens, he began to prepare, reviewing the best approaches to this problem.

Welch had told him of his concern that, despite clinical symptoms that looked like influenza, this might be a new disease. Avery's first step would still be to look for the presence of B. influenzae, everyone's chief suspect as the cause of influenza. Avery knew a fair amount about Pfeiffer's bacillus, including that it was exceptionally difficult to grow and that its chemistry made it difficult to stain and hence see in a smear under the microscope. The chemistry and metabolism of the bacteria interested him. He wondered how to make it grow better, how to make it easier to find, how to make it easier to identify. For he always did everything, down to washing the glassware, with precision and discipline.

Late that afternoon Avery arrived at the camp and immediately began laboratory tests. He was all but impervious to the chaos about him, impervious to the bodies of young men lying naked or in bloody sheets he had to step over—as Welch, Cole, Vaughan, Russell, and the others of that party had—to reach the autopsy room.

From the first he encountered difficulties, getting puzzling results from the Gram test. In this test, bacteria are stained with crystal violet, treated with iodine, washed with alcohol, and then stained again with a contrasting dye. Bacteria retaining the violet color are called "Gram-positive." Those that do not are "Gram-negative." The result of the Gram test is comparable to a witness identifying an assailant as white or black; the answer simply eliminates some possible suspects.

Unlike other investigators, Avery found no Gram-negative bacteria. *B. influenzae* is Gram-negative. The test eliminated *B. influenzae* as even a possibility. It eliminated all Gram-negative bacteria as possibilities. He repeated the experiment; again he found no Gram-negative bacteria, none at all.

Avery soon solved this particular puzzle. He discovered that all the liquid in the laboratory bottles labeled "alcohol" was actually water. Soldiers had apparently drunk the alcohol and replaced it with water. When he got alcohol, the test results came in as expected. He found Gram-negative bacteria.

Now he began his hunt in earnest. He began it with dead bodies, those of the men who had died most recently, some of whom so recently that their bodies remained warm to the touch. He felt the soggy sponginess of the still-warm lungs and respiratory tract with his gloved hands, seeking out areas of the most obvious infection from which to cut tissue samples, dipping into pockets of pus, seeking the organism responsible for the killing. Perhaps he was a little afraid, this tiny man surrounded by dead young soldiers, but he had courage and he was not hunting rabbits. He had no interest in hunting rabbits.

Smears across slides turned up several possible pathogens, all of them potential killers. He needed to know which one did the killing.

He stayed at Devens long enough to grow cultures of bacteria. Like Park and Lewis, Avery had initial difficulty but began to find Pfeiffer's bacillus. He discovered it in twenty-two of thirty dead soldiers and gave Welch his results. Meanwhile Burt Wolbach, the Harvard pathologist whom Welch had also asked to help at Devens, made a stronger statement: "Every case showed the influenza bacillus, in many instances pure cultures from one or more lobes. . . . Mixed cultures, usually pneumococcus, where bronchial dilation was marked. . . . Pure cultures of influenza bacillus in the more recent stages and therefore usually in the upper lobes." In an article in *Science,* another respected investigator also wrote, "The causative agent is believed to be the bacillus of Pfeiffer."

On September 27, Welch, Cole, and Victor Vaughan wired the surgeon general from Devens, "It is established that the influenza at Camp Devens is caused by the bacillus of Pfeiffer."

But it was not so established, at least not to Avery. Although he respected Wolbach, not to mention Park, Williams, and Lewis, all of whom were reaching the same conclusion at about the same time, he based conclusions only upon his own findings. And his findings did not convince him yet. In seven of the autopsies he found no sign of any bacterial invasion whatsoever, despite the devastation of the lungs. Also, although he found potentially lethal bacteria without any sign of Pfeiffer's in only a single instance, in roughly half the cases he was finding both Pfeiffer's and other organisms, including the pneumococcus, hemolytic streptococcus, and staphylococcus aureus, which although a lethal organism rarely caused pneumonia.

He could interpret these findings several ways. They might mean that Pfeiffer's *B. influenzae* did not cause the disease. But that was only one possible conclusion. Pfeiffer's might well be the cause of the disease, and, after it infected the victim, other bacteria took advantage of a weakened immune system to follow its lead. This would not be unusual. Finding several pathogens might even actually strengthen the case for Pfeiffer's. Pfeiffer's grew poorly in laboratory cultures whenever other bacteria, especially the pneumococcus or hemolytic streptococcus, were also present. So its existence at all in cultures with these other organisms might indicate that *B. influenzae* had been present in enormous numbers in the victim.

Methodically he ran through all this in his mind. By early October, he was back at Rockefeller hearing reports from dozens of other investigators around the country and the world that they too were finding the influenza bacillus. But there were also reports of failures to find *B. influenzae.* It would be easy to dismiss the failures to find it as failures of technique; Pfeiffer's was after all one of the most difficult organisms to grow. Still, Avery's own findings alone left too many unanswered questions for him to reach a conclusion, crisis or not. Unlike Park, Williams, and Lewis, Avery was not ready to reach even a tentative conclusion. Yes, Pfeiffer's might cause influenza. Oh yes it might. But he was not convinced. From Avery came no reports of finding influenza's cause, no phone calls or telegrams that he was sending cultures with which to infect horses and produce serum or vaccine.

He was pushing himself harder than he ever had at Devens—and he always pushed hard. He ate in the laboratory, ran dozens of experiments simultaneously, barely slept, bounced ideas by telephone off Rosenau and others. He bore into his experiments like a drill, breaking them apart and examining every fractured crack in the data for a clue. But if he pushed himself to work, he would not push himself toward a conclusion.

He was not convinced.

Oswald Avery was different. Pressure troubled him less than having to force the direction of his work, and that he could not pursue the trail wherever it led, could not move at his own pace, could not take the time to *think*. Make-do solutions were foreign to his nature. He worked on the vertical. He dove deeply into a thing, to the deepest depths, following down the narrowest pathways and into the tiniest openings, leaving no loose ends. In every way his life was vertical, focused, narrow, controlled.

He prepared . . . *everything*, wanting to control every effect. Even the drafts of his rare talks show marks denoting what words to emphasize, where to change the tone of his voice, where to use nuance. Even in casual conversation it sometimes seemed each word, indeed each hesitation, was carefully prepared, weighed, and perhaps staged. His personal office, adjacent to his laboratory, reflected focus as well. René Dubos, a prominent scientist, called it "small and bare, as empty as possible, without the photographs, mementos, pictures, unused books, and other friendly items that usually adorn and clutter a work place. The austerity symbolized how much he had given up all aspects of his life for the sake of utter concentration on a few chosen goals."

For in digging deep, Avery did not wish to be disturbed. He was not rude or unkind or ungenerous. Far from it. Young investigators who worked under him uniformly became his most loyal admirers. But he burrowed in, deeper and deeper into the world of his own making, a world—however narrow—that he could define and over which exert some control.

But narrow did not mean small. There was nothing small about his thinking. He used information like a springboard, a jumping-off point that allowed his mind to roam freely, indeed to race freely—even carelessly—to speculate. Colin MacLeod, like Dubos a brilliant Avery protégé, said that whenever an experiment yielded unexpected information Avery's "imagination was now fired. . . . He would explore theoretical implications exhaustively."

Dubos put it another way. He believed Avery uncomfortable in and possibly incapable of handling the chaos of social interaction. But he believed Avery comfortable with and capable of confronting the chaos of nature. Avery could do so because of his "uncanny sense of what was truly important" and "imaginative vision of reality. . . . He had the creative impulse to compose those facts into meaningful and elegant structures. . . . His scientific compositions had, indeed, much in common with artistic creations which do not imitate actuality but transcend it and illuminate reality."

Years after the pandemic, Avery's colleague and friend Alphonse Dochez received the Kober Medal, an award Avery himself had received earlier. In a tribute, Avery described Dochez's work ethic. He could have been describing his own: "[R]esults . . . are not random products of chance observations. They are the fruit of years of wise reflection, objective thinking, and thoughtful experimentation. I have never seen his laboratory desk piled high with Petri dishes and bristling with test tubes like a forest wherein the trail ends and the searcher becomes lost in dense thickets of confused thought. . . . I have never known him to engage in purposeless rivalries or competitive research. But often have I seen him sit calmly, lost in thought, while all around him others with great show of activity were flitting about like particles in Brownian motion; then, I have watched him rouse himself, smilingly saunter to his desk, assemble a few pipettes, borrow a few tubes of media, perhaps a jar of ice, and then do a simple experiment which answered the question."

But now, in the midst of a killing epidemic, everything and everyone around him—including even the pressure from Welch—shouldered thought aside, shouldered perspective and preparation aside, substituting for it what Avery so disdained: Brownian motion—the random movement of particles in a fluid. Others hated influenza for the death it caused. Avery hated it for that, too, but for a more personal assault as well, an assault upon his integrity. He would not yield to it.

When Avery experimented, a colleague said, "His attitude had many similarities with the hunter in search of his prey. For the hunter, all the components—the rocks, the vegetation, the sky—are fraught with information and meanings that enable him to become part of the intimate world of his prey." Avery had a hunter's patience. He could lie in wait, for an hour, a day, a week, a month, a season. If the prey mattered enough, he could wait through an entire season and then another and then another. But he did not simply wait; he wasted not a single hour, he plotted, he observed, he learned. He learned his prey's escape routes and closed them off; he found better and better vantage points; he bracketed the field through which the prey passed and kept tightening that field until, eventually, the prey had to pass through a noose. And he could lay traps: studying pneumococci by scratching it into the skin, for example, where the immune system could easily control the infection, but which still gave him the opportunity to experiment with the bacteria outside a test tube. He advised, "Whenever you fall, pick up something." And he often said, "Disappointment is my daily bread. I thrive on it."

He would not be rushed. There was pressure on him, pressure on everyone. But he would not be rushed. At Rockefeller he was hardly the only one devoting all his energies to influenza. Martha Wollstein, who had years before collaborated with Flexner on an unsuccessful effort to develop a serum for Pfeiffer's, was searching for antibodies in the blood of recovered patients. Dochez was making an intensive study of throats. Many others were working on the disease. But they had made little progress. Rufus Cole reported to Gorgas's office in mid-October, "We have been compelled to take care of the cases of influenza arising in the Hospital and Institute and these patients have occupied all of our space." Because of the time treating the patients took, he added, "I do not think we can add very much, so far, to the knowledge concerning the disease."

Everywhere the pressure was intense. Eugene Opie, another Hopkins product who was now a lieutenant colonel on the army's pneumonia commission, had been at Camp Pike in Arkansas when the epidemic broke out. He had gone there because, during the measles epidemic, Pike had had the highest rate of pneumonia of any cantonment in the country. Now of course his orders were to work entirely on influenza. Frederick Russell, speaking for Gorgas, demanded "daily . . . a statement of your findings, as you interpret them." Every *day* he was to report. If he found anything that gave the faintest hint of progress, Gorgas wanted to know it—instantly—so it could be shared. Opie would find no shortage of experimental material. Camp Pike held sixty thousand troops. At the crest of the epidemic thirteen thousand of them would be hospitalized simultaneously.

Investigators struggled to find something—anything—that could help, that could contain the explosion. Though no one had found anything certain, in Philadelphia following Lewis's methods, in New York following Park's, in Chicago following those developed at the Mayo Clinic, laboratories were producing enough vaccines and serum for hundreds of thousands and perhaps millions of people, while from Boston a huge and much-publicized shipment of vaccine was rushed across the country to San Francisco. On October 3, Gorgas's office in Washington offered all headquarters personnel the antipneumococcal vaccine that Cole and Avery had such hopes for, the one vaccine that had been tested—and with such success—that spring at Camp Upton.

Even in the midst of this death, this pressure, Avery would not be rushed. More and more reports came in that investigators around the world could not find the influenza bacillus. This in itself proved nothing. It was almost a test of a bacteriologist's skill to grow Pfeiffer's in the laboratory. At Camp Dodge in Iowa, for example, bacteriologists found Pfeiffer's *B. influenzae* in only 9.6 percent of the autopsied cases. An official army report blamed them: "The low incidence was undoubtedly due to poor technique in handling cultures. . . . [B]acteriologic methods . . . of this camp . . . were not to be depended upon." The laboratory chief at Camp Grant, whom Welch himself had pronounced "excellent" just three months before the epidemic struck, found Pfeiffer's bacillus in only six of 198 autopsies. Even so, his own report said, "We are inclined to take the stand that this study does not prove the lack of association between the Pfeiffer's bacillus and the epidemic owing to the irregular technique followed."

Perhaps that was the case, perhaps technical errors prevented those at

Dodge and Grant and elsewhere from identifying the bacillus. Or perhaps Pfeiffer's was not present to be identified.

In his usual methodical way Avery took the step most likely to settle the question. There was no drama to this step. He poured his energies into perfecting the tool, to find ways to make it easier to grow *B. influenzae.* If he succeeded, then everyone could learn whether the inability to find the bacillus was because of incompetence or the absence of the bacteria.

He filled his laboratory with petri dishes, prepared the culture media in dozens of different ways, isolated the different factors, and observed in which dishes the bacteria seemed to grow best. Then he pushed each element that seemed to encourage growth. A hypothesis lay behind each individual experiment. He had learned, for example, that the pneumococcus inhibited the growth of Pfeiffer's. So he wanted to prevent any pneumococci from growing. He already knew as much about the chemistry and metabolism of the pneumococcus as did any person living. He added a chemical, sodium oleate, to the medium to block pneumococcal growth. It worked. In cultures with sodium oleate the pneumococcus did not grow, and Pfeiffer's grew better.

Over a period of weeks he made significant progress. Pfeiffer's also required blood in the culture medium to grow, which was not so unusual. But blood serum inactivated the sodium oleate. So he centrifuged out only red blood cells and used them. And his experiments suggested that blood added to the culture at roughly body temperature inhibited growth. Avery found that *heated* blood, adding blood to media at nearly 200 degrees Fahrenheit, allowed the *B. influenzae* to flourish.

He promptly published the recipe for his preparation, which became known as "chocolate agar," in the *Journal of the American Medical Association,* writing, "It is possible that technical difficulties in the isolation and growth of this microorganism may be in part responsible for the discordant results obtained in different laboratories.... The use of this medium has led to an increase in positive findings of B. influenzae in actual cases of the disease and in convalescents."

With this information any reasonably competent scientist could grow and identify the bacteria. At least now they would know that if Pfeiffer's was not found it was because it was not there.

Avery himself still would not be rushed, would not discuss a conclusion he was not yet ready to support. But based on Avery's work Cole told Russell, "I feel less and less inclined to ascribe the primary infection to the influenza bacilli—although that possiblity cannot be excluded until the real cause of the infection is demonstrated. . . . I am very hopeful that the anti-pneumococcus vaccination can be pushed rapidly. While the anti-influenzal vaccination"—by this he meant vaccine against *B. influenzae*—"seems to me still doubtful we have very good evidence that the anti-pneumococcus vaccination is going to prove to be of a great help." He added, "It seems to me the influenza epidemic gives an opportunity for developing this in a way that could not have otherwise been done."

There was nothing easy about making either the antipneumococcus serum, which in tests had just cured twenty-eight of twenty-nine patients suffering infection with Type I pneumococcus, or the vaccine. It took two months to prepare the vaccine properly, two months of a difficult process: making 300-liter batches of broth—and the pneumococci themselves dissolved too often in ordinary broth, which meant adding chemicals that later had to be removed—concentrating it, precipitating some of it out with alcohol, separating out the additives, standardizing it. Avery and other Rockefeller investigators did make one important advance in production: by adjusting the amount of glucose in the media they increased the yield tenfold. But they could still move only twenty-five liters a day through centrifuges. It mocked the need.

In the meanwhile the killing continued.

■ Part VIII
THE TOLLING
OF THE BELL

CHAPTER TWENTY-SIX

WHILE SCIENCE was confronting nature, society began to confront the effects of nature. For this went beyond the ability of any individual or group of individuals to respond to. To have any chance in alleviating the devastation of the epidemic required organization, coordination, implementation. It required leadership and it required that institutions follow that leadership.

Institutions are a strange mix of the mass and the individual. They abstract. They behave according to a set of rules that substitute both for individual judgments and for the emotional responses that occur whenever individuals interact. The act of creating an institution dehumanizes it, creates an arbitrary barrier between individuals.

Yet institutions are human as well. They reflect the cumulative personalities of those within them, especially their leadership. They tend, unfortunately, to mirror less admirable human traits, developing and protecting self-interest and even ambition. Institutions almost never sacrifice. Since they live by rules, they lack spontaneity. They try to order chaos not in the way an artist or scientist does, through a defining vision that creates structure and discipline, but by closing off and isolating themselves from that which does not fit. They become bureaucratic.

The best institutions avoid the worst aspects of bureaucracy in two ways. Some are not really institutions at all. They are simply a loose confederation of individuals, each of whom remains largely a free agent whose achievements are independent of the institution but who also shares and benefits from association with others. In these cases the institution simply provides an infrastructure that supports the individual, allowing him or her to flourish so that the whole often exceeds the sum of the parts. (The Rockefeller Institute was such an institution.) Other institutions avoid the worst elements of bureaucracy by concentrating on a clearly defined purpose. Their rules have little to do with such procedural issues as a chain of command; instead rules focus on how to achieve a particular result, in effect offering guidance based on experience. This kind of institution even at its best can still stultify creativity, but such institutions can execute, can do a routine thing efficiently. They resemble professionals trying to do their jobs and duty; they accomplish their tasks.

In 1918 the institution of the federal government had more force than it had ever had—and in some ways more force than it has had since. But it was aiming all that force, all its vital energy, in another direction.

The United States had entered the war with little preparation in April 1917, and mobilizing the country took time. By the summer of 1918, however, Wilson had injected the government into every facet of national life and had created great bureaucratic engines to focus all the nation's attention and intent on the war.

He had created a Food Administration to control and distribute food, a Fuel Administration to ration coal and gasoline, a War Industries Board to oversee the entire economy. He had taken all but physical control over the railroads and had created a federally sponsored river barge line that brought commerce back to life on the Mississippi River, a commerce that had been killed by competition from those railroads. He had built many dozens of military installations, each of which held at least tens of thousands of soldiers or sailors. He had created industries that made America's shipyards teem with hundreds of thousands of laborers launching hundreds of ships, dug new coal mines to produce coal for the factories that weaned America's military from British and French weapons and munitions—for, unlike in World War II, America was no arsenal of democracy.

He had created a vast propaganda machine, an internal spy network, a bond-selling apparatus extending to the level of residential city blocks. He had even succeeded in stifling speech, in the summer of 1918 arresting and imprisoning—some for prison terms longer than ten years—not just radical labor leaders and editors of German-language newspapers but powerful men, even a congressman.

He had injected the government into American life in ways unlike any other in the nation's history. And the final extension of federal power had come only in the spring of 1918, after the first wave of influenza had begun jumping from camp to camp, when the government expanded the draft from males between the ages of twenty-one and thirty to those between the ages of eighteen and forty-five. Only on May 23, 1918, had Provost Marshal Enoch Crowder, who oversaw the draft, issued his "work or fight" order, stating that anyone not employed in an essential industry would be drafted—an order that caused major league baseball to shorten its season and sent many ballplayers scurrying for jobs that were "essential"—and promising that "all men within the enlarged age would be called within a year." *All* men, the government had said, with orders for an estimated thirteen million to register September 12. Crowder bragged about doing "in a day what the Prussian autocracy had been spending nearly fifty years to perfect."

All this enormous and focused momentum would not be turned easily.

It would not be turned even by the prospect of peace. In mid-August, as the lethal wave of the epidemic was gathering itself, Austria had already inquired about peace terms, an inquiry that Wilson rebuffed utterly. And as the epidemic was gathering full momentum, peace was only weeks away. Bulgaria had signed an armistice on September 29. On September 30, Kaiser Wilhelm had granted parliamentary government to the German nation; that same day Ludendorff had warned his government that Germany must extend peace feelers or disaster—immediate disaster—would follow. German diplomats sent out those feelers. Wilson ignored them. The Central Powers, Germany and her allies, were simultaneously breaking off one from one another and disintegrating internally as well. In the first week of October, Austria and Germany separately sent peace feelers to the Allies, and on October 7, Austria delivered a diplomatic note to Wilson formally seeking peace on any terms Wilson chose. Ten days later— days of battle and deaths—the Austrian note remained unanswered.

Earlier Wilson had spoken of a "peace without victory," believing only such a peace could last. But now he gave no indication that the war would soon be over. Although a rumor that the war had ended sent thrills through the nation, Wilson quickly renounced it. Nor would he relent. He was not now fighting to the death; he was fighting only to kill. *To fight you must be brutal and ruthless,* he had said. *Force!* he had demanded. *Force to the utmost! Force without stint or limit! The righteous and triumphant Force which shall make Right the law of the world, and cast every selfish dominion down in the dust.*

Reflecting his will, there was no letup in the ferocity and wrath of the Liberty Loan rallies, no letup in the frenzied pressure to produce in coal mines and shipyards, no letup among editorials or for that matter news stories exhorting people to insist upon total and complete German capitulation. Especially within the government itself, there was no letup. Instead Wilson pressed, pressed with all his might—and that meant all the nation's might—for total victory.

If Wilson and his government would not be turned from his end even by the prospect of peace, they would hardly be turned by a virus. And the reluctance, inability, or outright refusal of the American government to shift targets would contribute to the killing. Wilson took no public note of the disease, and the thrust of the government was not diverted. The relief effort for influenza victims would find no assistance in the Food Administration or the Fuel Administration or the Railroad Administration. From neither the White House nor any other senior administration post would there come any leadership, any attempt to set priorities, any attempt to coordinate activities, any attempt to deliver resources.

The military, especially the army, would confront the virus directly. Gorgas had done all that he could have, all that anyone could have, to prepare for an emergency. But the military would give no help to civilians. Instead it would draw further upon civilian resources.

The same day that Welch had stepped out of the autopsy room at Devens and called Gorgas's office, his warning had been relayed to the army chief of staff, urging that all transfers be frozen unless absolutely necessary and that under no circumstances transfers from infected camps be made: *The deaths at Camp Devens will probably exceed 500. . . . The experience at Camp Devens may be fairly expected to occur at other large cantonments. . . . New men will almost surely contract the disease.*

Gorgas's superiors ignored the warning. There was no interruption of movement between camps whatsoever; not until weeks later, with the camps paralyzed and, literally, tens of thousands of soldiers dead or dying, did the army make any adjustments.

One man did act, however. On September 26, although many training camps had not yet seen any influenza cases at all, Provost Marshal Enoch Crowder canceled the next draft (he would also cancel the draft after this one). It had been scheduled to send one hundred forty-two thousand men to the cantonments.

It was a bold move, made despite the unquenched appetite of General John J. Pershing, in charge of the American Expeditionary Force, for men. In France, Pershing was pressing forward, earlier that same day launching a major offensive in the Meuse-Argonne region. As the Americans charged out of their trenches, the Germans shredded their ranks. General Max von Gallwitz, the commander facing them, entered into his official record, "We [have] no more worries."

Despite this, Crowder had acted immediately and likely saved thousands of lives, but he did not cancel the draft to save lives. He did so because he recognized that the disease was utterly overwhelming and creating total chaos in the cantonments. There could be no training until the disease passed. He believed that sending more draftees into this chaos would only magnify it and delay the restoration of order and the production of soldiers. In *Murder in the Cathedral*, T. S. Eliot could call it "the greatest treason: to do the right thing for the wrong reason." The men who lived because of Crowder might disagree with the poet.

But Crowder's decision and the efforts of the Gorgas-led army medical corps would be the only bright spots in the response of the federal government. Other army decisions were not such good ones. Pershing still demanded fresh troops, troops to replace those killed or wounded in battle, troops to replace those killed by or recovering from influenza, troops to replace those who simply needed relief from the line. All the Allied powers were desperate for fresh American boys.

The army had to decide whether to continue to transport soldiers to France during the epidemic. They had information about the costs. The army knew the costs well.

On September 19 the acting army surgeon general, Charles Richard—Gorgas was in Europe—wrote General Peyton March, the commander of the army, urging him that "organizations known to be infected, or exposed to the disease, be not permitted to embark for overseas service until the disease has run its course within the organization."

March acknowledged the warning from Gorgas's deputy but did nothing. The chief medical officer at the port of embarkation in Newport News, Virginia, rephrased—more emphatically—the same warning: "The condition [on a troopship] is almost that of a powder magazine with troops unprotected by previous [influenza] attack. The spark will be applied sooner or later. On the other hand with troops protected by previous attack the powder has been removed." He too was ignored. Gorgas's office urged quarantining troops heading overseas for one week before departure, or eliminating overcrowding on board. March did nothing.

Meanwhile the *Leviathan* was loading troops. Once the pride of the German passenger fleet, built as the *Vaterland,* she was the largest ship in the world and among the fastest in her class. She had been in New York when America entered the war, and her captain could not bring himself to sabotage or scuttle her. Alone among all German ships confiscated in the United States, she was taken undamaged. In mid-September, on her voyage back from France she had buried several crew and passengers at sea, dead of influenza. Others arrived in New York sick, including Assistant Secretary of the Navy Franklin Roosevelt, who was taken ashore on a stretcher, then by ambulance to his mother's home on East Sixty-fifth Street, where he stayed for weeks too ill to speak with even his closest adviser, Louis Howe, who kept in almost hourly touch with his doctors.

The *Leviathan* and, over the course of the next several weeks, other troopships would ferry approximately one hundred thousand troops to Europe. Their crossings became much like that of the train that carried three thousand one hundred soldiers from Camp Grant to Camp Hancock. They became death ships.

Although the army had ignored most of the pleadings from its own medical corps, it did remove all men showing influenza symptoms before sailing. And to contain influenza on board, troops were quarantined. Military police carrying pistols enforced the quarantine—aboard the *Leviathan,* 432 MPs did so—sealing soldiers into separate areas of the ship behind shut watertight doors, sardining them into cramped quarters where they had little to do but lie on stacked bunks or shoot craps or play poker in the creases of open space available. Fear of submarines forced the portholes shut at night, but even during the day the closed doors and the massive overcrowding made it impossible for the ventilation system to keep pace. Access to the decks and open air was limited. The sweat and smells of hundreds of men—each room generally held up to four hundred—in close quarters quickly became a stench. Sound echoed off the steel bunks, the steel floors, the steel walls, the steel ceiling. Living almost like caged animals, they grew increasingly claustrophobic and tense. But at least they were safe, they thought.

For the plan to keep men quarantined in isolated groups had a flaw. They had to eat. They went to mess one group at a time, but they breathed the same air, their hands went from mouths to the same tables and doors that other soldiers had touched only minutes before.

Despite the removal before departure of men showing influenza symptoms, within forty-eight hours after leaving port, soldiers and sailors struck down with influenza overwhelmed the sick bay, stacked one on top of the other in bunks, clogging every possible location, coughing, bleeding, delirious, displacing the healthy from one great room after another. Nurses themselves became sick. Then the horrors began.

Colonel Gibson, commander of the Fifty-seventh Vermont, wrote of his regiment's experience on the _Leviathan_: "The ship was packed . . . [C]onditions were such that the influenza could breed and multiply with extraordinary swiftness. . . . The number of sick increased rapidly, Washington was apprised of the situation, but the call for men for the Allied armies was so great that we must go on at any cost. . . . Doctors and nurses were stricken. Every available doctor and nurse was utilized to the limit of endurance. The conditions during the night cannot be visualized by anyone who had not actually seen them . . . [G]roans and cries of the terrified added to the confusion of the applicants clamoring for treatment and altogether a true inferno reigned supreme."

It was the same on other ships. Pools of blood from hemorrhaging patients lay on the floor and the healthy tracked the blood through the ship, making decks wet and slippery. Finally, with no room in sick bay, no room in the areas taken over for makeshift sick bays, corpsmen and nurses began laying men out on deck for days at a time. Robert Wallace aboard the _Briton_ remembered lying on deck when a storm came, remembered the ship rolling, the ocean itself sweeping up the scuppers and over him and the others, drenching them, their clothes, their blankets, leaving them coughing and sputtering. And each morning orderlies carried away bodies.

At first the deaths of men were separated by a few hours: the log of the *Leviathan* noted, "12:45 P.M. Thompson, Earl, Pvt 4252473, company unknown died on board. . . . 3:35 P.M. Pvt O Reeder died on board of lobar pneumonia. . . ." But a week after leaving New York, the officer of the day was no longer bothering to note in the log "died on board," no longer bothering to identify the military organization to which the dead belonged, no longer bothering to note a cause of death; he was writing only a name and a time, two names at 2:00 A.M., another at 2:02 A.M., two more at 2:15 A.M., like that all through the night, every notation in the log now a simple recitation of mortality, into the morning a death at 7:56 A.M., at 8:10 A.M., another at 8:10 A.M., at 8:25 A.M.

The burials at sea began. They quickly became sanitary exercises more than burials, bodies lying next to one another on deck, a few words and a name spoken, then one at a time a corpse slipped overboard into the sea. One soldier aboard the *Wilhelmina* watched across the waves as bodies dropped into the sea from another ship in his convoy, the *Grant*: "I confess I was near to tears, and that there was tightening around my throat. It was death, death in one of its worst forms, to be consigned nameless to the sea."

The transports became floating caskets. Meanwhile, in France, by any standard except that of the cantonments at home, influenza was devastating troops. In the last half of October during the Meuse-Argonne offensive, America's largest of the war, more Third Division troops were evacuated from the front with influenza than with wounds. (Roughly the same number of troops were in the United States and Europe, but influenza deaths in Europe were only half those in America. The likely explanation is that soldiers at the front had been exposed to the earlier mild wave of influenza and developed some immunity to it.) One army surgeon wrote in his diary on October 17 that because of the epidemic, "Some hospitals are not even working. Evacuation 114 had no medical officer but hundreds of pneumonias, . . . dying by the score."

Shipping more men who required medical care into this maelstrom made little sense. It is impossible to state how many soldiers the ocean voyages killed, especially when one tries to count those infected aboard ship who died later on shore. But for every death at least four or five men were ill enough to be incapacitated for weeks. These men were a burden rather than a help in Europe.

Wilson had made no public statement about influenza. He would not shift his focus, not for an instant. Yet people he trusted spoke to him of the disease, spoke particularly of useless deaths on the transports. Chief among them was certainly Dr. Cary Grayson, a navy admiral and Wilson's personal physician, as he had been personal physician to Teddy Roosevelt and William Howard Taft when they were president. Highly competent and highly organized, Grayson had become a Wilson confidant who strayed into the role of adviser. (After Wilson's stroke in 1919, he would be accused of virtually running the country in concert with Wilson's wife.) He also had the confidence of and excellent relationships with Gorgas and Welch. It was likely that army medical staff had talked to Grayson, and Grayson had been urging army chief of staff General Peyton March to freeze the movement of troops to Europe. March had refused.

Grayson convinced Wilson to summon March to the White House on October 7 to discuss the issue. Late that night Wilson and March met. Wilson said, "General March, I have had representations sent to me by men whose ability and patriotism are unquestioned that I should stop the shipment of men to France until this epidemic of influenza is under control. . . . [Y]ou decline to stop these shipments."

March made no mention of any of the advice he had received from Gorgas's office. He insisted that every possible precaution was being taken. The troops were screened before embarking and the sick winnowed out. Some ships even put ashore in Halifax, Nova Scotia, those who fell seriously ill before the actual Atlantic crossing began. If American divisions stopped arriving in France, whatever the reason, German morale might soar. True, some men had died aboard ship, but, March said, "Every such soldier who has died just as surely played his part as his comrade who died in France."

The war would end in a little over a month. The epidemic had made virtually all training in cantonments impossible. A parliament—not the kaiser—had already taken over the German government and sent out peace feelers, while Germany's allies had already collapsed, capitulated, or, in the case of Austria, asked for peace on any terms Wilson dictated. But March insisted, "The shipment of troops should not be stopped for any cause."

March later wrote that Wilson turned in his chair, gazed out the window, his face very sad, then gave a faint sigh. In the end, only a single military activity would continue unaffected in the face of the epidemic. The army continued the voyages of troopships overseas.

If Wilson did nothing about influenza in the military but express concern about shipping troops to Europe, he did even less for civilians. He continued to say nothing publicly. There is no indication that he ever said anything privately, that he so much as inquired of anyone in the civilian arm of the government as to its efforts to fight the disease.

Wilson had appointed strong men to his administration, powerful men, and they took decisive actions. They dominated the nation's thought, and they dominated the nation's economy. But none of those appointees had any real responsibility for health. Surgeon General Rupert Blue, head of the United States Public Health Service, did. And Blue was not a strong man.

A square-faced man with a square thick athletic body, an amateur boxer, Blue was physically strong all right, even deep into middle age. But he was not strong in ways that mattered, in leadership. In a field that was largely new when he entered it, a field in which colleagues were cutting new paths into the wild in dozens of directions, he had broken no ground, demonstrated no professional courage, nor had he even showed real zeal. If he was by no means unintelligent, he lacked either real intellectual rigor or the creativity to ask important questions, and he had never manifested any truly special talents in or insights into public health.

As far as scientific public health issues went, the real leaders of the medical profession considered him a lightweight. Welch and Vaughan had not even trusted him to name the Public Health Service's representative to the National Research Council, and so they themselves had picked a PHS scientist they respected. Cary Grayson thought so little of him that he began to build an alternative national public health organization. (He abandoned his effort when Tammany took over the New York City Department of Health.) Blue became surgeon general simply by carrying out assigned tasks well, proving himself an adept and diplomatic maneuverer, and seizing his main chance. That was all.

After finishing his medical studies in 1892, Blue had immediately joined the Public Health Service and remained there his entire professional life. His assignments had moved him from port to port, to Baltimore, Galveston,

New Orleans, Portland, New York, Norfolk, where he worked in hospitals and quarantine stations and on sanitation issues. His opportunity came with an outbreak of bubonic plague in San Francisco in 1903. Another PHS officer, a highly regarded scientist, had engaged in a running battle with local government and business leaders, who denied plague existed in the city. Blue did not prove that it did—Simon Flexner did that, demonstrating the plague bacillus in the laboratory, as part of a scientific team brought in to settle the question—but Blue did win grudging cooperation from local authorities in efforts to control the disease. This was no easy task, and he both oversaw the killing of rats and kept, according to one laudatory report, "all interests in the State . . . harmonized."

This success won him powerful friends. (He was not successful enough, however, to prevent plague spreading from rats to wild rodent populations; today plague exists in squirrels, prairie dogs, and other animals in much of the Pacific Coast and inland to Arizona, New Mexico, and Colorado.) When plague resurfaced in San Francisco in 1907 he was called back. Another success won him more powerful friends. In 1912 he rose to surgeon general. That same year Congress expanded the Public Health Service's power. From that position he pushed for national medical insurance, which the medical profession then advocated, and in 1916 he became president of the American Medical Association. In his presidential address he declared, "There are unmistakable signs that health insurance will constitute the next great step in social legislation."

Wilson did not bother to choose a new surgeon general, but when the war began he did make the Public Health Service part of the military. It had consisted chiefly of several quarantine stations that inspected incoming ships, the Marine Hospital Service, which cared for merchant seamen and some federal workers, and the Hygienic Laboratory. Now it became responsible for protecting the nation's health, if only so the nation could produce more war matériel. Blue did not grow with the job.

In advance of the epidemic, Gorgas had used all means possible to protect the millions of soldiers from disease. His counterpart Navy Surgeon General William Braisted had done little to match Gorgas, but he was supporting work by such men as Rosenau in Boston and Lewis in Philadelphia.

Blue by contrast did, literally, less than nothing; he blocked relevant research. On July 28, 1918, Blue rejected a request from George McCoy, director of the Hygienic Laboratory, for $10,000 for pneumonia research designed to complement the efforts of the Rockefeller Institute. Although Congress in 1912 had given the agency authority to study "diseases of man and conditions affecting the propagation thereof," Blue determined that McCoy's "investigation is not immediately necessary to the enforcement of the law."

Blue knew of the possibility of influenza in the United States. On August 1, the *Memphis Medical Monthly* published comments by him warning of it. Yet he made no preparations whatsoever to try to contain it. Even after it began to show evidence of lethality, even after Rufus Cole prodded his office to collect data, neither he nor his office attempted to gather information about the disease anywhere in the world. And he made no effort whatsoever to prepare the Public Health Service for a crisis.

Many of those under him were no better. The Commonwealth Pier outbreak began late in August, and by September 9 newspapers were reporting that influenza victims filled "all the hospital beds at the forts at Boston harbor," Camp Devens had thirty-five hundred influenza cases, and Massachusetts hospitals were filling with civilians. Yet the local Public Health Service officer later insisted, "The first knowledge of the existence of the disease reached this officer September 10th."

The virus had reached New Orleans on September 4; the Great Lakes Naval Training Station on September 7; New London, Connecticut, on September 12.

Not until September 13 did the Public Health Service make any public comment, when it said, "Owing to disordered conditions in European countries, the bureau has no authoritative information as to the nature of the disease or its prevalence." That same day Blue did issue a circular telling all quarantine stations to inspect arriving ships for influenza. But even that order only advised delaying infected vessels until "the local health authorities have been notified."

Later Blue defended himself for not taking more aggressive action. *This was influenza, only influenza,* he seemed to be saying, "It would be manifestly unwarranted to enforce strict quarantine against . . . influenza."

No quarantine of shipping could have succeeded anyway. The virus was already here. But Blue's circular indicated how little Blue had done— in fact he had done nothing—to prepare the Public Health Service, much less the country, for any onslaught.

The virus reached Puget Sound on September 17.

Not until September 18 did Blue even seek to learn which regions of the United States the disease had penetrated.

On Saturday, September 21, the first influenza death occurred in Washington, D.C. The dead man was John Ciore, a railroad brakeman who had been exposed to the disease in New York four days earlier. That same day Camp Lee outside Petersburg, Virginia, had six deaths, while Camp Dix in New Jersey saw thirteen soldiers and one nurse die.

Still Blue did little. On Sunday, September 22, the Washington newspapers reported that Camp Humphreys (now Fort Belvoir), just outside the city, had sixty-five cases.

Now, finally, in a box immediately adjacent to those reports, the local papers finally published the government's first warning of the disease:

Surgeon General's Advice to Avoid Influenza

Avoid needless crowding. . . .

Smother your coughs and sneezes. . . .

Your nose not your mouth was made to breathe thru. . . .

Remember the 3 Cs, clean mouth, clean skin, and clean clothes. . . .

Food will win the war. . . . [H]elp by choosing and chewing your food
    well. . . .

Wash your hands before eating. . . .

Don't let the waste products of digestion accumulate. . . .

Avoid tight clothes, tight shoes, tight gloves—seek to make nature your
    ally not your prisoner. . . .

When the air is pure breathe all of it you can—breathe deeply.

Such generalizations hardly reassured a public that knew that the disease was marching from army camp to army camp, killing soldiers in large numbers. Three days later a second influenza death occurred in Washington; John Janes, like the first Washington victim, had contracted the disease in New York City. Also that day senior medical personnel of the army, navy, and Red Cross met in Washington to try to figure out how they could aid individual states. Neither Blue nor a representative of the Public Health Service attended the meeting. Twenty-six states were then reporting influenza cases.

Blue had still not laid plans for an organization to fight the disease. He had taken only two actions: publishing his advice on how to avoid the disease and asking the National Academy of Sciences to identify the pathogen, writing, "In view of the importance which outbreaks of influenza will have on war production, the Bureau desires to leave nothing undone. . . . The Bureau would deem it a valuable service if the Research Council arrange for suitable laboratory studies . . . as to the nature of the infecting organism."

Crowder canceled the draft. Blue still did not organize a response to the emergency. Instead, the senior Public Health Service officer in charge of the city of Washington reiterated to the press that there was no cause for alarm.

Perhaps Blue considered any further action outside the authority of the Public Health Service. Under him the service was a thoroughly bureaucratic institution, and bureaucratic in none of the good ways. Only a decade earlier he had been stationed in New Orleans, when the last yellow-fever epidemic to strike the United States had hit there, and the Public Health Service had required the city to pay $250,000—in advance—to cover the federal government's expenses in helping to fight that epidemic. Only a few weeks earlier, he had rejected the request from the service's own chief scientist for money to research pneumonia in concert with Cole and Avery at the Rockefeller Institute.

But governors and mayors were demanding help, beseeching everyone in Washington for help. Massachusetts officials in particular were begging for help from outside the state, for doctors from outside, for nurses from outside, for laboratory assistance from outside. The death toll there had climbed into the thousands. Governor Samuel McCall had wired governors for any assistance they could offer, and on September 26 he formally requested help from the federal government.

Doctors and nurses were what was needed. Doctors and nurses. And especially nurses. As the disease spread, as warnings from Welch, Vaughan, Gorgas, dozens of private physicians, and, finally, at last, Blue poured in, Congress acted. Without the delay of hearings or debate, it appropriated $1 million for the Public Health Service. The money was enough for Blue to hire five thousand doctors for emergency duty for a month—if he could somehow find five thousand doctors worth hiring.

Each day—indeed, each hour—was showing the increasingly explosive spread of the virus and its lethality. Blue, as if suddenly frightened, now considered the money too little. He had not complained to Congress about the amount; no record exists of his having asked for more. But the same day Congress passed the appropriation, he privately appealed to the War Council of the Red Cross both for more money and for its help.

The Red Cross did not get government funds or direction, although it was working in close concert with the government. Nor was its charge to care for the public health. Yet even before Blue asked, it had already allocated money to fight the epidemic and had begun organizing its own effort to do so—and do so on a massive scale. Its nursing department had already begun mobilizing "Home Defense Nurses," fully professional nurses, all of them women, who could not serve in the military because of age, disability, or marriage. The Red Cross had divided the country into thirteen divisions, and the nursing committee chief of each one had already been told to find all people with any nursing training, not only professionals or those who had dropped out of nursing schools—for the Red Cross checked with all nursing schools—but down to and including anyone who had ever taken a Red Cross course in caring for the sick at home. It had already instructed each division to form at least one mobile strike force of nurses to be ready to go to areas most in need. And before anyone within the government sought aid, the War Council of the Red Cross had designated a "contingent fund for the purpose of meeting the present needs in coping with the epidemic of Spanish influenza." Now the council agreed instantly to authorize expenditure of far more money than was in the contingency fund.

Finally, Blue began to organize the Public Health Service as well. Doctors and nurses were what was needed, doctors and nurses. But by then the virus had spanned the country, establishing itself on the perimeter, on the coasts, and it was working its way into the interior, to Denver, Omaha, Minneapolis, Boise. It was penetrating Alaska. It had crossed the Pacific to Hawaii. It had surfaced in Puerto Rico. It was about to explode across Western Europe, across India, across China, across Africa as well.

Science, then as now a journal written by scientists for their colleagues, warned, "The epidemics now occurring appear with electric suddenness, and, acting like powerful, uncontrolled currents, produce violent and eccentric effects. The disease never spreads slowly and insidiously. Wherever it occurs its presence is startling."

October, not April, would be the cruelest month.

CHAPTER TWENTY-SEVEN

NOTHING COULD HAVE STOPPED the sweep of influenza through
either the United States or the rest of the world—but ruthless intervention and quarantines might have interrupted its progress and created
occasional firebreaks.

Action as ruthless as that taken in 2003 to contain the outbreak
of a new disease called severe acute respiratory disorder, SARS, could
well have had effect.* Influenza could not have been contained as SARS
was—influenza is far more contagious. But any interruption in influenza's
spread could have had significant impact. For the virus was growing
weaker over time. Simply delaying its arrival in a community or slowing
its spread once there—just such minor successes—would have saved
many, many thousands of lives.

There was precedent for ruthless action. Only two years earlier several
East Coast cities had fought a polio outbreak with the most stringent
measures. Public health authorities wherever polio threatened had been
relentless. But that was before the United States entered the war. There
would be no comparable effort for influenza. Blue would not even attempt
to intrude upon war work.

The Public Health Service and the Red Cross still had a single chance
to accomplish something of consequence. By early October the first fall

*For more about SARS, see page 449.

outbreaks and the memory of those in the spring had already suggested
that the virus attacked in a cycle; it took roughly six weeks from the
appearance of the first cases for the epidemic to peak and then abate in
civilian areas, and from three to four weeks in a military camp with its
highly concentrated population. After the epidemic abated, cases still
occurred intermittently, but not in the huge numbers that overwhelmed
all services. So Red Cross and Public Health Service planners expected the
attack would be staggered just as the arrival of the virus was staggered,
peaking in different parts of the country at different times. During the
peak of the epidemic, individual communities would not be able to cope;
no matter how well organized they were they would be utterly overwhelmed. But if the Red Cross and Public Health Service could concentrate doctors, nurses, and supplies in one community when most needed,
they might be able to withdraw the aid as the disease ebbed and shift it to
the next area in need, and the next.

To manage this, Blue and Frank Persons, director of civilian relief and
head of the new influenza committee of the Red Cross, divided the labor.
The Public Health Service would find, pay, and assign all physicians. It
would decide when and where to send nurses and supplies, to whom
nurses would report, and it would deal with state and local public health
authorities.

The Red Cross would find and pay nurses, furnish emergency hospitals with medical supplies wherever local authorities could not, and take
responsibility for virtually everything else that came up, including distributing information. The Red·Cross did stipulate one limit on its
responsibility: it would not meet requests from military camps. This stip-
ulation was immediately forgotten; even the Red Cross soon gave the military precedence over civilians. Meanwhile, its War Council ordered each
one of its 3,864 chapters to establish an influenza committee even—
indeed, especially—where the disease had not yet hit. It gave instructions
on the organization of those committees, and it stated "each community
should depend upon its own resources to the fullest extent."

Persons had one model: Massachusetts. There James Jackson, the Red
Cross division director for New England, had done an amazing job, especially considering that the region was struck without warning by what was
originally an unknown disease. While chapters made gauze masks—the
masks that would soon be seen everywhere and would become a symbol

of the epidemic—Jackson first tried to supply nurses and doctors him-self. When he failed, he formed an ad hoc umbrella organization includ-ing the state Council of National Defense, the U.S. Public Health Service, state and local public health authorities, and the Red Cross. These groups pooled their resources and allocated to towns as needed.

Jackson had brought in nurses from Providence, New Haven, New York, even from Halifax and Toronto. He had succeeded at least some-what in alleviating the personnel shortage. But Massachusetts had been lucky. When the epidemic erupted there, no other locality needed help. In the fourth week of the epidemic, Jackson reported, "We have not yet reached the point where any community has been able to transfer its nurses or supplies. In Camp Devens . . . forty nurses ill there with many cases of pneumonia."

He also advised Red Cross headquarters in Washington: "The most important thing in this crisis is more workers to go into the homes quickly and aid the family. Consequently I have telegraphed to all my chapters twice regarding the mobilization of women who have had First Aid and Home Nursing training or any others who are willing to volun-teer their services."

And he confided, "The Federal public health service has been . . . unable to handle adequately the entire situation. . . . [They] have not been on the job."

It was October when he sent that wire. By then everyone needed nurses, or they were about to, and they knew it. By then everyone needed doc-tors, or they were about to, and they knew it. And they needed resources. The biggest task remained finding doctors, nurses, and resources. They needed all three.

Even in the face of this pandemic, doctors could help. They could save lives. If they were good enough, if they had the right resources, if they had the right help, if they had time.

True, no drug or therapy could alleviate the viral infection. Anyone who died directly from a violent infection of the influenza virus itself, from viral pneumonia progressing to ARDS, would have died anyway. In 1918, ARDS had virtually a 100 percent mortality rate.

But there were other causes of death. By far the most common was from pneumonia caused by secondary bacterial infections.

Ten days, two weeks, sometimes even longer than two weeks after the initial attack by the virus, after victims had felt better, after recovery had seemed to begin, victims were suddenly getting seriously ill again. And they were dying. The virus was stripping their lungs all but naked of their immune system; recent research suggests that the virus made it easier for some kinds of bacteria to lodge in lung tissue as well. Bacteria were taking advantage, invading the lungs, and killing. People were learning, and doctors were advising, and newspapers were warning, that even when a patient seemed to recover, seemed to feel fine, normal, well enough to go back to work, still that patient should continue to rest, continue to stay in bed. Or else that patient was risking his or her life.

Half a dozen years earlier medicine had been helpless here, so helpless that Osler in his most recent edition of his classic text on the practice of medicine had still called for bleeding of patients with pneumonia. But now, for some of those who developed a secondary bacterial infection, something could be done. The most advanced medical practice, the best doctors, could help—if they had the resources and the time.

Avery, Cole, and others at the Rockefeller Institute had developed the vaccine that had showed such promising result in the test at Camp Upton in the spring, and the Army Medical School was producing this vaccine in mass quantities. Avery and Cole had also developed the serum that slashed the mortality for pneumonias caused by Types I and II pneumococcus, which accounted for two-thirds or more of lobar pneumonias in normal circumstances. These were not normal circumstances; bacteria that almost never caused pneumonia were now making their way unopposed into the lungs, growing there, and thriving there. But Types I and II pneumococci were still causing many of the pneumonias, and in those cases this serum could help.

Other investigators had developed other vaccines and sera as well. Some, like the one developed by E. C. Rosenow at the Mayo Clinic and used in Chicago, were useless. But others may have done some good.

Physicians also had other assets to call upon. Surgeons developed new techniques during the epidemic that are still in use to drain empyemas, pockets of pus and infection that formed in the lung and poisoned the body. And doctors had drugs that alleviated some symptoms or stimulated the heart; major hospitals had x rays that could aid in diagnosis and triage; and some hospitals had begun administering oxygen to help victims breathe—a practice neither widespread nor administered nearly as effectively as it would be, but worth something.

Yet for a doctor to use these resources, any of them, that doctor had to have them—and also had to have time. The physical resources were hard to come by, but time was harder. There was no time. For that Rockefeller serum needed to be administered with precision and in numerous doses. There was no time. Not with patients overflowing wards, filling cots in hallways and on porches, not with doctors themselves falling ill and filling those cots. Even if they had resources, they had no time.

And the doctors found by the Public Health Service had neither resources nor time. Nor was it simple to find the doctors themselves. The military had already taken at least one-fourth—in some areas one-third—of all the physicians and nurses. And the army, itself under violent attack from the virus, would lend none of its doctors to civilian communities no matter how desperate the circumstances.

That left approximately one hundred thousand doctors in a labor pool to draw from—but it was a pool limited in quality. The Council of National Defense had had local medical committees secretly grade colleagues; those committees had judged roughly seventy thousand unfit for military service. Most of that number were unfit because they were judged incompetent.

The government had had a plan to identify the best of those remaining. As part of the mobilization of the entire nation, in January 1918 the Council of National Defense had created the "Volunteer Medical Service." This service tried to enlist every doctor in the United States, but it particularly wanted to track the younger physicians who were women or had a physical disability—in other words, those mostly likely to be good doctors who were not subject to and rejected by the draft.

The mass targeting succeeded. Within eight months, 72,219 physicians had joined this service. They had joined, however, only to prove their patriotism, not as a commitment to do anything real—for membership required of them nothing concrete, and they received an attractive piece of paper suitable for framing and office display.

But the plan to identify and have access to good doctors within this group collapsed. The virus was penetrating everywhere, doctors were needed everywhere, and no responsible doctor would abandon his (or, in a few instances, her) own patients in need, in desperate need. In addition, the federal government was paying only $50 a week—no princely sum even in 1918. Out of one hundred thousand civilian doctors, seventy-two thousand of whom had joined the Volunteer Medical Service, only 1,045 physicians answered the pleas of the Public Health Service. While a few were good young doctors who had not yet developed a practice and were waiting to be drafted, many of this group were the least competent or poorest trained doctors in the country. Indeed, so few doctors worked for the PHS that Blue would later return $115,000 to the Treasury from the the $1 million appropriation he had considered so insufficient.

The Public Health Service sent these 1,045 doctors to places where there were no doctors at all, to places so completely devastated by the disease that any help, any help at all, was embraced. But they sent them with almost no resources, certainly without Rockefeller vaccines and serum or the training to make or administer them, certainly without x rays, certainly without oxygen and the means to administer it. The huge caseloads overwhelmed them, weighed them down, kept them moving.

They diagnosed. They treated with all manner of materia medica. Yet in reality they could do nothing but advise. The best advice was this: stay in bed. And then the doctors moved on to the next cot or the next village.

What could help, more than doctors, were nurses. Nursing could ease the strains on a patient, keep a patient hydrated, resting, calm, provide the best nutrition, cool the intense fevers. Nursing could give a victim of the disease the best possible chance to survive. Nursing could save lives.

But nurses were harder to find than doctors. There were one-quarter fewer to begin with. The earlier refusal of the women who controlled the nursing profession to allow the training of large numbers either of nursing aides or of what came to be called practical nurses prevented the creation of what might have been a large reserve force. The plan had been to produce thousands of such aides; instead the Army School of Nursing had been established. So far it had produced only 221 student nurses and not a single graduate nurse.

Then, just before the epidemic struck, combat had intensified in France and with it so had the army's need for nurses. The need had in fact become so desperate that on August 1, Gorgas, just to meet existing requirements, transferred one thousand nurses from cantonments in the United States to hospitals in France and simultaneously issued a call for "one thousand nurses a week" for eight weeks.

The Red Cross was the route of supply for nurses to the military, especially the army. It had already been recruiting nurses for the military with vigor. After Gorgas's call, it launched an even more impassioned recruiting campaign. Each division, each chapter within a division, was given a quota. Red Cross professionals knew that their careers were at risk if they did not meet it. Already recruiters had a list of all nurses in the country, their jobs and locations. Those recruiters now pressured nurses to quit jobs and join the military, pressured doctors to let office nurses go, made wealthy patients who retained private nurses feel unpatriotic, pushed private hospitals to release nurses.

The drive was succeeding; it was removing from civilian life a huge proportion of those nurses mobile enough, unencumbered by family or other responsibilities, to leave their jobs. The drive was succeeding so well that it all but stripped hospitals of their workforce, leaving many private hospitals around the country so short-staffed that they closed, and remained closed until the war ended. One Red Cross recruiter wrote, "The work at National Headquarters has never been so difficult and is now overwhelming us. . . . [We are searching] from one end of the United States to the other to rout out every possible nurse from her hiding place. . . . There will be no nurses left in civil life if we keep on at this rate."

The recruiter wrote that on September 5, three days before the virus exploded at Camp Devens.

CHAPTER TWENTY-EIGHT

PHILADELPHIA STAGGERED under the influenza attack, isolated and alone. In Philadelphia no sign surfaced of any national Red Cross and Public Health Service effort to help. No doctors recruited by the Public Health Service were sent there. No nurses recruited by the Red Cross were sent there. Those institutions gave no help here.

Each day people discovered that friends and neighbors who had been perfectly healthy a week—or a day—earlier were dead. *What should I do?* People were panicked, desperate. *How long will it go on?*

The mayor, arrested in the early days of the epidemic and then himself ill, had done absolutely nothing. A review of five daily newspapers, the *Press, Inquirer, Bulletin, Public Ledger,* and *North American,* did not find even a single statement about the crisis from the mayor. The entire city government had done nothing. Wilmer Krusen, head of the city health department, no longer had the confidence of anyone. Someone had to do *something.*

Paul Lewis felt the pressures, felt the death all about him. He had felt at least some pressure since the sailors from the *City of Exeter* had been dying what seemed so long ago. In early September, with the virus killing 5 percent of all Philadelphia navy personnel who showed any symptoms of influenza at all, that pressure had intensified. Since then he and everyone under him had hardly left their laboratories to go home. Finding *B. influenzae* had begun his real work, not concluded it.

Never had he been so consumed with the laboratory. He had started his experiments with the pneumococcus. He had begun to explore the possibility that a filterable virus caused influenza. He had continued to look at the influenza bacillus. He and others had developed a vaccine. He was trying to make a serum. All of these he did simultaneously. For the one thing he did not have was time. No one had time.

If Lewis had a scientific weakness, it was that he too willingly accepted guidance from those he respected. Once when he asked for more direction from Flexner, Flexner had rebuffed him, saying, "I much prefer that you arrange plans. . . . I have not planned specifically for your time, but much prefer to leave the direction of it to you." Lewis respected Flexner. He respected Richard Pfeiffer as well.

In the overwhelming majority of cases he was now finding Pfeiffer's *B. influenzae* in swabs from living patients, in autopsied lungs. He was not finding it alone, necessarily, or always. It was not certain proof, but more and more he was coming to believe that this bacterium did in fact cause disease. And, under the pressure of time, he abandoned his investigation into the possibility that a filterable virus caused influenza.

Yet he loved this. Although he hated the disease he loved this. He believed he had been born to do this. He loved working deep into the night amid rows of glassware, monitoring the growth of bacteria in a hundred flasks and petri dishes, running a dozen experiments in staggered fashion; coordinating them like the conductor of a symphony. He even loved the unexpected result that could throw everything off.

The only thing Lewis disliked about his position as head of an institute was charming the fine families of Philadelphia out of philanthropic donations, attending their parties and performing as their pet scientist. The laboratory was where he had always belonged. Now he was in it hours and hours each day. He believed he had spent too much time mixing with the fine families of Philadelphia.

In fact, those fine families of the city deserved more respect. They were about to take charge.

The writer Christopher Morley once said that Philadelphia lies "at the confluence of the Biddle and Drexel families." In 1918 that description was not far wrong.

Of all the major cities in the United States, Philadelphia had a real claim to being the most "American." It certainly had the largest percentage of native-born Americans of major cities and, compared to New York, Chicago, Boston, Detroit, Buffalo, and similar cities, the lowest percentage of immigrants. Philadelphia was not unusual in that its oldest and wealthiest families controlled the charities, the social service organizations— including the local Red Cross—and the Pennsylvania Council of National Defense. But now, with the city government all but nonexistent, it was unusual in that these families considered it their duty to use the Council of National Defense to take charge.

Nationally that organization had been the vehicle through which, before the war, Wilson had laid plans to control the economy, using it to assemble data from across the country on factories, transportation, labor, and natural resources. But each state had its own council, which were often dominated by his political enemies. Once the war started, Wilson created new federal institutions, sidestepped this organization, and it lost power. The Pennsylvania council, however, retained extraordinary, although almost entirely unofficial, influence over everything from railroad schedules to profits and wages at every large company in the state even though it too was run by Wilson's enemies. It held this power chiefly because it was headed by George Wharton Pepper.

No one had better bloodlines. His great-great-grandfather had led the state militia in the Revolutionary War, his wife was a descendant of Benjamin Franklin, and a statue of his uncle William, who had worked closely with Welch to reform medical education and brought Flexner to the University of Pennsylvania, today sits astride the grand stairway of the Free Library in downtown Philadelphia. George Wharton Pepper had ability as well. An attorney who sat on the boards of half a dozen of the country's largest companies, he was not ruthless, but he knew how to command. An indication of his stature had come a few months earlier when he received one of three honorary degrees awarded by Trinity College in Hartford, Connecticut; his fellow honorees were J. P. Morgan and former president of the United States and soon-to-be chief justice of the Supreme Court William Howard Taft.

The Philadelphia office of the state Council of National Defense was run by Judge J. Willis Martin. His wife, Elizabeth, had organized the country's first garden club and was largely responsible for making Rittenhouse Square a green spot in the city. She also headed the council's Women's

Division as well as Emergency Aid, the most important private social agency in the city.

Nearly all the social agencies were run by women, strong women of intelligence and energy and born to a certain rank, but excluded from all pursuits beside charity. The mayor had created a committee of society women to respond to emergencies; it included Pepper's wife along with Mrs. John Wanamaker; Mrs. Edward Stotesbury, whose husband was the city's leading banker and head of Drexel & Co.; and Mrs. Edward Biddle, president of the Civic Club and whose husband was descended from Nicholas Biddle, creator of the first Bank of the United States, which to his nemesis Andrew Jackson embodied the sinister monied power of the nation. These women despised the Vare machine and had cooperated only to show unity during the war. But with city officials doing nothing whatsoever about the epidemic, the women resigned, effectively dissolving the committee. As Elizabeth Martin wrote the mayor, "Your committee has no real purpose. . . . I therefore hereby sever my connection with it."

Now, in place of the city government, Pepper, the Martins, and their colleagues summoned the heads of a dozen private organizations on October 7 to the headquarters of Emergency Aid at 1428 Walnut Street. There the women took charge, with Pepper adding his weight to theirs. To sell war bonds, they had already organized nearly the entire city, all the way down to the level of each block, making each residential block the responsibility of "a logical leader no matter what her nationality"—i.e., an Irishwoman in an Irish neighborhood, an African American woman in an African American neighborhood, and so on.

They intended to use that same organization now to distribute everything from medical care to food. They intended to inject organization and leadership into chaos and panic. In conjunction with the Red Cross—which here, unlike nearly everywhere else in the country, allowed its own efforts to be incorporated into this larger Emergency Aid—they also appealed for nurses, declaring, "The death toll for one day in Philadelphia alone was greater than the death toll from France for the whole American Army for one day."

The state Council of National Defense had already compiled a list of every physician in Pennsylvania, including those not practicing. Martin's ad hoc committee beseeched each one on the list for help. The committee had money, and access to more money, to pay for the help. It set up a twenty-four-hour telephone bank at Strawbridge & Clothier, which donated use of its phone lines; newspapers and placards urged people to call "Filbert 100" twenty-four hours a day for information and referrals. It transformed kitchens in public schools—which were closed—into soup kitchens that prepared meals for tens of thousands of people too ill to prepare their own. It divided the city into seven districts and, to conserve physicians' time, dispatched them according to geography, meaning that doctors did not see their own patients.

And it became a place that volunteers could come to. Nearly five hundred people offered to use their own cars either as ambulances or to chauffeur doctors—they were supplied with green flags that gave them right-of-way over all other vehicles. The organizers of the Liberty Loan drive diverted another four hundred cars to help. Thousands of individuals called the headquarters and offered to do what was needed.

Krusen had not attended the October 7 meeting of the private groups and had been slow to act before. Now he changed. Perhaps the deaths finally changed him. Perhaps the fact that someone else was taking charge forced him to move. But he seemed suddenly not to care about the Vares, or selling war bonds, or bureaucracy, or his own power. He just wanted to stop the disease.

He ceded to the group control over all nurses, hundreds of them, who worked for the city. He seized—in violation of the city charter—the city's $100,000 emergency fund and another $25,000 from a war emergency fund and used the money to supply emergency hospitals and hire physicians, paying them double what the Public Health Service was offering. He sent those physicians to every police station in South Philadelphia, the hardest-hit section. He wired the army and navy asking that no Philadelphia physicians be drafted until the epidemic abated, and that those who had already been drafted but had not yet reported to duty be allowed to remain in Philadelphia, because "the death rate for the past week [was] the largest in records of city."

The U.S. Public Health Service still had no presence in Philadelphia and had done nothing for it. Now Rupert Blue did the only thing he would do for the city in its distress: he wired the surgeon general of the navy to "heartily endorse" Krusen's request. The deaths spoke far more loudly than Blue. The military did allow Philadelphia to keep its doctors.

Krusen also cleaned the streets. The streets of South Philadelphia literally stank of rot and excrement. Victorians had considered it axiomatic
that filthy streets per se were linked to disease. The most modern public
health experts—Charles Chapin in Providence, Biggs in New York, and
others—flatly rejected that idea. But Dr. Howard Anders, who earlier had
been ignored by the press when he warned that the Liberty Loan parade
would spread influenza, was given page one by the *Ledger* on October 10 to
state, "Dirty streets, filth allowed to collect and stand until, germ-laden and
disease-breeding, it is carried broadcast with the first gust of wind—there
you have one of the greatest causes of the terrible epidemic." Other Philadelphia doctors agreed: "The condition of the streets spreads the epidemic."

So Krusen sent trucks and men down them with their water sprays
and sweepers almost daily, doing the job Vare had been paid for many
times but had never done. Krusen, Emergency Aid, and the Catholic
Church teamed up to do one more thing, the most important thing. They
began to clear the bodies.

The corpses had backed up at undertakers', filling every area of these
establishments and pressing up into living quarters; in hospital morgues
overflowing into corridors; in the city morgue overflowing into the
street. And they had backed up in homes. They lay on porches, in closets,
in corners of the floor, on beds. Children would sneak away from adults
to stare at them, to touch them; a wife would lie next to a dead husband,
unwilling to move him or leave him. The corpses, reminders of death and
bringers of terror or grief, lay under ice at Indian-summer temperatures.
Their presence was constant, a horror demoralizing the city; a horror that
could not be escaped. Finally the city tried to catch up to them.

Krusen sent police to clear homes of bodies that had remained there
for more than a day, piling them in patrol wagons, but they could not
keep up with the dying and fell further behind. The police wore their
ghostly surgical masks, and people fled them, but the masks had no effect
on the viruses and by mid-October thirty-three policemen had died, with
many more to follow. Krusen opened a "supplementary morgue" at a
cold-storage plant at Twentieth and Cambridge Streets; he would open
five more supplementary morgues. He begged military embalmers from
the army. Pepper and Martin convinced the Brill Company, which made
streetcars, to build thousands of simple boxes for coffins, and they gath-

ered students from embalming schools and morticians from as far as 150 miles away. More coffins came by rail, guarded by men with guns.

And graves were dug. First the families of the dead picked up shovels and dug into the earth, faces streaked with sweat and tears and grit. For gravediggers would not work. The city's official annual report notes that "undertakers found it impossible to hire persons willing to handle the bodies, owing to the decomposed nature of the same." When Anna Lavin's aunt died, "They took her to the cemetery. My father took me and the boy, who also had the flu, and he was wrapped—my father carried him—wrapped in a blanket to the cemetery to say the prayer for the dead. . . . The families had to dig their own graves. That was the terrible thing."

Pepper and Martin offered ten dollars a day to anyone who would touch a corpse, but that proved inadequate, and still the bodies piled up. Seminary students volunteered as gravediggers, but they still could not keep pace. The city and archdiocese turned to construction equipment, using steam shovels to dig trenches for mass graves. Michael Donohue, an undertaker, said, "They brought a steam shovel in to Holy Cross Cemetery and actually excavated. . . . They would begin bringing caskets in and doing the committal prayers right in the trench and they'd line them up right in, one right after another, this was their answer to helping the families get through things."

The bodies that were choking homes and lying in stacks in mortuaries were ready to go, finally, into the ground.

To collect them, Archbishop Denis Dougherty, installed in office only a few weeks earlier—later he became the first cardinal from the archdiocese—sent priests down the streets to remove bodies from homes. They joined the police and a few hardy others who were doing the same.

Sometimes they collected the bodies in trucks. "So many people died they were instructed to ask for wooden boxes and put the corpse on the front porches," recalled Harriet Ferrell. "An open truck came through the neighborhood and picked up the bodies. There was no place to put them, there was not room."

And sometimes they collected the bodies in wagons. Selma Epp's brother Daniel died: "[P]eople were being placed on these horse-drawn wagons and my aunt saw the wagons pass by and he was placed on the wagon; everyone was too weak to protest. There were no coffins in the wagon but the people who had died were wrapped in a sort of sackcloth and placed in the wagon. One was on top of the other, there were so many bodies. They were drawn by horses and the wagons took the bodies away."

No one could look at the trucks and carts carrying bodies—bodies wrapped in cloth stacked loosely on other bodies wrapped in cloth, arms and legs protruding, bodies heading for cemeteries to be buried in trenches—or hear the keening of the mourners and the call for the dead, and not think of another plague—the plague of the Middle Ages.

Under the initial burst of energy the city seemed at first to rally, to respond with vigor and courage now that leadership and organization seemed in place.

But the epidemic did not abate. The street cleaning accomplished nothing, at least regarding influenza, and the coroner—Vare's man— blamed the increasing death toll on the ban by the state public health commissioner on liquor sales, claiming alcohol was the best treatment for influenza.

In virtually every home, someone was ill. People were already avoiding each other, turning their heads away if they had to talk, isolating themselves. The telephone company increased the isolation: with eighteen hundred telephone company employees out, the phone company allowed only emergency calls; operators listened to calls randomly and cut off phone service of those who made routine calls. And the isolation increased the fear. Clifford Adams recalled, "They stopped people from communicating, from going to churches, closed the schools, . . . closed all the saloons. . . . Everything was quiet."

Very likely half a million—possibly more—Philadelphians fell sick. It is impossible to be more precise: despite the new legal requirement to report cases, physicians were far too busy to do so, and by no means did physicians see all victims. Nor did nurses.

People needed help and, notwithstanding the efforts of Emergency Aid, the Council of National Defense, and the Red Cross, help was impossible to get.

The *Inquirer* blared in headlines; "Scientific Nursing Halting Epidemic."

But there were no nurses.

The log of a single organization that sent out nurses noted without comment, "The number of calls received, 2,955, and calls not filled, 2,758." *Calls received, 2,955; calls not filled, 2,758.* And the report pointed out that even those numbers—93 percent of the calls unfilled, 7 percent filled—was an understatement, since the "'calls received' . . . does not represent the number of nurses required, for many of the calls were for several nurses to go to one place; two of the calls being for 50 nurses each."

Those nurses were needed, needed desperately. One study of fifty-five flu victims who were not hospitalized found that not one was ever seen by a nurse or a doctor. Ten of the fifty-five patients died.

It now seemed as if there had never been life before the epidemic. The disease informed every action of every person in the city.

The archbishop released nuns for service in hospitals, including Jewish hospitals, and allowed them to violate rules of their orders, to spend overnight away from the convent, to break vows of silence. They did not make a dent in the need.

By then many of those who had earlier rushed forward to volunteer had withdrawn. The work was too gruesome, or too arduous, or they themselves fell ill. Or they too were frightened. Every day newspapers carried new and increasingly desperate pleas for volunteers.

On the single *day* of October 10, the epidemic alone killed 759 people in Philadelphia. Prior to the outbreak, deaths from all causes—all illnesses, all accidents, all suicides, and all murders—averaged 485 a *week*.

Fear began to break down the community of the city. Trust broke down. Signs began to surface of not just edginess but anger, not just finger-pointing or protecting one's own interests but active selfishness in the face of general calamity. The hundreds of thousands sick in the city became a great weight dragging upon it. And the city began to implode in chaos and fear.

Pleas for volunteers became increasingly plaintive, and increasingly strident. Under the headline "Emergency Aid Calls for Amateur Nurses," newspapers printed Mrs. Martin's request: "In this desperate crisis the Emergency Aid calls on all . . . who are free from the care of the sick at home and who are in good physical condition themselves . . . to report at

1428 Walnut Street as early as possible Sunday morning. The office will be open all day and recruits will be enrolled and immediately sent out on emergency work."

Krusen declared, "It is the duty of every well woman in the city who can possibly get away from her duties to volunteer for this emergency."

But who listened to him anymore?

Mrs. Martin called for help from "all persons with two hands and a willingness to work."

Few came.

On October 13, the Bureau of Child Hygiene publicly begged for neighbors to take in, at least temporarily, children whose parents were dying or dead. The response was almost nil.

Elizabeth Martin pleaded, "We simply must have more volunteer helpers. . . . We have ceased caring for ordinary cases of the disease. . . . These people are almost all at the point of death. Won't you ask every able-bodied woman in Philadelphia whether or not she has any experience in nursing to come to our help?"

Few replied.

The need was not only for medical care, but for care itself. Entire families were ill and had no one to feed them. Krusen pleaded publicly; "Every healthy woman in the city who can possibly be spared from her home can be used in fighting the epidemic."

But by now the city had heard enough pleas, and had turned into itself. There was no trust, no trust, and without trust all human relations were breaking down.

The professionals had continued to do their duty. One physician at Philadelphia Hospital, a woman, had said she was certain she was going to die if she remained, and fled. But that was a rarity. Doctors died, and others kept working. Nurses died, and others kept working. Philadelphia Hospital had twenty student nurses from Vassar. Already two had died but the others "have behaved splendidly. . . . They say they will work all the harder."

Other professionals did their jobs as well. The police performed with heroism. Before the epidemic they had too often acted like a private army that owed its allegiance to the Vare machine. They had stood almost alone in the country against the navy's crackdown on prostitution near military facilities. Yet when the police department was asked for four volunteers to "remove bodies from beds, put them in coffins and load them in vehicles," when the police knew that many of those bodies had decomposed, 118 officers responded.

But citizens in general had largely stopped responding. Many women had reported to an emergency hospital for a single shift. They had never returned. Some had disappeared in the middle of a shift. On October 16 the chief nurse at the city's largest hospital told an advisory council, "[V]olunteers in the wards are useless. . . . [T]hey are afraid. Many people have volunteered and then refused to have anything to do with patients."

The attrition rate even where volunteers did not come into contact with the sick—in the kitchens, for example—was little better. Finally Mrs. Martin turned bitter and contemptuous: "Hundreds of women who are content to sit back . . . had delightful dreams of themselves in the roles of angels of mercy, had the unfathomable vanity to imagine that they were capable of great spirit of sacrifice. Nothing seems to rouse them now. They have been told that there are families in which every member is ill, in which the children are actually starving because there is no one to give them food. The death rate is so high and they still hold back."

Susanna Turner, who did volunteer at an emergency hospital and stayed, who went there day after day, remembered, "The fear in the hearts of the people just withered them. . . . They were afraid to go out, afraid to do anything. . . . You just lived from day to day, did what you had to do and not think about the future. . . . If you asked a neighbor for help, they wouldn't do so because they weren't taking any chances. If they didn't have it in their house, they weren't going to bring it in there. . . . You didn't have the same spirit of charity that you do with a regular time, when someone was sick you'd go and help them, but at that time they helped themselves. It was a horror-stricken time."

The professionals were heroes. The physicians and nurses and medical students and student nurses who were all dying in large numbers themselves held nothing of themselves back. And there were others. Ira Thomas played catcher for the Philadelphia Athletics. The baseball season had been shortened by Crowder's "work or fight" order, since sport was deemed unnecessary labor. Thomas's wife was a six-foot-tall woman, large-boned, strong. They had no children. Day after day he carried the sick in his car to hospitals and she worked in an emergency hospital. Of course there were others. But they were few.

"Help out?" said Susanna Turner. "They weren't going to risk it, they just refused because they were so panic-stricken, they really were, they feared their relatives would die because so many did die—they just dropped dead." No one could buy things. Commodities dealers, coal dealers, grocers closed "because the people who dealt in them were either sick or afraid and they had reason to be afraid."

During the week of October 16 alone, 4,597 Philadelphians died from influenza or pneumonia, and influenza killed still more indirectly. That would be the worst week of the epidemic. But no one knew that at the time. Krusen had too often said the peak had passed. The press had too often spoken of triumph over disease.

Even war industries, despite the massive propaganda campaigns telling workers victory depended upon their production, saw massive absences. Anna Lavin said, "We didn't work. Couldn't go to work. Nobody came into work." Even those who weren't sick "stayed in. They were all afraid."

Between 20 and 40 percent of the workers at Baldwin Locomotive, at Midvale Steel, at Sun Shipbuilding, each plant employing thousands, were absent. At virtually every large employer, huge percentages of employees were absent. Thirty-eight hundred Pennsylvania Railroad workers were out. The Baltimore and Ohio Railroad set up its own emergency hospitals along its tracks. The entire transportation system for the mid-Atlantic region staggered and trembled, putting in jeopardy most of the nation's industrial output.

The city was breaking apart. Orphans were already becoming a problem. Social service agencies that tried but fell short in their efforts to deliver food and transport people to hospitals began to plan for the orphans as well.

CHAPTER TWENTY-NINE

WHAT WAS HAPPENING in Philadelphia was happening everywhere. In that densely populated city, Isaac Starr had counted not a single other car on the road in his twelve-mile drive from the city center home. And on the other side of the world, the same experiences—the deaths, the terror, the reluctance to help, the silence—were replicated. Alfred Hollows was in Wellington, New Zealand: "I was detailed to an emergency hospital in Abel Smith Street. It was a hall . . . staffed by women volunteers." They had sixty beds. "Our death rate was really quite appalling—something like a dozen a day—and the women volunteers just disappeared, and weren't seen again. . . . I stood in the middle of Wellington City at 2 P.M. on a weekday afternoon, and there was not a soul to be seen—no trams running, no shops open, and the only traffic was a van with a white sheet tied to the side, with a big red cross painted on it, serving as an ambulance or hearse. It was really a City of the Dead."

In New York City at Presbyterian Hospital, each morning on rounds Dr. Dana Atchley was astounded, and frightened, to see that, for what seemed to him an eternity, every single patient—every one—in the critical section had died overnight.

The federal government was giving no guidance that a reasoning person could credit. Few local governments did better. They left a vacuum. Fear filled it.

The government's very efforts to preserve "morale" fostered the fear, for since the war began, morale—defined in the narrowest, most short-sighted fashion—had taken precedence in every public utterance. As California senator Hiram Johnson said in 1917, "The first casualty when war comes is truth."

It was a time when the phrase "brisk fighting" meant that more than 50 percent of a unit was killed or wounded; a time when the memoir of a nurse at the front, published in 1916, was withdrawn by her publisher after America entered the war because she told the truth about gruesome conditions; a time when newspapers insisted, "There is plenty of gasoline and oil for automobile use," even while gas stations were ordered to close "voluntarily" at night and Sundays and a national campaign was being waged against driving on "gasless Sundays"—and police pulled over motorists who did not "voluntarily" comply.

Newspapers reported on the disease with the same mixture of truth and half-truth, truth and distortion, truth and lies with which they reported everything else. And no national official ever publicly acknowledged the danger of influenza.

But in the medical community, deep concern had arisen. Welch of course had initially feared that it might be a new disease, although he soon recognized it as influenza. Many serious pathologists in Germany and Switzerland considered the possibility of plague. The director of the laboratory at Bellevue Hospital wondered in the *Journal of the American Medical Association* if "the world is facing" not a pandemic of an extraordinarily lethal influenza but instead a mild version of plague, noting, "The similarity of the two diseases is enforced by the clinical features, which are remarkably alike in many respects, and by the pathology of certain tissues other than the lungs."

What pathologists said in medical journals physicians muttered to each other, while laymen and -women watched a husband or wife turning almost black. And a great chill settled over the land, a chill of fear.

Meanwhile, William Park sat in his laboratory amid petri dishes, dissected mice, and cultures of pathogens, and quoted Daniel Defoe's *Journal of the Plague Year:* "In the whole the face of things, as I say, was much altered; sorrow and sadness sat upon every face; and though some parts were not yet overwhelmed, yet all looked deeply concerned; and as we saw it apparently coming on, so every one looked on himself and his family as in the utmost danger."

·   ·   ·

As terrifying as the disease was, the press made it more so. They terrified by making little of it, for what officials and the press said bore no relationship to what people saw and touched and smelled and endured. People could not trust what they read. Uncertainty follows distrust, fear follows uncertainty, and, under conditions such as these, terror follows fear.

When influenza struck in Massachusetts, the nearby *Providence Journal* reported; "All the hospital beds at the forts at Boston harbor are occupied by influenza patients. . . . There are 3,500 cases at Camp Devens." Yet the paper asserted, "Such reports may actually be reassuring rather than alarming. The soldier or sailor goes to bed if he is told to, just as he goes on sentry duty. He may not think he is sick, and he may be right about it, but the military doctor is not to be argued with and at this time the autocrat is not permitting the young men under his charge to take any chance."

As the virus infested the Great Lakes Naval Training Station, the Associated Press reported, "To dispel alarm caused throughout the country by exaggerated stories . . . Captain W. A. Moffat, commandant, gave out the statement today that while there are about 4,500 cases of the disease among the 45,000 blue jackets at the station, the situation in general is much improved. The death rate has been only one and one half per cent, which is below the death rate in the east."

That report was meant to reassure. It is unlikely that it did so, even though it omitted the fact that quarantines were being imposed upon the training station, the adjoining Great Lakes Aviation Camp, and the nearby Fort Sheridan army cantonment, which, combined, amounted to the largest military concentration in the country. And military authorities of course assured both civilians nearby as well as the country at large that "the epidemic is on the wane."

Over and over in hundreds of newspapers, day after day, repeated in one form or another people read Rupert Blue's reassurance as well: "There is no cause for alarm if precautions are observed."

They read the words of Colonel Philip Doane, the officer in charge of health at the country's shipyards, who told the Associated Press, "The so-called Spanish influenza is nothing more or less than old fashioned grippe."

Those words, too, ran in hundreds of newspapers. But people could smell death in them. Then they came to know that death.

Immediately outside Little Rock lay Camp Pike, where eight thousand

cases were admitted to the hospital in four days and the camp commandant stopped releasing the names of the dead. "You ought to see this hospital tonight," wrote Francis Blake, one of four members of the army's
pneumonia commission at Pike. "Every corridor and there are miles of
them with a double row of cots and every ward nearly with an extra row
down the middle with influenza patients and lots of barracks about the
camp turned into emergency infirmaries and the Camp closed. . . . There
is only death and destruction."

The camp called upon Little Rock for nurses, doctors, linens, and
coffins, all while within the city the *Arkansas Gazette* declared in headlines, "Spanish influenza is plain la grippe—same old fever and chills."

Outside Des Moines, Iowa, at Camp Dodge, also, influenza was killing
hundreds of young soldiers. Within the city a group called the Greater
Des Moines Committee, businessmen and professionals who had taken
charge during the emergency, included the city attorney who warned
publishers—and his warning carried the sting of potential prosecution—
"I would recommend that if anything be printed in regard to the disease
it be confined to simple preventive measures—something constructive
rather than destructive." Another committee member, a physician, said,
"There is no question that by a right attitude of the mind these people
have kept themselves from illness. I have no doubt that many persons
have contracted the disease through fear. . . . Fear is the first thing to be
overcome, the first step in conquering this epidemic."

The Bronxville, New York, *Review Press and Reporter* simply said
nothing at all about influenza, absolutely nothing, until October 4, when
it reported that the "scourge" had claimed its first victim there. It was as
if the scourge had come from nowhere; yet even the paper recognized
that, without its printing a word, everyone knew of it. And even as the
epidemic rooted itself in Bronxville, the paper condemned "alarmism"
and warned, "Fear kills more than the disease and the weak and timid
often succumb first."

Fear, that was the enemy. Yes, fear. And the more officials tried to control it with half-truths and outright lies, the more the terror spread.

The Los Angeles public health director said, "If ordinary precautions are
observed there is no cause for alarm." Forty-eight hours later he closed all
places of public gatherings, including schools, churches, and theaters.

The Illinois superintendent of public health had—privately, in a confidential meeting with other Illinois public health officials and Chicago politicians—suggested they close all places of business to save lives. Chicago Public Health Commissioner John Dill Robertson violently rejected that suggestion as unwarranted and very damaging to morale. In his official report on the epidemic, he bragged, "Nothing was done to interfere with the morale of the community." Later he explained to other public health professionals, "It is our duty to keep the people from fear. Worry kills more people than the epidemic."

The mortality rate at Cook County Hospital for all influenza cases—not just those who developed pneumonia—was 39.8 percent.

Literary Digest, one of the largest-circulation periodicals in the country, advised, "Fear is our first enemy."

"Don't Get Scared!" was the advice printed in virtually every newspaper in the country, in large, blocked-off parts of pages labeled "Advice on How to Avoid Influenza."

The *Albuquerque Morning Journal* issued instructions on "How to Dodge 'Flu.'" The most prominent advice was the usual: "Don't Get Scared." Almost daily it repeated, "Don't Let Flu Frighten You to Death," "Don't Panic."

In Phoenix the *Arizona Republican* monitored influenza from a distance. On September 22 it declared "Dr. W. C. Woodward of the Boston Health Department assumed an optimistic attitude tonight. . . . Dr. Woodward said the increase in cases today was not alarming." At Camp Dix "the camp medical authorities asserted they have the epidemic under control." And the paper noted the first influenza deaths in New Orleans two days before the New Orleans daily newspaper the *Item* mentioned any death in the city.

But after the first case appeared in Phoenix itself, the *Republican* fell silent, utterly silent, saying nothing about influenza anyplace in the country until the news was such that it could no longer keep silent. Its competitor the *Gazette* competed in reassurances, quoting local physician Herman Randall saying, "Ten people sit in the same draught, are exposed to the same microbes. Some will suffer and perhaps die, while the others go scot free. . . . The people during an epidemic who are most fearful are usually, on the testimony of physicians, the first ones to succumb to the disease." And in Phoenix, even after the war ended, the "Citizens' Committee" that had taken over the city during the emergency continued to impose silence, ordering that "merchants of the city refrain from mentioning the influenza epidemic directly or indirectly in their advertising."

Meanwhile, Vicks VapoRub advertisements in hundreds of papers danced down the delicate line of reassurance while promising relief, calling the epidemic, "Simply the Old-Fashioned Grip Masquerading Under a New Name."

Some papers experimented in controlling fear by printing almost nothing at all. In Goldsboro, North Carolina, recalls a survivor, "The papers didn't even want to publish the lists of names [of the dead]. . . . The information about who was dying had to come up through the grapevine, verbally, from one person to the other."

A historian studying Buffalo County, Nebraska, expressed puzzlement that "[t]he county newspapers manifested a curious reticence regarding the effects of influenza, perhaps most evident in the The *Kearney Hub*. It may be surmised that the editors played down the severity of the problem to discourage the onset of general panic in the face of what was a thoroughly frightening situation." As late as December 14 that paper was telling people not to "get panicky," telling them city officials were "not inclined to be as panicky as a great many citizens."

How could one not get panicky? Even before people's neighbors began to die, before bodies began to pile up in each new community, every piece of information except the newspapers told the truth. Even while Blue recited his mantra—*There is no cause for alarm if proper precautions are taken*—he was calling upon local authorities to "close all public gathering places, if their community is threatened with the epidemic. This will do much toward checking the spread of the disease." Even if Colonel Doane had said *Influenza is nothing more or less than old fashioned grippe*, newspapers also quoted him saying, "Every person who spits is helping the Kaiser."

And even while Blue and Doane, governors and mayors, and nearly all the newspapers insisted that this was influenza, only influenza, the Public Health Service was making a massive effort to distribute advice— nearly useless advice. It prepared ready-to-print plates and sent them to ten thousand newspapers, most of which did print them. It prepared—

the Red Cross paid for printing and distribution—posters and pamphlets, including six million copies of a single circular. Teachers handed them out in schools; bosses stacked them in stores, post offices, and factories; Boy Scouts stuffed them into tens of thousands of doorways; ministers referred to them on Sundays; mailmen carried them to rural free delivery boxes; city workers pasted posters to walls.

But a Public Health Service warning to avoid crowds came too late to do much good, and the only advice of any real use remained the same: that those who felt sick should go to bed immediately and stay there several days after all symptoms disappeared. Everything else in Blue's circulars was so general as to be pointless. Yet all over the country, newspapers printed again and again: "Remember the 3 Cs, clean mouth, clean skin, and clean clothes. . . . Keep the bowels open. . . . Food will win the war. . . . [H]elp by choosing and chewing your food well."

The *Journal of the American Medical Association* knew better. It dismissed the public reassurances and warned, "The danger to life from influenza in this epidemic is so grave that it is imperative to secure from the individual patient the most complete isolation." And it attacked "current advice and instructions to the public from the official and other sources"—Blue's advice, the advice from local public-health officials downplaying everything—as useless and dangerous.

"Don't Get Scared!" said the newspapers.

Meanwhile people read—those in the West seeing it before the virus reached them—the Red Cross appeals published in newspapers, often in half-page advertisements that said; "The safety of this country demands that all patriotic available nurses, nurses' aids [*sic*] or anyone with experience in nursing place themselves at once under the disposal of the Government. . . . Physicians are urgently requested to release from attendance on chronic cases and all other cases which are not critically ill every nurse working under their direction who can possibly be spared for such duty. Graduate nurses, undergraduates, nurses' aids, and volunteers are urged to telegraph collect at once . . . to their local Red Cross chapter or Red Cross headquarters, Washington, D.C."

"Don't Get Scared!" said the papers.

Be not afraid.

But not everyone was ready to trust in God.

.   .   .

In 2001 a terrorist attack with anthrax killed five people and transfixed America. In 2002 an outbreak of West Nile virus killed 284 people nationally in six months and sparked headlines for weeks, along with enough fear to change people's behavior. In 2003 SARS killed over eight hundred people around the world, froze Asian economies, and frightened millions of people in Hong Kong, Singapore, and elsewhere into wearing masks on the streets.

In 1918 fear moved ahead of the virus like the bow wave before a ship. Fear drove the people, and the government and the press could not control it. They could not control it because every true report had been diluted with lies. And the more the officials and newspapers reassured, the more they said, *There is no cause for alarm if proper precautions are taken,* or *Influenza is nothing more or less than old-fashioned grippe,* the more people believed themselves cast adrift, adrift with no one to trust, adrift on an ocean of death.

So people watched the virus approach, and feared, feeling as impotent as it moved toward them as if it were an inexorable oncoming cloud of poison gas. It was a thousand miles away, five hundred miles away, fifty miles away, twenty miles away.

In late September they saw published reports, reports buried in back pages, reports in tiny paragraphs, but reports nonetheless: eight hundred cases among midshipmen at Annapolis . . . in New York State coughing or sneezing without covering the face was now punishable by a year in jail and a $500 fine . . . thirty cases of influenza among students at the University of Colorado—but, of course, the Associated Press reassured, "None of the cases, it was said, is serious."

But then it *was* serious: four hundred dead in a day in Philadelphia . . . twenty dead in Colorado and New Mexico . . . four hundred now dead in Chicago . . . all social and amusement activities suspended in El Paso, where seven funerals for soldiers occurred in a single day (it would get much worse) . . . a terrible outbreak in Winslow, Arizona.

It was like being bracketed by artillery, the barrage edging closer and closer.

In Lincoln, Illinois, a small town thirty miles from Springfield, William Maxwell sensed it: "My first intimations about the epidemic was that it was something happening to the troops. There didn't seem to be any reason to think it would ever have anything to do with us. And yet in a gradual remorseless way it kept moving closer and closer. Rumors of the alarming situation reached this very small town in the midwest. . . . It was like, almost like an entity moving closer."

In Meadow, Utah, one hundred miles from Provo, Lee Reay recalled, "We were very concerned in our town because it was moving south down the highway, and we were next." They watched it kill in Payson, then Santaguin, then Nephi, Levan, and Mills. They watched it come closer and closer. They put up a huge sign on the road that ordered people to keep going, not to stop in Meadow. But the mailman stopped anyway.

Wherever one was in the country, it crept closer—it was in the next town, the next neighborhood, the next block, the next room. In Tucson the *Arizona Daily Star* warned readers not to catch "Spanish hysteria!" "Don't worry!" was the official and final piece of advice on how to avoid the disease from the Arizona Board of Health.

Don't get scared! said the newspapers everywhere. *Don't get scared!* they said in Denver, in Seattle, in Detroit; in Burlington, Vermont, and Burlington, Iowa, and Burlington, North Carolina; in Greenville. Rhode Island, and Greenville, South Carolina, and Greenville, Mississippi. And every time the newspapers said, *Don't get scared!* they frightened.

The virus had moved west and south from the East Coast by water and rail. It rose up in great crests to flood cities, rolled in great waves through the towns, broke into wild rivers to rage through villages, poured in swollen creeks through settlements, flowed in tiny rivulets into isolated homes. And as in a great flood it covered everything, varying in depth but covering everything, settling over the land in a great leveling.

Albert Camus wrote, "What's true of all the evils in the world is true of plague as well. It helps men to rise above themselves."

One who rose was Dr. Ralph Marshall Ward, who had abandoned medicine for cattle ranching. Leaving medicine had not been a business decision.

An intellectual, particularly interested in pharmacology, he was a prominent physician in Kansas City with an office and pharmacy in the Stockyard Exchange Building down by the bottoms. But Kansas City was a major railhead, with the yards near his office. Most of his practice involved treating railroad workers injured in accidents. He performed huge numbers of amputations, and seemed always to work on mangled men, men ripped into pieces by steel. To have a practice with so much human agony ripped him into pieces as well.

He had too much of doctoring, and, from treating cowboys hurt on cattle drives north to Kansas City, he had learned enough about the cattle business that he decided shortly before the war to buy a small ranch more than a thousand miles away, near San Benito, Texas, close to the Mexican border. On the long trip south, he and his wife made a pact never to utter a word that he had been a doctor. But in October 1918, influenza reached him. Some ranch hands got ill. He began treating them. Word spread.

A few days later his wife woke up to a disturbing and unrecognizable sound. She went outside and saw out there in the gloaming people, hundreds of people, on the horizon. They seemed to cover that horizon, and as they came closer, it was clear they were Mexicans, a few of them on mules, most on foot, women carrying babies, men carrying women, bedraggled, beaten down, a mass of humanity, a mass of horror and suffering. She yelled for her husband, and he came out and stood on the porch. "Oh my God!" he said.

The people had come with nothing. But they knew he was a doctor so they had come. The Wards later told their granddaughter it was like the hospital scene in *Gone With the Wind,* with rows of wounded and dying laid out on the ground in agony. These people had come with nothing, had nothing, and they were dying. The Wards took huge pots outside to boil water, used all their resources to feed them, treated them. Out on the empty harsh range near the Mexican border, they had no Red Cross to turn to for help, no Council of National Defense. They did what they could, and when it was over they went back to Kansas City; he had already gone back to being a doctor.

There were other men and women like the Wards. Physicians, nurses, scientists—did their jobs, and the virus killed them, killed them in such numbers that each week *JAMA* was filled with literally page after page after page after page after page of nothing but brief obituaries in tiny compressed type. Hundreds of doctors dying. Hundreds. Others helped too.

But as Camus knew, evil and crises do not make all men rise above themselves. Crises only make them discover themselves. And some discover a less inspiring humanity.

As the crest of the wave that broke over Philadelphia began its sweep across the rest of the country, it was accompanied by the same terror that had silenced the streets there. Most men and women sacrificed and risked their lives only for those they loved most deeply: a child, a wife, a husband. Others, loving chiefly themselves, fled in terror even from them.

Still others fomented terror, believing that blaming the enemy— Germany—could help the war effort, or perhaps actually believing that Germany was responsible. Doane himself charged that "German agents . . . from submarines" brought influenza to the United States. "The Germans have started epidemics in Europe, and there is no reason why they should be particularly gentle to America."

Others around the country echoed him. Starkville, Mississippi, a town of three thousand in the Mississippi hill country, was built around a sawmill, cotton farms—not the rich, lush plantations of the Delta but harsh land—and Mississippi A&M College (now Mississippi State University). It served as headquarters for Dr. M. G. Parsons, the U.S. Public Health Service officer for northeastern Mississippi, who proudly informed Blue that he had succeeded in getting local newspapers to run stories he made up that "aid in forming a proper frame of mind" in the public. That frame of mind was fear. Parsons wanted to create fear, believing it "prepared the public mind to receive and act on our suggestions."

Parsons got the local press to say, "The Hun resorts to unwanted murder of innocent noncombatants. . . . He has been tempted to spread sickness and death thru germs, and has done so in authenticated cases. . . . Communicable diseases are more strictly a weapon for use well back of the lines, over on French or British, or American land." Blue neither reprimanded Parsons for fomenting fear nor suggested that he take another tack. Another story read, "The Germs Are Coming. An epidemic of influenza is spreading or being spread, (we wonder which)." . . .

Those and similar charges created enough public sentiment to force Public Health Service laboratories to waste valuable time and energy investigating such possible agents of germ warfare as Bayer aspirin. Parsons's territory bordered on Alabama and there a traveling salesman from

Philadelphia named H. M. Thomas was arrested on suspicion of being a German agent and spreading influenza—death. Thomas was released, but on October 17, the day after influenza had killed 759 people in Philadelphia, his body was found in a hotel room with his wrists cut—and his throat slit. Police ruled it suicide.

Everywhere, as in Philadelphia, two problems developed: caring for the sick, and maintaining some kind of order.

In Cumberland, Maryland, a gritty railroad and industrial city in the heart of a coal-mining region—where one actually *could* throw a stone across the Potomac River into West Virginia—to prevent the spread of the disease schools and churches had already been closed, all public gathering places had been closed, and stores had been ordered to close early. Nonetheless, the epidemic exploded on October 5. At noon that day the local Red Cross chairman met with the treasurer of the Red Cross's War Fund and the head of the local Council of National Defense. Their conclusion: "The matter seemed far beyond control. . . . Reports were spreading fast that 'this one' or 'that one' had died without doctor or nurse and it was a panic indeed."

They decided to convert two large buildings on Washington Street to emergency hospitals. From there a handful of women took over, meeting barely an hour after the men had. Each woman had a task: to gather linens, or bathroom supplies, or cooking utensils, or flour. They worked fast. The next morning the hospitals filled with patients.

In Cumberland, 41 percent of the entire population got sick. But the emergency hospitals had only three nurses. The organizers begged for more: "We notified the Bd of Health we must have more nurses if we were to go on. . . . [Nurses] promised. However this help never materialized and up to date . . . 93 admissions, 18 deaths. The question of orderlies is difficult. They are just not to be found."

Back in Starkville, Parsons met with the president of the college, the army commander of the students—all the students had been inducted into the army—and physicians. "We had an open discussion of the dangers and best actions to take and they assured me everything possible would be done," he wired Blue. He asked for and received fifteen thousand pamphlets, posters, and circulars, more than the combined population of Starkville, Columbus, and West Point. But he, and they, accomplished little. Of eighteen hundred students, well over half would get influenza. On October 9 Parsons "found unbelievable conditions with everybody in power stunned." At that moment eight hundred students were sick and 2 percent of all students had already died, with many deaths to come. Parsons found "influenza is all thru the region, in town, hamlet, and single home. People are pretty well scared, with reason. . . ." In West Point, a town of five thousand, fifteen hundred were ill simultaneously. Parsons confessed, "Panic incipient."

In El Paso a U.S. Public Health Service officer reported to Blue, "I have the honor to inform you that from Oct 9th to date there have been 275 deaths from influenza in El Paso among civilians. This does not include civilians who are employed by the government and who died at the base hospital of Fort Bliss, nor does it include soldiers . . . [W]hole city in a panic."

In Colorado, towns in the San Juan Mountains did not panic. They turned grimly serious. They had time to prepare. Lake City guards kept the town entirely free of the disease, allowing no one to enter. Silverton, a town of two thousand, authorized closing businesses even before a single case surfaced. But the virus snuck in, with a vengeance. In a single week in Silverton, 125 died. The town of Ouray set up a "shot gun quarantine," hiring guards to keep miners from Silverton and Telluride out. But the virus reached Ouray as well.

It had not reached Gunnison. Neither tiny nor isolated, Gunnison was a railroad town, a supply center for the west-central part of the state, the home of Western State Teachers College. In early October—far in advance of any cases of influenza—Gunnison and most neighboring towns issued a closing order and a ban on public gatherings. Then Gunnison decided to isolate itself entirely. Gunnison lawmen blocked all through roads. Train conductors warned all passengers that if they stepped foot on the platform in Gunnison to stretch their legs, they would be arrested and quarantined for five days. Two Nebraskans trying simply to drive through to a town in the next county ran the blockade and were thrown into jail. Meanwhile, the nearby town of Sargents suffered six deaths in a single day—out of a total population of 130.

Early in the epidemic, back on September 27—it seemed like years before—the Wisconsin newspaper the *Jefferson County Union* had reported the truth about the disease, and the general in charge of the Army

Morale Branch decreed the report "depressant to morale" and forwarded it to enforcement officials for "any action which may be deemed appropriate," including criminal prosecution. Now, weeks later, after weeks of dying and with the war over, the *Gunnison News-Chronicle*, unlike virtually every other newspaper in the country, played no games and warned, "This disease is no joke, to be made light of, but a terrible calamity."

Gunnison escaped without a death.

In the United States, the war was something *over there*. The epidemic was *here*.

"Even if there was war," recalled Susanna Turner of Philadelphia, "the war was removed from us, you know . . . on the other side. . . . This malignancy, it was right at our very doors."

People feared and hated this malignancy, this alien thing in their midst. They were willing to cut it out at any cost. In Goldsboro, North Carolina, Dan Tonkel recalled, "We were actually almost afraid to breathe, the theaters were closed down so you didn't get into any crowds. . . . You felt like you were walking on eggshells, you were afraid even to go out. You couldn't play with your playmates, your classmates, your neighbors, you had to stay home and just be careful. The fear was so great people were actually afraid to leave their homes. People were actually afraid to talk to one another. It was almost like don't breathe in my face, don't look at me and breathe in my face. . . . You never knew from day to day who was going to be next on the death list. . . . That was the horrible part, people just died so quickly."

His father had a store. Four of eight salesgirls died. "Farmers stopped farming and the merchants stopped selling merchandise and the country really more or less just shut down holding their breath. Everyone was holding their breath." His uncle Benny was nineteen years old and had been living with him until he was drafted and went to Fort Bragg, which sent him home when he reported. The camp was refusing all new draftees. Tonkel recalls his parents not wanting to allow Benny back in the house. "'Benny we don't know what to do with you,'" they said. "'Well, what can I tell you. I'm here,'" his uncle replied. They let him in. "We were frightened, yes absolutely, we were frightened."

In Washington, D.C., William Sardo said, "It kept people apart. . . . It took away all your community life, you had no community life, you had no school life, you had no church life, you had nothing. . . . It completely destroyed all family and community life. People were afraid to kiss one another, people were afraid to eat with one another, they were afraid to have anything that made contact because that's how you got the flu. . . . It destroyed those contacts and destroyed the intimacy that existed amongst people. . . . You were constantly afraid, you were afraid because you saw so much death around you, you were surrounded by death. . . . When each day dawned you didn't know whether you would be there when the sun set that day. It wiped out entire families from the time that the day began in the morning to bedtime at night—entire families were gone completely, there wasn't any single soul left and that didn't happen just intermittently, it happened all the way across the neighborhoods, it was a terrifying experience. It justifiably should be called a plague because that's what it was. . . . You were quarantined, is what you were, from fear, it was so quick, so sudden. . . . There was an aura of a constant fear that you lived through from getting up in the morning to going to bed at night."

In New Haven, Connecticut, John Delano recalled the same isolating fear: "Normally when someone was sick in those days the parents, the mothers, the fathers, would bring food over to other families but this was very weird. . . . Nobody was coming in, nobody would bring food in, nobody came to visit."

Prescott, Arizona, made it illegal to shake hands. In Perry County, Kentucky, in the mountains where men either dug into the earth for coal or scratched upon the earth's surface trying to farm despite topsoil only a few inches deep, a county of hard people, where family ties bound tightly, where men and women were loyal and would murder for pride or honor, the Red Cross chapter chairman begged for help, reporting "hundreds of cases up in mountains that they were unable to reach." They were unreachable not just because the county had almost no roads; streambeds in dry weather substituted for them and when the streambeds filled, transport became impossible. It was more: "People starving to death not from lack of food but because the well were panic stricken and would not go near the sick; that in the stricken families the dead were lying uncared for." Doctors were offered $100 to come out and stay there one hour. None came. Even one Red Cross worker, Morgan Brawner, arrived in the county Saturday and left Sunday, himself terror stricken.

He had reason to fear: in some areas the civilian mortality rate reached 30 percent.

In Norwood, Massachusetts, a historian years later interviewed survivors. One man, a newsboy in 1918, remembered that his manager would "tell me to put the money on the table and he'd spray the money before he'd pick it up." Said another survivor; "There wasn't much visiting. . . . We stayed by ourselves." And another: "[H]e'd bring, you know, whatever my father needed and leave it on the doorstep. No one would go into each other's houses." And another: "Everything came to a standstill. . . . We weren't allowed out the door. We had to keep away from people." And another: "A cop, a big burly guy . . . came up to the house and nailed a big white sign and on the sign it said INFLUENZA in red letters. And they nailed it to the door." A sign made a family even more isolated. And another survivor: "I'd go up the street, walk up the street with my hand over my eyes because there were so many houses with crepe draped over the doors." And still another: "It was horrifying. Not only were you frightened you might come down with it but there was the eerie feeling of people passing away all around you."

In Luce County, Michigan, one woman was nursing her husband and three boys when she "came down with it herself," reported a Red Cross worker. "Not one of the neighbors would come in and help. I stayed there all night, and in the morning telephoned the woman's sister. She came and tapped on the window, but refused to talk to me until she had gotten a safe distance away. . . . I could do nothing for the woman . . . except send for the priest."

Monument and Ignacio, Colorado, went further than banning all public gatherings. They banned customers from stores; the stores remained open, but customers shouted orders through doors, then waited outside for packages.

Colorado Springs placarded homes with signs that read "Sickness."

In no industry did workers hear more about patriotism, about how their work mattered to the war effort as much as that of soldiers fighting at the front, than in shipbuilding. Nor were workers in any industry more carefully attended to. In all plants common drinking cups were immediately destroyed, replaced by tens of thousands of paper cups. Hospital and treatment facilities were arranged in advance, influenza vaccine supplied, and it was perhaps the only industry in which nurses and doctors remained available. As a result, claimed a Public Health Service officer, "There is no reason to believe that many men were absent from work through panic or fear of the disease, because our educational program took care to avoid frightening the men. The men were taught that they were safer at work than any where else."

They were also of course not paid unless they came to work. But at dozens of shipyards in New England, the absentee records were striking. At the L. H. Shattuck Company, 45.9 percent of the workers stayed home. At the George A. Gilchrist yard, 54.3 percent stayed home. At Freeport Shipbuilding, 57 percent stayed home. At Groton Iron Works, 58.3 percent stayed home.

Twenty-six hundred miles away was Phoenix, Arizona. At the beginning of the epidemic its newspapers had behaved as did those everywhere else, saying little, reassuring, insisting that fear was more dangerous than the disease. But the virus took its time there, lingered longer than elsewhere, lingered until finally even the press expressed fear. On November 8 the *Arizona Republican* warned, "The people of Phoenix are facing a crisis. The [epidemic] has reached such serious proportions that it is the first problem before the people. . . . Almost every home in the city has been stricken with the plague. . . . Fearless men and women [must] serve in the cause of humanity."

The war was three days from ending, and several false peaces had been announced. Still, for that newspaper to call influenza "the first problem" while the war continued was extraordinary. And finally the city formed a "citizens' committee" to take charge.

In Arizona, citizens' committees were taken seriously. A year earlier fifteen hundred armed members of a "Citizens Protective League" had put 1,221 striking miners into cattle and boxcars and abandoned them without food or water on a railroad siding in the desert, across the New Mexico line. In Phoenix another "citizens' committee" had been going after "bond slackers," hanging them in effigy on main streets. One man refused to buy a bond because of religious reasons. Nonetheless he was hung in effigy with a placard reading, "H. G. Saylor, yellow slacker. . . . Can, but won't buy a liberty bond!" Saylor was lucky. The committee also seized Charles Reas, a carpenter, tied his hands behind his back, painted his face yellow, put a noose around his neck, and dragged him through downtown Phoenix streets wearing a sign that read "with this exception we are 100%."

The influenza Citizens' Committee took similar initiatives. It deputized a special police force and also called upon all "patriotic citizens" to enforce anti-influenza ordinances, including requiring every person in public to wear a mask, arresting anyone who spit or coughed without covering his mouth, dictating that businesses (those that remained open) give twelve hundred cubic feet of air space to each customer, and halting all traffic into the city and allowing only those with "actual business here" to enter. Soon the *Republican* described "a city of masked faces, a city as grotesque as a masked carnival."

And yet—ironically—influenza touched Phoenix only lightly compared to elsewhere. The panic came anyway. Dogs told the story of terror, but not with their barking. Rumors spread that dogs carried influenza. The police began killing all dogs on the street. And people began killing their own dogs, dogs they loved, and if they had not the heart to kill them themselves, they gave them to the police to be killed. "At this death rate from causes other than natural," reported the *Gazette,* "Phoenix will soon be dogless." Back in Philadelphia Mary Volz lived near a church. She had always "loved to hear the church bells ringing, they were so jubilantly ringing." But now every few minutes people carried a casket into the church, left, "and there would be another casket." Each time the bells rang. "The bells were my joy and then this 'BONG! BONG! BONG!' I was terrified, lying sick in bed hearing 'BONG! BONG! BONG!' Is the bell going to bong for me?"

The war was over there. The epidemic was here. The war ended. The epidemic continued. Fear settled over the nation like a frozen blanket. "Some say the world will end in fire," wrote Robert Frost in 1920. "Ice is also great / and would suffice."

An internal American Red Cross report concluded, "A fear and panic of the influenza, akin to the terror of the Middle Ages regarding the Black Plague, [has] been prevalent in many parts of the country."

CHAPTER THIRTY

WIRES POURED INTO the Red Cross and the Public Health Service demanding, pleading, begging for help. From Portsmouth, Virginia: "Urgently need two colored physicians wire prospects obtaining same." From Carey, Kentucky: "Federal coal mines request immediate aid influenza. . . . Immediately rush answer." From Spokane, Washington; "urgent need of four nurses to take charge other nurses furnished by local Red Cross chapter."

The demands could not be met. Replies went back: "No colored physicians available." "It is almost impossible to send nurses all being needed locally." "Call for local volunteers with intelligence and practical experience."

The failure to meet demand was not from lack of trying. Red Cross workers went from house to house searching for anyone with nursing experience. And when they knew of a skilled nurse, the Red Cross tracked her down. Josey Brown was a nurse watching a movie in a St. Louis theater when the lights went on, the screen went blank, and a man appeared onstage announcing that anyone named Josey Brown should go to the ticket booth. There she found a telegram ordering her to the Great Lakes Naval Training Station.

The *Journal of the American Medical Association* repeatedly—sometimes twice in the same issue—published an "urgent call on physicians for help in localities where the epidemic is unusually severe. . . .

This service is just as definite a patriotic privilege as is that of serving in the Medical Corps of the Army or Navy. . . . As the call is immediate and urgent it is suggested that any physician who feels that he can do some of this work telegraph to the Surgeon General, USPHS, Washington, D.C."

There were never enough.

Meanwhile, physicians attempted everything—*everything*—to save lives. They could relieve some symptoms. Doctors could address pain with everything from aspirin to morphine. They could control coughing at least somewhat with codeine and, said some, heroin. They gave atropine, digitalis, strychnine, and epinephrine as stimulants. They gave oxygen.

Some treatment attempts that went beyond symptomatic relief had solid science behind them, even if no one had ever applied that science to influenza. There was Redden's approach in Boston based on Lewis's experiments with polio. That approach, with variations, was tried over and over again around the world.

And there were treatments less grounded in science. They sounded logical. They were logical. But the reasoning was also desperate, the reasoning of a doctor ready to try anything, the reasoning that mixed wild ideas or thousands of years of practice and a few decades of scientific method. First-rate medical journals rejected articles about the most outlandish and ridiculous so-called therapies, but they published anything that at least seemed to make sense. There was no time for peer review, no time for careful analysis.

JAMA published the work of a physician who claimed, "Infection was prevented in practically 100% of cases when [my] treatment was properly used." His approach had logic to it. By stimulating the flow of mucus, he hoped to help one of the first lines of defense of the body, to prevent any pathogen from attaching itself to any mucosal membrane. So he mixed irritating chemicals in powder form and blew them into the upper respiratory tract to generate large flows of mucus. The theory was sound; perhaps while mucus was actually flowing, it did some good.

One Philadelphia doctor had another idea, logical but more reaching, and wrote in *JAMA* that "when the system is saturated with alkalis, there is poor soil for bacterial growth." Therefore he tried to turn the entire body alkaline. "I have uniformly employed, and always with good results, potassium citrate and sodium bicarbonate saturation by mouth, bowel and skin. . . . Patients must be willing to forego [*sic*] the seductive relief by acetylsalicylic acid [aspirin]. . . . My very successful experience in this epidemic cannot be dismissed as accidental or unique. . . . I urge its immediate trial empirically. Further investigation in laboratory or clinic may follow later."

Physicians injected people with typhoid vaccine, thinking—or simply hoping—it might somehow boost the immune system in general even though the specificity of the immune response was well understood. Some claimed the treatment worked. Others poured every known vaccine into patients on the same theory. Quinine worked on one disease: malaria. Many physicians gave it for influenza with no better reasoning than desperation.

Others convinced themselves a treatment cured regardless of results. A Montana physician reported to the *New York Medical Journal* of his experimental treatment; "The results have been favorable." He tried the treatment on six people; two died. Still he insisted, "In the four cases that recovered the results were immediate and certain."

Two University of Pittsburgh researchers reasoned no better. They believed they had improved on the technique Redden had adopted from Flexner and Lewis. They treated forty-seven patients; twenty died. They subtracted seven deaths, arguing that the victims received the therapy too late. That still left thirteen dead out of forty-seven. Yet they claimed success.

One physician gave hydrogen peroxide intravenously to twenty-five patients in severe pulmonary distress, believing that it would get oxygen into the blood. Thirteen recovered; twelve died. This physician, too, claimed success: "The anoxemia was often markedly benefited, and the toxemia appeared to be overcome in many cases."

Many of his colleagues tried similarly outlandish treatments and likewise claimed success. Many of them believed it.

Homeopaths believed that the epidemic proved their superiority to "allopathic" physicians. The *Journal of the American Institute for Homeopathy* claimed that influenza victims treated by regular physicians had a mortality rate of 28.2 percent—an absurdity: if that were so, the United States alone would have had several million deaths—while also claiming that twenty-six thousand patients treated by homeopaths, chiefly with the herbal drug gelsemium, had a mortality rate of 1.05 percent, with many homeopaths claiming no deaths whatsoever among thousands of patients. But the results were self-reported, making it far too easy to rationalize away those under their care who did die—to remove, for instance, from their sample any patient who, against their advice, took aspirin, which homeopaths considered a poison.

It was no different elsewhere in the world. In Greece one physician used mustard plasters to create blisters on the skin of influenza victims, then drained them, mixed the fluid with morphine, strychnine, and caffeine and reinjected it. "The effect was apparent at once, and in 36 to 48 or even 12 hours the temperature declined and improvement progressed." But the mortality rate of his 234 patients was 6 percent.

In Italy one doctor gave intravenous injections of mercuric chloride. Another rubbed creosote, a disinfectant, into the axilla, where lymph nodes, outposts of white blood cells scattered through the body, lie beneath the skin. A third insisted that enemas of warm milk and one drop of creosote every twelve hours for every year of age prevented pneumonia.

In Britain the War Office published recommendations for therapy in *The Lancet*. They were far more specific than any guidance in the United States, and likely did relieve some symptoms. For sleep, twenty grains of bromide, opiates to relax cough, and oxygen for cyanosis. The recommendations warned that venesection was seldom beneficial, that alcohol was invaluable, but that little could be gained by giving food. For headache: antipyrin and salicylic acid—aspirin. To stimulate the heart: strychnine and digitalis.

In France, not until mid-October did the Ministry of War approach the Académie des Sciences for help. To prevent disease, some physicians and scientists advised masks. Others insisted arsenic prevented it. For treatment, the Pasteur Institute developed an antipneumococcus serum drawn as usual from horses, as well as a serum derived from the blood of patients who had recovered. (Comparisons proved the Cole and Avery serum far superior.) Anything that might lower fever was urged. Stimulants were recommended for the heart. So were "revulsions" that purged the body. Methylene blue, a dye used to stain bacteria to make them more visible under the microscope, was tried despite its known toxicity in the hopes of killing bacteria. Other doctors injected metallic solutions into muscle, so the body absorbed them gradually, or intravenously. (One doctor who injected it intravenously conceded that the treatment was "a little brutal.") Cupping was recommended—using a flame to absorb oxygen and thus create a vacuum in a glass container, then placing it on the body, in theory to draw out poisons. One prominent physician called for "prompt bleeding" of more than pint of blood at the first signs of pulmonary edema and cyanosis, along with acetylsalicylic acid. He was hardly alone in prescribing bleeding. One physician who recommended a return to "heroic medicine" explained that the more the doctor did, the more the body was stimulated to respond. In disease as in war, he said, the fighter must seize initiative.

Across the world hundreds of millions—very likely tens of millions in the United States alone—saw no doctor, saw no nurse, but tried every kind of folk medicine or fraudulent remedy available or imaginable. Camphor balls and garlic hung around people's necks. Others gargled with disinfectants, let frigid air sweep through their homes, or sealed windows shut and overheated rooms.

Advertisements filled the newspapers, sometimes set in the same small type as—and difficult to distinguish from—news articles, and sometimes set in large fonts blaring across a page. The one thing they shared: they all declared with confidence there *was* a way to stop influenza, there *was* a way to survive. Some claims were as simple as a shoe store's advertising, "One way to keep the flu away is to keep your feet dry." Some were as complex as "Making a Kolynos Gas Mask To Fight Spanish Influenza When Exposed to Infection."

They also all played to fear. "How To Prevent Infection From Spanish Influenza. . . . The Surgeon General of the U.S. Army urges you to keep your mouth clean. . . . [use] a few drops of liquid SOZODONT." "Help your Health Board Conquer Spanish influenza By Disinfecting your Home . . . Lysol Disinfectant." "For GRIP . . . You are Safe When You Take Father John's Medicine." "Influ-BALM Prevents Spanish Flu." "Special Notice to the Public. Telephone inquiries from Minneapolis physicians and the laity and letters from many parts of America are coming into our office regarding the use of Benetol, . . . a powerful bulwark for the prevention and treatment of Spanish influenza. . . ." "Spanish influenza—what it is and how it should be treated: . . . Always Call a Doctor/ No Occasion For Panic. . . . There is no occasion for panic—influenza itself has a very low percentage of fatalities. . . . Use Vicks VapoRub."

By the middle of October, vaccines prepared by the best scientists were appearing everywhere. On October 17 New York City Health Commissioner Royal Copeland announced that "the influenza vaccine discovered by Dr. William H. Park, director of the City Laboratories, had been tested sufficiently to warrant its recommendation as a preventive agency." Copeland assured the public that "virtually all persons vaccinated with it [were] immune to the disease."

In Philadelphia on October 19, Dr. C. Y. White, a bacteriologist with the municipal laboratory, delivered ten thousand dosages of a vaccine based on Paul Lewis's work, with tens of thousands of dosages more soon to come. It was "multivalent," made up of dead strains of several kinds of bacteria, including the influenza bacillus, two types of pneumococci, and several strains of other streptococci.

That same day a new issue of *JAMA* appeared. It was thick with information on influenza, including a preliminary evaluation of the experience with vaccines in Boston. George Whipple, another Welch product and later a Nobel laureate, concluded, "The weight of such statistical evidence as we have been able to accumulate indicates that the use of the influenza vaccine which we have investigated is without therapeutic benefit." By "therapeutic" Whipple meant that the tested vaccines could not cure. But he continued, "The statistical evidence, so far as it goes, indicates a probability that the use of this vaccine has some prophylactic value."

He was hardly endorsing Copeland's statement, but at least he provided some hope.

The Public Health Service made no effort to produce or distribute any vaccine or treatment for civilians. It received requests enough. It had nothing to offer.

The Army Medical School (now the Armed Forces Institute of Pathology) in Washington did mount a massive effort to make a vaccine. They needed one. At the army's own Walter Reed Hospital in Washington, the death rate for those with complicating pneumonia had reached 52 percent. On October 25 the vaccine was ready. The surgeon general's office informed all camp physicians, "The value of vaccination against certain of the more important organisms giving rise to pneumonia may be considered to be established. . . . The Army now has available for all officers, enlisted men, and civilian employees of the Army, a lipo vaccine containing pneumococcus Types I, II, and III."

The army distributed two million doses of this vaccine in the next weeks. This marked an enormous production triumph. Earlier a prominent British scientist had pronounced it impossible for the British government to produce even forty thousand doses on short notice. But the vaccine still protected only against pneumonias caused by Types I and II pneumococci, and it came too late; by then the disease had already passed through nearly all cantonments. When civilian physicians from New York to California begged for the vaccine from the army, the reply came back that the army had in fact produced "a vaccine for the prevention of pneumonia, but none is available for distribution." The army feared a recrudescence among troops; it had good reason to fear one.

The Army Medical School had also produced a vaccine against *B. influenzae,* but of this Gorgas's office spoke more cautiously: "In view of the possible etiologic importance of the bacillus influenzae in the present epidemic, a saline vaccine has been prepared by the Army and is available to all officers, enlisted men, and civilian employees of the Army. The effectiveness of bacillus influenzae vaccine . . . is still in the experimental stage."

That army statement was not a public one. Nor really was a cautionary *JAMA* editorial: "Unfortunately we as yet have no specific serum or other specific means for the cure of influenza, and no specific vaccine for its prevention. Such is the fact, all claims and propagandists in the newspapers and elsewhere to the contrary notwithstanding. . . . Consequently the physician must keep his head and not allow himself to make more promises than the facts warrant. This warning applies especially to health officers in their public relations." Nearly every issue contained a similar warning: "Nothing should be done by the medical profession that may arouse unwarranted hope among the public and be followed by disappointment and distrust of medical science and the medical profession."

JAMA represented the American Medical Association. AMA leaders had worked for decades to bring scientific standards and professionalism to medicine. They had only recently succeeded. They did not want to destroy the trust only recently established. They did not want medicine to become the mockery it had been not so long before.

In the meantime physicians continued to try the most desperate measures. Vaccines continued to be produced in great numbers—eighteen different kinds in Illinois alone. No one had any real idea whether any would work. They had only hope.

But the reality of the disease was expressed in a recitation of events during the epidemic at Camp Sherman, Ohio, the single camp with the highest death rate. Its doctors precisely followed the standard treatment for influenza Osler had recommended in the most recent edition of his textbook—aspirin, rest in bed, gargles, and "Dover's powders," which were a combination of ipecac to induce vomiting and opium to relieve pain and cough. For complicating but standard pneumonias they followed "the usual recommendations for diet, fresh air, rest, mild purgation and elimination. . . . All cases were digitalized"—digitalis given in maximum possible dosages to stimulate the heart—"and reliance placed on soluble caffeine salt for quick stimulation. Strychnin in large doses hypodermically had a distinct value in the existing asthenia."

Then, however, they reported their helplessness in the far too common "acute inflammatory pulmonary edema," what today would be called ARDS. "This presented a new problem in therapy. The principles of treatment employed in pulmonary edema incident to dilation of the heart, though seemingly not indicated by the condition in question, were employed. Digitalis, a double caffeine salt, morphin [sic], and venesection"—bleeding again—"were without significant value. . . . Oxygen was of temporary value. Posture accomplished drainage but did not influence the end result. Pituitary solution, hypodermically, was suggested by the similarity of this condition to the results of gassing. No benefits were gained by its use."

They tried everything, everything they could think of, until they finally took pity and stopped, abandoning some of the more brutal—and useless—treatments they had tried "on account of [their] heroic character." By then they had seen enough of heroism from dying soldiers. They were finally willing to let them go in peace. Against this condition they could only conclude, "No especial measure was of avail."

No medicine and none of the vaccines developed then could prevent influenza. The masks worn by millions were useless as designed and could not prevent influenza. Only preventing exposure to the virus could. Nothing today can cure influenza, although vaccines can provide significant—but nowhere near complete—protection, and several antiviral drugs can mitigate its severity.

Places that isolated themselves—such as Gunnison, Colorado, and a few military installations on islands—escaped. But the closing orders that most cities issued could not prevent exposure; they were not extreme enough. Closing saloons and theaters and churches meant nothing if significant numbers of people continued to climb onto streetcars, continued to go to work, continued to go to the grocer. Even where fear closed down businesses, where both store owners and customers refused to stand face-to-face and left orders on sidewalks, there was still too much interaction to break the chain of infection. The virus was too efficient, too explosive, too good at what it did. In the end the virus did its will around the world.

It was as if the virus were a hunter. It was hunting mankind. It found man in the cities easily, but it was not satisfied. It followed him into towns, then villages, then individual homes. It searched for him in the most distant corners of the earth. It hunted him in the forests, tracked him into jungles, pursued him onto the ice. And in those most distant corners of the earth, in those places so inhospitable that they barely allowed man to live, in those places where man was almost wholly innocent of civilization, man was not safer from the virus. He was more vulnerable.

In Alaska, whites in Fairbanks protected themselves. Sentries guarded all trails, and every person entering the city was quarantined for five days. Eskimos had no such luck. A senior Red Cross official warned that without "immediate medical assistance the race" could become "extinct."

Neither Red Cross nor territorial government funds were available. The governor of Alaska came to Washington to beg Congress for $200,000—compared to the $1 million given to the Public Health Service for the entire country. A senator asked why the territory couldn't spend any of the $600,000 in its treasury. The governor replied, "The people of Alaska consider that the money raised by taxes from the white people of Alaska should be spent for the improvements of the Territory. They need the money in roads a great deal. . . . They want to have the Indians in Alaska placed more on a parity with the Indians of other parts of the United States, where they are taken care of by the United States government."

He got $100,000. The navy provided the collier USS *Brutus* to carry a relief expedition. At Juneau the party divided and went in smaller boats to visit villages.

They found terrible things. Terrible things. In Nome, 176 of 300 Eskimos had died. But it would get worse. One doctor visited ten tiny villages and found "three wiped out entirely; others average 85% deaths. . . . Survivors generally children . . . probably 25% this number frozen to death before help arrived."

A later relief expedition followed, funded by the Red Cross, dividing itself in the Aleutian Islands into six groups of two doctors and two nurses each, then boarding other ships and dispersing.

The first group disembarked at a fishing village called Micknick. They arrived too late. Only half a dozen adults survived. Thirty-eight adults and twelve children had died. A small house had been turned into an orphanage for fifteen children. The group crossed the Naknek River to a village with a seafood cannery. Twenty-four adult Eskimos had lived there before the epidemic. Twenty-two had died; a twenty-third death occurred the day after the relief expedition arrived. Sixteen children, now orphans, survived. On Nushagak Bay the Peterson Packing Company had established a headquarters and warehouse. Nurses went hut to hut. "The epidemic of influenza had been most severe at this place, few adults living. On making a search Drs. Healy and Reiley found a few natives bedfast. . . . The doctors worked most faithfully but help arrived too late and five of the patients died."

There was worse. Another rescue team reported, "Numerous villages were found but no sign of life about except for packs of half-starved, semiwild dogs." The Eskimos there lived in what was called a "barabara." Barabaras were circular structures two-thirds underground; they were built like that to withstand the shrieking winds that routinely blew at hurricane force, winds that ripped conventional structures apart. One rescuer described a barabara as "roughed over with slabs of peat sod, . . . entrance to which is gained through a tunnel of from four to five feet in height, this tunnel being its only means of light and ventilation, in most cases; about the sides of these rooms are dug shelves and in these shelves, on mattresses of dried grasses and furs, the people sleep."

Entire family groups, a dozen people or more, lived in this one room. "On entering these barabaras, Dr. McGillicuddy's party found heaps of dead bodies on the shelves and floors, men, women, and children and the majority of the cases too far decomposed to be handled."

The virus probably did not kill all of them directly. But it struck so suddenly, with such simultaneity, it left no one well enough to care for any others, no one to get food, no one to get water. And those who could have survived, surrounded by bodies, bodies of people they loved, might well have preferred to go where their family had gone, might well have wanted to no longer be alone.

And then the dogs would have come.

"It was quite impossible to estimate the number of dead as the starving dogs had dug their way into many huts and devoured the dead, a few bones and clothing left to tell the story."

All the relief party could do was tie ropes around remains, drag them outside, and bury them.

On the opposite edge of the continent the story was the same. In Labrador man clung to existence with tenacity but not much more permanency than seaweed drying on a rock, vulnerable to the crash of surf at high tide. The Reverend Henry Gordon left the village of Cartwright in late October and returned a few days later, on October 30. He found "not a soul to be seen anywhere, and a strange, unusual silence." Heading home, he met a Hudson's Bay Company man who told him "sickness . . . has struck the place like a cyclone, two days after the Mail boat had left." Gordon went from house to house. "Whole households lay inanimate on their kitchen floors, unable even to feed themselves or look after the fire."

Twenty-six of one hundred souls had died. Farther up the coast, it was worse.

Of 220 people at Hebron, 150 died. The weather was already bitter cold. The dead lay in their beds, sweat having frozen their bedclothes to them. Gordon and some others from Cartwright made no effort to dig graves, consigning the bodies to the sea. He wrote, "A feeling of intense resentment at the callousness of the authorities, who sent us the disease by mail-boat, and then left us to sink or swim, filled one's heart almost to the exclusion of all else. . . ."

Then there was Okak. Two hundred sixty-six people had lived in

Okak, and many dogs, dogs nearly wild. When the virus came it struck so hard so fast people could not care for themselves or feed the dogs. The dogs grew hungry, crazed with hunger, devoured each other, and then wildly smashed through windows and doors, and fed. The Reverend Andrew Asboe survived with his rifle beside him; he personally killed over one hundred dogs.

When the Reverend Walter Perret arrived, only fifty-nine people out of 266 still lived. He and the survivors did the only work there was. "The ground was frozen hard as iron, and the work of digging was as hard as ever work was. It took about two weeks to do it, and when it was finished it was 32 feet long, 10 feet wide, and eight feet deep." Now began the task of dragging the corpses to the pit. They laid 114 bodies in the pit, each wrapped in calico, sprinkled disinfectants over them, and covered the trench, placing rocks on top to prevent the dogs from tearing it up.

In all of Labrador, at least one-third the total population died.

The virus pierced the ice of the Arctic and climbed the roadless mountains of Kentucky. It also penetrated the jungle.

Among Westerners the heaviest blows fell upon young adults densely packed together, civilian or military. Metropolitan Life Insurance found that 6.21 percent of *all* coal miners—not just those with influenza— whom it insured between the ages of twenty-five and forty-five died; in that same age group, 3.26 percent of *all* industrial workers it insured died—comparable to the worst rates in the army camps.

In Frankfurt the mortality rate of all those hospitalized with influenza— not all those with pneumonia—was 27.3 percent. In Cologne the mayor, Konrad Adenauer, who would become one of Europe's great statesmen, said the disease left thousands "too exhausted to hate."

In Paris the government closed only schools, fearing that anything else would hurt morale. The death rate there was 10 percent of influenza victims and 50 percent of those who developed any complications. "These cases," noted one French physician, "were remarkable for the severity of the symptoms and the rapidity with which certain forms progressed to death." Although the symptoms in France were typical of the disease elsewhere, deep into the epidemic physicians seemed to purposely misdiagnose it as cholera or dysentery and rarely reported it.

And populations whose immune systems were naive, whose immune systems had seen few if any influenza viruses of any kind, were not just decimated but sometimes annihilated. This was true not only of Eskimos but of all Native Americans, of Pacific Islanders, of Africans.

In Gambia, 8 percent of the Europeans would die, but from the interior one British visitor reported, "I found whole villages of 300 to 400 families completely wiped out, the houses having fallen in on the unburied dead, and the jungle having crept in within two months, obliterating whole settlements."

Even when the virus mutated toward mildness, it still killed efficiently in those whose immune systems had rarely or never been exposed to influenza. The USS *Logan* reached Guam on October 26. Nearly 95 percent of American sailors ashore caught the disease, but only a single sailor died. The same virus killed almost 5 percent of the entire native population in a few weeks.

In Cape Town and several other cities in South Africa, influenza would kill 4 percent of the entire population within four weeks of the first reported cases. Thirty-two percent of white South Africans and 46 percent of the blacks would be attacked; 0.82 percent of white Europeans would die, along with at least 2.72 percent—likely a far, far higher percentage—of black Africans.

In Mexico the virus swarmed through the dense population centers and through the jungles, overwhelming occupants of mining camps, slum dwellers and slum landlords, and rural peasants alike. In the state of Chiapas, 10 percent of the entire population—not 10 percent of those with influenza—would die.

The virus ripped through Senegal, Sierra Leone, Spain, and Switzerland, leaving each devastated and keening with a death toll that in some areas exceeded 10 percent of the overall population.

In Brazil—where the virus was relatively mild, at least compared with Mexico or for that matter Chile—Rio de Janeiro suffered an attack rate of 33 percent.

In Buenos Aires, Argentina, the virus attacked nearly 55 percent of the population.

In Japan it attacked more than one-third of the population.

The virus would kill 7 percent of the entire population in much of Russia and Iran.

In Guam, 10 percent of the population would die.

Elsewhere the mortality exceeded even that. In the Fiji Islands, 14 percent of the population would die *in the sixteen days between November 25 and December 10*. It was impossible to bury the dead. Wrote one observer, "day and night trucks rumbled through the streets, filled with bodies for the constantly burning pyres."

A very few—very few—isolated locations around the world, where it was possible to impose a rigid quarantine and where authorities did so ruthlessly, escaped the disease entirely. American Samoa was one such place. There not a single person died of influenza.

Across a few miles of ocean lay Western Samoa, seized from Germany by New Zealand at the start of war. On September 30, 1918, its population was 38,302, before the steamer *Talune* brought the disease to the island. A few months later, the population was 29,802. *Twenty-two percent of the population died.*

Huge but unknown numbers died in China. In Chungking one-half the population of the city was ill.

And yet the most terrifying numbers would come from India. As elsewhere, India had suffered a spring wave. As elsewhere, this spring wave was relatively benign. In September influenza returned to Bombay. As elsewhere, it was no longer benign.

Yet India was not like elsewhere. There influenza would take on truly killing dimensions. A serious epidemic of bubonic plague had struck there in 1900, and it had struck Bombay especially hard. In 1918 the peak daily influenza mortality in Bombay almost doubled that of the 1900 bubonic plague, and the case mortality rate for influenza reached 10.3 percent.

Throughout the Indian subcontinent, there was only death. Trains left one station with the living. They arrived with the dead and dying, the corpses removed as the trains pulled into station. British troops, Caucasians, in India suffered a case mortality rate of 9.61 percent. For Indian troops, 21.69 percent of those who caught influenza died. One hospital in Delhi treated 13,190 influenza patients; 7,044 of those patients died.

The most devastated region was the Punjab. One physician reported that hospitals were so "choked that it was impossible to remove the dead quickly enough to make room for the dying. The streets and lanes of the city were littered with dead and dying people. . . . Nearly every household was lamenting a death and everywhere terror reigned."

Normally corpses there were cremated in burning ghats, level spaces at the top of the stepped riverbank, and the ashes given to the river. The supply of firewood was quickly exhausted, making cremation impossible, and the rivers became clogged with corpses.

In the Indian subcontinent alone, it is likely that close to twenty million died, and quite possibly the death toll exceeded that number.

Victor Vaughan, Welch's old ally, sitting in the office of the surgeon general of the army and head of the army's Division of Communicable Diseases, watched the virus move across the earth. "If the epidemic continues its mathematical rate of acceleration, civilization could easily," he wrote in hand, "disappear . . . from the face of the earth within a matter of a few more weeks."

■ Part IX
LINGERER

CHAPTER THIRTY-ONE

VAUGHAN BELIEVED that the influenza virus came close to threatening the existence of civilization. In fact, some diseases depend upon civilization for their own existence. Measles is one example. Since a single exposure to measles usually gives lifetime immunity, the measles virus cannot find enough susceptible individuals in small towns to survive; without a new human generation to infect, the virus dies out. Epidemiologists have computed that measles requires an unvaccinated population of at least half a million people living in fairly close contact to continue to exist.

The influenza virus is different. Since birds provide a natural home for it, influenza does not depend upon civilization. In terms of its own survival, it did not matter if humans existed or not.

Twenty years before the great influenza pandemic, H. G. Wells published *War of the Worlds*, a novel in which Martians invaded the earth. They loosed upon the world their death ships, and they were indomitable. They began to feed upon humans, sucking the life force from them down to the marrow of the bone. Man, for all his triumphs of the nineteenth century, a century in which his achievements had reordered the world, had become suddenly impotent. No force known to mankind, no technology or strategy or effort or heroism that any nation or person on earth had developed, could stand against the invaders.

Wells wrote, "I felt the first inkling of a thing that presently grew quite clear in my mind, that oppressed me for many days, a sense of dethronement, a persuasion that I was no longer a master, but an animal among the animals. . . . The fear and empire of man had passed away."

But just as the destruction of the human race seemed inevitable, nature intervened. The invaders were themselves invaded; the earth's infectious pathogens killed them. Natural processes had done what science could not.

With the influenza virus, natural processes began to work as well.

At first those processes had made the virus more lethal. Whether it first jumped from an animal host to man in Kansas or in some other place, as it passed from person to person it adapted to its new host, became increasingly efficient in its ability to infect, and changed from the virus that caused a generally mild first wave of disease in the spring of 1918 to the lethal and explosive killer of the second wave in the fall.

But once this happened, once it achieved near-maximum efficiency, two other natural processes came into play.

One process involved immunity. Once the virus passed through a population, that population developed at least some immunity to it. Victims were not likely to be reinfected by the same virus, not until it had undergone antigen drift. In a city or town, the cycle from first case to the end of a local epidemic in 1918 generally ran six to eight weeks. In the army camps, with the men packed so densely, the cycle took usually three to four weeks.

Individual cases continued to occur after that, but the explosion of disease ended, and it ended abruptly. A graph of cases would look like a bell curve—but one chopped off almost like a cliff just after the peak, with new cases suddenly dropping to next to nothing. In Philadelphia, for example, in the week ending October 16 the disease killed 4,597 people. It was ripping the city apart, emptying the streets, sparking rumors of the Black Death. But new cases dropped so precipitously that only ten days later, on October 26, the order closing public places was lifted. By the armistice on November 11, influenza had almost entirely disappeared from that city. The virus burned through available fuel. Then it quickly faded away.

The second process occurred within the virus. It was only influenza. By nature the influenza virus is dangerous, considerably more dangerous than the common aches and fever lead people to believe, but it does not kill routinely as it did in 1918. The 1918 pandemic reached an extreme of virulence unknown in any other widespread influenza outbreak in history.

But the 1918 virus, like all influenza viruses, like all viruses that form mutant swarms, mutated rapidly. There is a mathematical concept called "reversion to the mean"; this states simply that an extreme event is likely to be followed by a less extreme event. This is not a law, only a probability. The 1918 virus stood at an extreme; any mutations were more likely to make it less lethal than more lethal. In general, that is what happened. So just as it seemed that the virus would bring civilization to its knees, would do what the plagues of the Middle Ages had done, would remake the world, the virus mutated toward its mean, toward the behavior of most influenza viruses. As time went on, it became less lethal.

This first became apparent in army cantonments in the United States. Of the army's twenty largest cantonments, the first five attacked saw roughly 20 percent of all soldiers who caught influenza develop pneumonia. And 37.3 percent of the soldiers who developed pneumonia died. The worst numbers came from Camp Sherman in Ohio, which suffered the highest percentage of soldiers killed and was one of the first camps hit: 35.7 percent of influenza cases at Sherman developed pneumonia. And 61.3 percent of those pneumonia victims died. Sherman doctors carried a stigma for this, and the army investigated but found them as competent as elsewhere. They did all that was being done elsewhere. They were simply struck by a particularly lethal strain of the virus.

In the last five camps attacked, hit on average three weeks later, only 7.1 percent of influenza victims developed pneumonia. And only 17.8 percent of the soldiers who developed pneumonia died.

One alternative explanation to this improvement is that army doctors simply got better at preventing and treating pneumonia. But people of scientific and epidemiological accomplishment looked hard for any evidence of that. They found none. The army's chief investigator was George Soper, later handpicked by Welch to oversee the nation's first effort to coordinate a comprehensive program of cancer research. Soper reviewed all written reports and interviewed many medical officers. He concluded that the only effective measure used against influenza in any of the camps had been to isolate both individual influenza victims and, if necessary, entire commands that became infected: these efforts "failed when and where they were carelessly applied" but "did some good. . . . when and where they were rigidly carried out." He found no evidence that anything else worked, that anything else affected the course of the disease, that anything else changed except the virus itself. The later the disease attacked, the less vicious the blow.

Inside each camp the same thing held true. Soldiers struck down in the first ten days or two weeks died at much higher rates than soldiers in the same camp struck down late in the epidemic or after the epidemic actually ended.

Similarly, the first cities invaded by the virus—Boston, Baltimore, Pittsburgh, Philadelphia, Louisville, New York, New Orleans, and smaller cities hit at the same time—all suffered grievously. And in those same places, the people infected later in the epidemic were not becoming as ill, were not dying at the same rate, as those infected in the first two to three weeks.

Cities struck later in the epidemic also usually had lower mortality rates. In one of the most careful epidemiological studies of the epidemic in one state, the investigator noted that, in Connecticut, "one factor that appeared to affect the mortality rate was proximity in time to the original outbreak at New London, the point at which the disease was first introduced into Connecticut. . . . The virus was most virulent or most readily communicable when it first reached the state, and thereafter became generally attenuated."

The same pattern held true throughout the country and, for that matter, the world. It was not a rigid predictor. The virus was never completely consistent. But places hit later tended to be hit more easily. San Antonio suffered one of the highest attack rates but lowest death rates in the country; the virus there infected 53.5 percent of the population, and 98 percent of all homes in the city had at least one person sick with influenza. But there the virus had mutated toward mildness; only 0.8 percent of those who got influenza died. (This death rate was still double that of normal influenza.) The virus itself, more than any treatment provided, determined who lived and who died.

A decade after the pandemic, a careful and comprehensive scientific review of findings and statistics not only in the United States but around the world confirmed, "In the later stages of the epidemic the supposedly characteristic influenza lesions were less frequently found, the share of secondary invaders was more plainly recognizable, and the differences of locality were sharply marked. . . . [I]n 1919 the 'water-logged' lungs"— those in which death came quickly from ARDS—"were relatively rarely encountered."

Despite aberrations, then, in general in youth the virus was violent and lethal; in maturity it mellowed. The later the epidemic struck a locality, and the later within that local epidemic someone got sick, the less lethal the influenza. The correlations are not perfect. Louisville suffered a violent attack in both spring and fall. The virus was unstable and always different. But a correlation does exist between the timing of the outbreak in a region and lethality. Even as the virus mellowed it still killed. It still killed often enough that in maturity it would have been, except for its own younger self, the most lethal influenza virus ever known. But timing mattered.

The East and South, hit earliest, were hit the hardest. The West Coast was hit less hard. And the middle of the country suffered the least. In Seattle, in Portland, in Los Angeles, in San Diego, the dead did not pile up as in the East. In St. Louis, in Chicago, in Indianapolis, the dead did not pile up as in the West. But if the dead did not pile up there as they had in Philadelphia and New Orleans, they did still pile up.

By late November, with few exceptions the virus had made its way around the world. The second wave was over, and the world was exhausted. And man was about to become the hunter.

But the virus, even as it lost some of its virulence, was not yet finished. Only weeks after the disease seemed to have dissipated, when town after town had congratulated itself on surviving it—and in some places where people had had the hubris to believe they had defeated it—after health boards and emergency councils had canceled orders to close theaters, schools, and churches and to wear masks, a third wave broke over the earth.

The virus had mutated again. It had not become radically different. People who had gotten sick in the second wave had a fair amount of immunity to another attack, just as people sickened in the first wave had fared better than others in the second wave. But it mutated enough, its antigens drifted enough, to rekindle the epidemic.

Some places were not touched by the third wave at all. But many—in fact most—were. By December 11, Blue and the Public Health Service issued a bulletin warning that "influenza has not passed and severe epidemic conditions exist in various parts of the country. . . . In California, increase; Iowa, a marked increase; Kentucky, decided recrudescence in Louisville and larger towns, and in contrast to earlier stage of epidemic disease now affects many schoolchildren; Louisiana, disease again increased in New Orleans, Shreveport, [in] Lake Charles height reached equalled last wave; . . . St. Louis 1,700 cases in three days; Nebraska very serious; Ohio recrudescences in Cincinnati, Cleveland, Columbus, Akron, Ashtabula, Salem, Medina . . . ; in Pennsylvania, conditions are worse than the original outbreak in Johnstown, Erie, Newcastle. The state of Washington shows a sharp increase. . . . West Virginia reports recrudescence in Charleston."

By any standard except that of the second wave, this third wave was a lethal epidemic. And in a few isolated areas—such as Michigan—December and January were actually worse than October. In Phoenix for three days in a row in mid-January, the new cases set a record exceeding any in the fall. Quitman, Georgia, issued twenty-seven epidemic ordinances that took effect December 13, 1918, after the disease had seemingly passed. Savannah on January 15 ordered theaters and public gathering places closed—for a third time—with even more rigid restrictions than before. San Francisco had gotten off lightly in the fall wave, as had the rest of the West Coast, but the third wave struck hard.

In fact, of all the major cities in the country, San Francisco had confronted the fall wave most honestly and efficiently. That may have had something to do with its surviving, and rebuilding itself after, the massive earthquake of only a dozen years before. Now on September 21 public health director William Hassler quarantined all naval installations, even before any cases surfaced in them or in the city. He mobilized the entire city in advance, recruiting hundreds of drivers and volunteers and dividing the city into districts, each with its own medical personnel, phones, transport and supply, and emergency hospitals in schools and churches. He closed public places. And far from the usual assurances that the disease was ordinary "la grippe," on October 22 the mayor, Hassler, the Red Cross, the Chamber of Commerce, and the Labor Council jointly declared in a full-page newspaper ad, "Wear a mask and save your life!" claiming that it was "99% proof against influenza." By October 26, the Red Cross had distributed one hundred thousand masks. Simultaneously, while local facilities geared up to produce vaccine, thousands of doses of a vaccine made by a Tufts scientist were raced across the continent on the country's fastest train.

In San Francisco, people felt a sense of control. Instead of the paralyzing fear found in too many other communities, it seemed to inspire. Historian Alfred Crosby has provided a picture of the city under siege, and his picture shows citizens behaving with heroism, anxious and fearful but accepting their duty. When schools closed, teachers volunteered as nurses, orderlies, telephone operators. On November 21, every siren in the city signaled that masks could come off. San Francisco had—to that point— survived with far fewer deaths than had been feared, and citizens believed that the masks deserved the credit. But if anything helped, it would have been the organization Hassler had set in place in advance.

The next day the *Chronicle* crowed that in the city's history "one of the most thrilling episodes will be the story of how gallantly the city of Saint Francis behaved when the black wings of war-bred pestilence hovered over the city."

They thought that *they* had controlled it, that *they* had stopped it. They were mistaken. The masks were useless. The vaccine was useless. The city had simply been lucky. Two weeks later, the third wave struck. Although at its peak it killed only half as many as did the second wave, it made the final death rates for the city the worst on the West Coast.

With the exception of a few small outposts that isolated themselves, there was by early in 1919 only one place the virus had missed.

Australia had escaped. It had escaped because of a stringent quarantine of incoming ships. Some ships arrived there with attack rates as high as 43 percent and fatality rates among *all* passengers as high as 7 percent. But the quarantine kept the virus out, kept the continent safe, until late December 1918 when, with influenza having receded around the world, a troopship carrying ninety ill soldiers arrived. Although they too were quarantined, the disease penetrated—apparently through medical personnel treating troops.

By then the strain had lost much of its lethality. In Australia the death rates from influenza were far less than in any other Westernized nation

on earth, barely one-third that of the United States, not even one-quarter
that of Italy. But it was lethal enough.

When it struck in January and February, the war had been over for more
than two months. Censorship had ended with it. And so in Australia the
newspapers were free to write what they wanted. And, more than in any
other English-language newspaper, what they wrote of was terror.

"We are told by some that the influenza is a return of the old 'Black
death,'" reported one Sydney newspaper. Another quoted the classic,
Daniel Defoe's *Journal of the Plague Year*—a work of fiction—for advice
on precautions to take to prevent "the influenza plague." And headlines of
terror ran day after day after day after day: "How They Fought Plagues in
the Old Days," "The Pneumonic Plague," "Fighting the Plague," "Plagues
in the Past," "The Pagans and the Plague," "Did the Plague Start in NSW?"
"Catholic Chaplains in Plague Stricken Camps," "Catholics as Plague
Fighters."

The pandemic itself—even in this its most mild incarnation in the
developed world—was terrifying enough that those who lived through it
as children remembered it not as influenza at all, but as plague. One Australian historian in the 1990s was recording oral histories. She was struck
when people she interviewed mentioned "Bubonic Plague," and she
explored the issue further.

One subject told her, "I can recall the Bubonic Plague, people dying by
the hundreds around us that was come back from the First World War."

Another: "We had to get vaccinated. . . . And I bear the scar today where
I was inoculated against the Bubonic Plague."

Another: "I can remember the Plague. There were doctors going
around in cabs with gowns and masks over their faces."

Another: "They all wore masks . . . after the war and how they used to
be worried here in Sydney . . . about the Plague."

Another: "We were quarantined, our food was delivered to the front
door. . . . We didn't read about the Bubonic Plague. We lived it."

Another: "[T]hey called it the Bubonic Plague. But in France they
called it bronchial pneumonia. See that's what they said my brother died
from. . . ."

Another: "The Plague. The Bubonic Plague. Yes, I can remember
that. . . . I always understood it was the same kind of flu that swept

Europe, the Black Death in the Middle Ages. I think it was the same kind of thing, it was carried by fleas on rats."

Another: "Bubonic Plague . . . I think it might have been called a form of influenza towards the finish. . . . The Bubonic Plague was a thing that stuck in my mind . . ."

Yet this was after all only influenza, and the influenza that struck Australia in 1919 was weaker than it was anywhere else in the world. Perhaps the measure of the extraordinary power of the 1918 virus was this: in Australia, without a censored press, the memory that stuck in the mind was not of influenza at all. It was of the Black Death.

The virus was still not finished. All through the spring of 1919 a kind of rolling thunder moved above the earth, intermittent, unleashing sometimes a sudden localized storm, sometimes even a lightning bolt, and sometimes passing over with only a rumble of threatened violence in the distant and dark sky.

It remained violent enough to do one more thing.

CHAPTER THIRTY-TWO

THE OVERWHELMING MAJORITY of victims, especially in the Western world, recovered quickly and fully. This was after all only influenza.

But the virus sometimes caused one final complication, one final sequela. The influenza virus affected the brain and nervous system. All high fevers cause delirium, but this was something else. An army physician at Walter Reed Hospital investigating serious mental disturbances and even psychoses that seemed to follow an attack of influenza specifically noted, "Delirium occurring at the height of the disease and clearing with the cessation of fever is not considered in this report."

The connection between influenza and various mental instabilities seemed clear. The evidence was almost entirely anecdotal, the worst and weakest kind of evidence, but it convinced the vast majority of contemporary observers that influenza could alter mental processes. What convinced them were observations such as these:

From Britain: ". . . profound mental inertia with intense physical prostration. Delirium has been very common. . . . It has varied from mere confusion of ideas through all grades of intensity up to maniacal excitement."

From Italy: ". . . influenzal psychoses of the acute period . . . as a rule subside in two or three weeks. The psychosis, however, may pass into a state of mental collapse, with stupor which may persist and become actual dementia. In other cases . . . depression and restlessness . . . to [which] can be attributed the large number of suicides during the pandemic of influenza."

From France: ". . . frequent and serious mental disturbances during convalescence from and as a result of influenza. . . . The mental disturbances sometimes took on the form of acute delirium with agitation, violence, fear and erotic excitation and at other times was of a depressive nature . . . fear of persecution."

From different U.S. Army cantonments:

". . . The mental condition was either apathetic or there was an active delirium. Cerebration was slow. . . . The patient's statements and assurances were unreliable, a moribund person stating he felt very well. . . . In other cases, apprehensiveness was most striking."

". . . The mental depression of the patient is often out of all proportion to the other symptoms."

". . . Nervous symptoms appeared early, restlessness and delirium being marked."

". . . melancholia, hysteria, and insanity with suicidal intent."

". . . Toxic involvement of the nervous system was evident in all the more severe cases."

". . . Many patients lay in muttering delirium which persisted after the temperature was normal."

". . . Symptoms referable to the central nervous system were seen at times, as twitching of the muscles of the fingers, forearms, and face, . . . an active, even maniacal occasional delirium, or more usually the low mumbling type."

". . . Infectious psychosis was seen in 18 cases, from simple transient hallucinations to maniacal frenzy with needed mechanical restraint."

Contemporary observers also linked influenza to an increase in Parkinson's disease a decade later. (Some have theorized that the patients in Oliver Sacks's *The Awakening* were victims of the 1918 influenza pandemic.) Many believed that the virus could cause schizophrenia, and in 1926, Karl Menninger studied links between influenza and schizophrenia. His study was considered significant enough that the *American Journal of Psychiatry* identified it as a "classic" article and reprinted it in 1994. Menninger spoke of the "almost unequalled neurotoxicity of influenza" and noted that two-thirds of those diagnosed with schizophrenia after an attack of influenza had completely recovered five years later. Recovery from schizophrenia is extremely rare, suggesting that some reparable process had caused the initial symptoms.

In 1927 the American Medical Association's review of hundreds of medical journal articles from around the world concluded, "There seems to be general agreement that influenza may act on the brain. . . . From the delirium accompanying many acute attacks to the psychoses that develop as 'post-influenzal' manifestations, there is no doubt that the neuropsychiatric effects of influenza are profound and varied. . . . The effect of the influenza virus on the nervous system is hardly second to its effect on the respiratory tract."

In 1934 a similar comprehensive review by British scientists agreed: "There would appear to be no doubt that influenza exerts a profound influence on the nervous system."

In 1992 an investigator studying the connection between suicide and the war instead concluded, "World War I did not influence suicide; the Great Influenza Epidemic caused it to increase."

A 1996 virology textbook said, "A wide spectrum of central nervous system involvement has been observed during influenza A virus infections in humans, ranging from irritability, drowsiness, boisterousness, and confusion to the more serious manifestations of psychosis, delirium, and coma."

The 1997 Hong Kong virus that killed six of the eighteen people infected provided some physical evidence. Autopsies of two victims showed "edematous brains." "Edema" means "swelling." "Most remarkably, bone marrow, lymphoid tissue, liver, and spleen of both patients were heavily infiltrated with [macrophages]. . . . One patient even had such cells on the meninges"—the membranes surrounding the brain and spinal cord—"and in the white matter of the cerebrum." The most likely reason for these macrophages to have infiltrated the brain was to follow the virus there, and kill it. And that 1997 pathology report echoes some from 1918: "*In cases accompanied by delirium, the meninges of the brain are richly infiltrated by serous fluid and the capillaries are injected. . . . Necropsy in the fatal cases demonstrated congestive lesions with small meningeal hemorrhages and especially in islands of edema in the cortical substance surrounding greatly dilated small vessels . . . hemorrhages into gray matter of the cord . . . [brain] tissue cells were altered in these zones of . . . edema.*"

In 2002 Robert Webster, one of the world's leading experts on the virus at St. Jude Children's Hospital in Memphis, observed, "These viruses do from time to time get across to central nervous systems and play hell." He recalled a child in Memphis who was an excellent student, got influenza, and became "a vegetable. I've seen enough examples in my lifetime to believe . . . influenza can get into the brain. It's tenuous but real. Put the virus into chickens, it can go up the olfactory nerve and the chicken's dead."

The 1918 virus did seem to reach the brain. The war fought on that battlefield could destroy brain cells and make it difficult to concentrate, or alter behavior, or interfere with thinking, or even cause temporary psychosis. If this occurred in only a minority of cases, the virus's impact on the mind was nonetheless real.

But that impact would, by terrible coincidence, have a profound effect indeed.

In January 1919 in France, Congressman William Borland of Kansas died, the third congressmen to be killed by the virus. That same month also in Paris, "Colonel" Edward House, Wilson's closest confidant, collapsed with influenza—again.

House had first gotten influenza during the first wave in March 1918, was confined to his home for two weeks, went to Washington and relapsed, and then spent three weeks in bed at the White House. Although a spring attack often conferred immunity to the virus, after the Armistice he was struck down a second time. He was in Europe then, and on November 30 he got up for the first time in ten days and met with French premier Georges Clemenceau for fifteen minutes. Afterward he noted, "Today is the first day I have taken up my official work in person for over a week. I have had influenza 10 days and have been exceeding miserable. . . . So many have died since this epidemic has scourged the world. Many of my staff have died and poor Willard Straight among them."

Now, in January 1919, he was attacked still a third time. He was sick enough that some papers reported him dead. House wryly called the obituaries "all too generous." But the blow was heavy: more than a month after his supposed recovery he wrote in his diary, "When I fell sick in January I lost the thread of affairs and I am not sure that I have ever gotten fully back."

There were affairs of some magnitude to attend to in Paris in early 1919.

Representatives of victorious nations, of weak nations, of nations hoping to be born from the splinters of defeated nations, had all come there to set the terms of peace. Several thousand men from dozens of countries circled around the edges of decision making. Germany would play no role in these decisions; Germany would simply be dictated to. And among this host of nations, this virtual Tower of Babel, a Council of Ten of the most powerful nations supposedly determined the agenda. Even within this tight circle was a tighter one, the "Big Four"—the United States, France, Britain, and Italy. And in reality only three of those four nations mattered. Indeed, only three men mattered.

French premier Georges Clemenceau, known as "the Tiger," negotiated with a bullet in his shoulder, put there by an assassination attempt during the peace conference on February 19. Prime Minister Lloyd George of Great Britain faced such political problems at home he was described as "a greased marble spinning on a glass table top." And there was Wilson, who arrived in Europe the most popular political figure in the world.

For weeks and then months the meetings dragged on, and tens of thousands of pages of drafts and memos and understandings went back and forth between ministers and staff. But Wilson, Clemenceau, and George did not much need these thousands of pages. They were not simply ratifying what foreign ministers and staffs had worked out, nor were they simply making decisions on options presented to them. They were themselves doing much of the actual negotiating. They were bargaining and wheedling, they were demanding and insisting, and they were rejecting.

Often only five or six men would be in a room, including translators. Often, even when Clemenceau and George had others present, Wilson represented the United States alone, with no staff, no secretary of state, no Colonel House, who by now had been all but discarded as untrustworthy by Wilson. Interrupted only by Wilson's relatively brief return to the United States, discussions were interminable. But they were deciding the future of the world.

In October, at the peak of the epidemic in Paris, 4,574 people had died there of influenza or pneumonia. The disease had never entirely left that city. In February 1919, deaths in Paris from influenza and pneumonia climbed back up to 2,676, more than half the peak death toll. Wilson's daughter Margaret had influenza in February; she was kept in bed in

Brussels at the American legation. In March another 1,517 Parisians died, and the *Journal of the American Medical Association* reported that in Paris "the epidemic of influenza which had declined has broken out anew in a most disquieting manner. . . . The epidemic has assumed grave proportions, not only in Paris but in several of the departments."

That month Wilson's wife, his wife's secretary, Chief White House Usher Irwin Hoover, and Cary Grayson, Wilson's personal White House physician and perhaps the single man Wilson trusted the most, were all ill. Clemenceau and Lloyd George both seemed to have mild cases of influenza.

Meanwhile the sessions with George and Clemenceau were often brutal. In late March Wilson told his wife, "Well, thank God I can still fight, and I'll win."

On March 29, Wilson said, "M. Clemenceau called me pro-German and left the room."

Wilson continued to fight, insisting, "The only principle I recognize is that of the consent of the governed." On April 2, after the negotiations for the day finished, he called the French "damnable"—for him, a deeply religious man, an extreme epithet. He told his press spokesman Ray Stannard Baker, "[W]e've got to make peace on the principles laid down and accepted, or not make it at all."

The next day, April 3, a Thursday, at three P.M., Wilson seemed in fine health, according to Cary Grayson. Then, very suddenly at six o'clock, Grayson saw Wilson "seized with violent paroxysms of coughing, which were so severe and frequent that it interfered with his breathing."

The attack came so suddenly that Grayson suspected that Wilson had been poisoned, that an assassination attempt had been made. But it soon became obvious the diagnosis was simpler, if only marginally more reassuring.

Joseph Tumulty, Wilson's chief of staff, had stayed in Washington to monitor political developments at home. Grayson and he exchanged telegrams daily, sometimes several times a day. But the information of the president's illness was too sensitive for a telegram. Grayson did wire him, "The President took very severe cold last night; confined to bed." Simultaneously he also wrote a confidential letter to be hand-delivered: "The President was taken violently sick last Thursday. He had a fever of over 103 and profuse diarrhoea. . . . [It was] the beginning of an attack of influenza. That night was one of the worst through which I have ever passed. I was able to control the spasms of coughing but his condition looked very serious."

Donald Frary, a young aide on the American peace delegation, came down with influenza the same day Wilson did. Four days later he died at age twenty-five.

For several days Wilson lay in bed, unable to move. On the fourth day, he sat up. Grayson wired Tumulty, "Am taking every precaution with him. . . . Your aid and presence were never needed more."

Wilson for the first time was well enough to have visitors. He received American commissioners in his bedroom and said, "Gentlemen, this is not a meeting of the Peace Commission. It is more a Council of War."

Just before getting sick Wilson had threatened to leave the conference, to return to the United States without a treaty rather than yield on his principles. He repeated that threat again, telling Grayson to order the *George Washington* to be ready to sail as soon as he was well enough to travel. The next day Gilbert Close, his secretary, wrote his wife, "I never knew the president to be in such a difficult frame of mind as now. Even while lying in bed he manifested peculiarities."

Meanwhile the negotiations continued; Wilson, unable to participate, was forced to rely on House as his stand-in. (Wilson had even less trust in Secretary of State Robert Lansing, whom he largely ignored, than in House.) For several days Wilson continued to talk about leaving France, telling his wife, "If I have lost the fight, which I would not have done had I been on my feet, I will retire in good order, so we will go home."

Then, on April 8, Wilson insisted upon personally rejoining the negotiations. He could not go out. Clemenceau and George came to his bedroom, but the conversations did not go well. His public threat to leave had infuriated Clemenceau, who privately called him "a cook who keeps her trunk ready in the hallway."

Grayson wrote that despite "that ill-omened attack of influenza, the insidious effects of which he was not in good condition to resist, . . . [the president] insisted upon holding conferences while he was still confined to his sickbed. When he was able to get up he began to drive himself as hard as before—morning, afternoon, and frequently evening conferences."

Herbert Hoover, not part of the American peace delegation but a large figure in Paris because he had charge of feeding a desolated and barren Europe, said, "Prior to that time, in all matters with which I had to deal, he was incisive, quick to grasp essentials, unhesitating in conclusions, and most willing to take advice from men he trusted. . . . [Now] others as well as I found we had to push against an unwilling mind. And at times, when I just had to get decisions, I suffered as much from having to mentally push as he did in coming to conclusions." Hoover believed Wilson's mind had lost "resiliency."

Colonel Starling of the Secret Service noticed that Wilson "lacked his old quickness of grasp, and tired easily." He became obsessed with such details as who was using the official automobiles. When Ray Stannard Baker was first allowed to see Wilson again, he trembled at Wilson's sunken eyes, at his weariness, at his pale and haggard look, like that of a man whose flesh has shrunk away from his face, showing his skull.

Chief Usher Irwin Hoover recalled several new and very strange ideas that Wilson suddenly believed, including one that his home was filled with French spies: "Nothing we could say could disabuse his mind of this thought. About this time he also acquired a peculiar notion he was personally responsible for all the property in the furnished place he was occupying. . . . Coming from the President, whom we all knew so well, these were very funny things, and we could but surmise that something queer was happening in his mind. One thing was certain: he was never the same after this little spell of sickness."

Grayson confided to Tumulty, "This is a matter that worries me."

"I have never seen the President look so worn and tired," Ray Baker said. In the afternoon "he could not remember without an effort what the council had done in the forenoon."

Then, abruptly, still on his sickbed, only a few days after he had threatened to leave the conference unless Clemenceau yielded to his demands, without warning to or discussion with any other Americans, Wilson suddenly abandoned principles he had previously insisted upon. He yielded to Clemenceau everything of significance Clemenceau wanted, virtually all of which Wilson had earlier opposed.

Now, in bed, he approved a formula Clemenceau had written demanding German reparations and that Germany accept all responsibility for starting the war. The Rhineland would be demilitarized; Germany would not be allowed to have troops within thirty miles of the east bank of the Rhine. The rich coal fields of the Saar region would be mined by France and the region would be administered by the new League of Nations for fifteen years, and then a plebiscite would determine whether the region would belong to France or Germany. The provinces of Alsace and Lorraine, which Germany had seized after the Franco-Prussian War, were moved from Germany back to France. West Prussia and Posen were given to Poland—creating the "Polish corridor" that separated two parts of Germany. The German air force was eliminated, its army limited to one hundred thousand men, its colonies stripped away—but not freed, simply redistributed to other powers.

Even Lloyd George commented on Wilson's "nervous and spiritual breakdown in the middle of the Conference."

Grayson wrote, "These are terrible days for the President physically and otherwise."

As Grayson made that notation, Wilson was conceding to Italy much of its demands and agreeing to Japan's insistence that it take over German concessions in China. In return the Japanese offered an oral—not written—promise of good behavior, a promise given not even to Wilson personally or, for that matter, to any chief of state, but to British Foreign Secretary Alfred Balfour.

On May 7 the Germans were presented with the treaty. They complained that it violated the very principles Wilson had declared were inviolate. Wilson left the meeting saying, "What abominable manners. . . . This is the most tactless speech I have ever heard."

Yet they had not reminded Wilson and the world that he had once said that a lasting peace could be achieved only by—and that he had once called for—"A peace without victory."

Wilson also told Baker, "If I were a German, I think I should never sign it."

Four months later Wilson suffered a major and debilitating stroke. For months his wife and Grayson would control all access to him and become arguably the de facto most important policy makers in the country.

In 1929 one man wrote a memoir in which he said that two doctors believed Wilson was suffering from arteriosclerosis when he went to Paris. In 1946 a physician voiced the same opinion in print. In 1958 a major biography of Wilson stated that experts on arteriosclerosis questioned Grayson's diagnosis of influenza and believed Wilson had instead suffered a vascular occlusion—a minor stroke. In 1960 a historian writing about the health of presidents said, "Present-day views are that [Wilson's disorientation] was based on brain damage, probably caused by arteriosclerotic occlusion of blood vessels." In 1964 another historian called Wilson's attack "thrombosis." In a 1970 article in the *Journal of American History,* titled "Woodrow Wilson's Neurological Illness," another historian called it "a little stroke."

Only one historian, Alfred Crosby, seems to have paid any attention to Wilson's actual symptoms—including high fever, severe coughing, and total prostration, all symptoms that perfectly fit influenza and have no association whatsoever with stroke—and the on-site diagnosis of Grayson, an excellent physician highly respected by such men as Welch, Gorgas, Flexner, and Vaughan.

Despite Crosby, the myth of Wilson's having suffered a minor stroke persists. Even a prize-winning account of the peace conference published in 2002 observes, "Wilson by contrast had aged visibly and the tic in his cheek grew more pronounced. . . . [It] may have been a minor stroke, a forerunner of the massive one he was to have four months later."

There was no stroke. There was only influenza. Indeed, the virus may have contributed to the stroke. Damage to blood vessels in the brain were often noted in autopsy reports in 1918, as they were in 1997. Grayson believed influenza was a cause of Wilson's "final breakdown." An epidemiological study published in 2004 demonstrates definite linkage between influenza and stroke.

It is of course impossible to say what Wilson would have done had he not become sick. Perhaps he would have made the concessions anyway, trading every principle away to save his League of Nations. Or perhaps he would have sailed home as he had threatened to do just as he was succumbing to the disease. Then either there would have been no treaty or his walkout would have forced Clemenceau to compromise.

No one can know what would have happened. One can only know what did happen.

Influenza did visit the peace conference. Influenza did strike Wilson. Influenza did weaken him physically, and—precisely at the most crucial point of negotiations—influenza did at the least drain from him stamina and the ability to concentrate. That much is certain. And it is almost certain that influenza affected his mind in other, deeper ways.

Historians with virtual unanimity agree that the harshness toward

Germany of the Paris peace treaty helped create the economic hardship, nationalistic reaction, and political chaos that fostered the rise of Adolf Hitler.

It did not require hindsight to see the dangers. They were obvious at the time. John Maynard Keynes quit Paris calling Wilson "the greatest fraud on earth." Later he wrote, "We are at the dead season of our fortunes. . . . Never in the lifetime of men now living has the universal element in the soul of man burnt so dimly." Herbert Hoover believed that the treaty would tear down all Europe, and said so.

Soon after Wilson made his concessions a group of young American diplomatic aides and advisers met in disgust to decide whether to resign in protest. They included Samuel Eliot Morison, William Bullitt, Adolf Berle Jr., Christian Herter, John Foster Dulles, Lincoln Steffens, and Walter Lippmann. All were already or would become among the most influential men in the country. Two would become secretary of state. Bullitt, Berle, and Morison did resign. In September, during the fight over ratifying the treaty, Bullitt revealed to the Senate the private comments of Secretary of State Robert Lansing that the League of Nations would be useless, that the great powers had simply arranged the world to suit themselves.

Berle, later an assistant secretary of state, settled for writing Wilson a blistering letter of resignation: "I am sorry that you did not fight our fight to the finish and that you had so little faith in the millions of men, like myself, in every nation who had faith in you. Our government has consented now to deliver the suffering peoples of the world to new oppressions, subjections and dismemberments—a new century of war."

Wilson had influenza, only influenza.

CHAPTER THIRTY-THREE

O N SEPTEMBER 29, 1919, Sir William Osler began coughing. One of the original "Four Doctors" in a famous portrait of the founding faculty of the Johns Hopkins Medical School, a portrait that symbolized the new primacy of science in American medicine, he was and still is regarded as one of the greatest clinicians in history. A man of wide interests, a friend of Walt Whitman, and author of the textbook that ultimately led to the founding of the Rockefeller Institute for Medical Research, Osler was then at Oxford.

Osler had already suffered one great loss with the death of his only child in the war. Now he suffered as well from a respiratory infection he diagnosed as influenza. In Oxford that fall, influenza was prevalent enough that the dons considered postponing the school term. To his sister-in-law, Osler wrote, "For two days I felt very ill & exhausted by the paroxysms" of coughing. He seemed to recover, but on October 13 his temperature rose to 102.5. He wrote a friend he had "one of those broncho-pneumonias so common after influenza." He tried to work on a talk about Whitman and also wrote Welch and John D. Rockefeller Jr. about giving a grant to his alma mater, McGill University. But on November 7, he felt "a stab and then fireworks" on his right side. Twelve hours later he began coughing again: "A bout arrived which ripped all pleural attachments to smithereens, & with it the pain."

After three weeks his physicans took him off morphine, gave him atropine, and said they were encouraged. On December 5 he received a local anesthetic and a needle was inserted into his lungs to drain fourteen ounces of pus. He gave up working on his Whitman talk and felt certain now of the end, joking, "I've been watching this case for two months and I'm sorry I shall not see the post mortem."

His wife did not like the joke. His pessimism was crushing her: "[W]hatever he says always does come true—so how can I hope for anything but a fatal ending?" She tried to remain optimistic as the disease dragged on. But one day she found him reciting a Tennyson poem: "Of happy men that have the power to die, / And grassy barrows of the happier dead. / Release me, and restore me to the ground. . . ."

He had turned seventy in July. A birthday tribute to him, a *Festschrift*—a collection of scientific articles in his honor—arrived on December 27, entitled, *Contributions to Medical and Biological Research, Dedicated to Sir William Osler*. Publication had been delayed because Welch was editing them. Welch never did anything on time.

His most recent biographer believes that had he been at the Johns Hopkins Hospital instead, he would have received better care. Physicians would have used x rays, electrocardiograms, earlier surgical intervention to drain an empyema, a pocket of pus from the lung. They might have saved him.

He died December 29, 1919, his last words being, "Hold up my head."

He had always held his head high.

If finally it seemed past, yet it wasn't past. In September 1919, as Osler was dying, Blue predicted that influenza would return: "Communities should make plans now for dealing with any recurrences. The most promising way to deal with a possible recurrence is, to sum it up in a single word, 'preparedness.' And now is the time to prepare."

On September 20, 1919, many of the best scientists in the country met to try to reach a consensus on the cause of the disease or course of therapy. They could not, but the *New York Times* stated that the conference marked the beginning of a joint federal, state, and city effort to prevent a recurrence. Two days later the Red Cross distributed its own confidential battle plan internally: "Proposed Staff Organization for Possible Influenza Emergency / Confidential / Note: No publicity is to be given this bulletin until . . . the first indication of a recurrence of influenza in epidemic form, but until such time there should be no public statement by a Red Cross Chapter or Division office."

By February 7, 1920, influenza had returned with enough ferocity that the Red Cross declared, "Owing to the rapid spread of influenza, the safety of the country demands, as a patriotic duty, that all available nurses or anyone with experience in nursing, communicate with the nearest Red Cross chapters or special local epidemic committees, offering their services."

In eight weeks in early 1920, eleven thousand influenza-related deaths occurred in just New York City and Chicago, and in New York City more cases would be reported on a single day than on any one day in 1918. In Chicago, Health Commissioner John Dill Robertson, who had been so concerned about morale in 1918, organized three thousand of the most professional nurses into regional squads that could range over the entire city. Whenever an influenza case developed, that victim's home was tagged.

The year 1920 would see either (sources differ) the second or third most deaths from influenza and pneumonia in the twentieth century. And it continued to strike cities sporadically. As late as January 1922, for example, Washington State's health director, Dr. Paul Turner, while refusing to admit the return of influenza, declared, "The severe respiratory infection which is epidemic at this time throughout the state is to be dealt with the same as influenza. . . . Enforce absolute quarantine."

Only in the next few years did it finally fade away in both the United States and the world. It did not disappear. It continued to attack, but with far less virulence, partly because the virus mutated further toward its mean, toward the behavior of most influenza viruses, partly because people's immune systems adjusted. But it left a legacy.

Even before the epidemic ended, New York City Health Commissioner Royal Copeland estimated that twenty-one thousand children in the city had been made orphans by the epidemic. He had no estimate of children who lost only one parent. Berlin, New Hampshire, a tiny town, had twenty-four orphaned children not counting, said a Red Cross worker, "in one street sixteen motherless children." Vinton County, Ohio, population thirteen thousand, reported one hundred children orphaned by the virus. Minersville, Pennsylvania, in the coal regions, had a population of six thousand; there the virus had orphaned two hundred children.

In March 1919 a senior Red Cross official advised district officers to help wherever possible on an emergency basis, because "the influenza epidemic not only caused the deaths of some six hundred thousand people, but it also left a trail of lowered vitality . . . nervous breakdown, and other sequella [*sic*] which now threaten thousands of people. It left widows and orphans and dependent old people. It has reduced many of these families to poverty and acute distress. This havoc is wide spread, reaching all parts of the United States and all classes of people."

Months after "recovering" from his illness, the poet Robert Frost wondered, "What bones are they that rub together so unpleasantly in the middle of you in extreme emaciation . . . ? I don't know whether or not I'm strong enough to write a letter yet."

Cincinnati Health Commissioner Dr. William H. Peters told the American Public Health Association meeting almost a year after the epidemic that "phrases like 'I'm not feeling right,' 'I don't have my usual pep,' 'I'm all in since I had the flu' have become commonplace." Cincinnati's public health agencies had examined 7,058 influenza victims since the epidemic had ended and found that 5,264 needed some medical assistance; 643 of them had heart problems, and an extraordinary number of prominent citizens who had had influenza had died suddenly early in 1919. While it was hardly a scientific sample, Peters believed that few victims had escaped without some pathological changes.

Throughout the world similar phenomena were noted. In the next few years a disease known as "encephalitis lethargica" spread through much of the West. Although no pathogen was ever identified and the disease itself has since disappeared—indeed, there is no incontrovertible evidence that the disease, in a clearly definable scientific sense, ever existed—physicians at the time did believe in the disease, and a consensus considered it a result of influenza.

There were other aftershocks impossible to quantify. There was the angry emptiness of a parent or a husband or a wife. Secretary of War Newton Baker—who had been criticized for being a pacifist when Wilson appointed him—particularly took to heart charges that War Department policies had in effect murdered young men. In several cases troops from Devens were transferred to a post whose commander protested receiving them because of the epidemic. The protests were futile, the troops came, and so did influenza. The father of one boy who died at such a camp wrote Baker, "My belief is that the heads of the War Department are responsible." Baker replied in a seven-page, single-spaced letter, a letter of his own agony.

The world was still sick, sick to the heart. The war itself . . . The senseless deaths at home, on top of all else . . . Wilson's betrayal of ideals at Versailles, a betrayal that penetrated the soul . . . The utter failure of science, the greatest achievement of modern man, in the face of the disease . . .

In January 1923 John Dewey wrote in the *New Republic*, "It may be doubted if the consciousness of sickness was ever so widespread as it is today. . . . The interest in cures and salvations is evidence of how sick the world is." He was speaking of a consciousness that went beyond physical disease, but physical disease was part of it. He was speaking of the world of which F. Scott Fitzgerald declared "all Gods dead, all wars fought, all faiths in man shaken."

The disease has survived in memory more than in any literature. Nearly all those who were adults during the pandemic have died now. Now the memory lives in the minds of those who only heard stories, who heard how their mother lost her father, how an uncle became an orphan, or heard an aunt say, "It was the only time I ever saw my father cry." Memory dies with people.

The writers of the 1920s had little to say about it.

Mary McCarthy got on a train in Seattle on October 30, 1918, with her three brothers and sisters, her aunt and uncle, and her parents. They arrived in Minneapolis three days later, all of them sick—her father had pulled out a gun when the conductor tried to put them off the train—met by her grandparents wearing masks. All the hospitals were full and so they went home. Her aunt and uncle recovered but her father, Roy, thirty-eight years old, died on November 6, and her mother, Tess, twenty-nine years old, died November 7. In *Memories of a Catholic Girlhood* she spoke of how deeply being an orphan affected her, made her desperate to distinguish herself, and she vividly remembered the train ride across two-thirds of the country, but she said almost nothing of the epidemic.

John Dos Passos was in his early twenties and seriously ill with influenza, yet barely mentioned the disease in his fiction. Hemingway, Faulkner, Fitzgerald said next to nothing of it. William Maxwell, a *New Yorker* writer and novelist, lost his mother to the disease. Her death sent his father, brother, and him inward. He recalled, "I had to guess what my older brother was thinking. It was not something he cared to share with me. If I hadn't known, I would have thought that he'd had his feelings hurt by something he was too proud to talk about. . . ." For himself, "[T]he ideas that kept recurring to me, perhaps because of that pacing the floor with my father, was that I had inadvertently walked through a door that I shouldn't have gone through and couldn't get back to the place I hadn't meant to leave." Of his father he said, "His sadness was of the kind that is patient and without hope." For himself, "the death of my mother . . . was a motivating force in four books."

Katherine Anne Porter was ill enough that her obituary was set in type. She recovered. Her fiancé did not. Years later her haunting novella of the disease and the time, *Pale Horse, Pale Rider,* is one of the best—and one of the few—sources for what life was like during the disease. And she lived through it in Denver, a city that, compared to those in the east, was struck only a glancing blow.

But the relative lack of impact it left on literature may not be unusual at all. It may not be that much unlike what happened centuries ago. One scholar of medieval literature says, "While there are a few vivid and terrifying accounts, it's actually striking how little was written on the bubonic plague. Outside of these few very well-known accounts, there is almost nothing in literature about it afterwards."

People write about war. They write about the Holocaust. They write about horrors that people inflict on people. Apparently they forget the horrors that nature inflicts on people, the horrors that make humans least significant. And yet the pandemic resonated. When the Nazis took control of Germany in 1933, Christopher Isherwood wrote of Berlin: "The whole city lay under an epidemic of discreet, infectious fear. I could feel it, like influenza, in my bones."

Those historians who have examined epidemics and analyzed how societies have responded to them have generally argued that those with power blamed the poor for their own suffering, and sometimes tried to stigmatize and isolate them. (The case of "Typhoid Mary" Mallon, an Irish immigrant in effect imprisoned for twenty-five years, is a classic instance of this attitude; if she had been of another class, the treatment of her might well have been different.) Those in power, historians have observed, often sought security in imposing order, which gave them some feeling of control, some feeling that the world still made sense.

In 1918 what might be considered a "power elite" did sometimes behave according to such a pattern. Denver Health Commissioner William Sharpley, for example, blamed the city's difficulties with influenza on "foreign settlements of the city," chiefly Italians. The *Durango Evening Herald* blamed the high death toll among Utes on a reservation on their "negligence and disobedience to the advice of their superintendent and nurses and physicians." One Red Cross worker in the mining regions of Kentucky took offense at uncleanliness: "When we reached the miserable shack it seemed deserted. . . . I went on in and there lying with her legs out of the bed and her head thrown way back on a filthy pillow was the woman, stone dead, her eyes staring, her mouth yawning, a most gruesome sight. . . . The mother of the woman's husband came in, an old woman living in an indescribable shack some 300 feet away. . . . I can still smell the terrible odor and will never forget the nauseating sight. The penalty for filth is death."

Yet, despite such occasional harshness, the 1918 influenza pandemic did not in general demonstrate a pattern of race or class antagonism. In epidemiological terms there was a correlation between population density and hence class and deaths, but the disease still struck down everyone. And the deaths of soldiers of such promise and youth struck home with everyone. The disease was too universal, too obviously not tied to race or class. In Philadelphia, white and black certainly got comparable treatment. In mining areas around the country, whether out of self-interest or not, mine owners tried to find doctors for their workers. In Alaska, racism notwithstanding, authorities launched a massive rescue effort, if too late, to save Eskimos. Even the very Red Cross worker so nauseated by filth continued to risk his own life day after day in one of the hardest-hit areas of the country.

During the second wave, many local governments collapsed, and those who held the real power in a community—from Philadelphia's bluebloods to Phoenix's citizens' committee—took over. But generally they exercised power to protect the entire community rather than to split it, to distribute resources widely rather than to guarantee resources for themselves.

Despite that effort, whoever held power, whether a city government or some private gathering of the locals, they generally failed to keep the community together. They failed because they lost trust. They lost trust because they lied. (San Francisco was a rare exception; its leaders told the truth, and the city responded heroically.) And they lied for the war effort, for the propaganda machine that Wilson had created.

It is impossible to quantify how many deaths the lies caused. It is impossible to quantify how many young men died because the army refused to follow the advice of its own surgeon general. But while those in authority were reassuring people that this was influenza, only influenza, nothing different from ordinary "la grippe," at least some people must have believed them, at least some people must have exposed themselves to the virus in ways they would not have otherwise, and at least some of these people must have died who would otherwise have lived. And fear really did kill people. It killed them because those who feared would not care for many of those who needed but could not find care, those who needed only hydration, food, and rest to survive.

It is also impossible to state with any accuracy the death toll. The statistics are estimates only, and one can only say that the totals are numbing.

The few places in the world that then kept reliable vital statistics under normal circumstances could not keep pace with the disease. In the United States, only large cities and twenty-four states kept accurate enough statistics for the U.S. Public Health Service to include them in their database, the so-called registration area. Even in them everyone from physicians to city clerks was trying to survive or help others survive. Record keeping had low priority, and even in the aftermath little effort was made to compile accurate numbers. Many who died never saw a doctor or nurse. Outside the developed world, the situation was far worse, and in the rural regions of India, the Soviet Union—which was engaged in a brutal civil war—China, Africa, and South America, where the disease was often most virulent, good records were all but nonexistent.

The first significant attempt to quantify the death toll came in 1927. An American Medical Association–sponsored study estimated that 21 million died. When today's media refers to a death toll of "more than 20 million" in stories on the 1918 pandemic, the source is this study.

But every revision of the deaths since 1927 has been upward. The U.S.

death toll was originally put at 550,000. Now epidemiologists have settled on 675,000 out of a population of 105 million. In the year 2004, the U.S. population exceeds 291 million.

Worldwide, both the estimated toll and the population have gone up by a far greater percentage.

In the 1940s Macfarlane Burnet, the Nobel laureate who spent most of his scientific life studying influenza, estimated the death toll at 50 to 100 million.

Since then various studies, with better data and statistical methods, have gradually moved the estimates closer and closer to his. First several studies concluded that the death toll on the Indian subcontinent alone may have reached 20 million. Other new estimates were presented at a 1998 international conference on the pandemic. And in 2002 an epidemiological study reviewed the data and concluded that the death toll was "in the order of 50 million, . . . [but] even this vast figure may be substantially lower than the real toll." In fact, like Burnet, it suggested that as many as 100 million died.

Given the world's population in 1918 of approximately 1.8 billion, the upper estimate would mean that in two years—and with most of the deaths coming in a horrendous twelve weeks in the fall of 1918—in excess of 5 percent of the people in the world died.

Today's world population is 6.3 billion. To give a sense of the impact in today's world of the 1918 pandemic, one has to adjust for population. If one uses the lowest estimate of deaths—the 21 million figure—that means a comparable figure today would be 73 million dead. The higher estimates translate into between 175 and 350 million dead. Those numbers are not meant to terrify—although they do. Medicine has advanced since 1918 and would have considerable impact on the mortality rate (see pages 450–452). Those numbers are meant simply to communicate what living through the pandemic was like.

Yet even those numbers understate the horror of the disease. The age distribution of the deaths brings that horror home.

In a normal influenza epidemic, 10 percent or fewer of the deaths fall among those aged between sixteen and forty. In 1918 that age group, the men and women with most vitality, most to live for, most of a future, accounted for more than half the death toll, and within that group the worst mortality figures fell upon those aged twenty-one to thirty.

The Western world suffered the least, not because its medicine was so advanced but because urbanization had exposed its population to influenza viruses, so immune systems were not naked to it. In the United States, roughly 0.65 percent of the total population died, with roughly double that percentage of young adults killed. Of developed countries, Italy suffered the worst, losing approximately 1 percent of its total population. The Soviet Union may have suffered more, but few numbers are available for it.

The virus simply ravaged the less developed world. In Mexico the most conservative estimate of the death toll was 2.3 percent of the entire population, and other reasonable estimates put the death toll over 4 percent. That means somewhere between 5 and 9 percent of all young adults died.

And in the entire world, although no one will ever know with certainty, it seems more than just possible that 5 percent—and in the less developed countries approaching 10 percent—of the world's young adults were killed by the virus.

In addition to the dead, in addition to any lingering complications among survivors, in addition to any contribution the virus made to the sense of bewilderment and betrayal and loss and nihilism of the 1920s, the 1918 pandemic left other legacies.

Some were good ones. Around the world, authorities made plans for international cooperation on health, and the experience led to restructuring public health efforts throughout the United States. The New Mexico Department of Public Health was created; Philadelphia rewrote its city charter to reorganize its public health department; from Manchester, Connecticut, to Memphis, Tennessee, and beyond, emergency hospitals were transformed into permanent ones. And the pandemic motivated Louisiana Senator Joe Ransdell to begin pushing for the establishment of the National Institutes of Health, although he did not win his fight until a far milder influenza epidemic in 1928 reminded Congress of the events of a decade earlier.

All those things are part of the legacy left by the virus. But the disease left its chief legacy in the laboratory.

■ Part X
ENDGAME

CHAPTER THIRTY-FOUR

BY WORLD WAR I, the revolution in American medicine led by William Welch had triumphed. That revolution had radically transformed American medicine, forcing its teaching, research, art, and practice through the filter of science.

Those in the United States capable of doing good scientific research remained a small, almost a tiny, cadre. The group was large enough to be counted in the dozens, and, counting the most junior investigators, by the mid-1920s it reached several dozen dozens, but no more.

They all knew each other, all had shared experiences, and nearly all had at least some connection to the Hopkins, the Rockefeller Institute, Harvard, or to a lesser extent the University of Pennsylvania, the University of Michigan, or Columbia. The group was so small that it still included the first generation of revolutionaries, with Welch and Vaughan and Theobald Smith and a few others still active. Then came their first students, men only a few years younger: Gorgas, who had reached mandatory retirement age from the army days before the war ended—the army could have allowed him to remain but he had no friends among army superiors—and who then shifted to international public health issues for a Rockefeller-funded foundation; Flexner and Park and Cole in New York; Milton Rosenau in Boston; Frederick Novy at Michigan; and Ludwig Hektoen in Chicago. Then came the next half generation of protégés: Lewis in Philadelphia; Avery, Dochez, Thomas Rivers, and others at

Rockefeller; George Whipple in Rochester, New York; Eugene Opie at Washington University in St. Louis; and a few dozen more. It was only in the next generation, and the next, that the numbers of true researchers began to multiply enormously and spread throughout the country.

The bonds that held these men together were not of friendship. Some of them—Park and Flexner, for example—had no love for each other, many had happily embarrassed a rival by finding flaws in his work, and they had no illusions about each other's virtues. The profession had grown large enough for maneuvering within it. If one listened closely, one could hear: "The appointment of Dr. Opie as the primary key man in this plan would be a fatal mistake." Or, "Jordan seems at first a rather dazzling possibility, but I am a little afraid . . . that he is not a man who can be absolutely certain to stand up for his convictions in a tight place." Or, "Of the names you suggest, I would distinctly prefer Emerson but I fear he would be particularly unacceptable to Russell and Cole, and perhaps to the [Rockefeller] Foundation group in general, as I have the impression that he has been somewhat at outs with them."

Yet these men also recognized that whatever each other's flaws might be, each of them also had strengths, remarkable strengths. Their work was good enough that, even if in error, one could often find in that error something new, something important, something to build upon. It was an exclusive group and, despite rivalries and dislikes, almost a brotherhood, a brotherhood that included a very few women, literally a handful, and in bacteriology these very few women did not extend far beyond Anna Williams and Martha Wollstein.*

All of these scientists had worked frenetically in their laboratories from the first days of the disease, and none of them had stopped. In those most desperate of circumstances, the most desperate circumstances in which they—and arguably any scientist—ever worked, most of them had willingly, hopefully, accepted less evidence than they would normally have to reach a conclusion. For of course as Miguel de Unamuno said, the more desperate one is, the more one hopes. But for all their frenzy of

---

*Florence Sabin was the leading female medical scientist in the United States, the first woman to graduate from the Hopkins Medical School, the first woman full professor at any medical school in the country (at the Hopkins), and the first woman elected to the National Academy of Sciences. Sabin was not a bacteriologist or involved in influenza research, and hence is not a part of this story.

activity, they had still always avoided chaos, they had always proceeded from well-grounded hypotheses. They had not, as Avery said with contempt, poured material from one test tube into another. They had not done the wild things that had no basis in their understanding of the workings of the body. They had not given quinine or typhoid vaccine to influenza victims in the wild hope that because it worked against malaria or typhoid it might work against influenza. Others had done these things and more, but they had not.

They also recognized their failures. They had lost their illusions. They had entered the first decades of the twentieth century confident that science, even if its victories remained limited, would triumph. Now Victor Vaughan told a colleague, "Never again allow me to say that medical science is on the verge of conquering disease." With the contempt one reserves for one's own failings, he also said, "Doctors know no more about this flu than 14th century Florentine doctors had known about the Black Death."

But they had not quit. Now this scientific brotherhood was beginning its hunt. It would take longer than they knew.

So far each laboratory had been working in isolation, barely communicating with the others. Investigators had to meet, to trade ideas, to trade laboratory techniques, to discuss findings not yet published or that one investigator thought unimportant that might mean something to another. They had to try to piece together some way to make concrete progress against this pestilence. They had to sift through the detritus of their failures for clues to success.

On October 30, 1918, with the epidemic on the East Coast fading to manageable proportions, Hermann Biggs organized an influenza commission of leading scientists. Biggs had a proud history, having made the New York City municipal health department the best in the world, but, fed up with Tammany politics, had left to become state commissioner of public health. His commission included Cole, Park, Lewis, Rosenau, epidemiologists, and pathologists. Welch, still recovering in Atlantic City, was too ill to attend. Biggs opened the first meeting by echoing Vaughan: "[T]here has never been anything which compares with this in importance . . . in which we were so helpless."

But unlike Vaughan he was angry, declaring their failures "a serious reflection upon public health administration and work and medical science that we should be in the situation we now are." They had seen the epidemic coming for months. Yet public health officials and scientists both had done nothing to prepare. "We ought to have been able to obtain all the scientific information available now or that can be had six months from now before this reached us at all."

He was determined that they would now address this problem, and solve it.

It would not be so easy. And even in that first meeting the problems presented themselves. They knew virtually nothing about this disease. They could not even agree upon its nature. The pathology was too confusing. The symptoms were too confusing.

Even this late Cole still wondered if it was influenza at all: "All who have seen cases in the early stage think we are dealing with a new disease. . . . One great difficulty for us is to find what influenza is and how to make the diagnosis. . . . We have been going over all case histories during this epidemic and it is almost as difficult to see which is influenza—a very complex picture."

A navy scientist observed, "In several places there has been a similarity of symptoms with the bubonic plague."

A Harvard investigator dismissed their observations: "It is the same old disease and does not change a bit in its character."

But it did change, changed constantly, from mild cases of influenza from which victims recovered quickly to cases with strange symptoms never associated with influenza, from sudden violent viral pneumonias or ARDS to secondary invaders causing bacterial pneumonias. All these conditions were being seen. Lewellys Barker, Cole's mentor at the Hopkins, noted, "The pneumonia specimens which came in from different areas are very different. Those from Devens are entirely different from those from Baltimore and they differ from several other camps. The lesions are quite different in different localities."

They reached no consensus about the disease and moved on to discuss the likely pathogen. There too they could reach not even a tentative conclusion. Investigators had found Pfeiffer's influenza bacillus, yes, but Cole reported that Avery had also discovered *B. influenzae* in 30 percent of healthy people at the Rockefeller Institute. That proved nothing. It might be commonly found now because of the epidemic and be an unusual finding in nonepidemic times. Besides, as they all knew, many healthy people carried pneumococci in their mouths and did not get pneumonia. And in the lungs of epidemic victims they had also found pneumococci, streptococci, staphylococci, and other pathogens. Park asked about the chances that a filterable virus caused the disease. Rosenau was conducting experiments pursuing that question.

They knew so little. So little. They knew only that isolation worked. The New York State Training School for Girls had quarantined itself, even requiring people delivering supplies to leave them outside. It had had no cases. The Trudeau Sanatorium in upstate New York had similar rules. It had no cases. Across the continent, a naval facility in San Francisco on an island that enforced rigid quarantine. It had no cases. All that proved was that the miasma theory, which none of them believed in anyway, could not account for the disease.

Yet they ended with agreement. They agreed on lines of approach, on the work that needed to be done. Only on that—in effect on how little they knew—they could agree.

They intended to proceed down two paths: one exploring the epidemiology of the disease, the other tracing clues in the laboratory. The first task in both lines of attack was to cut through the fog of data that was coming in.

They planned precise epidemiological investigations: correlating public health measures and deaths; performing extremely detailed studies in selected areas, for example, isolating small communities where they would account for the seventy-two hours before every single person who suffered from influenza felt the first symptoms; taking detailed personal histories of both victims and those who had not been attacked; looking for linkages with other diseases, with earlier influenza attacks, with diet.

The epidemiological studies would have the ancillary benefit of exciting and transforming another emerging field of medicine. In November 1918 the American Public Health Association created a Committee on Statistical Study of the Influenza Epidemic, funded largely by the Metropolitan Life Insurance Company. One committee member called this "an opportunity to show what statistics, especially vital statistics, and its methods can do for preventive medicine," while a colleague saw it as the "possible vindication of the theory of probabilities and the method of random sampling." In January 1919 the surgeons general of the army, the navy, and the Public Health Service also joined with the Census Bureau to form an influenza committee that grew into a permanent statistical office. Yet at the same time, an epidemiologist present at the first meeting of the Biggs group said, "I realize the problem has got to be solved ultimately in the laboratory."

Gorgas had had one goal: to make this war the first one in American history in which battle killed more troops than disease. Even with one out of every sixty-seven soldiers in the army dying of influenza, and although his superiors largely ignored his advice, he just barely succeeded— although when navy casualties and influenza deaths were added to the totals, deaths from disease did exceed combat deaths.

Gorgas had largely triumphed over every other disease. U.S. soldiers almost entirely escaped malaria, for example, even while it struck down tens of thousands of French, British, and Italians.

Now two million men were returning from Europe. After other wars, even in the late nineteenth century, returning troops had carried diseases home. British, French, and Russian troops had spread cholera after the Crimean War; Americans troops had spread typhoid, dysentery, and smallpox after the Civil War; Prussians had brought smallpox home from the Franco-Prussian War; and Americans had returned from the Spanish-American War carrying typhoid.

One of Gorgas's last acts was to set in motion plans to prevent any such happenings this time. Soldiers were kept isolated for seven days before they boarded ships home, and were deloused before embarking. Soldiers would be bringing no disease home.

Meanwhile, the most massive scientific inquiry ever undertaken was taking shape. Biggs's commission met three more times. By the last meeting, every member would be serving on other commissions as well. The American Medical Association, the American Public Health Association, the army, the navy, the Public Health Service, the Red Cross, and the Metropolitan Life Insurance Company all launched major studies in addition to those already begun, each of them designed to complement and not overlap with the others. At every meeting of every medical specialty, of

every public health organization, in every issue of every medical journal, influenza dominated the agenda. In Europe it was the same.

Every major laboratory in the United States continued to focus on the
disease. Lewis in Philadelphia kept after it, as did others at the University
of Pennsylvania. Rosenau in Boston led a team of Harvard researchers.
Ludwig Hektoen and Preston Kyes at the University of Chicago stayed
after it. Rosenow at the Mayo Clinic in Minnesota continued to work on
it. Every member of the army's pneumonia commission returned to civilian research and continued to investigate influenza. The Metropolitan
Life Insurance Company gave grants to university scientists and actually
subsidized both the city of New York and the federal government, giving
grants for research by Park and Williams in their New York laboratories
and by George McCoy of the Public Health Service's Hygienic Laboratory.

The army also made "every effort to collect . . . specimens representing pulmonary lesions due to the present influenza epidemic," not only
from army camps but from civilian sources. These specimens would
prove enormously important more than three-quarters of a century later,
when Jeffrey Taubenberger would extract the 1918 influenza virus from
them and successfully sequence its genome.

At the Rockefeller Institute, Cole put "every available man" to work on
it. He also put Martha Wollstein on it. When Captain Francis Blake, who
had been part of the army's pneumonia commission, visited his old colleagues at the institute at Christmas, he found everyone "working tooth
and nail on this influenza business with monkeys and everything else." A
week later, out of the army and back at Rockefeller, he said, "I shall be so
glad when we can get all this business off our hands and finished up and
I can to something else for a change, as it seems as though I have done
nothing but work on, and eat, and dream about and live with pneumonia
and influenza for six months."

He would not be free of it any time soon.

Slowly, over a period of months, a body of knowledge began to form.
Investigators began to learn about the firestorm that had roared around
the world and was continuing to smolder.

First, they confirmed what they had suspected: the lethal fall disease
was a second wave of the same disease that had hit in the spring. They

based their conclusion on the fact that those exposed to the spring wave had substantial immunity to the later one. The army had the best records. These records involved chiefly young men, so they were not useful in answering some questions. But they could speak to immunity, and clearly demonstrated it. Camp Shelby, for example, was home to the only division in the United States that remained in the United States from March through the fall. In April 1918 influenza sickened 2,000 of 26,000 troops there enough to seek treatment, many more probably had lesser or subclinical infections, and all 26,000 men were exposed to the disease. During the summer, 11,645 new recruits arrived. In October influenza "scarcely touched" the old troops but decimated the recruits. In Europe in the spring, influenza hit the Eleventh Regiment Engineers, making 613 men out of a command of 1,200 ill and killing two, but protecting them from the lethal wave: in the fall the regiment suffered only 150 "colds" and a single death. Camp Dodge had two units of seasoned troops; influenza had struck one group in the spring, and only 6.6 percent of this organization caught influenza in the fall; the other group escaped the spring wave, but 48.5 percent of them had influenza in the fall. And there were many other examples.

Statistics also confirmed what every physician, indeed every person, already knew. In the civilian population as well, young adults had died at extraordinary, and frightening, rates. The elderly, normally the group most susceptible to influenza, not only survived attacks of the disease but were attacked far less often. This resistance of the elderly was a worldwide phenomenon. The most likely explanation is that an earlier pandemic (later analysis of antibodies proved it was not the 1889–90 one), so mild as to not attract attention, resembled the 1918 virus closely enough that it provided protection.

Finally, a door-to-door survey in several cities also confirmed the obvious: people living in the most crowded conditions suffered more than those with the most space. It also seemed—although this was not scientifically established—that those who went to bed the earliest, stayed there the longest, and had the best care also survived at the highest rates. Those findings meant of course that the poor died in larger numbers than the rich. (Questions about race and the epidemic yielded contradictory information.)

But nearly everything else about the disease remained unsettled. Even the interplay between the germ theory of disease and other factors was at issue. As late as 1926, a respected epidemiologist still argued a version of the miasma theory, claiming "a correlation between . . . influenza and cyclic variation in air pressure."

In the laboratory, however, the fog remained dense. The pathogen remained unknown. Enormous resources were being poured into this research everywhere. In Australia, Macfarlane Burnet lived through the epidemic as a teenager, and it burned itself into his consciousness. As he said soon after receiving the Nobel Prize, "For me as for many others interested in bacteriology and infectious disease, the outstanding objective in medicine for years was . . . influenza."

Yet all this work had not penetrated the fog.

The problem did not lie in any lack of clues. The problem lay in distinguishing the few clues that led in the right direction from all those that led in the wrong direction. This was not bubonic plague. That was among the easiest pathogens to discover: the bacteria that caused it swarmed in the buboes. This was only influenza.

As the second wave of influenza had broken upon the world, thousands of scientists had attacked the problem. In Germany and France they had attacked it, in Britain and Italy, in Australia and Brazil, in Japan and China. But as 1919 wore away, then 1920, as the disease drifted toward mildness, one at a time these thousands began to peel off. They found the problem too difficult to conceptualize—to figure out a way to address it—or the techniques seemed too inadequate to address it, or it lay too far from their old interests or knowledge base. After two years of extraordinary—and continuing—efforts by many of the world's best investigators, in 1920 Welch made a frustrating prediction: "I think that this epidemic is likely to pass away and we are no more familiar with the control of the disease than we were in the epidemic of 1889. It is humiliating, but true."

Hundreds of investigators did continue to pursue the question but they could agree on little. Everything was in dispute. And central to those disputes were the old team of William Park and Anna Williams on one side, Paul Lewis and many of those at the Rockefeller Institute on another.

Lewis's research would end in irony and tragedy. The Rockefeller Institute would discover most of its own investigators in error.

But Oswald Avery would not be in error. Avery would make the most profound discovery of them all.

CHAPTER THIRTY-FIVE

THE GREATEST QUESTIONS remained the simplest ones: What caused influenza? What was the pathogen? Was Pfeiffer right when he identified a cause and named it *Bacillus influenzae*? And if he was not right, then what did cause it? What was the killer?

The pursuit of this question is a classic case of how one does science, of how one finds an answer, of the complexity of nature, of how one builds a solid scientific structure.

All through the epidemic bacteriologists had had mixed results looking for *B. influenzae*. People as skilled as Park and Williams in New York, Lewis in Philadelphia, and Avery had all been unable to isolate it from the first cases they studied. Then they adjusted their techniques, changed the medium in which they grew it, added blood heated to a particular temperature to the medium, changed the dyes used for staining, and they found it. Park and Williams soon found it so consistently that Park assured the National Research Council it was the etiological agent—the cause of the disease. The Public Health Service believed it to be the cause. Lewis, despite initial misgivings, thought it the cause.

At Rockefeller, Martha Wollstein had studied Pfeiffer's bacillus since 1906. After several years of work she still had not considered her experiments sufficiently "clean cut and stable to signify Pfeiffer's is the specific inciting agent." But she had continued to study the bacillus, and in the midst of the pandemic she had become convinced *B. influenzae* did cause the disease. She had been so confident that the vaccine she prepared included *only* Pfeiffer's bacillus. Her work convinced her Rockefeller colleagues as well; they all took her vaccine, even though they were among the few in the country with access to the Rockefeller antipneumococcus vaccine, which had proven itself effective.

Midway through the pandemic, failure to find Pfeiffer's seemed a mark not of good science but of incompetence. When one army bacteriologist failed to find it on "blood agar plates from 159 of the first patients," the army sent another scientist to the camp to undertake "an investigation of the bacteriologic methods employed in the laboratory of the base hospital." Typical of the institution Gorgas had built, it was a true investigation, not a witch-hunt, and it concluded that this particular laboratory had done "a splendid piece of work. If the influenza bacillus had been present . . . it would have been found." But that conclusion did not come out until long after the epidemic had passed.

In the meantime the existence of such an investigation told other army bacteriologists that inability to find *B. influenzae* meant they did not know their job. Simultaneously, Avery published the new techniques he had developed that made it much easier to grow the organism. Bacteriologists began to find what they were looking for. At Camp Zachary Taylor, bacteriologists had been unable to find Pfeiffer's bacillus. Now they reported, "More latterly Avery's oleate medium was used with very gratifying results." They found the bacteria everywhere: in 48.7 percent of samples of blood taken directly from the heart, in 54.8 percent of lungs, in 48.3 percent of spleens. At Camp Dix, "in every case studied the influenza bacillus was found either in the lungs or in the upper respiratory tract or nasal sinuses."

In camp after camp, bacteriologists fell into line. Bacteriologists at Camp MacArthur in Texas were not alone in their determination "to obtain the highest possible incidence of B. influenzae," and they found it in 88 percent of lungs. But they did so not through any irrefutable laboratory tests; they simply looked through a microscope and identified the bacteria by appearance. Such observations are subjective and not proof, only indications.

At Camp Sherman, where the mortality rate had been the highest in the country and the reputations of camp doctors had been called into question, the final report on the epidemic exemplified the tension. In a section written by the bacteriologist, the report said, "The persistent absence of influenza bacilli in the diverse materials examined militated against attributing the epidemic to the Pfeiffer organism." But the section written by the pathologist in effect accused the bacteriologist of incompetence. The pathologist said he had observed pathogens through the microscope that he believed *were* "Pfeiffer's organism" and that "all the bacteria which were present in this epidemic were not discovered as a result of the cultural methods used."

Civilian investigators isolated Pfeiffer's with similar regularity. Yet even with all the findings of Pfeiffer's *B. influenzae,* the picture remained confusing. For rarely—even though Avery's medium inhibited the growth of pneumococci and hemolytic streptococci, both of which had often been found in influenza cases—was Pfeiffer's found alone.

And sometimes *B. influenzae* was still not being found at all. Investigators were especially failing to find it in the lungs of victims who died quickly. In at least three camps—Fremont in California and Gordon and Wheeler in Georgia—the failure to find Pfeiffer's in an overwhelming majority of cases simply meant that the bacteriologists, instead of exposing themselves to possible criticism, diagnosed victims of the epidemic as suffering from "other respiratory diseases" instead of influenza. In some cases even the most experienced investigators found the bacillus rarely. In Chicago, D. J. Davis had studied Pfeiffer's for ten years, but found it in only five of sixty-two cases. In Germany, where Pfeiffer himself remained one of the most powerful figures in medical science, some researchers could not isolate the bacillus either, although he continued to insist it caused the disease.

These reports created increasing doubt about the Pfeiffer's influenza bacillus. Scientists did not doubt the word of those who found it. They did not doubt that the bacillus could cause disease and kill. But they began to doubt what finding it proved.

There were other questions. In the midst of the epidemic, under the greatest pressures, many bacteriologists had compromised the quality of their work in the hope of getting quick results. As one scientist said, "It requires at least three weeks of concentrated labor to investigate and identify the various species of streptococci from a single drop of normal sputum smeared on one plate of our culture medium. How then is it possible for two workers to investigate the bacteriology of the respiratory tract of, say, 100 cases of influenza and of 50 normal individuals in one year, except in the most slipshod manner?"

Park and Williams were anything but slipshod. They had been among the first to proclaim *B. influenzae* the likely cause of the epidemic. In mid-October, Park still held to that position, declaring, "The influenza bacilli have been found in nearly every case of clear-cut infectious influenza. In the complicating pneumonias, they have been found associated with either the hemolytic streptococcus or pneumococci. In one case the bronchopneumonia was due entirely to the influenza bacillus. The results of the Department of Health of the City of New York have closely agreed with those reported from Chelsea Naval Hospital."

They had prepared and distributed a vaccine based largely upon their conviction.

But even Park and Williams had made compromises. Now, as the epidemic waned, they continued their investigations with great deliberateness. They had always been best at testing hypotheses, looking for flaws, improving upon and expanding others' more original work. Now, chiefly to learn more about the organism in the hope of perfecting a vaccine and serum—but also to test their own hypothesis that *B. influenzae* caused influenza—they started an extensive series of experiments. They isolated the bacillus from one hundred cases and succeeded in growing twenty pure cultures of it. They then injected these cultures into rabbits, waited long enough for the rabbits to develop an immune response, then drew the rabbits' blood, centrifuged out the solids, and followed the other steps to prepare serum. When the serum from each rabbit was added in test tubes to the bacteria used to infect that rabbit, the antibodies in the serum agglutinated the bacteria—the antibodies bound to the bacteria and formed visible clumps.

They had expected that result, but not their next ones. When they tested these different sera against other cultures of Pfeiffer's, agglutination occurred only four of twenty times. The serum did not bind to the Pfeiffer's in the other sixteen cultures. Nothing happened. They repeated the experiments and got the same results. All the bacterial cultures were definitely Pfeiffer's bacillus, definitely *B. influenzae*. There was no mistake in that. All twenty of their sera would bind to and agglutinate bacteria from the same culture used to infect that particular rabbit. But only four of the twenty different sera would bind to any bacteria from another culture of Pfeiffer's.

For a decade scientists had tried to make vaccine and antiserum for Pfeiffer's influenza bacillus. Flexner himself had tried soon after Lewis left the institute. No one had succeeded.

Park and Williams believed they now understood why. They thought Pfeiffer's resembled the pneumococcus. There were dozens of strains of pneumococci. Types I, II, and III were common enough that a vaccine and serum had been made that could protect somewhat against all three, though with truly good effect only against Types I and II. So-called Type IV wasn't a type at all: it was a grab-bag designation of "other" pneumococci.

As they explored Pfeiffer's further, they became more and more convinced that *B. influenzae* similarly included dozens of strains, each different enough that an immune serum that worked against one would not work against the others. In fact, Williams found "ten different strains in ten different cases."

In early 1919, Park and Williams reversed their position. They stated, "This evidence of multiple strains seems to be absolutely against the influenza bacillus being the cause of the pandemic. It appears to us impossible that we should miss the epidemic strain in so many cases while obtaining some other strain so abundantly. The influenza bacilli, like the streptococci and pneumococci, are in all probability merely very important secondary invaders."

The influenza bacillus, they now said, did not cause influenza. Anna Williams wrote in her diary, "More and more, evidence points to a filterable virus being the cause."

Many others were also beginning to think that a filterable virus caused the disease. William MacCallum at the Hopkins wrote, "In Camp Lee we found practically no influenza bacilli. . . . At the Hopkins Hospital influenza bacilli was rarely found. . . . Since a great many different bacteria have been found producing pneumonia, often in complex mixtures, it would require very special evidence to prove that one of these is the universal cause of the primary disease. And since this particular organism is by no means always present it seems that the evidence is very weak.

Indeed, it appears probable that some other form of living virus not recognizable by our microscopic methods of staining, and not to be isolated or cultivated by methods currently in use, must be the cause of the epidemic."

But the subject remained controversial. No evidence pointed toward a filterable virus except negative evidence—the absence of proof of anything else. And the theory that a virus caused influenza had already been tested by excellent scientists. During the very first outbreak of the second wave in the United States, Rosenau had suspected a filterable virus. Indeed, he had suspected it at least since 1916. His instincts led him to conduct extensive and careful experiments with sixty-two human volunteers from the navy brig in Boston. He collected sputum and blood from living victims and emulsified lung tissue of the dead, diluted the samples in a saline solution, centrifuged them, drained off the fluid, and passed them through a porcelain filter, then tried various methods to communicate the disease to the volunteers. He used every imaginable method of injection, inhalation, dripping into nasal and throat passages, even into the eyes, using massive life-risking dosages. None of the volunteers got sick. One of the physicians conducting the experiments died.

In Germany a scientist had also tried, spraying the throats of volunteers with filtered nasal secretions, but none of the subjects got influenza. In Chicago a team of investigators failed to infect human volunteers with filtered secretions of influenza victims. Navy investigators in San Francisco failed.

Only one researcher in the world was reporting success in transmitting the disease with a filtrate: Charles Nicolle of the Pasteur Institute. But Nicolle's entire series of experiments involved fewer than a dozen people and monkeys. He tried four separate methods of transmitting the disease and claimed success for three of them. First he dripped filtrate into the nasal passages of monkeys and reported they got influenza. This was possible, although monkeys almost never get human influenza. He injected a filtrate into the mucosal membranes around the eyes of monkeys and reported they got influenza. This was theoretically possible, but even less likely. He also claimed to have given two human volunteers influenza by filtering the blood from an ill monkey and injecting the filtrate subcutaneously—under the men's skin. Both of the men may have gotten influenza. Neither of them could have gotten it by the method

Nicolle claimed. Nicolle was brilliant. In 1928 he won the Nobel Prize. But these experiments were wrong.

So, lacking other candidates, many scientists remained convinced Pfeiffer's did cause the disease, including most of those at the Rockefeller Institute. So did Eugene Opie, Welch's first star pupil at the Hopkins, who had gone to Washington University in St. Louis to model it after the Hopkins, and had led the laboratory work of the army's pneumonia commission. In 1922 he and several other commission members published their results in a book called *Epidemic Respiratory Disease*. One coauthor was Thomas Rivers, who by then had already begun working on viruses; in 1926 he defined the difference between viruses and bacteria—creating the field of virology and becoming one of the world's leading virologists. But he spent his first five years after the war continuing to research Pfeiffer's, writing many papers on it even while beginning his viral researches. He recalled, "We managed to get influenza bacilli out of every person that had an attack of influenza. . . . We found it and quickly jumped to the conclusion that the influenza bacillus was the cause of the pandemic."

What it came down to was that nearly all investigators believed their own work. If they had found the influenza bacillus in abundance, they believed it caused influenza. If they had not found it, they believed it did not cause influenza.

Only a very few saw beyond their own work and were willing to contradict themselves. Park and Williams were among these few. In doing so they demonstrated an extraordinary openness, an extraordinary willingness to look with a fresh eye at their own experimental results.

Park and Williams had convinced themselves—and many others— that the influenza bacillus did not cause influenza. Then they moved on. They stopped working on influenza, partly out of conviction, partly because the New York City municipal laboratory was losing the funding to do true research. And they were getting old now.

Through the 1920s, investigators continued to work on the problem. It was, as Burnet said, the single most important question in medical science for years.

In England, Alexander Fleming had, like Avery, concentrated on developing a medium in which the bacillus could flourish. In 1928 he left a petri dish uncovered with staphylococcus growing in it. Two days later he discovered a mold that inhibited the growth. He extracted from the mold the substance that stopped the bacteria and called it "penicillin." Fleming found that penicillin killed staphylococcus, hemolytic streptococcus, pneumococcus, gonococcus, diphtheria bacilli, and other bacteria, but it did no harm to the influenza bacillus. He did not try to develop penicillin into a medicine. To him the influenza bacillus was important enough that he used penicillin to help grow it by killing any contaminating bacteria in the culture. He used penicillin as he said, "for the isolation of influenza bacilli." This "special selective cultural technique" allowed him to find "B. influenzae in the gums, nasal space, and tonsils from practically every individual" he investigated.

(Fleming never did see penicillin as an antibiotic. A decade later Howard Florey and Ernst Chain, funded by the Rockefeller Foundation, did, and they developed Fleming's observation into the first wonder drug. It was so scarce and so powerful that in World War II, U.S. Army teams recovered it from the urine of men who had been treated with it, so it could be reused. In 1945, Florey, Chain, and Fleming shared the Nobel Prize.)

In 1929 at a major conference on influenza, Welch gave his personal assessment: "Personally I do feel there is very little evidence that [B. influenzae] can be the cause. But when such leading investigators as Dr. Opie, for example, feel that the evidence is altogether in favor of Pfeiffer's, and take the further exasperating position that the failure of other bacteriologists to find it was due to error in technique, to lack of skill, one cannot say there is not room for further investigation. . . . The fact has always appealed to me that influenza is possibly an infection due to an unknown virus . . . with this extraordinary effect of reducing the resistance so that the body, at least the respiratory tract, becomes such that any organisms are able to invade and produce acute respiratory trouble and pneumonia."

In 1931, Pfeiffer himself still argued that, of all organisms yet described, the pathogen he had called *Bacillus influenzae* and that informally bore his name had "the best claim to serious consideration as the primary etiologic agent, and its only competition is an unidentified filterable virus."

•   •   •

Avery continued to work on the influenza bacillus for several years after the pandemic. As his protégé René Dubos said, "His scientific problems were almost forced on him by his social environment." By that he meant that the Rockefeller Institute influenced his choice of problems. If something mattered to Flexner and Cole, Avery worked on it.

And he made remarkable progress, proving that passage in animals did make the bacillus more lethal and, far more importantly, isolating the factors in blood that *B. influenzae* needed to grow, initially identifying them as "X" and "V." It was extraordinary work, work that marked a milestone in understanding the nutritional needs and metabolism of all bacteria.

But as the likelihood of the influenza bacillus causing influenza began to fade, the pressure on him to work on it faded also. Although he had initially inclined toward the view that it caused influenza, he became one of the increasing number of scientists who believed *B. influenzae* had been misnamed. He had no inherent interest in the organism and had never abandoned his work on the pneumococcus. Far from it. And the epidemic had driven home more than ever the lethal nature of pneumonia. Pneumonia had done the killing. It remained the captain of the men of death. Pneumonia was the target. He returned to his work on the pneumococcus full-time. He would study it for the rest of his scientific life.

In fact, as first months and then years passed, Avery seemed to limit his entire world to the research he himself engaged in. He had always focused. Now his focus tightened. Even Dubos said, "I was often surprised and at times almost shocked by the fact that his range of scientific information was not as broad as could have been assumed from his fame and from the variety and magnitude of his scientific achievement." Another time Dubos observed, "He made little effort to follow modern trends in science or other intellectual fields, but instead focused his attention on subjects directly related to the precise problem he had under study. In the lab he was limited to a rather narrow range of techniques, which he rarely changed and to which he added little."

His interests increasingly narrowed to one interest, the one thing he was trying to comprehend: the pneumococcus. It was as if his mind became not only a filter but a funnel, a funnel that concentrated all the light and information in all the world on one point only. And at the bottom of this funnel he did not simply sit, sifting through data. He used its edges to dig deeper and deeper into the earth, tunneling so deep that the only light present was that which he carried with him. He could see nothing but what lay before him.

And, more and more, he began to narrow his focus even further, to a single aspect of the pneumococcus—to the polysaccharide capsule, the M&M-like sugar shell surrounding it. The immune system had great difficulty attacking pneumococci surrounded by capsules. Encapsulated pneumococci grew rapidly and unimpeded in the lungs; they killed. Pneumococci without capsules were not virulent. The immune system easily destroyed them.

At the lunch tables at the institute, sitting in the comfortable chairs, pulling apart baguettes of French bread, drinking an endless supply of coffee, scientists learned from each other. The tables were of eight, but usually one senior person would dominate a discussion. Avery spoke little, even as he grew in stature and seniority; yet he dominated in his own way, asking pointed questions about problems that confronted him, searching for any ideas that might help.

Constantly he tried to recruit people whose knowledge complemented his own. He wanted a biochemist, and, beginning in 1921, over and over he tried to lure Michael Heidelberger, a brilliant young biochemist, away from the laboratory of Nobel laureate Karl Landsteiner. Heidelberger recalled, "Avery would come upstairs from his lab and show me a little vial of dirty looking dark grey stuff and say, 'See, my boy, the whole secret of bacterial specificity is in this little vial. When are you going to work on it?'"

Inside the vial were dissolved capsules. Avery had isolated the material from the blood and urine of pneumonia patients. He believed that it held the secret to using the immune system to defeat pneumonia. If he could find that secret . . . Eventually Heidelberger did join Avery. So did others. And Avery settled into an unchanging routine. He lived on East Sixty-seventh Street and his laboratory was on Sixty-sixth and York. Every morning he walked in at the same time wearing what seemed the same gray jacket, took the elevator to his sixth-floor office, and traded the jacket for a light tan lab coat. Only if he was doing something unusual, if there was a special occasion, would he ever wear a white lab coat.

But there was nothing routine in this work. He conducted most experiments at the lab benches, actually wooden desks originally designed for an office. His equipment remained simple, almost primitive. Avery disliked gadgetry. When he experimented, remembered a colleague, he was "intensely focused . . . His movements were limited, but of extreme precision and elegance; his whole being appeared to be identified with the sharply defined aspect of the reality that he was studying. Confusions seemed to vanish, . . . perhaps simply because everything seemed so organized around his person."

Each experiment created its own world, with possibilities for joy and despair. He would leave cultures in an incubator overnight, and each morning he and his young colleagues would converge on the incubator not knowing what they would find. Quiet as he was, reserved as he was, he was always tense then, his expression simultaneously eager and fearful.

In 1923 he and Heidelberger turned the scientific world on its head by proving that the capsules did generate an immune response. The capsules were pure carbohydrate. Until then investigators had believed that only a protein or something containing proteins could stimulate the immune system to respond.

The finding only spurred Avery and his colleagues on. More than ever he concentrated on the capsule, forsaking practically everything else. He believed it to be the key to the specific reaction of the immune system, the key to making an effective therapy or vaccine, the key to killing the killer. And he believed that much of what he discovered about the pneumococcus would be applicable to all bacteria.

Then, in 1928, Fred Griffith in Britain published a striking and puzzling finding. Earlier Griffith had discovered that all known types of pneumococci could exist with or without capsules. Virulent pneumococci had capsules; pneumococci without capsules could be easily destroyed by the immune system. Now he found something much stranger. He killed virulent pneumococci, ones surrounded by capsules, and injected them into mice. Since the bacteria were dead, all the mice survived. He also injected living pneumococci that had no capsules, that were not virulent. Again the mice lived. Their immune systems devoured the unencapsulated pneumococci. But then he injected dead pneumococci surrounded by capsules and living pneumococci without capsules.

The mice *died*. Somehow the living pneumococci had acquired capsules. Somehow they had changed. And, when isolated from the mice, they continued to grow with the capsule—as if they had inherited it.

Griffith's report seemed to make meaningless years of Avery's work—and life. The immune system was based on specificity. Avery believed that the capsule was key to that specificity. But if the pneumococcus could change, that seemed to undermine everything Avery believed and thought he had proved. For months he dismissed Griffith's work as unsound. But Avery's despair seemed overwhelming. He left the laboratory for six months, suffering from Graves' disease, a disease likely related to stress. By the time he returned, Michael Dawson, a junior colleague he had asked to check Griffith's results, had confirmed them. Avery had to accept them.

His work now turned in a different direction. He had to understand how one kind of pneumococcus was transformed into another. He was now almost sixty years old. Thomas Huxley said, "A man of science past sixty does more harm than good." But now, more than ever, Avery focused on his task.

In 1931, Dawson, then at Columbia University but still working closely with Avery, and an assistant succeeded in changing—in a test tube—a pneumococcus that lacked a capsule into one that had a capsule. The next year people in Avery's own laboratory managed to use a cell-free extract from dead encapsulated pneumococci to do the same thing, to make bacteria without capsules change into ones with capsules.

One after another the young scientists in his laboratory moved on. Avery kept on. By the late 1930s he was working with Colin MacLeod and Maclyn McCarty, and they now turned all their energies to understanding how this happened. If Avery had demanded precision before, now he demanded virtual perfection, irrefutability. They grew huge amounts of virulent Type III pneumococci, and spent not just hours or days but months and years breaking the bacteria down, looking at each constituent part, trying to understand. The work was of the utmost tedium, and it was work that yielded failure after failure after failure after failure.

Avery's name was appearing on fewer and fewer papers. Much of that was because he put his name on papers of people in his laboratory only if he had physically performed an experiment included in the research the paper detailed, no matter how much he had contributed conceptually to the work, or how often he had talked over ideas with the investigator. (This was highly generous of Avery; usually a laboratory chief puts his or her name on virtually every paper anyone in his laboratory writes. Dubos recalled that he worked under Avery for fourteen years, that Avery influenced nearly all his work but only four times did Avery's name appear on his papers. Another young investigator said, "I had always felt so deeply that I was an associate of Avery that . . . with great astonishment I realized for the first time that we had never published a joint paper.")

But Avery was also publishing less because he had little to report. The work was extraordinarily difficult, pushing the limits of the technically possible. *Disappointment is my daily bread,* he had said. *I thrive on it.* But he did not thrive. Often he thought of abandoning the work, abandoning all of it. Yet every day he continued to fill nearly every waking hour with thinking about it. Between 1934 and 1941 he published nothing. *Nothing.* For a scientist to go through such a dry period is more than depressing. It is a refutation of one's abilities, of one's life. But in the midst of that dry spell, Avery told a young researcher there were two types of investigators: most "go around picking up surface nuggets, and whenever they can spot a surface nugget of gold they pick it up and add it to their collection. . . . [The other type] is not really interested in the surface nugget. He is much more interested in digging a deep hole in one place, hoping to hit a vein. And of course if he strikes a vein of gold he makes a tremendous advance."

By 1940 he had gone deep enough to believe he would find something, something of value. Between 1941 and 1944, he again published nothing. But now it was different. Now what he was working on excited him as nothing else had. He was gaining confidence that he would reach his destination. Heidelberger recalled, "Avery would come and talk about his work on the transforming substance. . . . There was something that told him that this transforming substance was something really fundamental to biology, . . . to the understanding of life itself."

Avery loved an Arab saying: "The dogs bark, the caravan moves on." He had nothing to publish because his work was being done chiefly by subtraction. But it was moving on. He had isolated whatever transformed the pneumococcus. Now he was analyzing that substance by eliminating one possibility after another.

First, he eliminated proteins. Enzymes that deactivated proteins had no effect on the substance. Then he eliminated lipids—fatty acids. Other enzymes that destroyed lipids had no effect on the ability of this substance to transform pneumococci. He eliminated carbohydrates. What he had left was rich in nucleic acids, but an enzyme isolated by Dubos that destroys ribonucleic acid had no effect on the transforming substance either. Each of these steps had taken months, or years. But he could see it now.

In 1943 he nominally retired and became an emeritus member of the institute. His retirement changed nothing. He worked exactly as he always had, experimenting, pushing, tightening. That year he wrote his younger brother, a physician, about extraordinary findings and in April informed the institute's Board of Scientific Directors. His findings would revolutionize all biology, and his evidence seemed beyond solid. Other scientists who had found what he had found would have published already. Still he would not publish. One of his junior colleagues asked, "Fess, what more do you want?"

But he had been burned so long ago in that very first work at Rockefeller, when he had published a sweeping theory encompassing bacterial metabolism, virulence, and immunity. He had been wrong, and he never forgot the humiliation. He did more work. Then, finally, in November 1943 he, MacLeod, and McCarty submitted a paper titled "Studies on the Chemical Nature of the Substance Inducing Transformation of Pneumococcal Types. Induction of Transformation by a Desoxyribonucleic Acid Fraction Isolated from Pneumoccus Type III" to the *Journal of Experimental Medicine,* the journal founded by Welch. In February 1944 the journal published the paper.

DNA, deoxyribonucleic acid, had been isolated in the late 1860s by a Swiss investigator. No one knew its function. Geneticists ignored it. The molecule seemed far too simple to have anything to do with genes or heredity. Geneticists believed that proteins, which are far more complex molecules, carried the genetic code. Avery, MacLeod, and McCarty wrote, "The inducing substance has been likened to a gene, and the capsular antigen which is produced in response to it has been regarded as a gene product."

Avery had found that the substance that transformed a pneumococcus from one without a capsule to one with a capsule was DNA. Once the pneumococcus changed, its progeny inherited the change. He had demonstrated that DNA carried genetic information, that genes lay within DNA.

His experiments were exquisite, elegant, and irrefutable. A Rockefeller colleague conducted confirming experiments on Pfeiffer's *B. influenzae*.

Among historians of science, there has been some controversy over how much immediate impact Avery's paper had, largely because one geneticist, Gunther Stent, wrote that it "had little influence on thought about the mechanisms of heredity for the next eight years." And Avery's conclusions were not immediately accepted as true by the broad scientific community.

But they were accepted as true by the scientists who mattered.

Prior to Avery's discovery—and proof—that DNA carried the genetic code, he was being seriously considered for the Nobel Prize for his lifetime of contributions to knowledge of immunochemistry. But then came his revolutionary paper. Instead of guaranteeing him the prize, the Nobel Committee found it too revolutionary, too startling. A prize would endorse his findings and the committee would take no such risk, not until others confirmed them. The official history of the organization that gives the prize states, "Those results were obviously of fundamental importance, but the Nobel Committee found it desirable to wait until more became known. . . ."

Others were determined to make more known.

James Watson, with Francis Crick the codiscoverer of the structure of DNA, wrote in his classic *The Double Helix* that "there was general acceptance that genes were special types of protein molecules" until "Avery showed that hereditary traits could be transmitted from one bacterial cell to another by purified DNA molecules. . . . Avery's experiments strongly suggested that future experiments would show that all genes were composed of DNA. . . . Avery's experiment made [DNA] smell like the essential genetic material. . . . Of course there were scientists who thought the evidence favoring DNA was inconclusive and preferred to believe that genes were protein molecules. Francis, however, did not worry about these skeptics. Many were cantankerous fools who always backed the wrong horses, . . . not only narrow-minded and dull, but also just stupid."

Watson and Crick were not the only investigators seeking the great prize, the greatest prize, the key to heredity and possibly to life, who immediately grasped the significance of Avery's work. Erwin Chargaff, a chemist whose findings were crucial to Watson and Crick's understanding enough about the DNA molecule to determine its structure, said, "Avery gave us the the first text of a new language, or rather he showed us where to look for it. I resolved to search for this text."

Max Delbruck, who was trying to use viruses to understand heredity, said, "He was very attentive to what we were doing and we were very attentive to what he was doing. . . . [I]t was obvious that he had something interesting there."

Salvador Luria, who worked with Delbruck—Watson was a graduate student under him—similarly rejected Stent's contention that Avery's findings were ignored. Luria recalled having lunch with Avery at the Rockefeller Institute and discussing the implications of his work with him: "I think it is complete nonsense to say that we were not aware."

Peter Medawar observed, "The dark ages of DNA came to an end in 1944 with" Avery. Medawar called the work "the most interesting and portentous biological experiment of the 20th century."

Macfarlane Burnet was, like Avery, studying infectious diseases, not genes, but in 1943 he visited Avery's laboratory and left astounded. Avery, he said, was doing "nothing less than the isolation of a pure gene in the form of desoxyribonucleic acid."

In fact, what Avery accomplished was a classic of basic science. He started his search looking for a cure for pneumonia and ended up, as Burnet observed, "opening . . . the field of molecular biology."

Watson, Crick, Delbruck, Luria, Medawar, and Burnet all won the Nobel Prize.

Avery never did.

Rockefeller University—the former Rockefeller Institute for Medical Research—did name a gate after him, the only such honor accorded to anyone. And the National Library of Medicine has produced a series of online profiles of prominent scientists; it made Avery the first to be so honored.

Oswald Avery was sixty-seven years old when he published his paper on "the transforming principle." He died eleven years later in 1955, two years after Watson and Crick unfolded DNA's structure. He died in

Nashville where he had gone to live to be near his brother, his family. Dubos compared his death to that of Welch, in 1934, and quoted Simon Flexner on Welch's exit from the stage: "While his body suffered, his mind struggled to maintain before the world the same placid exterior that had been his banner and his shield. Popsy, the physician who had been so greatly beloved, died as he had lived, keeping his own counsel and essentially alone."

CHAPTER THIRTY-SIX

I N THE FIRST YEARS after the pandemic, Paul Lewis continued to head the Henry Phipps Institute at the University of Pennsylvania.

Yet Lewis was not a happy man. He was one of those who continued to believe that *B. influenzae* caused the disease and continued to work on it after the epidemic passed. There was irony in that, since he had initially been reluctant to embrace its etiological role, suspecting instead a filterable virus. Perhaps the chief reason for his stubbornness was his own experience. He had not only found the bacillus with consistency, but he had produced a vaccine that seemed to work. True, the navy had administered a vaccine prepared according to his methods to several thousand men and it had proven ineffective, but he had not made that vaccine himself. A smaller batch that he had personally prepared and tested—during the peak of the epidemic, not in its later stages when many vaccines seemed to be working only because the disease itself was weakening—had given solid evidence of effectiveness. Only three of sixty people who received the vaccine developed pneumonia, and none died; a control group had ten pneumonias and three deaths.

Those results deceived him. In the past he had not always made the right scientific judgment—no investigator does—but this may have been his first significant scientific error. And it seemed to mark the beginning of a downhill slope for him.

That was not obvious at first. He had already built an international reputation. The German scientific journal *Zeitschrift für Tuberkulose* translated and reprinted his work. In 1917 he was invited to give the annual Harvey Lecture on tuberculosis, a great honor; Rufus Cole, for example, would not receive that invitation for another decade. Eighty-five years later, Dr. David Lewis Aronson, a scientist—whose father, a prize-winning scientist, had worked in the best European laboratories and considered Lewis the smartest man he ever met and gave his son Lewis's name—recalled reading that speech: "You could see Lewis's mind working, the depth of it, and vision, going well beyond what was going on at the time."

Lewis's views had broadened indeed. His interests now included mathematics and biophysics, and, with no resources of his own, he asked Flexner to "arrange for the support" of a physicist Lewis wanted to lure into medicine to examine fluorescent dyes and "the disinfectant power of light and the penetrating power of light for animal tissues." Flexner did so, and Flexner continued to be impressed by Lewis's own work, replying by return mail when Lewis sent him a paper, saying that he would publish it in the *Journal of Experimental Medicine,* calling it "interesting and important."

Yet Lewis's life after the war began pulling him away from the laboratory, frustrating him. Henry Phipps, the U.S. Steel magnate who had given his name to the institute Lewis headed, had not endowed it generously. Lewis's own salary had risen well enough, from $3,500 a year when he started in 1910 to $5,000 just before the war. Flexner still considered him vastly underpaid and saw to it that, immediately after the war, the University of California at Berkeley offered him a professorship. Lewis declined, but Penn raised his salary to $6,000, a substantial income at that time.

But if his own salary was more than adequate, he needed to fund an entire institute, even if a small one. He needed money for centrifuges, glassware, heating, not to mention "dieners"—the word still in use for technicians—and young scientists. He needed to raise the money for all that himself. As a result Lewis more and more found himself drawn into the social milieu of Philadelphia, raising money, being charming. More and more he was becoming a salesman, selling both the institute and himself. He hated it. He hated the time it took from the laboratory, the drain of his energies, the parties. And the country was in the midst of a deep recession, with four million soldiers suddenly thrown back onto the job market, with the government no longer building ships and tanks, with Europe desolate and unable to buy anything. Raising money was more than just difficult.

In 1921 the University of Iowa approached him. They wanted to become a first-class research institution, and they wanted him to run the program, to build the institution. The state would supply the money. Flexner was more than just a mentor to Lewis, and Lewis confided in him that the Iowa job seemed "heavy, safe and of limited inspiration. You know very well that I do not thrive on routine." And at Phipps, "Some of the work underway has great potential I believe. . . . You will see that I am trying to convince myself that I have a right to gamble here as against a rather dull safe outlook at Iowa City. A word from you would be much appreciated."

Flexner advised him to accept the offer: "All I have heard of the medical situation at Iowa City is favorable, . . . a pretty sharp contrast to the [situation] in Philadelphia. It is definite and has the elements of permanency. . . . I have no doubt under the influence of your vigorous guidance, the department—although quite large—over which you would preside would become so notable that the State would stand back of you in any enlargement."

He did not tell Lewis how well he thought the job might suit him, how extraordinary his gifts for a job like that were. But Flexner did tell a senior colleague that Lewis "might really come to exercise a real influence in medical teaching and research." There was perhaps some of what Welch had in him, that Lewis had "quite unusual gifts of exposition." He had broad knowledge, perhaps he even leaked knowledge, and, whether he realized it or not, he could inspire. Indeed, Flexner believed he could "be master of the field."

The University of Pennsylvania countered the offer: it gave him a new title, raised his salary to $8,000, guaranteed it for five years, and guaranteed funding for the institute itself for two years. He stayed. Flexner congratulated "you and the University especially on your new honor. Will the new chair add to your University responsibility?"

It would. Partly for that reason Lewis remained restless. He had rejected the Iowa position because, though it might allow him to build a major institution, it would keep him out of the laboratory. Now he found himself in much the same situation at Penn. He detested maneuvering with or around deans and he continued to play the role of social creature. Scientists were the new thing, Faustian figures able to create worlds and fashionable to show off on the Main Line. Lewis hated being shown off. There was tension at home with his wife as well. How much of that came from his research frustrations, how much because his wife liked the Philadelphia society that he wanted no part of, how much because his wife simply wanted more of him, it is impossible to know.

One research project in particular seemed to be going well, and he wanted to attend to it, and give up everything else. He envied not only Avery's ability to concentrate on one thing but also his opportunity to do so. For Lewis everything seemed to press upon him. Indeed, everything seemed ready to explode.

In 1922 Iowa offered him the position again. This time he accepted. He felt a responsibility to leave Phipps in good shape and recruited Eugene Opie from Washington University to replace him. Opie had if anything an even greater reputation than his own.

Flexner had always respected Lewis, yet there had always been a gap between them. They had been getting closer. At one point Flexner wrote him, "Some time do let me take a little trouble for you." Lewis confided in return, "You have stood in the light of 'father' to me." Now, when Opie agreed to replace Lewis at Phipps, Flexner seemed to see Lewis in a new light, capable not only as a scientist but as someone who could play another game well, telling him, "Opie surprised me. I supposed him a fixture in St. Louis. If you prepared the way for so good a man at the Phipps Institute, you may well feel gratified."

Lewis did not feel gratified. He remained restless and discontented. What he really wanted was to be shut of everything, everything except the laboratory. Perhaps without quite realizing it, he had been moving toward a crisis. Again he told Flexner that what he really wanted more than anything was to work at his laboratory bench. He was shut of Philadelphia. Now he had to get himself shut of Iowa.

In January 1923 he wrote Flexner, "It is quite clear to me today that I am entitled again for a short time at least to cultivate my personal interests. . . . I am giving up my place here and all of my plans for a future in Philadelphia. . . . I have written to President Jessop, of the University of Iowa, telling him of my change of plan and that that is also in the discard. . . . I am going to try my best to develop the opportunity for a year of study in some place as far removed from any question of 'affairs or position' as possible. . . . I cannot make it too plain that for the coming year I am seeking no position in the conventional sense of the word. What I really want is . . . the rehabilitation of a more or less vacant mind."

He was quitting everything, walking away from position, prestige, and money, walking into the wilderness with no guarantee of anything, stripping himself naked at the age of forty-four with a wife and two children. He was free.

Where he had been happiest in his life, where he had done the best science, had been at the Rockefeller Institute. The institute had created a Division of Animal Pathology in Princeton, close to Philadelphia. Theobald Smith, the same man who had rejected Welch's offer to become the first head of the Rockefeller Institute itself, had left Harvard and now headed this division. Smith had also been Lewis's first mentor, and had recommended him so many years before to Flexner. Lewis explored with Smith the possibility of going to Princeton. Smith first wanted assurances that Lewis wanted "to go to work again and . . . that all this advertising business had not gone to [his] head." Lewis eagerly gave them.

Flexner had urged him to take the Iowa job but replied, "I shall be rejoiced to see you return to the lab where you so naturally belong and in which you will do your best, most lasting, and effective work. It seems to me a crying pity that men who have given years to the necessary preparation for a lab career should be so ruthlessly drawn away from it and made to fill executive positions." He also told Lewis that Smith was "very pleased with the prospect of having you associated with him again."

Lewis asked for no salary whatsoever, just full access to the laboratories for a year. Flexner gave him $8,000, his salary at Phipps, and a budget for laboratory equipment, filing cabinets, 540 animal cages for breeding and experimenting, and three assistants. He told Lewis he would expect nothing whatsoever from him for the year, and then they could talk again about the future.

Lewis was ecstatic: "To start with Dr. Smith again on any possible basis, takes me back to 1905—on I hope certainly a new higher level. . . . You will not find me lacking in effort. . . . I am most fortunate and happy in being able to regard myself as entirely in the hands of you two men who, without distinction, and excepting only my parents, have given me the means and the education and the direction. Few have such a chance to renew their youth. My only hope is that I continue to deserve your confidence."

Princeton then was still surrounded by farms and countryside. It was peaceful, almost bucolic. The Rockefeller facility was not far from the campus of Princeton University, which was still transforming itself from the finishing school for gentlemen that F. Scott Fitzgerald described to the intellectual center that it would not fully become until a decade later, when Flexner's brother Abraham started the Institute for Advanced Study with Einstein as its first member. But if the setting was bucolic, if crops grew and assorted animals—not simply guinea pigs or rabbits but cattle, pigs, and horses—grazed only yards from the laboratories, the Rockefeller part of Princeton brewed intensity. Smith was continuing to produce world-class work. Just being around him energized Lewis. For the first time since he left the Rockefeller Institute, he felt at home. Yet he was alone. His wife and children stayed in Philadelphia. He was alone to work, alone to go to the laboratory in the middle of the night, alone with his thoughts.

In nearly a year, however, he produced nothing. Flexner and he did discuss his future. He was forty-five years old. His next move would likely be his last one. He could still return to the University of Pennsylvania if he chose. He did not so choose, telling Flexner, "I can only repeat that I am free of any entanglement there, even of sentiment." The University of Iowa had also extended its offer once again and once again raised the salary. But what he wanted was to stay at Rockefeller. He had made little progress on the tuberculosis project he had brought with him from Philadelphia, but, more importantly, he had, he assured himself as much as Flexner, rejuvenated himself. He informed Flexner that, despite the higher salary at Iowa, "My only interest in 'position' is [here]."

Lewis's presence fitted perfectly into Flexner's own plans. Flexner explained, "I have always believed that our departments should not be one man affairs." In New York a dozen or more extraordinary investigators led groups of younger researchers, each group working on a major problem. The Princeton location had not developed similarly; beyond

Smith's own operation, it had not filled out. Flexner told Lewis, "Your coming . . . [offers] the first chance to make a second center there."

Further, Smith would turn sixty-five that year. Flexner and Smith and even Welch hinted to Lewis that he might succeed Smith when he retired. Flexner suggested that Lewis stay one more year under a temporary arrangement, and then they would see.

Lewis told Flexner, "I am secure as I never was before." He believed he was home. It would be his last home.

If Lewis was going to build a department, he needed a young scientist— someone with more than just laboratory skills, someone with ideas. His contacts in Iowa urged him to try a young man they thought would make a mark.

Richard Shope was the son of a physician who was also a farmer. He had gotten his medical degree at the University of Iowa, then spent a year teaching pharmacology at the medical school and experimenting on dogs. An outstanding college track athlete, tall, a man's man at ease with himself—something Lewis never quite seemed to be—Shope always maintained contact with the wild, with the forest, with hunting, not only in the laboratory but with a gun in his hands. His mind had a certain wildness, too, like a small boy playing with a chemistry set hoping for an explosion; he had more than an inquiring mind, he had an original one.

Years later Thomas Rivers, the virologist who not only succeeded Cole as head of the Rockefeller Institute Hospital but served as president of four different scientific associations, said, "Dick Shope is one of the finest investigators I have ever seen. . . . A stubborn guy, and he is tough, . . . Dick would no sooner start to work on a problem than he would make a fundamental discovery. It never made one bit of difference where he was." In World War II, Rivers and Shope landed on Guam soon after combat troops secured it (in Okinawa they would come under fire) to investigate tropical diseases that might threaten soldiers. While there, Shope occupied himself by isolating an agent from a fungus mold that mitigated some viral infections. Ultimately he was elected to member-ship in the National Academy of Sciences.

Yet even with Shope's help, Lewis's work did not go well. It was not for lack of intelligence on Lewis's part. Shope knew Welch, Flexner, Smith, Avery and many Nobel laureates well, yet he considered Lewis a notch above; like Aronson, the prize-winning scientist who had worked at the Pasteur Institute and knew Lewis at Penn, Shope considered Lewis the smartest person he ever met.

Lewis had reached some tentative conclusions in Philadelphia about tuberculosis. He believed that three, and possibly four, inherited factors affected the natural ability of guinea pigs to produce antibodies—i.e., to resist infection. He had planned to unravel precisely what the nature of these factors was. This was an important question, one that potentially went far beyond tuberculosis to a deep understanding of the immune system.

But when he and Shope repeated the Philadelphia experiments they got different results. They examined every element of the experiments to see what might explain the differences and repeated them again. Then they repeated the process and the experiments again. Again they got differing results, results from which it was impossible to draw a conclusion.

Nothing in science is as damning as the inability of an outside experimenter to reproduce results. Now Lewis himself could not reproduce the results he had gotten in Philadelphia, results he had depended upon. Much less could he build upon and expand them. He had run into a wall.

He began plugging away at it. Shope too plugged away at it. Both of them had the tenacity to stay after a thing. But they made no progress.

More distressing to Smith and Flexner, who watched closely, was the way Lewis was approaching the problem. His failures seemed to confuse him. Unlike Avery, who broke his problems down into smaller ones that could be solved and who learned from each failure, Lewis seemed simply to be applying brute force, huge numbers of experiments. He sought to add other scientists with particular expertise to his team, but he did not define what precise role new people would play. Unlike Avery, who recruited people with specific skills to attack a specific question, Lewis seemed simply to want to throw resources at the problem, hoping someone would solve it.

He seemed desperate now. Desperate men can be dangerous, and even feared, but they are rarely respected. He was losing their respect, and with that would go everything.

As Lewis approached the end of his third year in Princeton, Smith confided his disappointment to Flexner: "He is perhaps aiming higher than his training and equipment warrant and this results in a demand to surround himself with technically trained chemists, etc. This is what Carrel"—Alexis Carrel at the Rockefeller Institute in New York, who had already received the Nobel Prize—"is doing but Carrel has another type of mind and gets results from his organization. A closely-knit group requires that the ideas come from the head man."

Nor did Lewis seem to recognize as worth pursuing potentially promising side questions his experiments raised. His explanation for his failures, for example, was that the diet of the guinea pigs was different in Princeton than it had been in Philadelphia. This was potentially significant, and it was possible he was correct. The relationship between diet and disease had been noted before but chiefly in terms of outright diet deficiencies that directly caused such diseases as scurvy and pellagra. Lewis was thinking about far more subtle and indirect linkages between diet and disease, including infectious disease. But instead of pursuing this line of inquiry, Lewis continued to pound away at his old one. He did so without result. He reported to the Board of Scientific Directors, "I have planned no change in my line of work for the coming year."

Flexner wanted to hear something different. Lewis was making himself a marked man, marked in no good way. It wasn't Lewis's failures that did so; it was the manner in which he was failing—dully, without imagination, and without the gain of knowledge elsewhere. Lewis had shown enough, or failed to show enough, that Flexner had already made one judgment. When Smith retired, Lewis would not replace him.

Flexner wrote him a chilling letter. In a draft Flexner was brutal: "There is no obligation expressed or implied in the Institute's relation to you, or your relation to the Institute, beyond this service year period. . . . As the Iowa chair is still open and you are very much wanted to fill it, and the University of Iowa would make a supreme effort to secure you, I believe it due you to be minutely informed just what the position the Board of Scientific Directors has taken with reference to you. . . . There was doubt expressed about your future in general."

Flexner did not send that letter. It was too harsh even for him. Instead he simply informed Lewis that the board was "unequivocally opposed to the appointment of one primarily a human pathologist"—which Lewis was—"to the directorship of the Department of Animal Pathology," and that therefore he would not replace Smith. But he also warned Lewis that the board would not elevate him to the rank of a "member" of the institute, the equivalent of a tenured full professor. He would remain only an associate. His appointment expired in six months, in mid-1926, and the board would give him a three-year appointment into 1929. Perhaps he should accept the Iowa offer after all.

In *Faust*, Goethe wrote, "Too old am I to be content with play, / Too young to live untroubled by desire."

Lewis was too old to play, too young to be untroubled by desire. Reading Flexner's letter had to have been a crushing blow. He had expected to be told he would succeed Smith. He had been certain he would be elevated to the rank of "member" of the institute. From the laboratory, he drew his identity, and yet now the laboratory gave him not sustenance but cold rebuff. The two men he most admired in the world, two men he had thought of as scientific fathers—one of whom he regarded as almost a father—had judged that he lacked something, lacked a thing that would entitle him to join their brotherhood, to become a member.

By now Lewis's family had moved to Princeton, but his marriage was no better. Perhaps the fault lay entirely within him, within what was now not so much a failing ambition as a failing love.

He declined the Iowa job once again. He had always been willing to gamble. Now he gambled on proving himself to Flexner and Smith.

For the next year and a half, he worked, at first feverishly but then . . . Something in him made him withdraw. His son Hobart, then fourteen years old, was having difficulties emotionally and difficulties in school, although a change of schools seemed to help. And Lewis had a car accident that broke his concentration.

He accomplished little. Again his failures were not like those that Avery would confront for nearly a decade. Avery was attacking the most fundamental questions of immunology and, ultimately, genetics. From each failed experiment he learned, perhaps not much but something. And what he was learning went beyond how to fine-tune an experiment. What he was learning from his failures had large ramifications that applied to entire fields of knowledge. One could argue that none of Avery's experiments failed.

Lewis was simply foundering. He had spent hour after hour in the laboratory. It had always been his favorite place, his place of rest, of peace. It gave him no peace now. He began to avoid it. His marriage was no better; his wife and he barely communicated. But he found other things to do, gardening, carpentry, things he had never attended to before. Perhaps he hoped getting away would clear his mind, allow him to see through the fog of data. Perhaps he thought that. But his mind never seemed to go back to the problem.

In August 1927, he confessed to Flexner, "I feel I have not been very productive—certainly I feel that I have had a meager return for a lot of hard work—but some way everything I have touched in the hope it would go faster than the very slow jobs I have been on for so long has either been a wash-out or turned into some other big [problem]."

Then he said something even more striking. He was no longer going to the laboratory: "I am spending most of my time on an old house and garden I have gotten hold of."

Flexner replied, for him, gently. Lewis was now more than a year into his three-year contract extension. Flexner warned that his tuberculosis work "has been under way as your major problem for four years. The outcome, even if continued many years longer, is uncertain and the yield of side issues, often the most fruitful of all, has been small. I do not believe in sticking to a rather barren subject. One of the requisites of an investigator is a kind of instinct which tells him quite as definitely when to drop, as well as when to take up a subject. Your time can be more promisingly employed along another major line."

Lewis rejected the advice.

On September 30, 1918, J. S. Koen, a veterinarian with the federal Bureau of Animal Industry, had been attending the National Swine Breeders Show in Cedar Rapids. Many of the swine were ill, some of them deathly ill. Over the next several weeks he tracked the spread of the disease, the deaths of thousands of swine, and concluded they had influenza—the same disease killing humans. Farmers attacked his diagnosis; it could cost them money. Nonetheless, a few months later he published his conclusion in the *Journal of Veterinary Medicine:* "Last fall and winter we were confronted with a new condition, if not a new disease. I believe I have as much to support this diagnosis in pigs as the physicians have to support a similar diagnosis in man. The similarity of the epidemic among people and the epidemic among pigs was so close, the reports so frequent, that an outbreak in the family would be followed immediately by an outbreak among the hogs, and vice versa, as to present a most striking coincidence if not suggesting a close relation between the two conditions."

The disease had continued to strike swine in the Midwest. In 1922 and 1923, veterinarians at the Bureau of Animal Industry transmitted the disease from pig to pig through mucus from the respiratory tract. They filtered the mucus and tried to transmit the disease with the filtrate. They failed.

Shope observed swine influenza during a trip home to Iowa. He began investigating it. Lewis helped him isolate a bacillus virtually identical to *B. influenzae* and named it *B. influenzae suis*. Shope also replicated the experiments by the veterinarians and began to move beyond them. He found this work potentially very interesting.

Lewis's own work, however, continued to founder. Flexner and Smith had kept their assessments of it confidential. As far as the rest of the world—even including Shope—knew, they held him in the highest regard. In June 1928, for the fourth time, the University of Iowa made Lewis still another offer, an outstanding offer. Flexner urged him to accept. Lewis replied that his "compelling" interest remained at Princeton.

Flexner called Smith to discuss "our future Lewis problem." They could not understand him. Lewis had produced nothing in five years. They in fact did have the highest regard for him—just no longer for his laboratory skills. Flexner still believed that Lewis had true gifts, broad and deep vision, an extraordinary ability to communicate and inspire. Flexner still believed that Lewis could become a dominant figure in medical teaching and research. Of that field, he could still be master.

Lewis had shown at least some of what Welch had. Perhaps he had much of it. And perhaps in the end he also lacked what Welch lacked, the creativity and organizational vision to actually run a major laboratory investigation.

Two days after Flexner and Smith talked, Flexner sat down with Lewis. He was blunt. But he assured Lewis the bluntness "was a conclusion placed before [you] in all kindness." The prospect of Lewis's becoming a member of the institute was a distant dream. His research had been "sterile" for the past five years. Unless it yielded something solid and important in the next year, he would not be reappointed even to a temporary position. He was approaching fifty years of age and Flexner told him, "The chances of [your] changing in the direction of more fertile ideas [are] small." He also said Lewis had not acted with "energy and determination." He had not *fought*. Then, most painfully, Flexner said he was "not essentially of the investigator type."

Flexner urged him—indeed, all but ordered him—to take the Iowa position. It was an extraordinary offer: $10,000 a year salary—more than double the median income for physicians—and a free hand in organizing a department. Flexner assured him that he still believed he had great gifts. Great gifts. He could still make a huge contribution, a significant and important contribution. At Iowa he could become a major figure, inspire respect, and be far happier.

Lewis listened quietly and said little. He did not remonstrate or argue. He was almost passive, yet firm. There was a cold, unreachable center within him. Regarding Iowa, that was settled. He would reject the offer. He had no interest in anything but the laboratory. He hoped in the next year to justify reappointment.

After the conversation Flexner was frustrated, frustrated and angry. "I put all the pressure I could upon him but without avail," he wrote Smith. "My notion is our obligations to Lewis are now fulfilled and that unless a great change takes place it will be our duty to act decisively next spring. He has been a real disappointment to me. . . . I left no doubt as to the risk he takes, and he left me no doubt that he understands and accepts that risk."

A few months before Flexner's brutal conversation with Lewis, Hideyo Noguchi had gone to Ghana to investigate yellow fever. Noguchi was as close to a pet as Flexner had. They had first met almost thirty years earlier, when Flexner was still at Penn and gave a speech in Tokyo. Uninvited, Noguchi had followed him to Philadelphia, knocked on his door, and announced he had come to work with him. Flexner found a position for him, then took him to the Rockefeller Institute. There Noguchi had developed an international reputation, but a controversial one.

He had done real science with Flexner, for example, identifying—and naming—neurotoxin in cobra venom. And he had claimed even more significant breakthroughs on his own, including the ability to grow polio and rabies viruses. (He could not have grown them with his techniques.) Rivers, also at Rockefeller and the first person to demonstrate that viruses were parasites on living cells, questioned those claims. Noguchi responded by telling him that a man who had done research for a long time had scars that he could never get rid of. Later Rivers discovered a significant unrelated mistake in his own work and confessed to Noguchi that he planned to retract his paper. Noguchi advised against it, saying it would take fifteen years for anyone else to find out he was wrong. Rivers was astounded, later saying, "I don't think Noguchi was honest."

Noguchi's most important claim, however, was to have isolated the pathogen that caused yellow fever. It was a spirochete, he said, a spiral-shaped bacterium. Years before, Walter Reed had seemed to prove that a filterable virus caused the disease. Reed was long dead, but others attacked Noguchi's findings. In response to one such attack, Noguchi wrote Flexner, "[H]is objections were very unreasonable. . . . I am not certain whether these Havana men are really interested in scientific discussion or not."

Noguchi did not lack courage. And so he went to Ghana to prove himself correct.

In May 1928 he died there, of yellow fever.

Noguchi's death came one month before Flexner and Lewis had their conversation. It attracted international attention, made the front pages of newspapers around the world, inspired glowing tributes in all the New York papers. For Noguchi, it was a Viking funeral, a blazing glory that obliterated all questions about the quality of his science.

The entire Rockefeller Institute reeled from the loss. Despite any scientific controversies, Noguchi had been buoyant, enthusiastic, always helpful, universally liked. Both Flexner and Lewis suffered in particular. Noguchi had been, literally, like a son to Flexner. Lewis had known him well, very well, going back to his first happy days in New York.

Noguchi's death also left open the question of whether he had in fact isolated the pathogen that caused yellow fever. The institute wanted that question answered.

Shope volunteered to do it. He was young and believed himself invulnerable. He wanted action. He wanted to investigate yellow fever.

Flexner refused to allow him to go. Shope was also only twenty-eight years old, with a wife and an infant son. It was too dangerous.

Then Lewis volunteered. The scientific question remained, and it was a major one. Who was more qualified to investigate it than he? He had proven himself expert at cultivating bacteria and, even more important, he had proven that polio was a viral disease. Noguchi notwithstanding, it seemed a virus did cause yellow fever. And, important as the question was, it also had built-in limits; it was the kind of narrow and focused science that Flexner still had faith in Lewis to answer.

Lewis's wife, Louise, objected. The laboratory had taken him away from her and their two children enough. She was already furious at him for once again declining the Iowa position. But *this* . . . this was something else.

Lewis had never listened to her. They had not had a real marriage for a long time. For him, this solved every problem. If he succeeded, he would restore himself in Flexner's eyes. Five years before he had resigned from the Phipps Institute and simultaneously withdrawn his acceptance of the Iowa offer without any other prospects. All that he had done in order to do the one thing he loved, return to the laboratory. He was willing to gamble again. He was energized again. And he was more desperate than ever.

Instead of Ghana, however, he would go to Brazil. A particularly virulent strain of yellow fever had surfaced there.

In late November 1928, Flexner came to Princeton to see Lewis off. Flexner's attitude toward him had already seemed to change. He was willing again to talk about the future. He also wanted, he said, to "learn about Shope's Iowa work." Shope had recently observed an extraordinarily violent influenza epizootic—an epidemic in animals—in swine. The overall mortality of the entire local pig population had reached 4 percent; in some herds mortality had exceeded 10 percent. That very much sounded like the influenza pandemic in humans a decade earlier.

A month later Lewis sailed for Brazil. On January 12, 1929, Frederick Russell, the colonel who had organized much of the army's scientific work for Gorgas and who now worked for a Rockefeller-sponsored international health organization, received a cable saying Lewis had arrived and was well. The institute relayed the news to his wife, who had been so angry at Lewis's departure that she had wanted nothing to do with the Rockefeller Institute and returned to Milwaukee, where both she and Lewis had grown up. Each week Russell was to receive news of Lewis and send it on to her.

Lewis located his laboratory in Belem, a port city on the Para River, seventy-two miles from the ocean but the main port of entry into the Amazon Basin. Europeans settled there in 1615, and a rubber boom in the nineteenth century had filled the city with Europeans while Indians went back and forth into the interior in dugout canoes. It was steamy, equatorial, and received as much precipitation as any area in the world.

On February 1, Lewis wrote Flexner, "Arrived here on Tuesday and went right to work. . . . [H]ave been setting up my own shop here, awaiting materials, having additional screening prepared, etc. . . . Should be started at something by early next week I hope."

He seemed the old Lewis, energetic and confident. And each week Russell received a two-word wire: "Lewis well." He received them through February, March, April, and May. But if Lewis was well, he sent no word about his research; he gave no sign that work was going well.

Then, on June 29, Russell sent a note hand-delivered by messenger to Flexner: "The following message from Rio de Janeiro, regarding Dr. Paul Lewis, was sent to me today, with the request that it be delivered to you. 'Lewis's illness began on June 25th. Doctors state it to be yellow fever. Condition of June 28th, temperature 103.8, pulse 80. . . .' The Foundation is sending the message to Dr. Theobald Smith and also to Mrs. Lewis at Milwaukee."

Even as Russell sent that note to Flexner, Lewis was in agony. He had vomited violently, the nearly black vomit of the severe cases; the virus attacked the mucosa in his stomach, which bled, giving the vomit the dark color; it attacked the bone marrow, causing violent aching. An intense, searing headache gave him no rest, except perhaps when he was delirious. He had seizures. His colleagues packed him in ice and tried to keep him hydrated but there was little else they could do.

The next day another wire came: "Lewis condition critical. Anuria supervened Saturday."

His kidneys were failing and he was producing no urine. All the toxins that the body normally rid itself of were now building up in his system. Later that same day, Russell received a second wire: "Lewis on fourth day of illness. Marked renal involvement." He was becoming jaundiced, taking on the classic color that gave the disease its name. Symptom by symptom, step by step his body was failing.

June 30, 1929, was a Sunday. All day Lewis suffered, writhed in delirium. He went into a coma. It was his only relief. It was the fifth day of his illness. There would not be a sixth.

Shortly before midnight Dr. Paul A. Lewis found release.

An unsigned wire to Russell reported, "Typical yellow fever. Probably laboratory infection. Wire instructions regarding body."

Shope walked down Maple Street on the edge of the Princeton campus to inform Lewis's wife, who had come back from Milwaukee, and son Hobart, now a college student who had remained in Princeton.

Lewis's widow gave simple and explicit instructions. She was returning immediately to Milwaukee and wanted the body shipped directly there, where those who cared about Paul were. She specifically stated that she wanted no memorial service held at the Rockefeller Institute, in either New York or Princeton.

There was none.

Shope accompanied the body to Wisconsin. The business manager of the Rockefeller Institute asked him, "I wonder if you could arrange when you arrive to order some flowers for the service for Dr. Lewis."

The flowers came, with a card signed "the Board of Scientific Directors of the Rockefeller Institute."

Lewis's daughter, Janet, wrote the thank you note, addressing it "Dear Sirs." Her mother could not bring herself to have any contact with the institute, particularly a thank you note. The institute paid Lewis's salary to her through June 1930 and also paid his son Hobart's college tuition. (Like his grandfather and aunt Marian, the first woman to graduate from Rush Medical College in Chicago, he became a physician—but a clinician, not a scientist.)

In the next report to the Board of Scientific Directors of the Rockefeller Institute—a board which now included Eugene Opie, whom Lewis had recruited as his successor at Phipps—Flexner noted that one scientist's resignation "which is much regretted, left the study of light phenomena unprovided for."

Lewis had originally suggested that work to Flexner. Flexner mentioned a "recrudescence of poliomyelitis." Lewis had proved that a filterable virus caused that disease.

Flexner went through item after item concerning the institute. He pointed out "a pressing problem was the one in connection with the still unfinished work of Dr. Noguchi." He made no mention of Paul A. Lewis, no mention of Dr. Lewis at all.

Later Flexner received Lewis's autopsy report and news that researchers at the institute in New York had succeeded in transmitting Lewis's virus—they called it "P.A.L."—to monkeys and were continuing experiments with it. Flexner wrote in reply, "Thank you for sending me the report on the comparison of the Rivas and P.A.L. strains of yellow fever virus. At your convenience I should like to talk over the report with you. Dr. Cole thinks white paint and some other improvements desirable in your animal quarters. Has he spoken with you about them?"

Lewis had worked with deadly pathogens his entire adult life and had never infected himself. Since Noguchi's death everyone working with yellow fever took special care.

In the five months Lewis worked in Brazil he did not report any details of his research and his laboratory notes provided almost no information about it. He died from a laboratory accident. Somehow he gave yellow fever to himself.

Shope later told his sons a rumor that Lewis, who smoked often, had somehow contaminated a cigarette with the virus and smoked it. The virus entered the bloodstream through a cut on his lip. David Lewis Anderson recalls that his father, Lewis's friend in Philadelphia, also blamed cigarettes for Lewis's death.

Three years earlier Sinclair Lewis, no relation, won the Pulitzer Prize for his bestselling novel *Arrowsmith,* a novel about a young scientist at a fictionalized version of the Rockefeller Institute. Everyone in medical science, especially at the institute, knew that novel. In it the main character's wife dies from smoking a cigarette contaminated by a deadly pathogen.

Flexner wrote an obituary of Lewis for *Science* in which he referred to "the important observations made by him in association with Sewall Wright on the hereditary factors in research in tuberculosis." Lewis's work with Wright had been carried out in Philadelphia; Flexner made no mention of anything Lewis had done in the five years since his return to the institute.

Meanwhile, Shope returned to Iowa to explore further this swine influenza, to observe still another epidemic among pigs.

. . .

In 1931, two years after Lewis's death, Shope published three papers in a single issue of the *Journal of Experimental Medicine*. His work appeared in good company. In that same issue were articles by Avery, one of the series on the pneumococcus that would lead to his discovery of the transforming principle; by Thomas Rivers, the brilliant virologist; and by Karl Landsteiner, who had just won the Nobel Prize. All of these scientists were at the Rockefeller Institute.

Each of Shope's articles was about influenza. He listed Lewis as the lead author on one. He had found the cause of influenza, at least in swine. It was a virus. We now know that the virus he found in swine descended directly from the 1918 virus, the virus that made all the world a killing zone. It is still unclear whether humans gave the virus to swine, or swine gave it to humans, although the former seems more likely.

By then the virus had mutated into mild form, or the swine's immune systems had adjusted to it, or both, since the virus alone seemed to cause only mild disease. Shope did demonstrate that with *B. influenzae* as a secondary invader it could still be highly lethal. Later he would show that antibodies from human survivors of the 1918 pandemic protected pigs against this swine influenza.

Shope's work was momentous and provocative. As soon as his articles appeared, a British scientist named C. H. Andrewes contacted him. Andrewes and several colleagues had been expending all their efforts on influenza, and they found Shope's articles compelling. Andrewes and Shope became close friends; Shope even took him hunting and fishing where he had vacationed since he was six years old, at Woman Lake, Minnesota.

In England in 1933, during a minor outbreak of human influenza, Andrewes, Patrick Laidlaw, and Wilson Smith, largely following Shope's methodology, filtered fresh human material and transmitted influenza to ferrets. They found the human pathogen. It was a filter-passing organism, a virus, like Shope's swine influenza.

Had Lewis lived, he would have coauthored the papers with Shope, and even added breadth and experience to them. He would have helped produce another of the seminal papers in virology. His reputation would have been secure. Shope was not perfect. For all his later accomplishments in influenza and in other areas, some of his ideas, including some of those pertaining to influenza, were mistaken. Lewis, if energized and once again painstaking, might have prevented those errors. But no matter.

Shope was soon made a member of Rockefeller Institute. Lewis would likely have also been made a member. He would have been invited into the inner sanctum. He would have maintained his membership in the community of those who do science. He would have belonged there. He would have had all that he wanted.

William Park, Oswald Avery, and Paul Lewis each approached science in his own way.

Park, a man who almost became a medical missionary, saw it as a means to a larger end; he saw it as a tool to relieve suffering. Disciplined and methodical, his interest lay chiefly in immediate results that he could apply to his purpose. His contributions, particularly those made with Anna Williams, were enormous; their improvement of diphtheria anti-toxin alone doubtless saved hundreds of thousands of lives over the past century. But his purpose also limited him, narrowed him, and limited the kind of findings he and those under him would make.

Avery was driven and obsessive. Part artist and part hunter, he had vision, patience, and persistence. His artist's eye let him see a landscape from a new perspective and in exquisite detail, the hunter in him told him when something, no matter how seemingly trivial, was out of place, and he wondered. The wonder moved him to the sacrifice of all else. He had no choice but to sacrifice. It was his nature. Cutting a Gordian knot gave him no satisfaction. He wanted to unfold and understand mysteries, not cut through them. So he tugged at a thread and kept tugging, untangling it, following where it led, until he unraveled an entire fabric. Then others wove a new fabric for a different world. T. S. Eliot said any new work of art alters slightly the existing order. Avery accomplished that all right, and far more.

Paul Lewis was a romantic, and a lover. He wanted. He wanted more and loved more passionately than Park or Avery. But like many romantics, it was the idea of the thing as much or more than the thing itself that he loved. He loved science, and he loved the laboratory. But it did not yield to him. The deepest secrets of the laboratory showed themselves to Lewis when he was guided by others, when others opened a crack for him. But when he came alone to the laboratory, that crack closed. He could not find the right loose thread to tug at, the way to ask the question. To him the laboratory presented a stone face, unyielding to his pleadings. And whether his death was a suicide or a true accident, his failure to win what he loved killed him. One could consider Lewis, in a way meaningful only to him, the last victim of the 1918 pandemic.

AFTERWORD

WHEN I BEGAN work on this book early in 1997, my plan was to use the events of 1918 as a narrative vehicle, a case study, and a probe to explore several questions that did not even necessarily involve influenza. I had no interest in frightening anyone or advocating anything. I wanted to see how American society reacted to an immense challenge, a war nature launched against man imposed on a war of man against man. And I wanted to explore how individuals who had at least some power to deal with this challenge reacted.

This meant examining not only those with political power on the national or local level, but also scientists, for they exercise power as well. I particularly wanted to examine how investigators did science under the most stressful conditions, and to explore epistemological questions that confront anyone making a decision. What process does one follow to collect information that most likely leads to a good choice? How does, or should, a crisis affect the decision-making process? At what point should people have confidence that they have enough data? In short, how do you know when you know? And I wanted to see what lessons we might take from such an examination.

Those are, I believe, important areas of inquiry, and the reader can judge whether this book sheds any light on them.

But my original intent in writing this book has been somewhat overtaken by events, as new avian influenza viruses infect humans at an increasing rate—and hence threaten to spark a new pandemic, which many experts fear is imminent. The evolving status of this threat has led me to make several adjustments in the body of this book, and to write this new afterword.

The avian virus that has gotten the most attention is known as H5N1. It first appeared in 1997, just a few months after I began researching this book, killing six of eighteen people it infected in Hong Kong, and leading to the slaughter of more than one million poultry in an attempt to exterminate it. Seven years later, just as the book was being published, the virus exploded in the southeast Asian poultry population and also killed several dozen people, then briefly went underground when public health officials in several countries slaughtered well over 100 million fowl in another attempt to wipe out the virus.

This attempt failed. H5N1 established itself in wild bird populations in much of Asia, and in December 2004 resurfaced with a vengeance, devastating poultry and killing more people as well as other mammals, including domestic cats and tigers. Though at this writing (and hopefully forever) it has not adapted to person-to-person transmission, it seems to kill the people it sickens at a rate that dwarfs that of even the 1918 virus.

So the questions to address here are:

1. Will another influenza pandemic occur?
2. If so, how dangerous will it be and what threat does the H5N1 virus present?
3. How prepared are we for it and what can we do to better prepare?

The answer to the first question is a simple yes. The World Health Organization, the National Academy of Sciences (through its medical arm, the Institute of Medicine), and the U.S. Centers for Disease Control and Prevention all agree that influenza pandemics are virtually certain to recur.

Of greater concern, the WHO, CDC, and other health organizations have also used such words as "likely" and "probable" to warn of the chances of a pandemic in the *immediate* future. They base these warnings on concrete and sobering information.

The threat of new reassorted viruses crossing the species barrier has always existed, but it is increasing as the direct infection of humans by avian viruses increases.

Of course, every time the virus infects a person it has a new opportunity to jump species. As anyone who has read the chapters in this book about the virus itself knows, all influenza viruses originate in birds, but they mutate with extraordinary speed and can trade genes with other influenza viruses. Whenever a bird virus infects a person—or possibly another mammal, especially a pig—and then either reassorts with an existing human influenza virus or, conceivably, mutates directly to create a new virus capable of passing from person to person, a new influenza pandemic may erupt.

Between 1959 and 1997, only two people suffered documented infections by avian viruses; each instance was isolated and neither victim died.

By contrast, between 1997 and the spring of 2005, three different avian viruses have caused illness in more than two hundred people. These infections have often occurred in clusters, and two of the three viruses have killed people.

The most persistent and seemingly the most dangerous of these three viruses is H5N1. It has caused well over half of all known avian viral infections in humans, with a mortality rate ranging from 33 to 70 percent of those with confirmed infections. Because it is now endemic in Asian bird populations, it will likely continue to infect people for the foreseeable future.

Still another threat is the virus that caused the 1957 pandemic—the H2N2 virus. Many virologists consider it the most likely next pandemic virus because, unlike the avian viruses, it has proved its ability to pass from person to person. In addition, this virus was driven into virtual extinction by the 1968 pandemic virus, the dominant influenza virus today. That means an increasing majority of today's population has never been exposed to it, leaving them vulnerable to infection should it return. (A mild and distant relative of the H1N1 virus of 1918 does still circulate, hence people should have some protection against any H1 virus.)

For these reasons, virologists and public health officials consider new pandemics almost inevitable. But they cannot predict when one will occur. As one influenza expert has said, "The clock is ticking. We just don't know what time it is."

·   ·   ·

So, how bad will the next pandemic be? Will it kill two million, twenty million, two hundred million? How many will die in the United States?

No one can say. But if one compares the 1918–1919 pandemic to AIDS, one sees how threatening influenza can be. Today the world population exceeds six billion. Worldwide, in the roughly twenty-four years since AIDS was recognized (it now appears that the virus entered the human population several decades earlier), the total death toll is estimated at 23 million with an estimated 39.4 million people in 2005 infected with HIV. In the United States the cumulative death toll from AIDS is roughly 500,000.

In 1918 the world's population was 1.8 billion, only 28 percent of today's. Yet the 1918 influenza virus killed a likely 50 million and possibly as many as 100 million people. The AIDS deaths reported above occurred over twenty-four years; most of the influenza deaths occurred in less than twenty-four weeks.

But what really demonstrates the power of influenza is not a worst case scenario. A best case scenario, a mild pandemic, serves well enough.

The 1968 pandemic was a mild pandemic, with approximately 34,000 deaths in the United States (equivalent to about 55,000 in today's population). This death toll was only a tiny fraction of that in 1918, but not because medical science had mastered the virus. Antibiotics did cut deaths from complicating bacterial pneumonias, but vaccines did not become available until the pandemic was far advanced. The 1968 pandemic killed relatively few people only because the virus itself was mild.

Nonetheless, the World Health Organization estimates that a virus akin to that of 1968 would, in today's world, kill between 2 million and 7.4 million people worldwide. And in developed countries, ironically, even a mild pandemic today would probably hit harder than one has in the past. In fact, the CDC has produced a study of what would likely happen if a new pandemic virus—much like 1968's—struck the United States. Even with a mild virus, it projected a most likely death toll between 89,000 and 207,000. The reason for this high toll is the same reason that the CDC has concluded that, despite medical advances, *more* Americans are now dying from ordinary, endemic influenza than in the past: in 1918, 1957, and even 1968 relatively few people alive had impaired immune systems. Today a large and growing number of people do—primarily the elderly, but also cancer survivors who have undergone chemotherapy or radiation, transplant recipients, those infected with HIV, and others.

In addition, even in advanced countries a pandemic would stretch the health care system to the point of collapse, and possibly beyond it. Hospitals, like every other industry, have gotten more efficient and cut costs—which means virtually no excess capacity. Hence the United States now has far fewer hospital beds available on a per capita basis than it did in 1968. (This was driven home to me in a personal way on my book tour; when I reached Kansas City, a flare-up of ordinary influenza forced eight hospitals to close emergency rooms. The disease forced similar closings in many other cities. Yet the mildest pandemic would put infinitely more pressure on health care.) In developing countries the health care system would all but disintegrate.

Similarly, the United States has 105,000 mechanical respirators, three-quarters of which are normally in use. During a routine influenza season, usage rises to nearly 100 percent. During a pandemic, most people who needed a mechanical respirator would not get one. This and similar issues—such as an exhausted stock of antibiotics, a resistant secondary bacterial invader, or even a run on hypodermic needles—could easily make moot all medical advances since 1918.

Deaths are, however, not the full measure of the impact of a pandemic. Even a mild pandemic would cause massive economic losses and social disruption.

As Michael Osterholm of the University of Minnesota has pointed out, society has changed radically since 1918, and these changes have created new vulnerabilities.

The most obvious change is the expansion of international trade. The SARS outbreak in 2003 only briefly shut down trade with parts of China, yet, because so many computer chips come from China, it still impacted the computer industry worldwide. A pandemic would disrupt trade far more, forcing, at best, major dislocations in many domestic industries.

Social behavior has altered, too. In 1957 only 10 percent of meals were eaten outside the home, and only 20 percent of food items sold were perishables—fresh vegetables instead of canned. Today 38 percent of meals are eaten outside the home, and 48 percent of food items are perishable. These new habits would affect both the spread of the virus and the degree of social dislocation it would cause.

Meanwhile, American business' adoption of "just-in-time" delivery of inventory means that if a single supplier had so many workers out sick it couldn't ship a key item, an entire industry might all but shut down. The briefest disruption of the transportation system—sick railroad workers or air traffic controllers—could also dislocate the entire economy. Even the funeral business would be caught short. In 1968 coffins were used on average five months after manufacture; now they are used three and a half weeks after manufacture, making it almost certain that anything beyond the most mild conceivable pandemic will leave undertakers without coffins, re-creating at least one of 1918's horrors.

These are the best case scenarios, in a mild pandemic.

A worst case scenario could be beyond imagining. One need not use H5N1 with its extraordinary mortality rate to terrify. The 2003 outbreak of an H7N7 avian virus in the Netherlands will suffice. This virus surfaced in poultry farms, sickened eighty-nine people, and killed one. One death in eighty-nine may not sound terrifying, but a new influenza virus makes between 15 and 40 percent of the population ill enough to show symptoms. It would make between 44 and 115 million Americans sick. And, in the United States alone, a mortality rate of just over 1 percent would translate into roughly 500,000 to 1.3 million dead.

The only good news seems to be that an increasing number of virologists now doubt that H5N1 will be the next pandemic virus. (And if it does provide the seed for the next pandemic virus, it might become mild after adapting to humans.) Their reasoning is simple. Large numbers of people—vastly more than the confirmed infections—have by now been exposed to it. Yet the virus has not become easily transmissible from person to person. These virologists believe if H5N1 could transmit this way, it would have done so already.

But never before in history has there been such a combination of so many people and animals. In 1968, for example, China had only 5.2 million pigs and 12.3 million poultry; now it has 508 million pigs and 13 *billion* poultry. And H5N1 is adapting itself to more and more animals.

How prepared are we for a new pandemic?

At this writing, we are not prepared. At all.

Vaccines are a good answer, but at this point only a theoretical one.

First, it is almost physically impossible to produce, distribute, and administer hundreds of millions of doses, and possibly a billion or more, within six months after the emergence of a new pandemic virus. It is also likely that protection against a new virus will require two doses of vaccine, not the usual one. So even under a best case scenario a vaccine would probably not be available in any quantity until the pandemic was deep into its second wave.

And present production techniques and facilities are far, far from a best case scenario. This was demonstrated dramatically in 2004, when contamination in a single plant in Britain cut the U.S. vaccine supply by roughly 50 million doses, nearly half the total. Finally, it is quite likely that, in the face of a new pandemic, no country in the world would allow the export of any vaccine until its entire population is protected—and only half the vaccine used in the United States is made in the United States.

Science has developed several antiviral drugs, particularly oseltamivir, that cut down the duration and severity of the illness (although, oddly, it remains uncertain whether it cuts the mortality rate). More important in terms of a pandemic, these antivirals also work as a prophylactic, preventing people from getting the disease while they are taking it. This makes it of absolutely critical importance in the months that would pass before a vaccine could be made. The United States and several other governments have just begun—but only just begun—to stockpile oseltamivir, but the single manufacturer making oseltamivir cannot meet demand. If a pandemic struck in the near future, supplies would quickly run out. And of course, there is always the fear that the virus would become resistant to it or any other drug.

The threat of H5N1 has, however, focused the minds of scientists and public health officials around the world. They are quietly, and sometimes not so quietly, warning those with the power to spend money that, if they do not prepare for a pandemic now, some time in the near future an investigative commission will write the equivalent of a 9/11 Commission Report, asking why they failed to act. Only this time, instead of a few thousand dead, the toll will be in the millions.

What needs to be done?

Influenza has to be seen as a lethal threat. A pandemic would prove more deadly than even a major bioterrorism attack, and it is more likely to occur. In addition, according to the CDC, every year influenza kills

36,000 Americans, almost triple the country's AIDS death toll, and, as stated earlier, despite medical advances influenza's annual death toll is trending up, not down. Only after the 2004 vaccine fiasco did Congress begin to take the need for a vaccine supply seriously, yet, based on the money it is spending, it still does not take influenza seriously enough.

The first step in preparing for a pandemic is surveillance. The earlier we identify a new virus, the better chance we have to develop and distribute a vaccine. For several decades now, the World Health Organization has monitored influenza.

Surveillance has two purposes: to track mutations of existing viral subtypes in order to adjust each year's vaccine, and to search for any sign of a new pandemic strain. Of course, one must know where to look, so the origin of the 1918 virus becomes vitally important.

This book hypothesizes that the 1918 virus emerged in Haskell County, Kansas, but there are other theories. Since influenza is both an endemic and epidemic disease, without virus samples and modern molecular biology techniques, it is impossible to state with absolute certainty which theory, if any yet advanced, is correct. The only evidence is epidemiologic.

Most pandemics whose origin is known began in Asia. The reason is simple: larger numbers of people live in close contact with pigs and birds in Asia than elsewhere, so more opportunities exist for a virus to cross over from animals to humans. Some medical historians and epidemiologists believe that the 1918 pandemic also began in China.

Another recent theory, suggested by British virologist J. S. Oxford, suggests that the 1918 pandemic originated in a British Army post in France, where a disease British physicians called "purulent bronchitis" erupted in 1916. Autopsy reports of soldiers killed by this outbreak do bear a striking resemblance to those killed by influenza in 1918.

But in the immediate wake of the pandemic, many scientists and organizations searched for the source of the disease. The American Medical Association sponsored what is generally considered the best of several comprehensive international studies conducted by Dr. Edwin Jordan, editor of *The Journal of Infectious Disease*. He spent years reviewing evidence from all over the world.

Jordan first considered China. Influenza did surface there in early

1918, but the outbreaks seemed minor and did not spread. Hong Kong had only twenty-two influenza hospital admissions in the first five months of 1918, and in Canton the first case of influenza did not surface until June 4. Some medical historians have suggested that one particular outbreak of deadly pulmonary disease in China in 1918 was actually influenza, but Chinese scientists, trained by the Rockefeller Institute, diagnosed it as pneumonic plague, which by then could be easily and conclusively identified in the laboratory. These Chinese scientists also believed no evidence connected any of these outbreaks to the pandemic. Jordan also concluded that no known outbreak in China "could be reasonably regarded as the true forerunner of the European epidemic."

Jordan then considered the evidence for Oxford's hypothesis. He rejected it for several reasons. The "purulent bronchitis" did not seem to spread rapidly or widely, and a new influenza virus almost always does both. In fact, the outbreak seemed so contained that at least some members of the British medical corps did not even consider the infection contagious.

(And, we now know a sudden mutation in an existing influenza virus can account for a sudden virulent outbreak. In the summer of 2002, for example, an influenza epidemic erupted in parts of Madagascar with an extremely high death rate; in some towns it also struck an outright majority—in one instance 67 percent—of the population. But the virus causing this lethal epidemic was an old one, an H3N2 virus of a subtype isolated in 1999 that normally caused mild disease. It had simply mutated in a violent direction, then reverted to its normal mild status. The epidemic affected only 13 of 111 health districts in Madagascar before fading away. If the outbreak Oxford points to was in fact influenza, it could have followed a path similar to that of the Madagascar virus.)

Jordan considered as possible sources other early outbreaks of influenza elsewhere in the world. But they too behaved like local eruptions of endemic influenza, and he concluded that it was highly unlikely that any of them marked the pandemic's site of origin.

That left the United States. Given a series of spring outbreaks there, the evidence seemed far stronger. One could see influenza jumping from army camp to army camp, then traveling with troops into cities, and with them on to Europe. His conclusion: the United States was the site of origin.

A later equally comprehensive, multivolume British study of the pandemic agreed with Jordan. It too found no evidence for the influenza's origin in Asia, it too rejected the outbreak of "purulent bronchitis" among British troops, and it too concluded, "The disease was probably carried from the United States to Europe."

Australian Macfarlane Burnet, quoted earlier on this point, studied the pandemic for years and also found the evidence "strongly suggestive" that the disease started in the United States and spread with "the arrival of American troops in France."

Molecular biology provides more evidence. Jeffrey Taubenberger at the Armed Forces Institute of Pathology has extracted several samples of the 1918 virus, some obtained from lung tissue preserved after autopsy, some from bodies buried in permafrost in the Arctic. He sequenced the genomes and, based on their rates of mutation, he believes that the virus jumped to humans in the winter of 1917–1918, roughly six to nine months prior to the lethal wave of the pandemic.

This timing perfectly fits the Haskell hypothesis. As does that outbreak's unusual nature and the difficulty in explaining how the virus got to Haskell if it did not originate there. And, one can trace with precision the route the Haskell virus took to the outside world: draftees carried it to Camp Funston (in fact, several histories of the pandemic begin their story there), and from there one can easily track the disease outward, to other cantonments, to the United States civilian population, and to Europe.

Epidemiological research is ongoing. Since the initial publication of this book, investigators reviewing more historical data have detected an increase in mortality among young adults in New York City in February and March 1918, which could indicate an influenza outbreak there. The lead investigator in this work does not believe that these findings, even if the deaths are from influenza, eliminate the Haskell hypothesis, but they do not strengthen it. For now, however, the thesis that Haskell County, Kansas, is the site of origin remains the most consistent with all available evidence.

This tells investigators where to look for a new virus. It—along with the 2003 outbreak in Europe—tells them they must look everywhere.

We do not live in a perfect world, and the World Health Organization lacks the resources to look everywhere. Its surveillance program sounds strong: currently more than one hundred laboratories in eighty-two countries participate. Four collaborating WHO influenza centers—the CDC in Atlanta and laboratories in Britain, Japan, and Australia—provide detailed analysis.

And although the WHO is, overall, a typical bureaucracy, its influenza arm has demonstrated decisiveness and competence in meeting difficult tests. It identified and contained the 1997 H5N1 outbreak; in 2003 it did the same for both SARS, a virus initially feared to be a new pandemic influenza threat, and the H7N7 avian influenza outbreak in the Netherlands. So far it has performed at a high level on H5N1.

Yet fewer than half the countries in the world participate in the surveillance system at all, while enormous regions of such participating nations as China go uncovered. This is an enormous weakness. Although the WHO is trying to address it, it is virtually impossible to convince an African government with much of its population infected with HIV to divert resources to a potential threat of influenza. Meanwhile, the WHO itself lacks the resources it needs to devote even to the immediate threat of H5N1 in southeast Asia.

So the surveillance system, while useful and worth trying to improve, will not be adequate any time soon, if ever.

Two things can be done.

We need to get more out of current surveillance. Although the SARS experience is and should be counted as a success, many of those directly involved in that work report that some labs withheld information. That needs to change.

On a larger scale, and far more difficult, will be getting governments to tell the truth about the disease. This is perhaps the biggest lesson of 1918, and it is a lesson not yet learned.

China lied about SARS for months; had SARS been a new influenza virus, the delay would have made it impossible to contain, or to develop a vaccine in advance of a worldwide onslaught. A year after SARS, Thailand and Indonesia also lied about H5N1 outbreaks, while Vietnam cooperates only reluctantly with the WHO on H5N1, carefully controlling all samples of material and absorbing information itself before releasing it to WHO personnel. (And when the Vietnamese wanted to share information, U.S. visa policies prevented their scientists from participating in an international workshop at the National Academy of Sciences.)

Getting open communication on this issue will take a serious diplomatic commitment. It may also take the creation of an insurance system that compensates countries and individual farmers for the financial losses that telling the truth can bring. No one is going to volunteer information that they know will destroy their economy or livelihood.

Communication matters. If communication is open enough, surveillance good enough, and leadership decisive enough, there is a slight but real chance a new pandemic virus could be snuffed out at the source by isolating cases, quarantining the area, and giving antivirals.

The most important actions we can take, however, can be taken immediately. The United States and other governments with a scientific infrastructure can launch, either in concert or unilaterally, a major effort to investigate influenza. It is time to make a rational decision about resources—about where we spend money.

Consider for a moment that total annual spending on the West Nile virus until 2005 exceeded spending on influenza. In its deadliest year, West Nile killed 284 Americans, and in five years killed a total of less than 900. More important, it is not a disease that is ever likely to explode through the human population. Even if we spend nothing—not a single penny—to fight it, it is far more likely that it will all but disappear by itself, just as happened with St. Louis encephalitis, a disease that is almost a twin to West Nile.

Comparing this to the tens of thousands of U.S. citizens killed annually by ordinary influenza—not to mention the threat of a pandemic—demonstrates more than the irrationality of those who make spending decisions. It demonstrates their irresponsibility.

Comparing a pandemic influenza threat to terrorism is also useful. The Department of Homeland Security views pandemic influenza as both the most likely and the most lethal of all threats facing the United States.

The WHO believes forty-three infectious organisms could be used as weapons. While influenza is on the list, the three most serious infectious threats are anthrax, plague, and smallpox, while botulinum toxin is considered the most dangerous poison. But vaccines can prevent smallpox, anthrax, and plague—antibiotics also work against anthrax and plague—and antitoxin can neutralize botulinum. Also, neither anthrax nor botulinum toxin can spread from person to person. The WHO has also studied what it called a worst case scenario of an attack with pneumonic plague on a city of 5 million, and concluded it would make 150,000 ill and kill 36,000. Adjusted for population, this worst case of bioterrorism represents considerably fewer fatalities than occurred in Philadelphia in 1918.

It's time to start spending serious money on influenza.

We need to invest in vaccine manufacture, and create surge capacity for when a pandemic does come. The federal government is already spending some money to address this, but problems remain. Vaccine makers say that their chief concern in expanding production is low demand and unpredictability. Some policy makers believe that an increase in the number of people the CDC recommends should get vaccinated annually might build enough demand to create adequate manufacturing facilities. Even if that worked, however, it would not address a second problem: our reliance on companies overseas for 50 percent of our supply. Americans have to decide whether they want, as a national security measure, to build that capacity here. Doing that could require government involvement, either through guarantees or subsidies. Also, although manufacturers consider liability exposure more of an irritant than a significant factor in the lack of production, the government might need to legislate limited protection for them as an incentive.

Second, we need to invest in improving the technology of vaccine production itself. Most people get injected with vaccines using killed viruses, but in 2003 a new vaccine was introduced that uses a live virus and is inhaled. This is a better delivery system for people at low risk because it stimulates the immune response in the throat's mucosal membranes. But the basics of the manufacturing process used for both vaccines are decades old and dependent on eggs. Taking advantage of molecular biology techniques could cut several weeks off the time it takes to produce vaccine—and in a pandemic a few weeks could save hundreds of thousands of lives. More research money might also yield more and better antiviral drugs.

Better yet, more investment in basic research might yield a vaccine effective against all influenza viruses. Work is under way targeting "conserved" portions of the genome, i.e., parts of the genetic structure that are common to all influenza viruses.

In the meantime, money must be spent to stockpile oseltamivir. At the moment this antiviral drug is the only weapon we have against H5N1. But it is no magic potion; H3N2, the influenza virus that causes most illness today, has demonstrated some ability to develop resistance to it. So far, H5N1 has not developed a resistance to it in laboratories, but there is no guarantee that it and other viruses won't.

Meanwhile, as we wait for science, as we wait for the next Rufus Cole or Oswald Avery, international organizations, national governments, and state governments in the United States are preparing for the next pandemic. Only if one erupts will we know how thorough these planners have been.

There was terror afoot in 1918. The randomness of death, its speed, and its tendency to kill off the healthiest brought that terror home.

The media and public officials helped create that terror—not by exaggerating the disease but by minimizing it, in their attempts to reassure the public.

Terror rises in the dark of the mind, an unknown beast tracking us in the jungle. All good horror movies build upon the fear of the unknown, the uncertain threat that we cannot see, do not know, and from which we can find no safe haven. In every horror movie, once the monster appears, terror condenses into the concrete and diminishes. Fear remains. But the edge of panic created by the unknown dissipates.

In 1918 the lies of officials and of the press prevented the terror from becoming concrete. The public could trust nothing and so they knew nothing. And this terror prevented one woman from caring for her sister, prevented volunteers from bringing food to families too ill to feed themselves and who then starved to death, prevented trained nurses from responding to the most urgent calls for their services. The fear, not the disease, threatened to break the society apart. As Victor Vaughan—a man who did not overstate to make a point—warned, "Civilization could have disappeared within a few more weeks."

So the final lesson of 1918, a simple one yet the one most difficult to execute, is that those who occupy positions of authority must lessen the panic that can alienate the members of a society. A society that takes as its motto, "every man for himself" is no longer a civilized society.

Those in authority must retain the public's trust. The way to do that is to distort nothing, to put the best face on nothing, to try to manipulate no one. Lincoln said that first, and best.

A leader must make whatever horror exists concrete. Only then will people be able to break it apart.

Acknowledgments

THIS BOOK was initially supposed to be a straightforward story of the deadliest epidemic in human history, told from the perspectives of both scientists who tried to fight it and political leaders who tried to respond to it. I thought it would take me two and a half years to write, three at the most.

That plan didn't work. Instead this book took seven years to write. It has evolved (and, I hope, grown) into something rather different than originally conceived.

It took so long partly because it didn't seem possible to write about the scientists without exploring the nature of American medicine at this time, for the scientists in this book did far more than laboratory research. They changed the very nature of medicine in the United States.

And, finding useful material on the epidemic proved remarkably difficult. It was easy enough to find stories of death, but my own interests have always focused on people who try to exercise some kind of control over events. Anyone doing so was far too busy, far too overwhelmed, to pay any attention to keeping records.

In the course of these seven years, many people helped me. Some shared with me their own research or helped me find material, others helped me understand the influenza virus and the disease it causes, and some offered advice on the manuscript. None of them, of course, is responsible for any errors of commission or omission, whether factual or of judgment, in the book. (Wouldn't it be entertaining to once read an acknowledgment in which the author blames others for any mistakes?)

Two friends, Steven Rosenberg and Nicholas Restifo at the National Cancer Institute, helped me understand how a scientist approaches a problem and also read parts of the manuscript and offered comments. So did Peter Palese at Mount Sinai Medical Center in New York, one of the world's leading experts on the influenza virus, who gave very generously of his time and expertise. Robert Webster, at St. Jude Medical Center, like Palese a world leader in influenza research, offered his insights and criticisms as well. Ronald French checked the manuscript for accuracy on the clinical course of the disease. Vincent Morelli introduced me to Warren Summers, who along with the entire pulmonary section of the Louisiana State University Health Sciences Center in New Orleans helped me understand much of what happens in the lung during an influenza attack; Warren was extremely patient and repeatedly helpful. Mitchell Freidman at the Tulane Medical School also explained events in the lung to me.

Jeffrey Taubenberger at the Armed Forces Institute of Pathology kept me abreast of his latest findings. John Yewdell at the National Institutes of Health also explained much about the virus. Robert Martensen at Tulane made valuable suggestions on the history of medicine. Alan Kraut at American University also read and commented on part of the manuscript.

I also particularly thank John MacLachlan of the Tulane-Xavier Center for Bioenvironmental Research, who very much helped make this book possible. William Steinmann, head of the Center for Clinical Effectiveness and Life Support at the Tulane Medical Center, gave generously of his office space, knowledge of disease, and friendship.

All of the above have M.D.s or Ph.D.s or both. Without their assistance I would have been lost trying to understand my own cytokine storm.

People who write books are always thanking librarians and archivists. They have good reason to. Virtually everyone at the Rudolph Matas Medical Library at Tulane University was extraordinarily helpful to me, but Patsy Copeland deserves truly special mention. So do Kathleen Puglia, Sue Dorsey, and Cindy Goldstein.

I also want to thank Mark Samels of WGBH's *American Experience,* who made available all the material collected for its program on the pandemic; Janice Goldblum at the National Academy of Sciences, who did more than just her job; Gretchen Worden at the Mutter Museum in Philadelphia; Jeffrey Anderson, then a graduate student at Rutgers, and Gery Gernhart, then a graduate student at American University, both of whom generously offered me their own research; and Charles Hardy of West Chester University, who gave me oral histories he had collected; and Mitch Yockelson at the National Archives, who gave me the benefit of his knowledge. Eliot Kaplan, then the editor of *Philadelphia Magazine,* also supported the project. I also want to thank Pauline Miner and Catherine Hart in Kansas. For help with photos I want to especially thank Susan Robbins Watson at the American Red Cross, Lisa Pendergraff at the Dudley Township Library in Kansas, Andre Sobocinski and Jan Herman at the Bureau of Navy Medicine, Darwin Stapleton at the Rockefeller University archives, and Nancy McCall at the Alan Mason Chesney archives at Johns Hopkins. I also want to thank Pat Ward Friedman for her information about her grandfather.

Now we come to my editor, Wendy Wolf. Although this is only my fifth book, counting magazine articles I've worked with literally dozens of editors. Wendy Wolf very much stands out. She edits the old-fashioned way; she works at it. On this manuscript she worked particularly hard, and working with her has been a pleasure. It is a true statement to say that, for better or worse (and I hope better), this book wouldn't exist without her. I'd also like to thank Hilary Redmon for her diligence, reliability, and just general assistance.

Thanks also to my agent Raphael Sagalyn, as good a professional as there is. I've had many editors but only one agent, a fact that speaks for itself.

Finally I thank my brilliant wife, Margaret Anne Hudgins, who helped me in too many ways to enumerate, including both in concept and in the particular—but chiefly by being herself. And then there are the cousins.

Notes

Abbreviations

APS	American Philosophical Society, Philadelphia
HSP	Historical Society of Philadelphia
JHU	Alan Mason Chesney Medical Archives, the Johns Hopkins University
LC ·	Library of Congress
NA	National Archives
NAS	National Academy of Sciences Archives
NLM	National Library of Medicine
RG	Record group at National Archives
RUA	Rockefeller University Archives
SG	Surgeon General William Gorgas
SLY	Sterling Library, Yale University
UNC	University of North Carolina, Chapel Hill
WP	Welch papers at JHU

PROLOGUE

Page

   2 *the smartest man:* Personal communication with Dr. David Aronson, Jan. 31, 2002, and Dr. Robert Shope, Sept. 9, 2002.

   4 *fifty million deaths:* Niall Johnson and Juergen Mueller, "Updating the Accounts: Global Mortality of the 1918–1920 'Spanish' Influenza Pandemic," *Bulletin of the History of Medicine* (2002), 105–15.

   4 *"doubly dead":* Sherwin Nuland, *How We Die* (1993), 202.

   6 *college degree:* Kenneth M. Ludmerer, *Learning to Heal: The Development of American Medical Education* (1985), 113.

7 *"vibrate and shake"*: William James, "Great Men, Great Thoughts, and Environment" (1880); quoted in Sylvia Nasar, *A Beautiful Mind* (1998), 55.
7 *"'Tis writ, 'In the beginning'"*: Johann Wolfgang Goethe, *Faust, Part One* (1949), 71.

Part I: The Warriors

CHAPTER ONE

11 *"the hostile Sioux"*: *Washington Star*, Sept. 12, 1876.
12 *"For God's sake"*: *New York Times*, Sept. 12, 1876.
13 *"great change in human thought"*: H. L. Mencken, "Thomas Henry Huxley
   1825–1925," *Baltimore Evening Sun* (1925).
13 *"voice was low, clear and distinct"*: For accounts of this speech, see *New York
   Times, Washington Post, Baltimore Sun*, Sept. 13, 1876.
14 *endowed chairs of theology*: Simon Flexner and James Thomas Flexner, *William
   Henry Welch and the Heroic Age of American Medicine* (1941), 237.
16 *theories that attributed epilepsy*: Roy Porter, *The Greatest Benefit to Mankind*
   (1997), 56.
16 *"a theory is a composite memory"*: Quoted in Charles-Edward Amory Winslow,
   The Conquest of Epidemic Disease: A Chapter in the History of Ideas (1943), 63.
17 *four kinds of bodily fluids*: For a discussion of the theory, see Porter, *The Greatest
   Benefit to Mankind*, 42–66, passim.
17 *"the true path of medicine"*: Ibid., 77.
18 *"recognizable only by logic"*: Vivian Nutton, "Humoralism," in *Companion Encyclopedia to the History of Medicine* (1993).
19 *"our own observation of nature"*: Quoted in Winslow, *Conquest of Epidemic Disease*, 126.
19 *"unequalled . . . between Hippocrates and Pasteur"*: Ibid., 142.
20 *"Don't think. Try."*: Ibid., 59.
20 *"I placed it upon a rock"*: Quoted in Milton Rosenau's 1934 presidential address
   to the Society of American Bacteriologists, Rosenau papers, UNC.
21 *"more simple and consistent system"*: For an excellent review of this see Richard
   Shryock, *The Development of Modern Medicine*, 2nd ed. (1947), 30–31.
21 *"sagacity and judgment"*: Ibid., 4.
22 *still seen as a manifestation*: Charles Rosenberg, "The Therapeutic Revolution,"
   in *Explaining Epidemics and Other Studies in the History of Medicine* (1992), 13–14.
23 *natural healing process*: Ibid., 9–27, passim.
23 *"profuse perspiration"*: Benjamin Coates practice book, quoted in ibid., 17.
24 *never had a peaceful bath again*: Steven Rosenberg in personal communication
   to the author.
25 *"withered arm of science"*: Quoted in Richard Shryock, *American Medical
   Research* (1947), 7.
26 *Michel Foucault condemned*: John Harley Warner, *Against the Spirit of the System: The French Impulse in Nineteenth-Century American Medicine* (1998), 4.
26 *"The practice of medicine"*: Ibid., 183–84.
28 *"Why think?"*: See Richard Walter, *S. Weir Mitchell, M.D., Neurologist: A Medical
   Biography* (1970), 202–22.
28 *"Nature answers only"*: Winslow, *Conquest of Epidemic Disease*, 296.

29 *"if all disease were left to itself"*: Quoted in Paul Starr, *The Social Transformation of American Medicine* (1982), 55.

29 *In 1862 in Philadelphia*: Charles Rosenberg, *Explaining Epidemics and Other Studies in the History of Medicine* (1992), 14.

29 *"popular crafts of every description"*: *Thomsonian Recorder* (1832), 89; quoted in Charles Rosenberg, *The Cholera Years: The United States in 1832, 1849, and 1866* (1962), 70–71.

29 *"False theory and hypothesis"*: John Harley Warner, "The Fall and Rise of Professional Mystery," in *The Laboratory Revolution in Medicine* (1992), 117.

30 *"priests' and Doctors' slavery"*: Quoted in Rosenberg, *Cholera Years*, 70–71.

30 *"a greater humbug"*: John King, "The Progress of Medical Reform," *Western Medical Reformer* (1846); quoted in Warner, "The Fall and Rise of Professional Mystery," 113.

30 *only thirty-four licensed physicians*: Burton J. Bledstein, *The Culture of Professionalism: The Middle Class and the Development of Higher Education in America* (1976), 33.

30 *"the Diminished Respectability"*: Shryock, *Development of Modern Medicine*, 264.

30 *court-martialed and condemned*: Ludmerer, *Learning to Heal*, 10, 11, 23, 168.

31 *not to treat malaria*: Rosenberg, "The Therapeutic Revolution," 9–27, passim.

31 *"all the worse for the fishes"*: Bledstein, *Culture of Professionalism*, 33.

31 *"a vast deal to be done"*: Quoted in Donald Fleming, *William Welch and the Rise of American Medicine* (1954), 8.

31 *7,000 to 226,000*: Edwin Layton, *The Revolt of the Engineers: Social Responsibility and the American Engineering Profession* (1971), 3.

32 *fail four of nine courses*: Ludmerer, *Learning to Heal*, 37 (re: Harvard), 12 (re: Michigan).

32 *"truths that lie about me so thick"*: Quoted in ibid., 25.

32 *not know how to use a microscope*: Ibid., 37.

32 *"something horrible to contemplate"*: Ibid., 48.

33 *"can't pass written examinations"*: Bledstein, *Culture of Professionalism*, 275–76.

33 *"No medical school has thought"*: Ludmerer, *Learning to Heal*, 15.

33 *"simply horrible"*: Ibid., 25.

33 *Against the advice*: James Thomas Flexner, *An American Saga: The Story of Helen Thomas and Simon Flexner* (1984), 125; see also ibid., 294.

34 *"strongest evidence of this demand"*: Benjamin Gilman, quoted in Flexner, *American Saga*, 125.

CHAPTER TWO

36 *eightieth-birthday celebration*: Flexner and Flexner, *William Henry Welch*, 3–8, passim.

37 *fifteen hundred stores*: Ezra Brown, ed., *This Fabulous Century, The Roaring Twenties 1920–1930* (1985), 105, 244.

37 *"beyond the capacity of an individual parent"*: Quoted in Sue Halpern, "Evangelists for Kids," *New York Review of Books* (May 29, 2003), 20.

38 *work of Rudolph Virchow*: Flexner and Flexner, *William Henry Welch*, 33.

38 *"accurate observation of facts"*: Ibid.

38 *filled him with repugnance*: Ibid., 29.

38 *begged his cousins:* Fleming, *William Welch*, 15.

39 *"every noble and good quality":* Flexner and Flexner, *William Henry Welch*, 50.

40 *"the light of his own mind":* Quoted in ibid., 49.

41 *"the labyrinths of Chemistry":* Ibid., 62–63.

41 *scientists had met in Berlin:* Shryock, *Development of Modern Medicine*, 206.

41 *"I can only admire":* Flexner and Flexner, *William Henry Welch*, 64, see also 71.

42 *"the easiest examination":* Ibid, 62.

42 *"a voyage of exploration":* Ibid., 76.

43 *fifteen thousand American doctors:* Thomas Bonner, *American Doctors and German Universities: A Chapter in International Intellectual Relations, 1870–1914* (1963), 23.

43 *"those who have studied abroad":* Welch to father, March 21, 1876, WP.

43 *"a source of pleasure and profit":* Welch to stepmother, March 26, 1877, WP.

43 *"Germany has outstripped":* Flexner and Flexner, *William Henry Welch*, 83.

44 *"certain important methods":* Welch to father, Oct. 18, 1876, WP.

44 *"carry on investigations hereafter":* Welch to father, Feb. 25, 1877, WP.

44 *"observe closely and carefully":* Welch to father, Oct. 18, 1876, WP.

44 *"He is almost the founder":* Welch to father, Sept. 23, 1877, WP.

44 *"The facts of science":* Quoted in Flexner and Flexner, *William Henry Welch*, 87.

45 *"constantly astonished at the wealth of experience":* Quoted in Shryock, *Development of Modern Medicine*, 181–82.

45 *"the greatest and most useful":* Quoted in ibid., 182.

46 *"the first men to be secured":* Quoted in Flexner and Flexner, *William Henry Welch*, 93.

46 *"a modest livelihood":* Ibid., 106.

47 *"cannot make much of a success":* Ibid., 112.

47 *"the drudgery of life":* Ibid.

CHAPTER THREE

48 *"leak knowledge":* Ibid., 70.

48 *"a larger circle of hearers":* Quoted in ibid., 117.

50 *"poisoning of half the population":* John Duffy, *A History of Public Health in New York City 1866–1966* (1974), 113.

51 *the zymote theory:* For more on zymotes see Phyllis Allen Richmond, "Some Variant Theories in Opposition to the Germ Theory of Disease," *Journal of the History of Medicine and Allied Sciences* (1954), 295.

53 *laurel wreath "such are given to the brave":* Paul De Kruif, *Microbe Hunters* (1939), 130.

53 *"What was theory":* Charles Chapin, "The Present State of the Germ Theory of Disease," Fists Fund Prize Essay (1885), unpaginated, Chapin papers, Rhode Island Historical Society.

53 *"powerless to create an epidemic":* Michael Osborne, "French Military Epidemiology and the Limits of the Laboratory: The Case of Louis-Felix-Achille Kelsch," in Andrew Cunningham and Perry Williams, eds., *The Laboratory Revolution in Medicine* (1992), 203.

54 *"however bright the prospect":* Flexner and Flexner, *William Henry Welch*, see 128–32.

55 *"not be so cheaply earned"*: Welch to stepmother, April 3, 1884, WP.

55 *"in no way discuss with him"*: Ibid.

55 *"on a high plane of loneliness"*: Flexner and Flexner, *William Henry Welch*, 136, see also 153.

56 *"deliberately break off relationships"*: According to Dr. Allen Freeman, quoted in ibid., 170.

57 *"already has a German reputation"*: Welch to father, Jan. 25, 1885, WP.

57 *the greatest name in science:* Florence Sabin, *Franklin Paine Mall: The Story of a Mind* (1934), 70.

58 *"a small chemical lab"*: Sabin, *Franklin Paine Mall,* 24.

58 *"What we shall consider success"*: Flexner and Flexner, *William Henry Welch,* 225.

58 *"which will cost $200,000"*: Sabin, *Franklin Paine Mall,* 112.

58 *"You make the opportunities"*: Ibid.

59 *"the real pioneer of modern"*: Martha Sternberg, *George Sternberg: A Biography* (1925), see 5, 68, 279, 285.

61 *build a theory on the right ones:* An anecdote related by Dr. Steven Rosenberg, July 1991.

61 *"keystone of the arch"*: Flexner and Flexner, *William Henry Welch,* 165.

62 *"putting an opponent down"*: Ibid., 151.

63 *"the richness of the world"*: Ibid., 230.

63 *"atmosphere of achievement"*: Ibid., 165.

64 *"never anything quite like it"*: John Fulton, *Harvey Cushing* (1946), 118.

CHAPTER FOUR

65 *"no evidence of preliminary education"*: Flexner and Flexner, *William Henry Welch,* 222.

66 *"long and painful controversy"*: Ludmerer, *Learning to Heal,* 53.

66 *"The talk was of pathology"*: Fulton, *Harvey Cushing,* 121.

66 *"what was true of Harvard"*: Shryock, *Unique Influence of Johns Hopkins,* 8.

66 *"and want no others"*: Quoted in Ludmerer, *Learning to Heal,* 75.

66 *"to one man—Franklin P. Mall"*: Shryock, *Unique Influence,* 20.

67 *"whether they were saved"*: Michael Bliss, *William Osler: A Life in Medicine* (1999), 216.

67 *fifty-three became professors:* Bonner, *American Doctors and German Universities,* 99.

67 *"the whole still concert"*: William G. MacCallum, *William Stewart Halsted* (1930), 212.

68 *"violate all the best precedents"*: Flexner and Flexner, *William Henry Welch,* 263.

68 *"flick of a wrist"*: Ludmerer, *Learning to Heal,* 128.

68 *endowments totaled $500,000:* Shryock, *Unique Influence,* 37.

70 *marvelous curative agent:* Victor A. Vaughan, *A Doctor's Memories* (1926), 153.

71 *"an epoch in the history of medicine"*: Flexner and Flexner, *William Henry Welch,* 207.

71 *"a body of research"*: Wade Oliver, *The Man Who Lived for Tomorrow: A Biography of William Hallock Park, M.D.* (1941), 238.

72 *"little less than lunatic"*: Frederick T. Gates to Starr Murphy, Dec. 31, 1915, WP.

72 *"to become a pioneer"*: Ibid.

73 *accepting the Jew:* James Thomas Flexner, *American Saga,* 241–42.

73 *"every letter handwritten":* Ibid., 278.

74 *"not have anything to do with":* Benison and Nevins, "Oral History, Abraham Flexner," Columbia University Oral History Research Office; Flexner, *American Saga,* see 30–40.

74 *"never heard a heart or lung":* James Thomas Flexner, *American Saga,* 133.

74 *"great gaps":* Ibid., 421.

74 *"He read . . . as he ate":* Benison and Nevins, "Oral History, Abraham Flexner."

74 *"days of acute fear":* James Thomas Flexner, *American Saga,* 239.

74 *"a museum in print":* Peyton Rous comments, Simon Flexner Memorial Pamphlet, Rockefeller Institute of Medical Research, 1946.

75 *"His mind was like a searchlight":* Corner, *History of the Rockefeller Institute,* 155.

75 *"final as a knife":* Ibid.

75 *"or they can be bled further":* Flexner to Cole, Jan. 21, 1919, Flexner papers, APS.

75 *"Individuals were as nothing":* Peyton Rous comments, Simon Flexner Memorial Pamphlet.

76 *mortality rate fell to 31.4 percent:* Simon Flexner, "The Present Status of the Serum Therapy of Epidemic Cerebro-spinal Meningitis," *JAMA* (1909), 1443; see also Abstract of Discussion, 1445.

76 *"Remarkable results were obtained":* Ibid.

76 *a shouting match ensued:* Wade Oliver, *Man Who Lived for Tomorrow,* 300.

76 *"mortality rate of 25 percent":* M. L. Durand et al., "Acute Bacterial Meningitis in Adults—A Review of 493 Episodes," *New England Journal of Medicine* (Jan. 1993), 21–28.

76 *"I advise the publication":* Flexner to Wollstein, March 26, 1921, Flexner papers.

77 *"Before night your discovery":* Corner, *History of the Rockefeller Institute,* 159.

77 *"frequent ballyhoo of unimportant stuff":* Ibid., 158.

77 *"he also was tender":* Saul Benison, *Tom Rivers: Reflections on a Life in Medicine and Science, An Oral History Memoir* (1967), 127.

77 *"made to believe":* Corner, *History of the Rockefeller Institute,* 155.

77 *"I won't expect anything":* Ibid., 158.

78 *"a great inspiration":* Heidelberger, oral history, 1968, NLM, 66.

78 *"an organism, not an establishment":* Peyton Rous comments, Simon Flexner Memorial Pamphlet.

78 *"science isolated Dr. Koch":* For an account of this meeting see Wade Oliver, *Man Who Lived for Tomorrow,* 272–76.

CHAPTER FIVE

80 *"wasn't afraid to fight":* Benison, *Tom Rivers,* 30, 70, 204.

81 *"quite remarkable in that way":* Heidelberger, oral history, 83.

81 *"Cole was adamant":* Benison, *Tom Rivers,* 70.

81 *"urged to undertake experimental work":* Benison, *Tom Rivers,* 68.

82 *"results were better than the system":* Quoted in Flexner and Flexner, *William Henry Welch,* 61.

83 *Not until 1912 would Harvard:* Fleming, *William Welch,* 4.

83 *a blistering . . . report:* Vaughan, *A Doctor's Memories,* 440.

83 *fifty-seven medical schools:* Ludmerer, *Learning to Heal,* 116.

83 *only eight thousand members:* Paul Starr, *The Social Transformation of American Medicine* (1982), 109.

84 *"my initial visit to Baltimore":* Ludmerer, *Learning to Heal,* 172.

84 *"make better farmers":* Ibid., see 169–73.

84 *6,843 locations:* Meirion Harries and Susie Harries, *The Last Days of Innocence: America at War, 1917–1918* (1997), 15.

85 *"to . . . legitimize . . ." capitalism:* E. Richard Brown, *Rockefeller's Medicine Men* (1979), quoted in Starr, *Social Transformation,* 227.

85 *thirty-one states denied licensing:* Ludmerer, *Learning to Heal,* 238–43.

85 *still 25 percent less:* Shryock, *Development of Modern Medicine,* 350; Ludmerer, *Learning to Heal,* 247.

85 *"The AMA deserved . . . the credit":* Fulton, *Harvey Cushing,* 379.

86 *$154 million into medicine:* Ludmerer, *Learning to Heal,* 192–93.

87 *"the sole argument for putting":* Charles Eliot to Abraham Flexner, Feb. 1 and Feb. 16, 1916, WP.

Part II: The Swarm

CHAPTER SIX

92 *"A slow rain fell":* Santa Fe Monitor, Feb. 28, 1918.

92 *didn't suffer fools:* Material on L. V. Miner comes from an interview with his daughter-in-law Mrs. L. V. Miner Jr. on Aug. 27, 1999, and granddaughter Catherine Hart in July 2003, and from *Kansas and Kansans* (1919).

93 *hold the train for him:* For a description of a typical western practice, especially in Kansas, see Arthur E. Hertzler, *The Horse and Buggy Doctor* (1938) and Thomas Bonner, *The Kansas Doctor* (1959).

94 *"sick with pneumonia":* Santa Fe Monitor, Feb. 14, 1918.

94 *"influenza of severe type":* Public Health Reports 33, part 1 (April 5, 1918), 502.

95 *"Most everybody over the country":* Santa Fe Monitor, Feb. 21, 1918.

95 *"John will make an ideal soldier":* Santa Fe Monitor, Feb. 28, 1918.

96 *"animosity towards me":* Maj. John T. Donnelly, 341st Machine Gun Battalion, Camp Funston, RG 393, NA.

96 *"to exercise command":* Commanding General C. G. Ballou, Camp Funston, to Adjutant General, March 12, 1918, Camp Funston, RG 393.

96 *"overcrowded and inadequately heated":* Maj. General Merritt W. Ireland, ed., *Medical Department of the United States Army in the World War,* v. 9, *Communicable Diseases* (1928), 415.

CHAPTER SEVEN

98 *"arrival of American troops in France":* F. M. Burnet and Ellen Clark, *Influenza: A Survey of the Last Fifty Years* (1942), 70.

102 *"a special instance" among infectious diseases:* Bernard Fields, *Fields' Virology,* (1996), 265.

105 *mutate much faster:* Ibid., 114.

105 *"mutant swarm"*: J. J. Holland, "The Origin and Evolution of Viruses," in *Microbiology and Microbial Infections* (1998), 12.

105 *"certain randomness to the disease"*: Ibid., 17.

CHAPTER EIGHT

107 *resist putrefaction:* Quoted in Milton Rosenau notebook, Dec. 12, 1907, Rosenau papers, UNC.

110 *influenza kills more people:* Harvey Simon and Martin Swartz, "Pulmonary Infections," and R. J. Douglas, "Prophylaxis and Treatment of Influenza," in section 7, Infectious Diseases, in Edward Rubenstein and Daniel Feldman, *Scientific American Medicine* (1995).

112 *"It's equally likely"*: Peter Palese, personal communication with the author, Aug. 2, 2001.

113 *"attacked at once"*: W. I. B. Beveridge, *Influenza: The Last Great Plague: An Unfinished Story of Discovery* (1977), 26.

113 *"entirely depopulated"*: Ibid.

113 *"as in a plague"*: John Duffy, *Epidemics in Colonial America* (1953), 187–88, quoted in Dorothy Ann Pettit, "A Cruel Wind: America Experiences the Pandemic Influenza, 1918–1920, A Social History" (1976), 31.

113 *"youngest as well as the oldest"*: Beveridge, *Influenza,* 26.

113 *"all weer sick"*: Quoted in Pettit, "Cruel Wind," 32.

114 *more people died from influenza:* Beveridge, *Influenza,* 26–31.

Part III: The Tinderbox

CHAPTER NINE

119 *"The rat serves one useful function"*: Major George Crile, "The Leading War Problems and a Plan of Organization to Meet Them," draft report, 1916, NAS.

120 *"The war sentiment"*: Randolph Bourne, "The War and the Intellectuals," *The Seven Arts* (June 1917), 133–46.

121 *"I am sure that my heart"*: Arthur Walworth, *Woodrow Wilson,* v. 2 (1965), 63.

121 *"I will not cry 'peace'"*: Walworth, *Woodrow Wilson,* v. 1, 344.

121 *"Once lead this people into war"*: Walworth, *Woodrow Wilson,* v. 2, 97.

122 *"It isn't an army we must shape"*: Stephen Vaughn, *Holding Fast the Inner Lines: Democracy, Nationalism, and the Committee on Public Information* (1980), 3.

122 *"the poison of disloyalty"*: David Kennedy, *Over Here: The First World War and American Society* (1980), 24.

123 *"Thank God for Abraham Lincoln"*: Walworth, *Woodrow Wilson,* v. 2, 101.

123 *"an imperative necessity"*: Walworth, *Woodrow Wilson,* v. 2, 97.

123 *"governed by public opinion"*: Kennedy, *Over Here,* 47.

123 *"casual or impulsive disloyal utterances"*: Vaughn, *Holding Fast the Inner Lines,* 226; Kennedy, *Over Here,* 81.

123 *"from good motives"*: Richard W. Steele, *Free Speech in the Good War* (1999), 153.

124 *two hundred thousand APL members:* Joan Jensen, *The Price of Vigilance* (1968), 115.

124 *"seditious street oratory"*: Ibid., 96.

124 *"ninety percent of all the men"*: Kennedy, *Over Here,* 54.

125 *"What the nation demands"*: Quoted in Jensen, *Price of Vigilance,* 79.

125 *"Every German or Austrian"*: Ibid., 99.

125 *"What had been folly"*: Kennedy, *Over Here,* 74.

125 *"spreads pessimistic stories"*: Vaughn, *Holding Fast the Inner Lines,* 155.

125 *"sinister intrigue"*: Jensen, *Price of Vigilance,* 51.

125 Two Communist parties: Robert Murray, *Red Scare: A Study in National Hysteria* (1955), 16, 51–53.

125 *"That community is already in the process"*: Learned Hand speech, Jan. 27, 1952, quoted in www.conservativeforum.org/authquot.asp?ID915.

126 *"Truth and falsehood are arbitrary"*: Vaughn, *Holding Fast the Inner Lines,* 3.

126 most citizens were *"mentally children"*: Kennedy, *Over Here,* 91–92.

126 climbed onto a chandelier: Interview with Betty Carter, April 1997.

126 *"one white-hot mass"*: Vaughn, *Holding Fast the Inner Lines,* 3.

127 *"intellectual cohesion—herd-instinct"*: Bourne, "War and the Intellectuals," 133.

127 *"the noblest of all mottoes"*: Vaughn, *Holding Fast the Inner Lines,* 141.

127 *"I am Public Opinion"*: Ibid., 169.

127 *"every printed bullet"*: Murray, *Red Scare,* 12.

127 *"To fight for an ideal"*: Vaughn, *Holding Fast the Inner Lines,* 126.

128 *"questionable jokes"*: *Philadelphia Inquirer,* Sept. 1, 1918.

128 *"Force to the utmost!"*: Walworth, *Woodrow Wilson,* v. 2, 168.

129 *"exert itself in any way"*: Red Cross news release, Aug. 23, 1917, entry 12, RG 52, NA.

129 *"delivered at any point"*: Aug. 24, 1917 memo, entry 12, RG 52, NA.

130 *"Confectioners and restaurants"*: See, for example, the *Arizona Gazette,* Sept. 26, 1918.

130 *"go down to roll bandages"*: William Maxwell, unaired interview re Lincoln, Illinois, Feb. 26, 1997, for "Influenza 1918," *American Experience.*

131 *"Military instruction under officers"*: *Committee on Education and Training: A Review of Its Work,* by the advisory board, unpaginated, appendix. C. R. Mann, chairman, RG 393, NA.

131 *"mobilization of all physically fit registrants"*: Memo to the Colleges of the U.S. from Committee on Education and Training, Aug. 28, 1918; copy found in Camp Grant files, RG 393, NA.

CHAPTER TEN

133 *"The Academy now considers"*: Quoted in Simon Flexner and James Thomas Flexner, *William Henry Welch and the Heroic Age of American Medicine* (1941), 366.

135 More soldiers had died of disease: United States Civil War Center, www.cwc.lsu.edu/cwc/other/stats/warcost.htm.

136 not a single microscope: Victor Vaughan, *A Doctor's Memories* (1926), 410.

136 *"virgin"* human population: Interview with Dr. Peter Palese, March 20, 2001.

136 killing 5 percent of all the men: Memo on measles, undated, RG 112, NA; see also Maj. General Merritt W. Ireland, ed., *Medical Department of the United States Army in the World War,* v. 9, *Communicable Diseases* (1928), 409.

137 rotating his attention: David McCullough, *The Path Between the Seas: The Creation of the Panama Canal, 1870–1914* (1977), 425–26.

138 *"extremes the sexual moralist can go"*: William Allen Pusey, M.D., "Handling of the Venereal Problem in the U.S. Army in Present Crisis," *JAMA* (Sept. 28, 1918), 1017.

139 *"A Soldier who gets a dose"*: Kennedy, *Over Here*, 186.

139 *"no longer a danger"*: C. P. Knight, "The Activities of the USPHS in Extra-Cantonment Zones, with Special Reference to the Venereal Disease Problem," *Military Surgeon* (Jan. 1919), 41.

139 *test the antitoxin*: Flexner and Flexner, *William Henry Welch*, 371.

140 *"[U]nit will be arranged"*: Colonel Frederick Russell to Flexner, June 11, 1917, Flexner papers, APS.

140 *no mere cosmetic change*: George A. Corner, *A History of the Rockefeller Institute: 1901–1953, Origins and Growth* (1964), 141.

141 *"best from these classes"*: Notes on meeting of National Research Council executive committee, April 19, 1917, NAS.

141 *half of all those . . . fit for service*: Arthur Lamber, "Medicine: A Determining Factor in War," *JAMA* (June 14, 1919), 1713.

141 *army had fifty-eight dentists*: Franklin Martin, *Fifty Years of Medicine and Surgery* (1934), 379.

141 *replaced labels on drug bottles*: Lavinia Dock, 1909, quoted in Soledad Mujica Smith, "Nursing as Social Responsibility: Implications for Democracy from the Life Perspective of Lavinia Lloyd Dock (1858–1956)" (2002), 78.

142 *"at once sever my connection"*: Lavinia Dock et al., *History of American Red Cross Nursing* (1922), 958.

142 *"carry out the plans"*: Ibid., 954.

CHAPTER ELEVEN

144 *"Every single activity"*: Editorial, *Military Surgeon* 43 (Aug. 1918), 208.

144 *"The consideration of human life"*: John C. Wise, "The Medical Reserve Corps of the U.S. Navy," *Military Surgeon* (July 1918), 68.

145 *"they should be bayonetted"*: "Review of *Offensive Fighting* by Major Donald McRae," *Military Surgeon* (Feb. 1919), 86.

145 *"I was very glad"*: Flexner and Flexner, *William Henry Welch*, 371.

146 *lowered the death rate*: H. J. Parish, *A History of Immunization* (1965), 3.

147 *banned all sales*: Wade Oliver, *The Man Who Lived for Tomorrow: A Biography of William Hallock Park, M.D.* (1941), 378.

147 *enough typhoid vaccine for five million*: Vaughan to George Hale, March 21, 1917, Executive Committee on Medicine and Hygiene, general file, NAS.

147 *"sent to any one of the camps"*: Flexner to Russell, Nov. 28, 1917, Flexner papers.

147 *"prevention of infectious disease"*: Flexner to Vaughan, June 2, 1917, Flexner papers.

147 *"Although pneumonia occurs"*: Rufus Cole et al., "Acute Lobar Pneumonia Prevention and Serum Treatment" (Oct. 1917), 4.

148 *"as if the men had pooled their diseases"*: Flexner and Flexner, *William Henry Welch*, 372.

148 *"How many lives were sacrificed"*: Vaughan, *A Doctor's Memories*, 428–29.

149 *"Not a troop train"*: Ibid., 425.

149 *three thousand were sick enough*: Ireland, *Communicable Diseases*, 415.

149 *complications of measles*: Vaughan, *A Doctor's Memories*, 57.

149 *average death rate from pneumonia:* Dorothy Ann Pettit, "A Cruel Wind: America Experiences the Pandemic Influenza, 1918–1920, A Social History" (1976), 56.

150 *"never in their confidence":* Ibid., 3.

150 *"seem to have deserted me":* John M. Gibson, *Physician to the World: The Life of General William C. Gorgas* (1989), 242.

150 *"send directions for Avery's":* Welch diary, Jan. 2, 1918, WP.

CHAPTER TWELVE

153 *evidence that the influenza virus:* J. A. McCullers and K. C. Bartmess, "Role of Neuraminidase in Lethal Synergism Between Influenza Virus and Streptococcus Pneumoniae," William Osler, *Osler's Textbook Revisited* (1967), *Journal of Infectious Diseases* (2003), 1000–1009.

154 *"To bleed at the very onset":* 00.

154 *"Pneumonia is a self-limited disease":* Ibid.

156 *"true inwardness of research":* Quoted in McLeod, "Oswald Theodore Avery, 1877–1955," *Journal of General Microbiology* (1957), 540.

156 *"An acute need for privacy":* René Dubos, "Oswald Theodore Avery, 1877–1955," *Biographical Memoirs of Fellows of the Royal Society,* 35.

156 *"as if a mask dropped":* Ibid.

157 *"a natural born comedian":* Donald Van Slyke, oral history, NLM.

157 *about Landsteiner's personal life:* René Dubos, *The Professor, the Institute, and DNA* (1976), 47.

157 *notified he'd won the Nobel:* Saul Benison, *Tom Rivers: Reflections on Life in Medicine and Science, an Oral History Memoir* (1967), 91–93.

158 *"motives that lead persons to art or science":* Quoted in Dubos, *Professor,* 179.

158 *"a sweeping metabolic theory":* Ibid., 95.

CHAPTER THIRTEEN

162 *"Protection in man is inferior":* Rufus Cole et al., "Acute Lobar Pneumonia," 4.

162 *"lead all diseases":* Ibid.

163 *"diseases amongst the troops":* See, for example, Gorgas to Commanding Officer, Base Hospital, Camp Greene, Oct. 26, 1917, entry 29, file 710, RG 112, NA.

163 *All of them had negative reactions:* Scientific reports of the Corporation and Board of Scientific Directors of Rockefeller Institute, April 20, 1918.

163 *Camp Gordon outside Atlanta:* Ireland, *Communicable Diseases,* 442.

163 *"the matter of prophylactic vaccination":* Cole to Russell, Dec. 14, 1917, entry 29, RG 112, NA.

164 *controls suffered 101:* Memo from Flexner to Russell, Oct. 3, 1918, entry 29, RG 112, NA.

164 *Pasteur Institute was also testing:* Ireland, *Communicable Diseases,* 125.

164 *to meet Gorgas and Welch:* Welch to Flexner wire, April 15, 1918; Flexner to Cole, April 16, 1918, Flexner papers.

164 *"really a privilege":* Michael Heidelberger, oral history, NLM, 83.

165 *checking on everything:* Ibid.

165 *"chiefly in epidemic form":* Rufus Cole, "Prevention of Pneumonia," *JAMA* (Aug. 1918), 634.

166 *the Canadian army:* W. David Parsons, "The Spanish Lady and the Newfoundland Regiment" (1998).
166 *"detention camps for new recruits":* Welch diary, Dec. 28, 1917, WP.

Part IV: It Begins

CHAPTER FOURTEEN

169 *Thirty of the fifty largest cities:* Edwin O. Jordan, *Epidemic Influenza* (1927), 69.
170 *"convenient to follow":* F. M. Burnet and Ellen Clark, *Influenza: A Survey of the
Last Fifty Years* (1942), 70.
170 *of 172 marines:* W. J. MacNeal, "The Influenza Epidemic of 1918 in the AEF in
France and England," *Archives of Internal Medicine* (1919), 657.
170 *appearance in the French army:* Burnet and Clark, *Influenza,* 70.
170 *36,473 hospital admissions:* Quoted in Jordan, *Epidemic Influenza,* 78.
170 *"At the end of May":* Ibid.
171 *"broken clean through":* Harvey Cushing, *A Surgeon's Journal 1915–18* (1934), 311.
171 *"The expected third stage":* Ibid.
171 *"the epidemic of grippe":* Ibid.
171 *"a grievous business":* Ray Stannard Baker, *Woodrow Wilson: Life and Letters/
Armistice March 1–November 11, 1918* (1939), 233.
172 *"abuts on the harbor":* Jordan, *Epidemic Influenza,* 85.
172 *"swept over the whole country":* Ibid., 87.
172 *10,313 sailors fell ill:* David Thomson and Robert Thomson, *Annals of the Pickett-
Thomson Research Laboratory,* v. 9, *Influenza* (1934), 178.
172 *"of a mild form":* Jordan, *Epidemic Influenza,* 93.
172 *doubt that it was influenza:* MacNeal, "Influenza Epidemic," *Archives of Internal
Medicine* (1919), 657.
172 *"not influenza":* From *Policlinico* 25, no. 26 (June 30, 1918), quoted in *JAMA* 71,
no. 9, 780.
172 *"very short duration":* T. R. Little, C. J. Garofalo, and P. A. Williams, "B Influenzae and Present Epidemic," *The Lancet* (July 13, 1918), quoted in *JAMA* 71, no.
8 (Aug. 24, 1918), 689.
173 *"fatal in from 24 to 48 hours":* Major General Merritt W. Ireland, ed., *Medical
Department of the United States Army in the World War,* v. 9, *Communicable Disease* (1928), 132.
173 *"a new disease":* Jordan, *Epidemic Influenza,* 36.
173 *688 men were ill:* George Soper, M.D., "The Influenza Pandemic in the Camps,"
undated draft report, RG 112, NA.
174 *"any definite information":* Cole to Pearce, July 19, 1918, NAS.
174 *put more resources:* Cole to Pearce, July 24, 1918, NAS.
174 *declared the epidemic over:* "The Influenza Pandemic in American Camps, September 1918," memo to Col. Howard from Office of the Army Surgeon General,
Oct. 9, 1918, Red Cross papers, War Council notes, RG 200, NA.
174 *"completely disappeared":* Letter from London of Aug. 20, 1918, quoted in *JAMA*
71, no. 12 (Sept. 21, 1918), 990.
174 *"mistaken for meningitis":* Late summer report quoted in *JAMA* 71, no. 14 (Oct.
5, 1918), 1136.

174 *"No letter from my beloved"*: Dorothy Ann Pettit, "A Cruel Wind: America Experiences the Pandemic Influenza, 1918–1920, A Social History" (1976), 97, 98.

175 *"some interesting cases"*: Ibid., 67.

CHAPTER FIFTEEN

176 *most influenza experts:* Interview with Robert Webster, June 13, 2002.

177 *At the fifteenth passage:* William Bulloch, *The History of Bacteriology* (1938, reprinted 1979), 143.

177 *Changing the environment:* Jordan, *Epidemic Influenza*, 511.

177 *As the bacteria adapted to rabbits:* Richard Shryock, *The Development of Modern Medicine,* 2nd edition (1947), 294–95.

178 *1 million pigs:* Bulloch, *History of Bacteriology,* 246.

178 *"primarily virus influenza"*: Burnet and Clark, *Influenza,* 40.

178 *"We must suppose"*: Ibid., 69, 70.

179 *a ward was sealed off:* Soper, "Influenza Pandemic in the Camps."

179 *"they had influenza"*: Ibid.

180 *"not like the common broncho-pneumonia"*: Adolph A. Hoehling, *The Great Epidemic* (1961), 21.

180 *"an outbreak of epidemic influenza"*: *Public Health Reports,* 33, part 2 (July 26, 1918), 1259.

180 *"I am confidentially advised"*: Entry 12, index card 126811, RG 52, NA.

181 *"a progressive increase in cases"*: Ireland, *Communicable Diseases,* 83, 135.

181 *"indistinguishably blend with"*: Ibid., 135.

181 *"the seamen were prostrate"*: Jordan, *Epidemic Influenza,* 114.

181 *"a well-nourished people"*: John Duffy, *A History of Public Health in New York City 1866–1966* (1974), 286.

181 *children were malnourished:* Ibid., 287.

181 *two steamships from Norway:* Soper, "The Influenza Pandemic in the Camps."

182 *outbreak with high mortality:* Ireland, *Communicable Diseases,* 137.

182 *overwhelmed the naval hospital:* Director of Labs, AEF, to SG, Dec. 10, 1918, entry 29, RG 112, NA.

182 *"number of American negroes"*: Quoted in Pettit, "Cruel Wind," 94.

182 *two natives died:* Burnet and Clark, *Influenza,* 72.

183 *five hundred of the six hundred laborers:* A. W. Crosby, *America's Forgotten Pandemic: The Influenza of 1918* (1989), 37.

183 *7 percent of the entire crew died:* Burnet and Clark, *Influenza,* 72.

183 *struck down nine hundred:* Ibid.

183 *115 more deaths:* Director of Labs, AEF, to SG, Dec. 10, 1918, entry 29, RG 112, NA.

183 *"grossly overcrowded"*: Crosby, *America's Forgotten Pandemic,* 38.

184 *"The Bible"*: From Medical Officers Training Camp at Camp Greenleaf, Georgia, Nov. 18, 1918, Rosenau papers, UNC.

CHAPTER SIXTEEN

185 *"mess officer is well informed"*: Major R. C. Hoskins, "Report of Inspection on Sept. 30, 1918," Oct. 9, 1918, RG 112, NA.

185 *inoculating a series of human volunteers:* Undated report by Major Andrew Sellards, entry 29, RG 112, NA.

186 *only eighty-four patients:* "Influenza Pandemic in American Camps, September 1918"; see also Paul Wooley to SG, Aug. 29, 1918, RG 112, NA.

186 *"very significant increase":* Boston Health Department Monthly Bulletin, Sept. 1918, 183, quoted in Jordan, *Epidemic Influenza,* 115.

186 *diagnosed as having meningitis:* Major Paul Wooley, "Epidemiological Report on Influenza and Pneumonia, Camp Devens, August 28 to October 1, 1918," entry 29, RG 112, NA.

187 *"which attacked so many":* Ibid.

187 *"occurred as an explosion":* Ibid.

187 *Eight of the twelve collapsed:* "Steps Taken to Check the Spread of the Epidemic," undated, unsigned, entry 29, RG 112, NA; see also Katherine Ross, "Battling the Flu," *American Red Cross Magazine* (Jan. 1919), 11.

187 *"These men start with what appears to be":* Dr. Roy N. Grist to "Burt," *British Medical Journal* (Dec. 22–29, 1979).

188 *"only a matter of a few hours":* Ibid.

188 *"we are all well":* Russell to Flexner, Sept. 18, 1918, Flexner papers, APS.

189 *"You will proceed immediately":* Victor Vaughan, *A Doctor's Memories* (1926), 431.

189 *"hundreds of young stalwart men":* Ibid., 383–84.

189 *in excess of six thousand:* Vaughan and Welch to Gorgas, Sept. 27, 1918, entry 29, RG 112, NA.

190 *"dead bodies are stacked":* Vaughan, *A Doctor's Memories,* 383–84.

190 *"step amongst them":* Cole to Flexner, May 26, 1936, file 26, box 163, WP.

190 *"too much for Dr. Welch":* Ibid.

191 *"influenza be kept out of the camps":* "Memo for Camp and Division Surgeons," Sept. 24, 1918, entry 710, RG 112, NA.

191 *"New men will almost surely":* Brigadier General Richard to adjutant general, Sept. 25, 1918, entry 710, RG 112, NA; see also Charles Richard to chief of staff, Sept. 26, 1918, entry 710, RG 112, NA.

192 *"spread rapidly across":* J. J. Keegan, "The Prevailing Epidemic of Influenza," *JAMA* (Sept. 28, 1918), 1051.

193 *Around the world from Boston:* I. D. Mills, "The 1918–1919 Influenza Pandemic—The Indian Experience," *The Indian Economic and Social History Review* (1986), 27, 35.

Part V: Explosion

CHAPTER SEVENTEEN

197 *three hundred sailors arrived:* "Sanitary Report for Fourth Naval District for the Month of September 1918," entry 12, file 584, RG 52, NA.

197 *tenements still had outhouses:* "Philadelphia—How the Social Agencies Organized to Serve the Sick and Dying," *The Survey* 76 (Oct. 19, 1918); oral history of Anna Lavin, July 14, 1982, courtesy of Charles Hardy, West Chester University.

198 *"death rate . . . has gone up":* Mrs. Wilmer Krusen reports, Feb. 4, 1918, entries 13B-D2, RG 62.

198 *no high school until 1934:* Allen Davis and Mark Haller, eds., *The Peoples of Philadel-phia: A History of Ethnic Groups and Lower-Class Life, 1790–1940* (1973), 256.

198 *"worst-governed city":* Quoted in Russell Weigley, ed., *Philadelphia: A 300-Year History* (1982), 539.

200 *"took control of police":* Major William Snow and Major Wilbur Sawyer, "Vene-real Disease Control in the Army," *JAMA* (Aug. 10, 1918), 462.

200 *left Philadelphia for Puget Sound:* Annual Report of the Surgeon General of the U.S. Navy for Fiscal Year 1918, Government Printing Office.

202 *put the body on a stretcher:* Robert St. John, *This Was My World* (1953), 49–50, quoted in Dorothy Ann Pettit, "A Cruel Wind: America Experiences the Pan-demic Influenza, 1918–1920" (1976), 103.

202 *"33 caskets to Naval":* "Journal of the Medical Department, Great Lakes," entry 22a, RG 52, NA.

202 *toe tags on the boys':* Carla Morrisey, transcript of unaired interview for "Influenza 1918," *American Experience*, Feb. 26, 1997.

202 *"what it would feel like":* Ibid.

202 *"this threat of influenza invasion":* Howard Anders to William Braisted, Sept. 12, 1918, RG 52, NA.

203 *refused to release six:* Board of Trustees minutes, Sept. 9 and Sept. 30, 1918, Jef-ferson Medical College, Philadelphia.

204 *"When obliged to cough or sneeze":* *Philadelphia Inquirer,* Sept. 19, 1918.

204 *"No concern whatever":* *The Evening Bulletin,* Sept. 18, 1918.

205 *"can successfully be prevented":* Department of Public Health and Charities min-utes, Sept. 21 and Oct. 3, 1918.

205 *"ideas of whole populations":* Quoted in Victoria De Grazia, "The Selling of America, Bush Style," *New York Times* (Aug. 25, 2002).

205 *"world lives by phrases":* Quoted in Joan Hoff Wilson, *Herbert Hoover: Forgotten Progressive* (1974), 59.

206 *"'Every Scout to Save a Soldier'":* Quoted in ibid., 105 fn.

206 *"If you find a disloyal":* Gregg Wolper, "The Origins of Public Diplomacy: Woodrow Wilson, George Creel, and the Committee on Public Information" (1991), 80.

206 *"The IWW agitators":* Kennedy, *Over Here,* 73.

207 *"nobody can say we aren't loyal":* Ellis Hawley, *The Great War and the Search for a Modern Order: A History of the American People and Their Institutions, 1917–1933* (1979), 24.

207 *"In spite of excesses such as lynching":* Ibid.

207 *"most powerful of human motives":* William McAdoo, *Crowded Years* (1931), 374–79, quoted in David Kennedy, *Over Here* (1980), 105.

207 *"Every person who refuses":* David Kennedy, *Over Here,* 106.

208 *"a ready-made inflammable mass":* Howard Anders, letter to *Public Ledger,* Oct. 9, 1918, in which he cites his earlier opposition to the rally; quoted in Jeffrey Anderson, "Influenza in Philadelphia 1918" (1998).

CHAPTER EIGHTEEN

211 *"excellent chief of service":* Frederick Russell and Rufus Cole, Camp Grant inspection diary, June 15–16, 1918, WP.

211 *"keep our eye on him"*: Welch to Dr. Christian Herter, treasurer, Rockefeller Institute for Medical Research, Jan. 13, 1902, WP.

211 *"different type of pneumonia"*: Ibid.

211 *"an important contribution"*: Richard Pearce to Major Joseph Capps, July 10, 1918, Camp Grant, influenza file, NAS.

211 *"a very important matter"*: Rufus Cole to Richard Pearce, July 24, 1918, influenza file, NAS.

211 *"vital measures in checking contagion"*: Joseph Capps, "Measures for the Prevention and Control of Respiratory Disease," *JAMA* (Aug. 10, 1918), 448.

212 *"one of the most brilliant"*: *Chicago Tribune*, Oct. 9, 1918.

212 had issued warnings: George Soper, M.D., "The Influenza Pandemic in the Camps," undated draft report, entry 29, RG 112, NA.

213 *"None of these diseases"*: A. Kovinsky, Camp Grant epidemiologist, report to SG, Sept. 4, 1918, entry 31, RG 112, NA.

213 *"Until further notice"*: Quoted in Kovinsky, report to SG, Nov. 5, 1918, entry 29, RG 112, NA.

213 *"crowding of troops"*: Charles Hagadorn, Sept. 20, 1918, entry 29, box 383, RG 112, NA.

214 *"No visitors will be permitted"*: Kovinsky, report to SG, Nov. 5, 1918.

214 the first soldier died: "Bulletin of the Base Hospital," Camp Grant, Sept. 28, 1918, RG 112, NA.

215 *"except under extraordinary circumstances"*: "Bulletin of the Base Hospital," Oct. 3 and Oct. 4, 1918, RG 112, NA.

215 *"formalin should be added"*: Ibid.

216 *"Devoting special personal care"*: "Bulletin of the Base Hospital," Oct. 6, 1918, RG 112, NA.

216 escorts of the dead . . . be prohibited: Dr. H. M. Bracken, Executive Director, Minnesota State Board of Health, Oct. 1, 1918, entry 31, RG 112, NA.

216 *"No power on earth"*: Victor Vaughan, *A Doctor's Memories,* 425.

216 *"movements of officers and men"*: See telegram from adjutant general, Oct. 3, 1918, RG 92.

217 two thousand of the 3,108 troops: "Analysis of the Course and Intensity of the Epidemic in Army Camps," unsigned, undated report, 4, entry 29, RG 112, NA.

217 likely that the death toll: Camp Hancock, Georgia, entry 29, RG 112, NA.

217 twenty-eight hundred troops would report ill: Soper, "The Influenza-Pneumonia Pandemic in the American Army Camps, September and October 1918," *Science* (Nov. 8, 1918), 451.

217 *"very carefully controlled"*: Stone to Warren Longcope, July 30, 1918, entry 29, RG 112, NA.

218 only 16.7 percent died: Alfred Gray, "Anti-pneumonia Serum (Kyes') in the Treatment of Pneumonia," entry 29, RG 112, NA.

218 Desperate efforts were being made: Maj. General Merritt W. Ireland, ed., *Medical Department of the United States Army in the World War,* v. 9, *Communicable Diseases* (1928), 448.

218 *"the duty of the Ward Surgeon"*: "Bulletin of the Base Hospital," Oct. 7 and 8, 1918, RG 112, NA.

218 *"friends of persons dying"*: "Bulletin of the Base Hospital," Oct. 3 and 4, 1918, RG 112, NA.

218 *"winning their fight"*: *Chicago Tribune,* Oct. 7, 1918.

219 *"verandas must be used"*: "Bulletin of the Base Hospital," Oct. 5, 1918, RG 112, NA.

219 *"too early to foretell"*: George Soper, "The Influenza-Pneumonia Pandemic in the American Army Camps, September and October 1918," *Science* (Nov. 8, 1918), 451.

CHAPTER NINETEEN

220 *$100 bribes:* Visiting Nurse Society minutes, Oct. and Nov., 1918, Center for the Study of the History of Nursing, University of Pennsylvania.

220 *"no doctors available"*: Selma Epp, transcript of unaired interview for "Influenza 1918," *American Experience,* Feb. 28, 1997.

220 *average* weekly *death toll: Public Health Reports* 33, part 2, (July 26, 1918), 1252.

222 *"Don't get frightened"*: *Public Ledger,* Oct. 8, 1918.

223 *"another crepe and another door"*: Anna Milani, transcript of unaired interview for "Influenza 1918," *American Experience,* Feb. 28, 1997.

223 *"People were dying like flies"*: Oral history of Clifford Adams, June 3, 1982, provided by Charles Hardy of West Chester University.

223 *"My uncle died there"*: Anna Lavin oral history, June 3, 1982, Charles Hardy oral history tapes.

223 *"caskets stacked up outside"*: Michael Donohue, transcript of unaired interview for "Influenza 1918," *American Experience* interview, Feb. 28, 1997.

223 *"'Let me get a macaroni box'"*: Louise Apuchase, June 3, 1982, Charles Hardy oral history tapes. June 24, 1982.

223 *"They couldn't bury them"*: Clifford Adams, Charles Hardy oral history tapes, June 3, 1982.

224 *"may also die of the plague"*: *North American,* Oct. 7, 1918.

224 *"cyanosis reached an intensity"*: Isaac Starr, "Influenza in 1918: Recollections of the Epidemic in Philadelphia," *Annals of Internal Medicine* (1976), 517.

224 *"no truth in the black plague assertion"*: Unidentified newspaper clipping in epidemic scrapbook, Dec. 29, 1918, College of Physicians Library, Philadelphia.

225 *ports and naval facilities: Public Health Reports,* Sept. 13, 1918, 1554.

225 *"an influenza-like disease"*: Ibid., Sept. 20, 1918, 1599.

227 *did not come again:* Charles Scott to William Walling, Oct. 1, 1918, RG 200, NA.

227 *"After gasping for several hours"*: Starr, "Influenza in 1918," 517.

227 *"the city had almost stopped"*: Ibid, 518.

Part VI: The Pestilence

CHAPTER TWENTY

232 *"two groups of symptoms"*: Edwin O. Jordan, *Epidemic Influenza* (1927), 260, 263.

232 *"In nonfatal cases"*: Maj. General Merritt W. Ireland, ed., *Medical Department of the United States Army in the World War,* v. 9, *Communicable Diseases* (1928), 159.

232 *"didn't care if I died"*: Clifford Adams, Charles Hardy oral history tapes, West Chester University, June 3, 1982.

233 *"sick as a dog"*: Bill Sardo, transcript of unaired interview for "Influenza 1918," *American Experience,* Feb. 27, 1997.

233 *"time was a blur"*: William Maxwell, transcript of unaired interview for "Influenza 1918," *American Experience,* Feb. 26, 1997.

233 *"ice would rattle"*: Carla Morrisey, transcript of unaired interview for "Influenza 1918," *American Experience,* Feb. 26, 1997.

233 *"happened to my hind legs"*: John Fulton, *Harvey Cushing* (1946), 435.

233 *"something like typhoid"*: Dorothy Ann Pettit, "A Cruel Wind: America Experiences the Pandemic Influenza, 1918–1920, A Social History" (1976), 91.

234 *"on a narrow ledge over a pit"*: Katherine Anne Porter, "Pale Horse, Pale Rider" (1965), 310–12.

235 *"pain above the diaphragm"*: Richard Collier, *The Plague of the Spanish Lady: The Influenza Pandemic of 1918–1919* (1974), 35.

235 *"Many had vomiting"*: Ireland, ed., *Medical Department of the United States Army in the World War,* v. 12, *Pathology of the Acute Respiratory Diseases, and of Gas Gangrene Following War Wounds* (1929), 13.

235 *In Paris, while some:* Diane A. V. Puklin, "Paris," in Fred Van Hartesfeldt, ed., *The 1918–1919 Pandemic of Influenza: The Urban Impact in the Western World* (1992), 71.

235 *"general throughout Spain"*: *Public Health Reports* 33, part 2 (Sept. 27, 1918), 1667.

235 *"beginning in the neck"*: W. S. Thayer, "Discussion of Influenza," *Proceedings of the Royal Society of Medicine* (Nov. 1918), 61.

235 *bowl of rice crispies:* Carla Morrisey, transcript of unaired interview for "Influenza 1918," *American Experience,* Feb. 26, 1997.

235 *"rupture of the drum membrane"*: Ireland, ed., *Medical Department of the United States Army in the World War,* v. 9, *Communicable Diseases* (1928), 448.

235 *"bulging eardrums"*: Ireland, *Pathology of Acute Respiratory Diseases,* 13.

235 *"destructive action on the drum"*: Burt Wolbach to Welch, Oct. 22, 1918, entry 29, RG 112, NA.

236 *eye involvement with special frequency:* David Thomson and Robert Thomson, *Annals of the Pickett-Thomson Research Laboratory,* v. 10, *Influenza* (1934), 751.

236 *ability to smell:* Ibid., 773.

236 *"symptoms of exceeding variety"*: Ireland, *Pathology of Acute Respiratory Diseases,* 13.

236 *"Intense cyanosis"*: Ibid., 56, 141–42.

236 *"even to an indigo blue"*: Ireland, *Communicable Diseases,* 159.

237 *Many mechanisms can cause bleeding:* Interview with Dr. Alvin Schmaier, University of Michigan, Oct. 2, 2002; J. L. Mayer and D. S. Beardsley, "Varicella-associated Thrombocytopenia: Autoantibodies Against Platelet Surface Glycoprotein V," *Pediatric Research* (1996), 615–19.

237 *"suffered from epistaxis"*: Ireland, *Pathology of Acute Respiratory Diseases,* 13, 35.

237 *"pint of bright red blood"*: Jordan, *Epidemic Influenza,* 260.

237 *"died from loss of blood"*: Ireland, *Pathology of Acute Respiratory Diseases,* 13.

237 *"hemorrhages . . . interior of the eye"*: Thomson and Thomson, *Influenza,* v. 9, 753.

237 *"subconjunctional hemorrhage"*: Ireland, *Pathology of Acute Respiratory Diseases,* 13.

237 *"uterine mucosa"*: Ibid., 76.

238 *chief diagnostician . . . diagnosed:* Jordan, *Epidemic Influenza,* 265.

238 *47 percent of all deaths:* Thomson and Thomson, *Influenza,* v. 9, 165.

238 *average life expectancy:* Jeffrey K. Taubenberger, "Seeking the 1918 Spanish Influenza Virus," *American Society of Microbiology News* 65, no. 3 (July 1999).

239 South African cities: J. M. Katzenellenbogen, "The 1918 Influenza Epidemic in Mamre," *South African Medical Journal* (Oct. 1988), 362–64.

239 In Chicago the deaths: Fred R. Van Hartesveldt, *The 1918–1919 Pandemic of Influenza: The Urban Impact in the Western World* (1992), 121.

239 A Swiss physician: E. Bircher, "Influenza Epidemic," *Correspondenz-Blatt fur Schweizer Aerzte, Basel* (1918), 1338, quoted in *JAMA* 71, no. 23 (Dec. 7, 1918), 1946.

239 "doubly dead in that": Sherwin Nuland, *How We Die* (1993), 202.

240 from 23 percent to 71 percent: Jordan, *Epidemic Influenza,* 273.

240 26 percent lost the child: John Harris, "Influenza Occurring in Pregnant Women: A Statistical Study of 130 Cases," *JAMA* (April 5, 1919), 978.

240 "interesting pathological experience": Wolbach to Welch, Oct. 22, 1918, entry 29, RG 112, NA.

240 "convolutions of the brain": Douglas Symmers, M.D. "Pathologic Similarity Between Pneumonia of Bubonic Plague and of Pandemic Influenza," *JAMA* (Nov. 2, 1918), 1482.

240 "relaxed and flabby": Ireland, *Pathology of Acute Respiratory Diseases,* 79.

240 damage to the kidneys: Ireland, *Communicable Diseases,* 160.

240 "necrotic areas, frank hemorrage": Ireland, *Pathology of Acute Respiratory Diseases,* 392.

241 "comparable findings . . . death from toxic gas": Ireland, *Communicable Diseases,* 149.

241 "inhalation of poison gas": Edwin D. Kilbourne, M.D., *Influenza* (1987), 202.

CHAPTER TWENTY-ONE

242 "died within twelve hours": Transcript of influenza commission appointed by governor of New York, meeting at New York Academy of Medicine, Oct. 30, 1918, SLY.

242 "One robust person": E. Bircher, "Influenza Epidemic," *JAMA* (Dec. 7, 1918), 1338.

242 the conductor collapsed, dead: Collier, *Plague of the Spanish Lady,* 38.

243 "a new disease": Jordan, *Epidemic Influenza,* 36.

245 "Physical signs were confusing": Ireland, *Communicable Diseases,* 160.

245 "old classification . . . was inappropriate": Ireland, *Pathology of Acute Respiratory Diseases,* 10.

245 "little evidence of bacterial action": F. M. Burnet and Ellen Clark, *Influenza: A Survey of the Last Fifty Years,* (1942), 92.

245 "lesion of characterization": Ireland, *Communicable Diseases,* 150.

247 inhibits the release of interferon: Fields, *Fields' Virology,* 196.

247 weakened immune responses: Thomson and Thomson, *Influenza,* v. 9, 604.

249 "acute inflammatory injection": Ibid., 92.

250 "not previously described": P. K. S. Chan et al., "Pathology of Fatal Human Infection Associated with Avian Influenza A H5N1 Virus," *Journal of Medical Virology* (March 2001), 242–46.

250 had seen the same thing: Jordan, *Epidemic Influenza,* 266–68, passim.

250 mortality rate for ARDS: Lorraine Ware and Michael Matthay, "The Acute Respiratory Distress Syndrome," *New England Journal of Medicine* (May 4, 2000), 1338.

251 *Recent research also suggests:* J. A. McCullers and K. C. Bartmess, "Role of Neuraminidase in Lethal Synergism Between Influenza Virus and Streptococcus Pneumoniae," *Journal of Infectious Diseases* (March 15, 2003), 1000–1009.

252 *almost half the autopsies:* Ireland, *Communicable Diseases,* 151.

252 *the same conclusion:* Milton Charles Winternitz, *The Pathology of Influenza,* (1920).

252 *deaths came from complications:* Frederick G. Hayden and Peter Palese, "Influenza Virus" in Richman et al., *Clinical Virology* (1997), 926.

252 *still roughly 7 percent:* Murphy and Werbster, "Orthomyxoviruses," in Fields, *Fields' Virology,* 1407.

252 *35 percent of pnemococcal infections:* "Pneumococcal Resistance," Clinical Updates IV, issue 2, January 1998, National Foundation for Infectious Diseases, www.nfid.org/publications/clinicalupdates/id/pneumococcal.html.

Part VII: The Race

CHAPTER TWENTY-TWO

258 *Three Hopkins medical students:* Dorothy Ann Pettit, "A Cruel Wind: America Experiences the Pandemic Influenza, 1918–1920" (1976), 134.

258 *"could not have dreamed":* Comments at USPHS conference on influenza, Jan. 10, 1929, file 11, box 116, WP.

258 *went to bed immediately:* Welch to Walcott, Oct. 16, 1918, Frederic Collin Walcott papers, SLY.

258 *"the Flip-flap railroad":* Simon Flexner and James Thomas Flexner, *William Henry Welch and the Heroic Age of American Medicine* (1941), 251.

259 *"temperature has been normal":* Welch to Walcott, Oct. 16, 1918, Walcott papers.

261 *"astonishing numbers":* Quoted in David Thomson and Robert Thomson, *Annals of the Pickett-Thomson Research Laboratory,* v. 9, *Influenza* (1934), 265.

261 *the cause of influenza:* William Bulloch, *The History of Bacteriology* (1938), 407–8.

264 *"Surely there is a time":* Quoted in Wade Oliver, *The Man Who Lived for Tomorrow: A Biography of William Hallock Park, M.D.,* (1941), 218.

264 *"Everyone believed it":* Saul Benison, *Tom Rivers: Reflections on a Life in Medicine and Science, An Oral History Memoir* (1967), 237–40, 298.

265 *"No influenza bacilli":* A. Montefusco, *Riforma Medica* 34, no. 28 (July 13, 1918), quoted in *JAMA* 71, no. 10, 934.

CHAPTER TWENTY-THREE

267 *"a new bronchopneumonia":* Pettit, "Cruel Wind," 98.

269 *Copeland was sworn in:* Ibid., 9: 555.

269 *his loyalty to Tammany:* Ernest Eaton, "A Tribute to Royal Copeland," *Journal of the Institute of Homeopathy* 9: 554.

269 *perform it within thirty minutes:* Charles Krumwiede Jr. and Eugenia Valentine, "Determination of the Type of Pneumococcus in the Sputum of Lobar Pneumonia, A Rapid Simple Method," *JAMA* (Feb. 23, 1918), 513–14; Oliver, *Man Who Lived for Tomorrow,* 381.

270 *"so-called Spanish influenza":* "New York City letter," *JAMA* 71, no. 12 (Sept. 21,

1918): 986; see also John Duffy, *A History of Public Health in New York City 1866–1966* (1974), 280–90, passim.

270 *"prepared to compel"*: "New York City letter," *JAMA* 71, no. 13 (Sept. 28, 1918), 1076–77.

270 *"We mourn for him"*: Letter of Jan. 5, 1890, quoted in Oliver, *Man Who Lived for Tomorrow*, 26.

272 *despite their animosity*: Benison, *Tom Rivers*, 183.

272 *"secret of course"*: Oliver, *Man Who Lived for Tomorrow*, 149.

272 *"wanted to go places"*: Anna Williams, diary, undated, chap. 26, pp. 1, 17, carton 1, Anna Wessel Williams papers, Schlesinger Library, Radcliffe College.

272 *"no one particular friend"*: "Marriage" folder, undated, Williams papers.

273 *"degrees to everything, including friendship"*: "Religion" folder, March 24, 1907, Williams papers.

273 *"if we were sure, oh!"*: "Religion" folder, Aug. 20, 1915, Williams papers.

273 *"discontent rather than happiness"*: "Affections, longing, desires, friends" folder, Feb. 23, 1908, Williams papers.

273 *"I have had thrills"*: "Marriage" folder, undated, Williams papers.

273 *no advice to give*: Diary, Sept. 17, 1918, Williams papers.

273 *"Death occurring so quickly"*: Diary, undated, chap. 22, p. 23, Williams papers.

275 *quadrupled the number of horses*: Oliver, *Man Who Lived for Tomorrow*, 378.

275 *"Will your lab undertake"*: Pearce wire to Park, Sept. 18, 1918, influenza files, NAS.

275 *"Will undertake work"*: Park wire to Pearce, Sept. 19, 1918, influenza files, NAS.

275 *dismissed most of it*: William Park et al., "Introduction" (entire issue devoted to his laboratory's findings, divided into several articles), *Journal of Immunology* 6, no. 2 (Jan. 1921).

276 *in fifteen minutes could fill three thousand tubes*: *Annual Report of the Department of Health*, New York City, 1918, 86.

276 *arbitrarily stopped counting*: Mortality figures for the epidemic were no longer tabulated after March 31, 1919. By then the disease had died out in every major city in the country except New York City.

277 *Nurses were literally being kidnapped*: Permillia Doty, "A Retrospect on the Influenza Epidemic," *Public Health Nurse* (1919), 953.

277 *"we are justified in"*: William Park and Anna Williams, *Pathogenic Microroganisms* (1939), 281.

277 *"our methods . . . did not take into account"*: Park et al., "Introduction," 4.

277 *"We had plenty of material"*: Diary, undated, chap. 22, p. 23, Williams papers.

278 *220,488 test tubes*: *Annual Report of the Department of Health*, New York City, 1918, 88.

278 *"only results so far"*: Park to Pearce, Sept. 23, 1918, NAS.

279 *she would find it*: Edwin O. Jordan, *Epidemic Influenza* (1927), 391.

279 *"the most delicate test"*: Park et al., "Introduction," 4.

279 *"the starting point of the disease"*: Park to Pearce, Sept. 26, 1918, NAS.

CHAPTER TWENTY-FOUR

281 *"[h]is heart lies in research"*: Smith to Flexner, April 5, 1908, Lewis papers, RUA.

282 *"one of the best"*: Flexner to Eugene Opie, Feb. 13, 1919, Flexner papers, APS.

282 *the smartest man:* Interview with Dr. Robert Shope, Jan. 31, 2002; interview with Dr. David Lewis Aronson, May 16, 2002.

282 *"special service in connection":* Lewis to Flexner, June 19, 1917, Flexner papers.

282 *"no onerous routine duties":* Lewis to Flexner, Oct. 24, 1917, Flexner papers.

282 *"capacity to inhibit growth":* See assorted correspondence between Flexner and Lewis, esp. Lewis to Flexner, Nov. 13, 1916, Flexner papers.

283 *only one had died:* W. R. Redden and L. W. McQuire, "The Use of Convalescent Human Serum in Influenza Pneumonia" *JAMA* (Oct. 19, 1918), 1311.

284 *suspected a virus:* On Dec. 9, 1918, Lewis received permission from the navy to publish "The Partially Specific Inhibition Action of Certain Aniline Dyes for the Pneumococcus," entry 62, RG 125, NA; see also polio clipping in epidemic scrapbook, College of Physicians Library, Philadelphia, which mistakenly referred to a vaccine used by the city as being produced according to methods used in New York for polio. The specificity of this error almost certainly came from a misunderstanding of Lewis's work.

284 *"badly decomposed" bodies:* Transcript of New York influenza commission, meeting, Nov. 22, 1918, Winslow papers, SLY.

284 *"armed the medical profession":* *Philadelphia Inquirer,* Sept. 22, 1918.

285 *only three people developed pneumonia:* Transcripts of New York influenza commission, first session, Oct. 30, 1918; second session, Nov. 22, 1918; and fourth session, Feb. 14, 1919, Winslow papers.

286 *failed to cure:* Thomson and Thomson, *Influenza,* v. 10, (1934), 822.

286 *"Technically, I am not well-trained":* James Thomas Flexner, *An American Saga: The Story of Helen Thomas and Simon Flexner* (1984), 421.

287 *"cleanliness of the glassware":* Steven Rosenberg was the student. See Rosenberg and John Barry, *The Transformed Cell: Unlocking the Secrets of Cancer* (1992).

CHAPTER TWENTY-FIVE

290 *"Every case showed":* Wolbach to Welch, Oct. 22, 1918, entry 29, RG 112, NA.

290 *"causative agent":* George Soper, M.D., "The Influenza-Pneumonia Pandemic in the American Army Camps, September and October 1918," *Science* (Nov. 8, 1918), 455.

290 *"It is established":* Vaughan and Welch to Gorgas, Sept. 27, 1918, entry 29, RG 112, NA.

291 *"utter concentration on a few chosen goals":* Dubos, *The Professor, the Institute, and DNA* (1976), 78.

292 *"explore theoretical implications":* McLeod, "Oswald Theodore Avery, 1877–1955," *Journal of General Microbiology* (1957), 541.

292 *"imaginative vision of reality":* Dubos, *Professor,* 177, 179.

292 *"not random products of chance":* Quoted in McLeod, "Oswald Theodore Avery," 544–46.

293 *"hunter in search of his prey":* Dubos, *Professor,* 173.

293 *"Disappointment is my daily bread":* Ibid., 91.

293 *"compelled to take care of the cases":* Cole to Russell, Oct. 23, 1918, entry 710, RG 112, NA.

294 *the highest rate of pneumonia:* "Annual Morbidity Rate per 1000 Sept. 29, 1917 to March 29, 1918," entry 710, RG 112, NA.

294 *"as you interpret them"*: Callender to Opie, Oct. 16, 1918, entry 710, RG 112, NA.

294 *thirteen thousand . . . hospitalized simultaneously:* "Red Cross Report on Influenza, Southwestern Division," undated, RG 200, NA, 9.

294 *offered all headquarters:* Memo from Russell, Oct. 3, 1918, entry 29, RG 112, NA.

294 *"not to be depended on"*: Maj. General Merritt W. Ireland, ed., *Medical Department of the United States Army in the World War,* v. 12, *Pathology of the Acute Respiratory Diseases, and of Gas Gangrene Following War Wounds* (1929), 73, 75.

294 *six of 198 autopsies:* Unsigned Camp Grant report, 6–7, entry 31d, RG 112, NA.

294 *"inclined to take the stand"*: Ibid., 8.

295 *"technical difficulties in the isolation"*: Oswald Theodore Avery, "A Selective
Medium for B. Influenzae, Oleate-hemoglobin Agar," *JAMA* (Dec. 21, 1918),
2050.

296 *"seems to me still doubtful"*: Cole to Russell, Oct. 23, 1918, entry 710, RG 112, NA.

296 *had just cured twenty-eight:* Cole, "Scientific Reports of the Corporation and
Board of Scientific Directors 1918," Jan. 18, 1918, NLM.

296 *took two months:* Heidelberger oral history in Sanitary Corps, 84, NLM.

296 *twenty-five liters a day:* "Scientific Reports of the Corporation and Board of Scientific Directors 1918," April 20, 1918, RUA.

Part VIII: The Tolling of the Bell

CHAPTER TWENTY-SIX

301 *"what the Prussian autocracy"*: David Kennedy, *Over Here: The First World War
and American Society* (1980), 166.

303 *"no more worries"*: John Eisenhower and Joanne Eisenhower, *Yanks: The Epic
Story of the American Army in World War I* (2001), 221.

304 *"not permitted to embark"*: Richard to March, Sept. 19, 1918, entry 29, RG 112, NA.

304 *"that of a powder magazine"*: Surgeon, Port of Embarkation, Newport News, to
Surgeon General, Oct. 7, 1918, entry 29, RG 112, NA.

304 *quarantining . . . for one week:* See Richard to Adjutant General, various corre-
spondences and cables, Sept. 25 through Oct. 10, 1918, entry 29, RG 112, NA.

304 *Franklin Roosevelt . . . on a stretcher:* Eleanor Roosevelt, *This Is My Story* (1937),
268.

305 *"a true inferno reigned supreme"*: A. A. Hoehling, *The Great Epidemic* (1961), 63.

305 *tracked the blood through the ship:* John Cushing and Arthur Stone, eds., *Vermont and the World War, 1917–1919* (1928), 6, quoted in A. W. Crosby, *America's
Forgotten Pandemic: The Influenza of 1918* (1989), 130.

306 *orderlies carried away bodies:* Crosby, *America's Forgotten Pandemic,* 130.

306 *"died on board"*: Log of *Leviathan,* RG 45, NA.

306 *"death in one of its worst forms"*: Quoted in Crosby, *America's Forgotten Pandemic,* 138.

306 *more Third Division:* Ibid., 163.

306 *"dying by the score"*: George Crile, *George Crile, An Autobiography,* v. 2 (1947),
350–51, quoted in Crosby, *America's Forgotten Pandemic,* 166.

307 *to freeze the movement:* Undated *Washington Star* clipping in Tumulty papers, box
4, LC; see also Arthur Walworth, *Woodrow Wilson,* v. 2 (1965), 183–89, 462–63.

307 *"decline to stop these shipments"*: Walworth, *Woodrow Wilson,* v. 2, 462–63.

307 *"Every such soldier who has died"*: Ibid.

308 *continued the voyages:* Ibid.

308 *picked a PHS scientist:* Vaughan to George Hale, Aug. 23, 1917, Council National Defense papers, NAS.

308 *when Tammany took over:* Haven Anderson to Rosenau, Dec. 24, 1917, Rosenau papers, UNC.

309 *"interests in the State . . . harmonized":* Morris Fishbein, *A History of the American Medical Association, 1847 to 1947* (1947), 736.

309 *"health insurance will constitute":* Blue, presidential address, reprinted in *JAMA* 66, no. 25 (June 17, 1916), 1901.

310 *"not immediately necessary to the enforcement":* Blue's office to McCoy, July 28, 1918, entry 10, file 2119, RG 90, NA.

310 *"Owing to disordered conditions":* Cole to Pearce, July 19, 1918, NAS.

310 *"local health authorities":* Public Health Reports, Sept. 13, 1918, 1340.

310 *"manifestly unwarranted":* Blue, undated draft report, entry 10, file 1622, RG 90, NA.

311 *first influenza death: Washington Post,* Sept. 22, 1918.

311 *"Surgeon General's Advice to Avoid Influenza": Washington Evening Star,* Sept. 22, 1918.

312 *"arrange for suitable laboratory studies":* Blue to Pearce, Sept. 9, 1919, NAS.

312 *last yellow-fever epidemic:* John Kemp, ed., *Martin Behrman of New Orleans: Memoirs of a City Boss,* (1970), 143.

313 *appealed to the War Council:* "Minutes of War Council," Oct. 1, 1918, 1573, RG 200, NA.

313 *"contingent fund for . . . influenza":* "Minutes of War Council," Sept. 27, 1918, RG 200.

313 *"appear with electric suddenness":* George Soper, M.D., "The Influenza-Pneumonia Pandemic in the American Army Camps, September and October 1918," *Science* (Nov. 8, 1918), 454, 456.

CHAPTER TWENTY-SEVEN

315 *"depend upon its own resources":* Quoted in "Summary of Red Cross Activity in Influenza Epidemic" (undated), 6, box 688, RG 200; see also Evelyn Berry, "Summary of Epidemic 1918–1919," July 8, 1942, RG 200, NA.

316 *"forty nurses ill":* Jackson to W. Frank Persons, Oct. 4, 1918, box 688, RG 200, NA.

316 *"telegraphed to all my chapters":* Ibid.

316 *"unable to handle adequately":* Ibid.

318 *72,219 physicians:* Franklin Martin, *Fifty Years of Medicine and Surgery,* (1934), 384.

320 *stripped hospitals of their workforce:* Lavinia Dock et al., *History of American Red Cross Nursing* (1922), 969.

320 *"no nurses left in civil life":* Ibid.

CHAPTER TWENTY-EIGHT

322 *"not planned specifically for your time":* Flexner to Lewis, July 8, 1908, RUA.

324 *"sever my connection":* Mrs. J. Willis Martin to Mayor Thomas Smith, Oct. 8, 1918, Council of National Defense papers, HSP.

324 *use that same organization:* Undated memo, entries 13B–D2, RG 62, NA.

324 *"death toll for one day"*: Ibid.

325 *ceded to the group control:* "Minutes of Visiting Nurse Society for October and November, 1918," Center for the Study of the History of Nursing, University of Pennsylvania.

325 *"death rate for the past week"*: Krusen to Navy Surgeon General William Braisted, Oct. 6, 1918, entry 12, RG 52, NA.

325 *"heartily endorse"*: Blue to Braisted, Oct. 7, 1918, entry 12, RG 52, NA.

326 *"filth allowed to collect"*: *Philadelphia Public Ledger,* Oct. 10, 1918.

326 *"condition . . . spreads the epidemic"*: Ibid.

327 *"undertakers found it impossible"*: *Mayor's Annual Report for 1918,* 40, Philadelphia City Archives.

327 *"took her to the cemetery"*: Anna Lavin, June 3, 1982, Charles Hardy oral history tapes, West Chester University.

327 *"brought a steam shovel"*: Michael Donohue, transcript of unaired interview for "Influenza 1918," *American Experience,* Feb. 28, 1997.

327 *"corpse on the front porches"*: Harriet Ferrell, transcript of unaired interview for "Influenza 1918," *American Experience,* Feb. 27, 1997.

328 *"drawn by horses"*: Selma Epp, transcript of unaired interview for "Influenza 1918," *American Experience,* Feb. 28, 1997.

328 *"Everything was quiet"*: Clifford Adams, Charles Hardy oral history tapes.

328 *"Nursing Halting Epidemic"*: *Philadelphia Inquirer,* Oct. 16, 1918.

329 *"calls not filled, 2,758"*: "Directory of Nurses," College of Physicians of Philadelphia papers.

329 *Ten of the fifty-five:* Joseph Lehman, "Clinical Notes on the Recent Epidemic of Influenza," *Monthly Bulletin of the Department of Public Health and Charities* (March 1919), 38.

329 *"Calls for Amateur Nurses"*: In at least three Philadelphia newspapers, including the *Philadelphia Inquirer* and two unidentified newspaper clippings in epidemic scrapbook, Oct. 6, 1918, College of Physicians Library, Philadelphia.

330 *"all persons with two hands"*: Unidentified newspaper clipping in epidemic scrapbook, Oct. 9, 1918, College of Physicians Library, Philadelphia.

330 *"must have more volunteer helpers"*: *Philadelphia Inquirer,* Oct. 14, 1918.

330 *"they will work all the harder"*: "Minutes of Philadelphia General Hospital Woman's Advisory Council," Oct. 16, 1918, HSP.

331 *118 officers responded:* *Mayor's Annual Report for 1918,* 40, City Archives, Philadelphia.

331 *"[V]olunteers . . . are useless"*: "Minutes of Philadelphia General Hospital Woman's Advisory Council," Oct. 16, 1918, HSP.

331 *"they still hold back"*: Undated clipping in epidemic scrapbook, College of Physicians Library.

331 *"fear in the hearts"*: Susanna Turner, transcript of unaired interview for "Influenza 1918," *American Experience,* Feb. 27, 1997.

331 *Day after day he carried:* Ibid.

CHAPTER TWENTY-NINE

333 *"not a soul to be seen"*: Geoffrey Rice, *Black November: The 1918 Influenza Epidemic in New Zealand* (1988), 51–52.

333 *had died overnight:* See "Reminiscences Dana W. Atchley, M.D." (1964), 94–95, Columbia oral history, quoted in Dorothy Ann Pettit, "A Cruel Wind: America Experiences the Pandemic Influenza, 1918–1920," (1976), 109.

334 *"first casualty when war comes":* Many citations of this comment originally made in 1917, including *Newsday,* June 15, 2003.

334 *"plenty of gasoline":* See, for example, *Arizona Republican,* Sept. 1, 1918.

334 *possibility of plague:* E. Bircher, "Influenza Epidemic," *Correspondenz-Blatt fur Schweizer Aertze,* Basel (Nov. 5, 1918), 1338, quoted in *JAMA* 71, no. 24 (Dec. 7, 1918), 1946.

334 *"similarity of the two diseases":* Douglas Symmers, M.D., "Pathologic Similarity Between Pneumonia of Bubonic Plague and of Pandemic Influenza," *JAMA* (Nov. 2, 1918), 1482.

334 *"sorrow and sadness sat":* Wade Oliver, *The Man Who Lived for Tomorrow: A Biography of William Hallock Park, M.D.* (1941), 384.

335 *"may actually be reassuring":* Providence Journal, Sept. 9, 1918.

335 *"To dispel alarm":* Run in many newspapers, for example, *Arizona Republican,* Sept. 23, 1918.

335 *"epidemic is on the wane":* JAMA 71, no. 13 (Sept. 28, 1918): 1075.

335 *"no cause for alarm":* Washington Evening Star, Oct. 13, 1918.

336 *"ought to see this hospital tonight":* Quoted in Pettit, "A Cruel Wind," 105.

336 *"Spanish influenza is plain la grippe":* Arkansas Gazette, Sept. 20, 1918.

336 *"something constructive rather than destructive":* Report from *Christian Science Monitor* reprinted in *Arizona Gazette,* Oct. 31, 1918.

336 *said nothing at all:* See *Review Press and Reporter,* Feb. 1972 clipping, RG 200, NA.

336 *"Fear kills more than the disease":* Ibid.

336 *"If ordinary precautions":* Quoted in Crosby, *America's Forgotten Pandemic,* 92.

337 *"Nothing was done":* John Dill Robertson, *Report of an Epidemic of Influenza in Chicago Occurring During the Fall of 1918,* (1919) City of Chicago, 45.

337 *"Worry kills more":* The Survey 41 (Dec. 21, 1918), 268, quoted in Fred R. Van Hartesveldt, *The 1918–1919 Pandemic of Influenza: The Urban Impact in the Western World* (1992), 144.

337 *mortality rate at Cook County:* Riet Keeton and A. Beulah Cusman, "The Influenza Epidemic in Chicago," *JAMA* (Dec. 14, 1918), 2000–2001. Note the 39.8 percent corrects an earlier report in *JAMA* by Nuzum on Nov. 9, 1918, 1562.

337 *"Fear is our first enemy":* Literary Digest 59 (Oct. 12, 1918), 13–14, quoted in Van Hartesveldt, *1918–1919 Pandemic of Influenza,* 144.

337 *"Don't Get Scared":* Albuquerque *Morning Journal,* Oct. 1, 1918, quoted in Bradford Luckingham, *Epidemic in the Southwest, 1918–1919* (1984), 18.

337 *"epidemic under control":* Arizona Republican, Sept. 23, 1918.

337 *deaths in New Orleans:* Compare *Arizona Republican,* Sept. 19, 1918, to *New Orleans Item,* Sept. 21, 1918.

337 *utterly silent:* See *Arizona Republican* of Sept. 25, 26, 27, 28, 1918.

337 *"most fearful are . . . first to succumb":* Arizona Gazette, Jan. 9, 1919.

338 *"refrain from mentioning the influenza":* Arizona Gazette, Nov. 26, 1918.

338 *"Simply the Old-Fashioned Grip":* See Vicks VapoRub ad run repeatedly all over the country, for example, in *Seattle Post-Intelligencer,* Jan. 7, 1919.

338 *"come up through the grapevine":* Dan Tonkel, transcript of unaired interview for "Influenza 1918," *American Experience,* March 3, 1997.

338 *"not inclined to be as panicky"*: Gene Hamaker, "Influenza 1918," *Buffalo County, Nebraska, Historical Society* 7, no. 4.

338 *"do much toward checking the spread"*: See, for example, *Washington Evening Star,* Oct. 3, 1918.

338 *"Every person who spits"*: Unidentified, undated clipping in epidemic scrapbook, College of Physicians Library.

339 *"Remember the 3 Cs"*: For example, *Rocky Mountain News,* Sept. 28, 1918, quoted in Stephen Leonard, "The 1918 Influenza Epidemic in Denver and Colorado," *Essays and Monographs in Colorado History,* essays no. 9, (1989), 3.

339 *"The danger . . . is so grave"*: *JAMA* 71, no. 15 (Oct. 12, 1918), 1220.

340 *"None of the cases . . . serious"*: *Arizona Republican,* Sept. 23, 1918.

340 *"My first intimations"*: William Maxwell, "Influenza 1918," *American Experience.*

341 *"we were next"*: Lee Reay, "Influenza 1918," *American Experience.*

341 *"Spanish hysteria"*: Luckingham, *Epidemic in the Southwest,* 29.

341 *"What's true of all the evils"*: Quoted in Sherwin Nuland, *How We Die* (1993), 201.

342 *gone back to being a doctor:* interview with Pat Ward, Feb. 13, 2003.

342 *nothing but brief obituaries:* See, for example, *JAMA* 71, no. 21 (Nov. 16, 1918).

343 *"Germans have started epidemics"*: Doane made the statement in Chicago and was quoted by the *Chicago Tribune,* Sept. 19, 1918. The story appeared in many papers nationally, for example, the *Arizona Republican,* same date.

343 *"prepared the public mind"*: Parsons to Blue, Sept. 26, 1918, entry 10, file 1622, RG 90, NA.

343 *"well back of the lines"*: Ibid.

343 *"we wonder which"*: Ibid.

344 *Police ruled it a suicide:* Associated Press, Oct. 18, 1918; see also *Mobile Daily Register,* Oct. 18, 1918.

344 *41 percent of the entire population:* U.S. Census Bureau, *Mortality Statistics 1919,* 30–31; see also W. H. Frost, "Statistics of Influenza Morbidity," Public Health Reports (March 1920), 584–97.

344 *"this help never materialized"*: A. M. Lichtenstein, "The Influenza Epidemic in Cumberland, Md," *Johns Hopkins Nurses Alumni Magazine* (1918), 224.

344 *"everything possible would be done"*: Parsons to Blue, Oct. 13, 1918, entry 10, file 1622, RG 90, NA.

345 *"Panic incipient"*: Parsons to Blue, Oct. 13, 1918, entry 10, file 1622, RG 90, NA.

345 *"[W]hole city in a panic"*: J. W. Tappan to Blue, Oct. 22 and Oct. 23, 1918, entry 10, file 1622, RG 90.

345 *125 died:* Leonard, "1918 Influenza Epidemic," 7.

345 *"shot gun quarantine"*: *Durango Evening Herald,* Dec. 13, 1918, quoted in Leonard, "1918 Influenza Epidemic," 8.

346 *"which may be deemed appropriate"*: Memo by E. L. Munson, Oct. 16, 1918, entry 710, RG 112.

346 *"a terrible calamity"*: *Gunnison News-Chronicle,* Nov. 22, 1918, quoted in Leonard, "1918 Influenza Epidemic," 8.

346 *"right at our very doors"*: Susanna Turner, transcript of unaired interview for "Influenza 1918," *American Experience,* Feb. 27, 1997.

346 *"almost afraid to breathe"*: Dan Tonkel, transcript of unaired interview for "Influenza 1918," *American Experience,* March 3, 1997.

346 *"Farmers stopped farming"*: Ibid.

346 *"It kept people apart"*: William Sardo, transcript of unaired interview for "Influenza 1918," *American Experience,* Feb. 27, 1997.

347 *"Nobody was coming in"*: Joe Delano, transcript of unaired interview for "Influenza 1918," *American Experience,* March 3, 1997.

347 *illegal to shake hands:* Jack Fincher, "America's Rendezvous with the Deadly Lady," *Smithsonian Magazine* (Jan. 1989), 131.

347 *"starving to death not from lack of food"*: "An Account of the Influenza Epidemic in Perry County, Kentucky," unsigned, Aug. 14, 1919, box 689, RG 200, NA.

347 *arrived . . . Saturday and left Sunday:* Shelley Watts to Fieser, Nov. 11, 1918, box 689, RG 200, NA.

348 *mortality reached 30 percent:* Nancy Baird, "The 'Spanish Lady' in Kentucky," *Filson Club Quarterly,* 293.

348 *"he'd spray the money"*: Patricia J. Fanning, "Disease and the Politics of Community: Norwood and the Great Flu Epidemic of 1918" (1995), 139–42.

348 *"send for the priest"*: From Red Cross pamphlet: "The Mobilization of the American National Red Cross During the Influenza Pandemic 1918–1919" (1920), 24.

348 *"shouted orders through doors"*: Leonard, "1918 Influenza Epidemic," 9.

349 *"taught that they were safer at work"*: C. E. Turner, "Report Upon Preventive Measures Adopted in New England Shipyards of the Emergency Fleet Corp," undated, entry 10, file 1622, RG 90, NA.

349 *absentee records were striking:* Ibid.

349 *"the first problem"*: *Arizona Republican,* Nov. 8, 1918.

349 *"H. G. Saylor, yellow slacker"*: *Arizona Gazette,* Oct. 11, 1918.

350 *"a city of masked faces"*: *Arizona Republican,* Nov. 27, 1918.

350 *"Phoenix will soon be dogless"*: *Arizona Gazette,* Dec. 6, 1918.

350 *"BONG! BONG! BONG!"*: Mrs. Volz, transcript of unaired interview "Influenza 1918," *American Experience,* Feb. 26, 1997.

350 *"Ice is also great"*: Robert Frost, "Fire and Ice," originally published in *Harper's,* 1920.

350 *"akin to the terror of the Middle Ages"*: "Mobilization of the American National Red Cross," 24.

CHAPTER THIRTY

351 *"two colored physicians"*: Converse to Blue, Oct. 8, 1918, entry 10, file 1622, RG 90, NA.

351 *"urgent need of four nurses"*: Rush wire to Blue, Oct. 14, 1918, entry 10, file 1622. RG 90, NA.

351 *"No colored physicians"*: Blue to Converse, Oct. 10, 1918, entry 10, file 1622, RG 90.

351 *"impossible to send nurses"*: Rush wire to Blue, Oct. 14, 1918, entry 10, file 1622, RG 90, NA.

351 *house to house searching:* Report, Oct. 22, 1918, box 688, RG 200, NA.

351 *go to the ticket booth:* Carla Morrisey, transcript of unaired interview for "Influenza 1918," *American Experience,* Feb. 26, 1997.

351 *"urgent call on physicians"*: See, for example, *JAMA* 71, no. 17 (Oct. 26 1918): 1412, 1413.

352 *"Infection was prevented"*: James Back, M.D., *JAMA* 71 no. 23, (Dec. 7, 1918), 1945.

352 *"saturated with alkalis"*: Thomas C. Ely, M.D., letter to editor, *JAMA* 71, no. 17, (Oct. 26, 1918): 1430.

353 *injected people with typhoid vaccine*: D. M. Cowie and P. W. Beaven, "Nonspecific Protein Therapy in Influenzal Pneumonia," *JAMA* (April 19, 1919), 1170.

353 *"results were immediate and certain"*: F. B. Bogardus, "Influenza Pneumonia Treated by Blood Transfusion," *New York Medical Journal* (May 3, 1919), 765.

353 *forty-seven patients; twenty died*: W. W. G. MacLachlan and W. J. Fetter, "Citrated Blood in Treatment of Pneumonia Following Influenza," *JAMA* (Dec. 21, 1918), 2053.

353 *hydrogen peroxide intravenously*: David Thomson and Robert Thomson, *Annals of the Pickett-Thomson Research Laboratory*, v. 10, *Influenza* (1934), 1287.

354 *homeopaths claiming no deaths*: T. A. McCann, "Homeopathy and Influenza," *The Journal of the American Institute for Homeopathy* (May 1921).

354 *"effect was apparent"*: T. Anastassiades, "Autoserotherapy in Influenza," *Grece Medicale*, reported in *JAMA* (June 1919), 1947.

354 *therapy in* The Lancet: Quoted in Thomson and Thomson, *Influenza*, v. 10, 1287.

355 *"prompt bleeding"*: "Paris Letter," Oct. 3, 1918, in *JAMA* 71, no. 19 (Nov. 9, 1918).

355 *In disease as in war*: Quoted in Van Hartesveldt, *1918–1919 Pandemic of Influenza*, 82.

355 *"keep your feet dry"*: *Arizona Gazette,* Nov. 26, 1918.

355 *"a powerful bulwark for the prevention"*: All these and others reproduced under title "Propaganda for Reform" in *JAMA* 71, no. 21 (Nov. 23, 1918), 1763.

356 *"Use Vicks VapoRub"*: *Seattle Post-Intelligencer,* Jan. 3, 1919.

356 *"vaccinated . . . immune to the disease"*: Numerous papers both in and outside New York City, see, for example, Philadelphia *Public Ledger,* Oct. 18, 1918.

356 *thousands of dosages more*: John Kolmer, M.D., "Paper Given at the Philadelphia County Medical Society Meeting, Oct. 23, 1918," *Pennsylvania Medical Journal* (Dec. 1918), 181.

356 *"some prophylactic value"*: George Whipple, "Current Comment, Vaccines in Influenza," *JAMA* (Oct. 19, 1918), 1317.

356 *death rate . . . 52 percent*: Egbert Fell, "Postinfluenzal Psychoses," *JAMA* (June 7, 1919), 1658.

357 *"now has available"*: E. A. Fennel, "Prophylactic Inoculation against Pneumonia," *JAMA* (Dec. 28, 1918), 2119.

357 *"none is available for distribution"*: Major G. R. Callender to Dr. W. B. Holden, Oct. 7, 1918, entry 29, RG 112, NA.

357 *"still in the experimental stage"*: Acting surgeon general to camp and division surgeons, Oct. 25, 1918, entry 29, RG 112, NA.

357 *"health officers in their public relations"*: Editorial, *JAMA* 71, no. 17, (Oct. 26, 1918), 1408.

357 *"may arouse unwarranted hope"*: Editorial, *JAMA* 71, no. 19 (Nov. 9, 1918), 1583.

358 *eighteen different kinds*: Fincher, "America's Rendezvous," 134.

358 *"large doses hypodermically"*: Friedlander et al., "The Epidemic of Influenza at Camp Sherman" *JAMA* (Nov. 16, 1918), 1652.

358 *"No benefits were gained"*: Ibid.

359 *Sentries guarded all trails: Engineering News-Record* 82 (1919), 787, quoted in Jordan, *Epidemic Influenza,* 453.

359 *could become "extinct":* Kilpatrick to FC Monroe, Aug. 7, 1919; see also Mrs. Nichols, "Report of Expedition," July 21, 1919, RG 200.

359 *"people of Alaska consider":* U.S. Congress, Senate Committee on Appropriations, "Influenza in Alaska" (1919).

360 *176 of 300 Eskimos:* W. I. B. Beveridge, *Influenza: The Last Great Plague: An Unfinished Story of Discovery* (1977), 31.

360 *"frozen to death before help arrived":* U.S. Congress, Senate Committee on Appropriations, "Influenza in Alaska."

360 *"few adults living":* Mrs. Nichols, "Report of Expedition."

361 *"heaps of dead bodies":* Ibid.

361 *"starving dogs dug their way":* Ibid.

361 *"Whole households lay inanimate":* Eileen Pettigrew, *The Silent Enemy: Canada and the Deadly Flu of 1918* (1983), 28.

361 *"left us to sink or swim":* Ibid., 31.

362 killed over one hundred dogs: Richard Collier, *The Plague of the Spanish Lady: The Influenza Pandemic of 1918–1919* (1974), 300.

362 *laid 114 bodies in the pit:* Pettigrew, *Silent Enemy,* 30.

362 *one-third of the population died:* Ibid., 33.

362 *Metropolitan Life Insurance:* Jordan, *Epidemic Influenza,* 251.

362 *In Frankfurt the mortality:* Van Hartesveldt, *1918–1919 Pandemic of Influenza,* 25.

362 *"too exhausted to hate":* Fincher, "America's Rendezvous," 134.

362 *"remarkable for the severity":* Pierre Lereboullet, *La grippe, clinique, prophylaxie, traitement* (1926), 33, quoted in Diane A. V. Puklin, "Paris," in Van Hartesveldt, *1918–1919 Pandemic of Influenza,* 77.

363 *"obliterating whole settlements":* Jordan, *Epidemic Influenza,* 227.

363 *only a single sailor died:* Crosby, *America's Forgotten Pandemic,* 234.

363 *46 percent of the blacks would be attacked:* Jordan, *Epidemic Influenza,* 204–5.

363 *the state of Chiapas:* Thomson and Thomson, *Influenza,* v. 9, 165.

363 *attack rate of 33 percent:* "Rio de Janeiro Letter," *JAMA* 72 no. 21, May 24, 1919, 1555.

363 *In Buenos Aires:* Thomson and Thomson, *Influenza,* v. 9, 124.

363 *In Japan:* Ibid., 124.

364 die *in the sixteen days:* Jordan, *Epidemic Influenza,* 224.

364 *"filled with bodies":* Ibid., 225.

364 *Talune brought the disease:* Rice, *Black November,* 140.

364 *In Chungking one-half the population: Public Health Reports,* Sept. 20, 1918, 1617.

364 *doubled that of the:* Jordan, *Epidemic Influenza,* 222.

364 *case mortality rate:* Mills, "The 1918–19 Influenza Pandemic—The Indian Experience," *The Indian Economic and Social History Review* (1986), 27.

364 *arrived with the dead and dying:* Richard Gordon, M.D., *Great Medical Disasters* (1983), 87; Beveridge, *Influenza: The Last Great Plague,* 31.

364 *For Indian troops:* Jordan, *Epidemic Influenza,* 246.

364 *7,044 of those patients died:* Memo to Dr. Warren from Dr. Armstrong, May 2, 1919, entry 10, file 1622, RG 90, NA.

365 *"littered with dead and dying"*: "London Letter," *JAMA* 72, no. 21 (May 24, 1919), 1557.

365 *firewood was quickly exhausted:* Mills, "The 1918–19 Influenza Pandemic," 35.

365 *Close to twenty million:* Ibid., 4; Kingsley Davis, *The Population of India and Pakistan* (1951), 36.

365 *"civilization could easily . . . disappear":* Collier, *Plague of the Spanish Lady,* 266.

Part IX: Lingerer

CHAPTER THIRTY-ONE

369 *measles requires an unvaccinated:* Quoted in William McNeill, *Plagues and Peoples* (1976), 53.

370 *"no longer a master":* H. G. Wells, *War of the Worlds,* online edition, www.fourmilab.ch/etexts/www/warworlds/b2c6.html.

371 *worst numbers came from Camp Sherman:* George Soper, M.D., "The Influenza Pandemic in the Camps," undated, unpaginated, RG 112, NA.

371 *last five camps attacked:* Ibid.

372 *"failed when . . . carelessly applied":* Ibid.

372 *"when it first reached the state":* Wade Frost quoted in David Thomson and Robert Thomson, *Annals of the Pickett-Thomson Research Laboratory,* v. 9, *Influenza* (1934), 215.

373 *"relatively rarely encountered":* Edwin O. Jordan, *Epidemic Influenza* (1927), 355–56.

374 *"influenza has not passed":* "Bulletin of the USPHS," Dec. 11, 1918, quoted in *JAMA* 71, no. 25 (Dec. 21, 1918), 2088.

374 *twenty-seven epidemic ordinances:* Dorothy Ann Pettit, "A Cruel Wind: America Experiences the Pandemic Influenza, 1918–1920, A Social History" (1976), 162.

374 *places closed—for a third time:* Ibid., 177.

375 *"99% proof against influenza":* June Osborn, ed., *Influenza in America, 1918–1976: History, Science, and Politics* (1977), 11.

375 *teachers volunteered as nurses:* See Alfred W. Crosby, *America's Forgotten Pandemic: The Influenza of 1918* (1989), 91–116, passim.

375 *"how gallantly the city":* Quoted in ibid., 106.

375 *worst on the West Coast:* Osborn, *Influenza in America,* 11.

375 *quarantine of incoming ships:* W. I. B. Beveridge, *Influenza: The Last Great Plague: An Unfinished Story of Discovery* (1977), 31.

376 *not even one-quarter that of Italy:* K. D. Patterson and G. F. Pyle, "The Geography and Mortality of the 1918 Influenza Pandemic," *Bulletin of the History of Medicine* (1991), 14.

376 *"the influenza plague":* Quoted in Lucy Taksa, "The Masked Disease: Oral History, Memory, and the Influenza Pandemic," in *Memory and History in Twentieth Century Australia* (1994), 86.

376 *"I can recall the Bubonic Plague":* Ibid., 79.

376 *"inoculated against the Bubonic Plague":* Ibid., 83.

376 *"I can remember that":* Ibid., 79–85, passim.

CHAPTER THIRTY-TWO

378 *"not considered in this report"*: Egbert Fell, "Postinfluenzal Psychoses," *JAMA* (June 1919), 1658.

378 *"profound mental inertia"*: Thomson and Thomson, *Influenza*, v. 10, 772.

378 *"influenzal psychoses"*: G. Draggoti, "Nervous Manifestations of Influenza," *Policlinico* (Feb. 8, 1919), 161, quoted in *JAMA* 72 (April 12, 1919), 1105.

379 *"serious mental disturbances"*: Henri Claude M.D., "Nervous and Mental Disturbances Following Influenza," *JAMA* (May 31, 1919), 1635.

379 *"an active delirium"*: Martin Synnott, "Influenza Epidemic at Camp Dix" *JAMA* (Nov. 2, 1918), 1818.

379 *"mental depression"*: Jordan, *Epidemic Influenza*, 35.

379 *"Nervous symptoms"*: Maj. General Merritt W. Ireland, ed., *Medical Department of the United States Army in the World War*, v. 9, *Communicable Diseases* (1928), 159.

379 *"melancholia, hysteria, and insanity"*: Thomson and Thomson, *Influenza*, v. 10, 263.

379 *"involvement of the nervous"*: Ireland, *Influenza*, 160.

379 *"muttering delirium which persisted"*: Ireland, ed., *Medical Department of the United States Army in the World War*, v. 12, *Pathology of the Acute Respiratory Diseases, and of Gas Gangrene Following War Wounds* (1929), 141–42.

379 *"central nervous system"*: Ibid., 119.

379 *"Infectious psychosis"*: Ibid., 13.

379 *increase in Parkinson's*: Frederick G. Hayden and Peter Palese, "Influenza Virus," in *Clinical Virology* (1997), 928.

380 *"influenza may act on the brain"*: Jordan, *Epidemic Influenza*, 278–80.

380 *"profound influence on the nervous system"*: Thomson and Thomson, *Influenza*, v. 10, 768.

380 *"influence suicide"*: I. M. Wasserman, "The Impact of Epidemic, War, Prohibition and Media on Suicide: United States, 1910–1920," *Suicide and Life Threatening Behavior* (1992), 240.

380 *"wide spectrum of central nervous system"*: Brian R. Murphy and Robert G. Webster, "Orthomyxoviruses" (1996), 1408.

380 *"membranes surrounding the brain"*: P. K. S. Chan et al., "Pathology of Fatal Human Infection Associated With Avian Influenza A H5N1 Virus," *Journal of Medical Virology* (March 2001), 242–46.

380 *"meninges of the brain"*: Douglas Symmers, M.D., "Pathologic Similarity Between Pneumonia of Bubonic Plague and of Pandemic Influenza," *JAMA* (Nov. 2, 1918), 1482.

380 *"hemorrhages into gray matter"*: Claude, "Nervous and Mental Disturbances," 1635.

381 *"across to central nervous systems"*: Interview with Robert Webster, June 13, 2002.

381 *"have been exceeding miserable"*: Diaries, House collection, Nov. 30, 1918, quoted in Pettit, "Cruel Wind," 186.

381 *"all too generous"*: *New York Telegram*, Jan. 14, 1919, quoted in Ibid.

381 *"lost the thread of affairs"*: Quoted in Arthur Walworth, *Woodrow Wilson*, v. 2 (1965), 279.

382 *"a greased marble"*: Tasker Bliss, quoted in Bernard Baruch, *Baruch: The Public Years* (1960), 119, quoted in Crosby, *America's Forgotten Pandemic*, 186.

383 *1,517 Parisians died:* From Great Britain Ministry of Health, "Report on the Pandemic of Influenza" (1920), 228, quoted in Crosby, *America's Forgotten Pandemic,* 181.

383 *"grave proportions . . . in Paris":* "Paris Letter," March 2, 1919, *JAMA* 72, no. 14 (April 5, 1919), 1015.

383 *"the principles laid down":* Walworth, *Woodrow Wilson,* v. 2, 294.

383 *"severe cold last night":* Grayson wire to Tumulty, 8:58 A.M., April 4, 1919, box 44, Tumulty papers, LC.

383 *"The President was taken violently sick":* Grayson to Tumulty, April 10, 1919, marked PERSONAL AND CONFIDENTIAL, box 44, Tumulty papers.

384 *"taking every precaution":* Grayson wire to Tumulty, 11:00 A.M., April 8, 1919, box 44, Tumulty papers.

384 *"he manifested peculiarities":* Walworth, *Woodrow Wilson,* v. 2, 297.

384 *"we will go home":* Edith Wilson, *My Memoir* (1939), 249, quoted in Crosby, *America's Forgotten Pandemic,* 191.

384 *"a cook who keeps her trunk":* Quoted in Walworth, *Woodrow Wilson,* v. 2, 398.

384 *"began to drive himself":* Cary Grayson, *Woodrow Wilson: An Intimate Memoir* (1960), 85.

385 *"push against an unwilling mind":* Herbert Hoover, *America's First Crusade* (1942), 1, 40–41, 64, quoted in Crosby, *America's Forgotten Epidemic,* 193.

385 *"lacked his old quickness":* Hugh L'Etang, *The Pathology of Leadership* (1970), 49.

385 *obsessed with such details:* Elbert Smith, *When the Cheering Stopped: The Last Years of Woodrow Wilson* (1964), 49.

385 *"never the same after":* Irwin H. Hoover, *Forty-two Years in the White House,* (1934) 98.

385 *"so worn and tired":* Grayson to Tumulty, April 10, 1919, box 44, Tumulty papers.

385 *"could not remember":* Margaret Macmillan, *Paris 1919: Six Months That Changed the World* (2002), 276.

386 *"nervous and spiritual breakdown":* Lloyd George, *Memoirs of the Peace Conference,* (1939) quoted in Crosby, *America's Forgotten Epidemic,* 193.

386 *"terrible days for the President":* Grayson to Tumulty, April 30, 1919, box 44, Tumulty papers.

386 *"What abominable manners":* Walworth, *Woodrow Wilson,* v. 2, 319.

386 *"I should never sign it":* Ibid.

387 *suffering from arteriosclerosis:* Archibald Patterson, *Personal Recollections of Woodrow Wilson* (1929), 52.

387 *"arteriosclerotic occlusion":* Rudolph Marx, *The Health of the Presidents* (1961), 215–16.

387 *"thrombosis":* Elbert Smith, *When the Cheering Stopped: The Last Years of Woodrow Wilson* (1964), 105–6.

387 *"a little stroke":* Edward Weinstein, "Woodrow Wilson's Neurological Illness," *Journal of American History* (1970–71), 324.

387 *"a minor stroke":* Macmillan, *Paris 1919,* 276.

387 *"final breakdown":* Grayson, *Woodrow Wilson,* 82.

388 *"the dead season of our fortunes":* John Maynard Keynes, *Economic Consequences of the Peace* (1920), 297.

388 *"you did not fight":* "Papers Relating to the Foreign Relations of the United

States, The Paris Peace Conference" (1942–1947), 570–74, quoted in Schlesinger, *The Age of Roosevelt*, v. 1, *Crisis of the Old Order 1919–1933*, (1957), 14.

CHAPTER THIRTY-THREE

389 *"felt very ill":* Quoted in Michael Bliss, *William Osler: A Life in Medicine* (1999), 469. For more on Osler's illness, see Bliss 468–76, passim.

389 *"broncho-pneumonias so common after influenza":* Ibid., 469.

389 *"with it the pain":* Ibid., 470.

390 *"shall not see the post mortem":* Ibid., 472.

390 *"how can I hope":* Ibid., 470.

390 *"might have saved him":* Ibid., 475.

390 *"Hold up my head":* Ibid., 476

390 *"dealing with any recurrences":* Pettit, "Cruel Wind," 234.

390 *"No publicity is to be given":* Red Cross files, undated, RG 200, NA.

391 *"rapid spread of influenza":* Memo to division managers from chairman of influenza committee, Feb. 7, 1920, RG 200, NA.

391 *more cases would be reported:* Pettit, "Cruel Wind," 248.

391 *victim's home was tagged:* Ibid., 241.

391 *"Enforce absolute quarantine":* R. E. Arne to W. Frank Persons, Jan. 30, 1922, RG 200, NA.

391 *twenty-one thousand children . . . made orphans:* Associated Press wire, appearing in *Arizona Republican,* Nov. 9, 1918.

391 *"sixteen motherless children":* Alice Latterall to Marjorie Perry, Oct. 17, 1918, RG 200, NA.

391 *one hundred children orphaned:* "Report of Lake Division," Aug. 12, 1919, RG 200, NA.

391 *orphaned two hundred children: JAMA* 71, no. 18 (Nov. 2, 1918), 1500.

392 *"havoc is wide spread":* General manager to division managers, March 1, 1919, RG 200, NA.

392 *"What bones are they":* Quoted in Pettit, "A Cruel Wind," 173.

393 *"how sick the world is":* John Dewey, *New Republic* (Jan. 1923), quoted in Dewey, *Characters and Events: Popular Essays in Social and Political Philosophy,* v. 2 (1929), 760–61.

393 *"all faiths in man shaken":* F. Scott Fitzgerald, *This Side of Paradise* (1920), 304.

394 *"a motivating force in four books":* William Maxwell, "A Time to Mourn," *Pen America* (2002), 122–23, 130.

394 *"almost nothing in literature":* Personal communication from Donald Schueler, July 5, 2003.

394 *"an epidemic of discreet, infectious fear":* Christopher Isherwood, *Berlin Stories* (New York: New Directions, 1951), 181.

395 *"foreign settlements of the city":* Rocky Mountain News, Oct. 31, 1918, quoted in Stephen Leonard, "The 1918 Influenza Epidemic in Denver and Colorado," *Essays and Monographs in Colorado History* (1989), 7–8.

395 *"negligence and disobedience":* Durango Evening Herald, Nov. 26, 1918, quoted in Leonard, "1918 Influenza Epidemic in Denver and Colorado," 7.

395 *"penalty for filth is death":* Shelley Watts to Fieser, Nov. 13, 1918, RG 200, NA.

397 *may have reached 20 million:* Kingsley Davis, *The Population of India and Pakistan* (1951), 36, cited in and see also I. D. Mills, "The 1918–19 Influenza Pandemic—The Indian Experience" (1986), 1–40, passim.

397 *"in the order of 50 million":* Niall Johnson and Juergen Mueller, "Updating the Accounts: Global Mortality of the 1918–1920 'Spanish' Influenza Pandemic," *Bulletin of the History of Medicine* (spring 2002), 105–15, passim.

397 *as many as 100 million:* Ibid.

397 *those aged twenty-one to thirty:* Virtually all studies showed similar results. See, for example, Thomson and Thomson, *Influenza*, v. 9, 21.

398 *most conservative estimate:* Ibid., 165.

Part X: Endgame

CHAPTER THIRTY-FOUR

402 *"The appointment of Dr. Opie":* Winslow to Wade Frost, Feb. 1, 1930, Winslow papers, SLY.

402 *"Jordan seems at first":* Winslow to Frost, Jan. 16, 1930, Winslow papers.

402 *"distinctly prefer Emerson":* Frost to Winslow, Jan. 20, 1930, Winslow papers.

403 *"the Black Death":* Quoted in Michael Levin, "An Historical Account of the Influence," *Maryland State Medical Journal* (May 1978), 61.

403 *"we were so helpless":* Transcript of Influenza Commission minutes, Oct. 30, 1918, Winslow papers.

405 *precise epidemiological investigations:* "Association Committee Notes on Statistical Study of the 1918 Epidemic of So-called Influenza" presented at American Public Health Association meeting, Dec. 11, 1918, entry 10, file 1622, RG 90, NA.

405 *"an opportunity to show":* Ibid.

406 *"ultimately in the laboratory":* Transcript of Influenza Commission minutes, Feb. 4, 1919, Winslow papers.

406 *isolated for seven days:* George Soper, M.D., "Epidemic After Wars," *JAMA* (April 5, 1919), 988.

407 *"every effort to collect":* Russell to Flexner, Nov. 25, 1918, Flexner papers, APS.

407 *"this business off our hands":* Quoted in Dorothy Ann Pettit, "A Cruel Wind: America Experiences the Pandemic of Influenza, 1918–1920, A Social History" (1976), 229.

408 *two units of seasoned troops:* Maj. General Merritt W. Ireland, ed., *Medical Department of the United States Army in the World War*, v. 9, *Communicable Diseases* (1928), 127–29.

409 *"cyclic variation in air pressure":* David Thomson and Robert Thomson, *Annals of the Pickett-Thomson Research Laboratory*, v. 9, *Influenza* (1934), 259.

409 *"the outstanding objective":* F. M. Burnet, "Portraits of Viruses: Influenza Virus A," *Intervirology* (1979), 201.

409 *"humiliating but true":* Comments by Welch on influenza bacillus paper, undated, file 17, box 109, WP.

CHAPTER THIRTY-FIVE

411 *"the specific inciting agent":* Thomson and Thomson, *Influenza*, v. 9, 499.

412 "blood agar plates": Capt. Edwin Hirsch to SG, Oct. 7, 1919, entry 31D, RG 112.

412 "investigation of the bacteriologic methods": J. Wheeler Smith Jr. to Callender, Feb. 20, 1919, entry 31D, RG 112, NA.

412 They found the bacteria everywhere: Maj. General Merritt W. Ireland, ed., *Medical Department of the United States Army in the World War,* v. 12, *Pathology of the Acute Respiratory Diseases, and of Gas Gangrene Following War Wounds* (1929), 180–81.

412 "in every case": Ibid., 58.

413 "absence of influenza bacilli": Ibid., 140.

413 "were not discovered": Ibid., 144.

413 "other respiratory diseases": Ireland, *Communicable Diseases,* 62.

413 only five of sixty-two cases: Edwin O. Jordan, *Epidemic Influenza* (1927), 393.

414 "the most slipshod manner": Thomson and Thomson, *Influenza,* v. 9, 512.

414 "found in nearly every case": William H. Park, "Anti-influenza Vaccine as Pro-phylactic," *New York Medical Journal* (Oct. 12, 1918), 621.

415 "ten different strains": Park comments, transcript of Influenza Commission minutes, Dec. 20, 1918, Winslow papers.

415 "important secondary invaders": Thomson and Thomson, *Influenza,* v. 9, 498.

415 "evidence points to a filterable virus": Carton 1, chapter 22, p. 24, Anna Wessel Williams papers, Schlesinger Library, Radcliffe College.

416 "not recognizable by our microscopic methods": William MacCallum, "Pathologi-cal Anatomy of Pneumonia Following Influenza," *Johns Hopkins Hospital Reports* (1921), 149–51.

416 failed to infect: Thomson and Thomson, *Influenza,* v. 9, 603–8.

416 claimed success for three: Charles Nicolle and Charles LeBailly, "Recherches experimentales sur la grippe," *Annales de l'Institut Pasteur* (1919), 395–402, translated for the author by Eric Barry.

417 "jumped to the conclusion": Saul Benison, *Tom Rivers: Reflections on a Life in Medicine and Science, An Oral History Memoir* (1967), 59.

418 Fleming found: Thomson and Thomson, *Influenza,* v. 9, 287, 291, 497.

418 "reducing the resistance": Welch comments, USPHS Conference on Influenza, Jan. 10, 1929, box 116, file 11, WP. Conference itself reported in *Public Health Reports* 44, no. 122.

418 "the best claim to serious consideration": Thomson and Thomson, *Influenza,* v. 9, 512.

419 "scientific problems were almost forced on him": René Dubos, *The Professor, the Institute and DNA* (1976), 174.

419 "not as broad": Ibid., 74.

419 "narrow range of techniques": Dubos, "Oswald Theodore Avery, 1877–1955," *Biographical Memoirs of Fellows of the Royal Society* (1956), 40.

420 "'the whole secret . . . in this little vial'": Michael Heidelberger, oral history, 70, NLM.

421 "extreme precision and elegance": Dubos, *Professor, Institute and DNA,* 173.

423 "never published a joint paper": Ibid., 82.

423 "digging a deep hole": Ibid., 175.

423 "fundamental to biology": Heidelberger, oral history, 129.

424 "what more do you want": Dubos, *Professor, Institute and DNA,* 143.

424 "likened to a gene": Oswald Avery, Colin McLeod, and Maclyn McCarty, "Stud-ies on the Chemical Nature of the Substance Inducing Transformation of Pneumococcal Types," *Journal of Experimental Medicine* (Feb. 1, 1944, reprinted Feb. 1979), 297–326.

425 *"little influence on thought"*: Gunther Stent, Introduction, *The Double Helix: A Norton Critical Edition* by James Watson (1980), xiv.

425 *"obviously of fundamental importance"*: Nobelstiftelsen, *Nobel, the Man, and his Prizes* (1962), 281.

425 *"Avery showed"*: James Watson, *The Double Helix: A Norton Critical Edition,* See 12, 13, 18.

426 *"Avery gave us"*: Horace Judson, *Eighth Day of Creation: The Makers of the Revolution in Biology* (1979), 94.

426 *"we were very attentive"*: Ibid., 59.

426 *"nonsense to say that we were not aware"*: Ibid., 62–63.

426 *"dark ages of DNA"*: Watson, *Double Helix,* 219.

426 *"opening . . . the field of molecular biology"*: Dubos, *Professor, Institute and DNA,* 156.

427 *"keeping his own counsel"*: Ibid., 164.

CHAPTER THIRTY-SIX

428 *solid evidence:* Transcript of Influenza Commission minutes, first session, Oct. 30, 1918; second session, Nov. 22, 1918; fourth session, Feb. 14, 1919, Winslow papers.

429 *"Lewis's mind working, the depth of it"*: Interview with Dr. David Aronson, Jan. 31, 2002, and April 8, 2003.

429 *"disinfectant power of light"*: Lewis to Flexner, Nov. 29, 1916, Flexner papers, APS.

429 *"interesting and important"*: Flexner to Lewis, Jan. 29, 1919, Flexner papers, APS.

430 *"I do not thrive on routine"*: Lewis to Flexner, April 21, 1921, Flexner papers, APS.

430 *"All I have heard"*: Flexner to Lewis, April 22, 1921, Flexner papers, APS.

430 *"your new honor"*: Flexner to Lewis, Jan. 21, 1921, Flexner papers, APS.

431 *"let me take a little trouble for you"*: Flexner to Lewis, Dec. 21, 1921, Flexner papers, APS.

431 *"'father' to me"*: Lewis to Flexner, Sept. 8, 1924, Flexner papers, APS.

431 *"you may well feel gratified"*: Flexner to Lewis, Jan. 26, 1923, Flexner papers, APS.

432 *"rehabilitation of a . . . mind"*: Lewis to Flexner, Jan. 20, 1923, Flexner papers, APS.

432 *"to go to work again"*: Lewis to Flexner, Jan. 24, 1923, Lewis papers, RUA.

432 *"I shall be rejoiced"*: Flexner to Lewis, undated response to Lewis's Jan. 20, 1923, letter, Flexner papers, APS.

433 *"to deserve your confidence"*: Lewis to Flexner, Jan. 24, 1923, Lewis to Flexner, Jan. 30, 1923, Lewis papers, RUA.

433 *"free of any entanglement"*: Lewis to Flexner, June 26, 1924, Lewis papers, RUA.

434 *"the first chance to make a second center"*: Flexner to Lewis, summer 1924 (probably late June or July), Lewis papers, RUA.

434 *"I am secure"*: Lewis to Flexner, Sept. 8, 1924, Lewis papers, RUA.

434 *"one of the finest investigators"*: Benison, *Tom Rivers,* 341, 344.

435 *understanding of the immune system:* "Scientific Reports of the Corporation and Board of Scientific Directors" (1927–28), RUA, 345–47; see also George A. Corner, *A History of the Rockefeller Institute: 1901–1953 Origins and Growth* (1964), 296.

435 *"aiming higher than his training":* Smith to Flexner, Nov. 2, 1925, Lewis papers, RUA.

436 *diet of the guinea pigs:* Lewis and Shope, "Scientific Reports of the Corporation" (1925–26), 265, RUA.

436 *"no change in my line of work":* Ibid.

436 *"doubt expressed about your future":* Flexner to Lewis, draft letter, Dec. 1, 1925, Lewis papers, RUA.

436 *"unequivocally opposed":* Flexner to Lewis, Dec. 1, 1925, Lewis papers, RUA.

438 *"have not been very productive":* Lewis to Flexner, Aug. 4, 1927, Lewis papers, RUA.

438 *"rather barren subject":* Flexner to Lewis, Sept. 22, 1927, Lewis papers, RUA.

438 *"this diagnosis in pigs":* Richard Collier, *The Plague of the Spanish Lady: The Influenza Epidemic of 1918–1919* (1974), 55; W. I. B. Beveridge, *Influenza: The Last Great Plague: An Unfinished Story of Discovery* (1977), 4; J. S. Koen, "A Practical Method for Field Diagnosis of Swine Diseases," *Journal of Veterinary Medicine* (1919), 468–70.

439 *filtered the mucus:* M. Dorset, C. McBryde, and W. B. Niles, *Journal of the American Veterinary Medical Association* (1922–23), 62, 162.

439 *"our future Lewis problem":* Flexner to Smith, phone message, June 21, 1928, Lewis papers, RUA.

439 *he could still be master:* Flexner to Smith, June 20, 1928, Lewis papers, RUA.

439 *"in all kindness":* Flexner to Smith, June 22, 1928, Lewis papers, RUA.

440 *"not essentially . . . investigator type":* Flexner to Smith, June 29, 1928, Lewis papers, RUA.

440 *double the median income:* Paul Starr, *The Social Transformation of American Medicine* (1982), 142.

440 *"no doubt as to the risk":* Flexner to Smith, June 29, 1928, Lewis papers, RUA.

441 *"I don't think Noguchi was honest":* Benison, *Tom Rivers,* 95.

441 *"objections were very unreasonable":* Corner, *History of Rockefeller Institute,* 191.

442 *"learn about Shope's Iowa work":* Flexner to Lewis, Nov. 21, 1928, Lewis papers, RUA.

442 *in some herds:* Richard E. Shope, "Swine Influenza I. Experimental Transmission and Pathology," *Journal of Infectious Disease* (1931), 349.

443 *"went right to work":* Lewis to Flexner, Feb. 1, 1929, Lewis papers, RUA.

443 *"Lewis well":* Russell to Smith, Jan. 28 through May 23, 1929, "our weekly cable arrived containing the words 'Lewis well,'" each with notation "copy mailed to Mrs. Lewis," Lewis papers, RUA.

443 *"'Lewis's illness began'":* Russell to Flexner, June 29, 1929, Lewis papers, RUA.

443 *"Lewis condition critical":* George Soper to Russell, June 29, 1929, Lewis papers, RUA.

443 *"Marked renal involvement":* Davis to Russell, June 28, 1929, Lewis papers, RUA.

444 *"Probably laboratory infection":* unsigned to Russell, July 1, 1929, Lewis papers, RUA.

444 *Shope walked down Maple:* Lewis to David Aronson, Aug. 21, 1998, provided by Robert Shope.

444 *"order some flowers"*: Smith to Shope, July 16, 1929, Lewis papers, RUA.

444 *"Dear Sirs"*: Janet Lewis to Board of Scientific Directors, July 30, 1929, Lewis papers, RUA.

444 *"study of light phenomena"*: "Scientific Reports of the Corporation" (1929), 6, RUA.

444 *"recrudescence of poliomyelitis"*: Ibid., 11.

445 *"unfinished work of Dr. Noguchi"*: Ibid., 10.

445 *"white paint and some other improvements"*: Flexner to Sawyer, March 17, 1930, Lewis papers, RUA.

445 *blamed cigarettes:* Interview with Robert Shope, Jan. 2002; interview with David Aronson, April 8, 2003.

445 *"in association with Sewall Wright"*: Simon Flexner, "Paul Adin Lewis," *Science* (Aug. 9, 1929), 133–34.

446 *Shope did demonstrate:* Paul A. Lewis and Richard E. Shope, "Swine Influenza II. Hemophilic Bacillus from the Respiratory Tract of Infected Swine," *Journal of Infectious Disease* (1931), 361; Shope, "Swine Influenza I," 349; Shope, "Swine Influenza III. Filtration Experiments and Etiology," *Journal of Infectious Disease* (1931), 373.

446 *took him hunting and fishing:* C. H. Andrewes, *Biographical Memoirs, Richard E. Shope* (1979), 363.

Afterword

452 *death toll . . . 23 million:* www.avert.org/worldstats.htm.

452 *In the United States . . . 500,000:* Centers for Disease Control, "AIDS Surveillance Report" v. 13, no. 2 (Sept. 24, 2002). www.cdc.gov/hiv.stats.htm#ddaids.

452 *if a new pandemic:* personal communication from Martin Meltzer May 9, 2005, and Martin Meltzer et al., "Modeling the Economic Impact of Pandemic Influenza in the United States: Implications for Settling Priorities for Intervention," background paper accompanying publication of article of same title in *Emerging Infectious Disease* (1999). www.cdc.gov/ncidod/eid/vol5no5/melt_back.htm.

453 *In 1957 only 10 percent of meals:* Michael Osterholm, personal communication, June 20, 2005.

456 *a striking resemblance:* J. S. Oxford, "The So-called Great Spanish Influenza Pandemic of 1918 May Have Originated in France in 1916" (Dec. 2001), 1857.

457 *but Chinese scientists:* Ibid., 73.

457 *These Chinese scientists:* Edwin O. Jordan, *Epidemic Influenza* (1927), 73.

457 *"could be reasonably regarded"*: Ibid., 73.

457 *"purulent bronchitis"*: Ibid., 62.

457 *in parts of Madagascar:* "Outbreak of Influenza, Madagascar, July–August 2002," *Weekly Epidemiological Report* (2002), 381–87, passim.

457 *highly unlikely that any of them:* Jordan, *Epidemic Influenza,* 73.

457 *"probably carried from the United States"*: David Thomson and Robert Thomson, *Annals of the Pickett-Thomson Research Laboratory,* v. 10, *Influenza* (1934), 1090.

458 *studied the pandemic for years:* Burnet and Clark, *Influenza* (1942), 70.

458 *extracted several samples:* personal communication with the author from Taubenberger, June 5, 2003.

Selected Bibliography

Primary Sources

ARCHIVES AND COLLECTIONS

Alan Mason Chesney Archives, Johns Hopkins University
Stanhope Bayne-Jones papers
Wade Hampton Frost papers
William Halsted papers
Christian Herter papers
Franklin Mall papers
Eugene Opie papers
William Welch papers

American Philosophical Society
Harold Amoss papers
Rufus Cole papers
Simon Flexner papers
Victor Heiser papers
Peter Olitsky papers
Eugene Opie papers
Raymond Pearl papers
Peyton Rous papers

City Archive, Philadelphia
Alms House, Philadelphia General Hospital Daily Census, 1905–1922 Census Book

Coroner's Office, Interments in Potters Field, 1914–1942
Department of Public Health and Charities Minutes
Journal of the Board of Public Education
Journal of the Common Council
Journal of Select Council
Letterbook of Chief of Electrical Bureau, Department of Public Safety

College of Physicians, Philadelphia
William N. Bradley papers
Arthur Caradoc Morgan papers
Influenza papers

Columbia University, Butler Library, Oral History Research Office
A. R. Dochez oral history
Abraham Flexner oral history

Historical Society of Philadelphia
The Advisory Committee on Nursing, Philadelphia Hospital for Contagious Disease,
    Report for Feb. 1919
Council of National Defense papers
Benjamin Hoffman collection
Dr. William Taylor collection
Herbert Welsh collection
Woman's Advisory Council, Philadelphia General Hospital collection

Jefferson Medical College
Annual Report, Jefferson Hospital, year ended May 31, 1919

Library of Congress
Newton Baker papers
Ray Stannard Baker papers
George Creel papers
Joseph Tumulty papers
Woodrow Wilson papers

National Academy of Sciences
Executive Committee of Medicine 1916–1917 files
Medicine and Related Sciences, 1918 Activities Summary
Committee on Medicine and Hygiene 1918 files
Committee on Psychology/Propaganda Projects files
Influenza files
Biographical files for Oswald Avery, Rufus Cole, Alphonse Dochez, Eugene Opie,
    Thomas Rivers, Hans Zinsser

National Archives
Red Cross records
U.S. Army Surgeon General records
U.S. Navy Surgeon General records
U.S. Public Health Service records

National Library of Medicine
Stanhope Bayne-Jones papers and oral history
Michael Heidelberger oral history
Frederick Russell papers
Donald Van Slyke oral history
Shields Warren oral history

New York City Municipal Archives
Annual Report of the Department of Health of the City of New York for 1918
Collected Studies of the Bureau of Laboratories of the Department of Health of the City of New York for the Years 1916–1919, v. 9
Collected Reprints of Dr. William H. Park, v. 3, 1910–1920

Rhode Island Historical Society
Charles Chapin papers

Rockefeller University Archives
Paul Lewis papers
Reports to the Board of Scientific Directors

Sterling Library, Yale University
Gordon Auchincloss papers
Arthur Bliss Lane papers
Vance C. McCormick papers
Frederic Collin Walcott papers
Charles-Edward Winslow papers

Temple University Special Collections
Thomas Whitehead papers

Temple University Urban Archives
Carson College for Orphan Girls
Children's Hospital, Bainbridge
Clinton Street Boarding Home
Housing Association of Delaware Valley papers
Rabbi Joseph Krauskopf papers
Pennsylvania Hospital
Pennsylvania Society to Protect Children from Cruelty
Philadelphia Association of Day Nurseries
Whosoever Gospel Mission of Germantown
Young Women's Boarding Home Association of Philadelphia
Report of the Hospital of the Women's Medical College of Pennsylvania, 1919

Tennessee Historical Society
Oswald Avery papers

University of North Carolina, Chapel Hill
Milton Rosenau papers

University of Pennsylvania Archives
George Wharton Pepper papers

Secondary Sources

NEWSPAPERS

Arizona Gazette
Arizona Republican
Boston Globe
Chicago Tribune
London Times
Los Angeles Times
New Orleans Item
New Orleans Times-Picayune
New York Times
Philadelphia Inquirer
Philadelphia North American
Philadelphia Public Ledger
Providence Journal
San Francisco Chronicle
Santa Fe Monitor (Kansas)
Seattle Post-Intelligencer
Seattle Times
Washington Post
Washington Star

ARTICLES

"Advertisements in the Laryngoscope: Spanish Influenza—1918." Laryngoscope 106, no. 9, part 1 (Sept. 1996): 1058.

Anastassiades, T. "Autoserotherapy in Influenza." Grece Medicale, reported in JAMA 72, no. 26 (June 28, 1919): 1947.

Andrewes, C. H. "The Growth of Virus Research 1928–1978." Postgraduate Medical Journal 55, no. 64 (Feb. 1979): 73–77.

Ashford, Bailey K. "Preparation of Medical Officers of the Combat Division in France at the Theatre of Operations." Military Surgeon 44 (Feb. 1919): 111–14.

Austrian, R. "The Education of a 'Climatologist.'" Transactions of the American Clininical Climatolology Association 96 (1984): 1–13.

Avery, Oswald Theodore. "A Selective Medium for B. Influenzae, Oleate-hemoglobin Agar." JAMA 71, no. 25 (Dec. 21, 1918): 2050–52.

Avery, Oswald Theodore, Colin MacLeod, and Maclyn McCarty. "Studies on the Chemical Nature of the Substance Inducing Transformation of Pneumococcal Types." Journal of Experimental Medicine (1979, originally published Feb. 1, 1944): 297–326.

Baer, E. D. "Letters to Miss Sanborn: St. Vincent's Hospital Nurses' Accounts of World War I." Journal of Nursing History 2, no. 2 (April 1987): 17–32.

Baird, Nancy. "The 'Spanish Lady' in Kentucky." *Filson Club Quarterly* 50, no. 3: 290–302.

Barnes, Frances M. "Psychoses Complicating Influenza." *Missouri State Medical Association* 16 (1919): 115–20.

Benison, Saul. "Poliomyelitis and the Rockefeller Institute: Social Effects and Institutional Response." *Journal of the History of Medicine and Allied Sciences* 29 (1974): 74–92.

Bernstein, B. J. "The Swine Flu Immunization Program." *Medical Heritage* 1, no. 4 (July–Aug. 1985): 236–66.

Bircher, E. "Influenza Epidemic." *Correspondenz-Blatt fur Schweizer Aerzte, Basel.* 48, no. 40, (Nov. 5, 1918): 1338, quoted in *JAMA* 71, no. 24 (Dec. 7, 1918): 1946.

Bloomfield, Arthur, and G. A. Harrop Jr. "Clinical Observations on Epidemic Influenza." *Johns Hopkins Hospital Bulletin* 30 (1919).

Bogardus, F. B. "Influenza Pneumonia Treated by Blood Transfusion." *New York Medical Journal* 109, no. 18 (May 3, 1919): 765–68.

Bourne, Randolph. "The War and the Intellectuals." *The Seven Arts* 2 (June 1917): 133–46.

Brown P., J. A. Morris, and D. C. Gajdusek. "Virus of the 1918 Influenza Pandemic Era: New Evidence About Its Antigenic Character." *Science* 166, no. 901 (Oct. 3, 1969): 117–19.

Burch, M. "'I Don't Know Only What We Hear': The Soldiers' View of the 1918 Influenza Epidemic." *Indiana Medical Quarterly* 9, no. 4 (1983): 23–27.

Burnet, F. M. "The Influence of a Great Pathologist: A Tribute to Ernest Goodpasture." *Perspectives on Biology and Medicine* 16, no. 3 (spring 1973): 333–47.

———. "Portraits of Viruses: Influenza Virus A." *Intervirology* 11, no. 4 (1979): 201–14.

Capps, Joe. "Measures for the Prevention and Control of Respiratory Disease." *JAMA* 71, no. 6 (Aug. 10, 1918): 571–73.

Centers for Disease Control. *AIDS Surveillance Report* 13, no. 2 (Sept. 24, 2002).

Chan, P. K. S. et al. "Pathology of Fatal Infection Associated with Avian Influenza A H5N1 Virus." *Journal of Medical Virology* 63, no. 3 (March 2001), 242–46.

Charles, A. D. "The Influenza Pandemic of 1918–1919: Columbia and South Carolina's Response." *Journal of the South Carolina Medical Association* 73, no. 8 (Aug. 1977): 367–70.

Chesney, Alan. "Oswald Theodore Avery." *Journal of Pathology and Bacteriology* 76, no. 2 (1956): 451–60.

Christian, Henry. "Incorrectness of Diagnosis of Death from Influenza." *JAMA* 71 (1918).

Claude, Henri, M.D. "Nervous and Mental Disturbances Following Influenza." Quoted in *JAMA* 72, no. 22 (May 31, 1919): 1634.

Clough, Paul. "Phagocytosis and Agglutination in the Serum of Acute Lobar Pneumonia." *Johns Hopkins Hospital Bulletin* 30 (1919): 167–70.

Cole, Rufus. "Pneumonia as a Public Health Problem." *Kentucky Medical Journal* 16 (1918): 563–65.

———. "Prevention of Pneumonia." *JAMA* 71, no. 8 (August 24, 1918): 634–36.

Cole, Rufus, et al. "Acute Lobar Pneumonia Prevention and Serum Treatment." Monograph of the Rockefeller Institute for Medical Research 7 (Oct. 1917).

Cowie, D. M., and P. W. Beaven. "Nonspecific Protein Therapy in Influenzal Pneumonia." *JAMA* 72, no. 16 (April 19, 1919).

Cumberland, W. H. "Epidemic! Iowa Battles the Spanish Influenza." *Palimpsest* 62, no. 1 (1981): 26–32.

Davenport, F. M. "The Search for the Ideal Influenza Vaccine." *Postgraduate Medical Journal* 55, no. 640 (Feb. 1979): 78–86.

Davenport, R. M., G. N. Meiklejohn, and E. H. Lennette. "Origins and Development of the Commission on Influenza." *Archives of Environmental Health* 21, no. 3 (Sept. 1970): 267–72.

De Grazia, Victoria. "The Selling of America, Bush Style." *New York Times,* Aug. 25, 2002.

Dingle, J. H., and A. D. Langmuir. "Epidemiology of Acute Respiratory Disease in Military Recruits." *American Review of Respiratory Diseases* 97, no. 6 (June 1968): 1–65.

Doty, Permillia. "A Retrospect on the Influenza Epidemic." *Public Health Nurse,* 1919.

Douglas, R. J. "Prophylaxis and Treatment of Influenza." In *Scientific American's Medicine,* edited by E. Rubinstein and D. Federman. New York: Scientific American Inc., 1994.

Dowdle, W. R., and M. A. Hattwick. "Swine Influenza Virus Infections in Humans." *Journal of Infectious Disease* 136, supp. S (Dec. 1977): 386–89.

Draggoti, G. "Nervous Manifestations of Influenza." *Policlinico* 26, no. 6 (Feb. 8, 1919) 161, quoted in *JAMA* 72, no. 15 (April 12, 1919): 1105.

Dubos, René. "Oswald Theodore Avery, 1877–1955." *Biographical Memoirs of Fellows of the Royal Society* 2 (1956): 35–48.

Durand, M. L. et al. "Acute Bacterial Meningitis in Adults: A Review of 493 Episodes." *New England Journal of Medicine* 328, no. 1 (Jan. 1993) 21–28.

Eaton, Ernest. "A Tribute to Royal Copeland." *Journal of the Institute of Homeopathy* 31, no. 9: 555–58.

Ebert, R. G. "Comments on the Army Venereal Problem." *Military Surgeon* 42 (July–Dec. 1918), 19–20.

Emerson, G. M. "The 'Spanish Lady' in Alabama." *Alabama Journal of Medical Science* 23, no. 2 (April 1986): 217–21.

English, F. "Princeton Plagues: The Epidemics of 1832, 1880 and 1918–19." *Princeton History* 5 (1986): 18–26.

Ensley, P. C. "Indiana and the Influenza Pandemic of 1918." *Indiana Medical History* 9, no. 4 (1983): 3–15.

"Epidemic Influenza and the United States Public Health Service." *Public Health Reports* 91, no. 4 (July–Aug. 1976): 378–80.

Feery, B. "1919 Influenza in Australia." *New England Journal of Medicine* 295, no. 9 (Aug. 26, 1976): 512.

Fell, Egbert. "Postinfluenzal Psychoses." *JAMA* 72, no. 23 (June 7, 1919): 1658–59.

Fennel, E. A. "Prophylactic Inoculation Against Pneumonia." *JAMA* 71, no. 26, (Dec. 28, 1918): 2115–18.

Fincher, Jack. "America's Rendezvous with the Deadly Lady." *Smithsonian Magazine,* Jan. 1989: 131.

Finland, M. "Excursions into Epidemiology: Selected Studies During the Past Four Decades at Boston City Hospital." *Journal of Infectious Disease* 128, no. 1 (July 1973): 76–124.

Flexner, Simon. "Paul Adin Lewis." *Science* 52 (Aug. 9, 1929): 133–34.

———. "The Present Status of the Serum Therapy of Epidemic Cerebro-spinal Meningitis." *JAMA* 53 (1909) 53: 1443–46.

Flexner, Simon, and Paul Lewis. "Transmission of Poliomyelitis to Monkeys: A Further Note." *JAMA* 53 (1909): 1913.

Friedlander et al. "The Epidemic of Influenza at Camp Sherman." *JAMA* 71, no. 20 (Nov. 16, 1918): 1650–71.

Frost, W. H. "Statistics of Influenza Morbidity." *Public Health Reports* 7 (March 12, 1920): 584–97.

Galishoff, S. "Newark and the Great Influenza Pandemic of 1918." *Bulletin of the History of Medicine* 43, no. 3 (May–June 1969): 246–58.

Gear, J. H. "The History of Virology in South Africa." *South African Medical Journal* (Oct. 11, 1986, suppl): 7–10.

Glezen, W. P. "Emerging Infections: Pandemic Influenza." *Epidemiology Review* 18, no. 1 (1996): 64–76.

Goodpasture, Ernest W. "Pathology of Pneumonia Following Influenza." *U.S. Naval Bulletin* 13, no. 3 (1919).

Grist, N. R. "Pandemic Influenza 1918." *British Medical Journal* 2, no. 6205 (Dec. 22–29, 1979): 1632–33.

Guerra, F. "The Earliest American Epidemic: The Influenza of 1493." *Social Science History* 12, no. 3 (1988): 305–25.

Halpern, Sue. "Evangelists for Kids." *New York Review of Books,* May 29, 2003.

Hamaker, Gene. "Influenza 1918." *Buffalo County, Nebraska, Historical Society* 7, no. 4.

Hamilton, D. "Unanswered Questions of the Spanish Flu Pandemic." *Bulletin of the American Association of the History of Nursing* 34 (spring 1992): 6–7.

Harris, John. "Influenza Occuring in Pregnant Women: A Statistical Study of 130 Cases." *JAMA* 72, no. 14 (April 5, 1919): 978–80.

Harrop, George A. "The Behavior of the Blood Toward Oxygen in Influenzal Infections." *Johns Hopkins Hospital Bulletin* 30 (1919): 335.

Hayden, Frederick G., and Peter Palese. "Influenza Virus." In *Clinical Virology,* edited by Douglas Richman, Richard Whitley, and Frederick Hayden, 911–30. New York: Churchill Livingstone, 1997.

Heagerty, J. J. "Influenza and Vaccination." *Canadian Medical Association Journal* 145, no. 5 (Sept. 1991, originally published 1919): 481–82.

Herda, P. S. "The 1918 Influenza Pandemic in Fiji, Tonga and the Samoas. In *New Countries and Old Medicine: Proceedings of an International Conference on the History of Medicine and Health,* edited by L. Bryder and D. A. Dow, 46–53. Auckland, New Zealand: Pyramid Press, 1995.

Hewer, C. L. "1918 Influenza Epidemic." *British Medical Journal* 1, no. 6157 (Jan. 1979): 199.

Hildreth, M. L. "The Influenza Epidemic of 1918–1919 in France: Contemporary Concepts of Aetiology, Therapy, and Prevention." *Social History of Medicine* 4, no. 2 (Aug. 1991): 277–94.

Holladay, A. J. "The Thucydides Syndrome: Another View." *New England Journal of Medicine* 315, no. 18 (Oct. 30, 1986): 1170–73.

Holland, J. J. "The Origin and Evolution of Chicago Viruses." In *Microbiology and Microbial Infections,* v. 1, *Virology,* edited by Brian W. J. Mahy and Leslie Collier, 10–20. New York: Oxford University Press, 1998.

Hope-Simpson, R. E. "Andrewes Versus Influenza: Discussion Paper." *Journal of the Royal Society of Medicine* 79, no. 7 (July 1986): 407–11.

———. "Recognition of Historic Influenza Epidemics from Parish Burial Records: A Test of Prediction from a New Hypothesis of Influenzal Epidemiology." *Journal of Hygiene* 91, no. 2 (Oct. 1983): 293–308.

"How to Fight Spanish Influenza." *Literary Digest* 59 (Oct. 12, 1918).

Hyslop, A. "Old Ways, New Means: Fighting Spanish Influenza in Australia, 1918–1919." In *New Countries and Old Medicine: Proceedings of an International Conference on the History of Medicine and Health,* edited by L. Bryder and D. A. Dow, 54–60. Auckland, New Zealand: Pyramid Press, 1995.

Irwin, R. T. "1918 Influenza in Morris County." *New Jersey Historical Community Newsletter* (March 1981): 3.

Jackson, G. G. "Nonbacterial Pneumonias: Contributions of Maxwell Finland Revisited." *Journal of Infectious Disease* 125, supp. (March 1972): 47–57.

Johnson, Niall, and Juergen Mueller. "Updating the Accounts: Global Mortality of the 1918–1920 'Spanish' Influenza Pandemic." *Bulletin of the History of Medicine* 76 (spring 2002): 105–15.

Kass, A. M. "Infectious Diseases at the Boston City Hospital: The First 60 Years." *Clinical Infectious Disease* 17, no. 2 (Aug. 1993): 276–82.

Katz, R. S. "Influenza 1918–1919: A Further Study in Mortality." *Bulletin of the History of Medicine* 51, no. 4 (winter 1977): 617–19.

———. "Influenza 1918–1919: A Study in Mortality." *Bulletin of the History of Medicine* 48, no. 3 (fall 1974): 416–22.

Katzenellenbogen, J. M. "The 1918 Influenza Epidemic in Mamre." *South African Medical Journal* 74, no. 7 (Oct. 1, 1988), 362–64.

Keating, Peter. "Vaccine Therapy and the Problem of Opsonins." *Journal of the History of Medicine* 43 (1988), 275–96.

Keegan, J. J. "The Prevailing Epidemic of Influenza." *JAMA* 71 (Sept. 28, 1918), 1051–52.

Keeton, Riet, and A. Beulah Cusman. "The Influenza Epidemic in Chicago." *JAMA* 71, no. 24 (Dec. 14, 1918): 2000–2001.

Kerson, T. S. "Sixty Years Ago: Hospital Social Work in 1918." *Social Work Health Care* 4, no. 3 (spring 1979): 331–43.

Kilbourne, E. D., M.D. "A History of Influenza Virology." In *Microbe Hunters—Then and Now,* edited by H. Koprowski and M. B. Oldstone, 187–204. Bloomington, Ill.: Medi-Ed Press, 1996.

———. "In Pursuit of Influenza: Fort Monmouth to Valhalla (and Back)." *Bioessays* 19, no. 7 (July 1997): 641–50.

———. "Pandora's Box and the History of the Respiratory Viruses: A Case Study of Serendipity in Research." *History of the Philosophy of Life Sciences* 14, no. 2 (1992): 299–308.

King, John. "The Progress of Medical Reform." *Western Medical Reformer* 6, no. 1846: 79–82.

Kirkpatrick, G. W. "Influenza 1918: A Maine Perspective." *Maine Historical Society Quarterly* 25, no. 3 (1986): 162–77.

Knight, C. P. "The Activities of the USPHS in Extra-Cantonment Zones, With Special Reference to the Venereal Disease Problem." *Military Surgeon* 44 (Jan. 1919): 41–43.

Knoll, K. "When the Plague Hit Spokane." *Pacific Northwest Quarterly* 33, no. 1 (1989): 1–7.

Koen, J. S. "A Practical Method for Field Diagnosis of Swine Diseases." *Journal of Veterinary Medicine* 14 (1919): 468–70.

Kolmer, John, M.D., "Paper Given at the Philadelphia County Medical Society Meeting, Oct. 23, 1918." *Pennsylvania Medical Journal,* Dec. 1918.

Krumwiede, Charles, Jr., and Eugenia Valentine. "Determination of the Type of Pneumococcus in the Sputum of Lobar Pneumonia, A Rapid Simple Method." *JAMA* 70 (Feb. 23, 1918): 513–14.

Kyes, Preston. "The Treatment of Lobar Pneumonia with an Anti-pneumococcus Serum." *Journal of Medical Research* 38 (1918): 495–98.

Lachman, E. The German Influenza of 1918–19: Personal Recollections and Review of the German Medical Literature of that Period." *Journal of the Oklahoma State Medical Association* 69, no. 12 (Dec. 1976): 517–20.

Lamber, Arthur. "Medicine: A Determining Factor in War." *JAMA* 21, no. 24 (June 14, 1919): 1713.

Langmuir, A. D. "The Territory of Epidemiology: Pentimento." *Journal of Infectious Disease* 155, no. 3 (March 1987): 349–58.

Langmuir, A. D., et al. "The Thucydides Syndrome: A New Hypothesis for the Cause of the Plague of Athens." *New England Journal of Medicine* 313, no. 16 (Oct. 17, 1985): 1027–30.

Lautaret, R. L. "Alaska's Greatest Disaster: The 1918 Spanish Influenza Epidemic." *Alaska Journal* 16 (1986): 238–43.

Lehman, Joseph. "Clinical Notes on the Recent Epidemic of Influenza." *Monthly Bulletin of the Department of Public Health and Charities* (Philadelphia), March 1919.

Leonard, Stephen, "The 1918 Influenza Epidemic in Denver and Colorado." *Essays and Monographs in Colorado History,* essays no. 9, 1989.

Levin, M. L. "An Historical Account of 'The Influence.'" *Maryland State Medical Journal* 27, no. 5 (May 1978): 58–62.

Lewis, Paul A., and Richard E. Shope. "Swine Influenza II. Hemophilic Bacillus from the Respiratory Tract of Infected Swine." *Journal of Infectious Disease* 54, no. 3 (1931): 361–372.

Lichtenstein, A. M. "The Influenza Epidemic in Cumberland, Md." *Johns Hopkins Nurses Alumni Magazine* 17, no. 4 (Nov. 1918): 224–27.

Lyons, D., and G. Murphy. "Influenza Causing Sunspots?" *Nature* 344, no. 6261 (March 1, 1990): 10.

MacCallum, William G. "Pathological Anatomy of Pneumonia Following Influenza." *Johns Hopkins Hospital Reports* 20 fasciculus II (1921): 149–51.

———. "The Pathology of Pneumonia in the U.S. Army Camps During the Winter of 1917–18." *Monographs of the Rockefeller Institute for Medical Research* (10), 1919.

McCann, T. A. "Homeopathy and Influenza." *Journal of the American Institute for Homeopathy,* May 1921.

McCord, C. P. "The Purple Death: Some Things Remembered About the Influenza Epidemic of 1918 at One Army Camp." *Journal of Occupational Medicine* 8, no. 11 (Nov. 1966): 593–98.

McCullers, J. A., and K. C. Bartmess. "Role of Neuraminidase in Lethal Synergism Between Influenza Virus and Streptococcus Pneumoniae." *Journal of Infectious Diseases* 187, no. 6 (March 15, 2003): 1000–1009.

McCullum, C. "Diseases and Dirt: Social Dimensions of Influenza, Cholera, and Syphilis." *Pharos* 55, no. 1 (winter 1992): 22–29.

Macdiarmid, D. "Influenza 1918." *New Zealand Medical Journal* 97, no. 747 (Jan. 1984): 23.

McGinnis, J. D. "Carlill v. Carbolic Smoke Ball Company: Influenza, Quackery, and the Unilateral Contract." *Bulletin of Canadian History of Medicine* 5, no. 2 (winter 1988): 121–41.

MacLachlan, W. W. G., and W. J. Fetter. "Citrated Blood in Treatment of Pneumonia Following Influenza." *JAMA* 71, no. 25 (Dec. 21, 1918): 2053–54.

MacLeod, Colin. "Theodore Avery, 1877–1955." *Journal of General Microbiology* 17 (1957): 539–49.

McMichael, A. J. et al. "Declining T-cell Immunity to Influenza, 1977–82. *Lancet* 2, no. 8353 (Oct. 1, 1983): 762–64.

MacNeal, W. J. "The Influenza Epidemic of 1918 in the AEF in France and England." *Archives of Internal Medicine* 23 (1919).

McQueen, H. "Spanish 'Flu"—1919: Political, Medical and Social Aspects." *Medical Journal of Australia* 1, no. 18 (May 3, 1975): 565–70.

Maxwell, William. "A Time to Mourn." *Pen America* 2, no. 4 (2002).

Mayer, J. L., and D. S. Beardsley. "Varicella-associated Thrombocytopenia: Autoantibodies Against Platelet Surface Glycoprotein V." *Pediatric Research* 40 (1996): 615–19.

Meiklejohn, G. N. "History of the Commission on Influenza." *Social History of Medicine* 7, no. 1 (April 1994): 59–87.

Meltzer, Martin, Nancy Cox, and Keiji Fukuda. "Modeling the Economic Impact of Pandemic Influenza in the United States: Implications for Setting Priorities for Intervention." In *Emerging Infectious Diseases,* CDC, 1999, www.cdc.gov/ncidod/eid/vol5no5/melt back.htm.

Mencken, H. L. "Thomas Henry Huxley 1825–1925." *Baltimore Evening Sun,* May 4, 1925.

Mills, I. D. "The 1918–19 Influenza Pandemic—The Indian Experience." *Indian Economic and Social History Review* 23 (1986): 1–36.

Morens, D. M., and R. J. Littman. "'Thucydides Syndrome' Reconsidered: New Thoughts on the 'Plague of Athens.'" *American Journal of Epidemiology* 140, no. 7 (Oct. 1, 1994): 621–28, discussion 629–31.

Morton, G. "The Pandemic Influenza of 1918." *Canadian Nurse* 69, no. 12 (Dec. 1973): 25–27.

Mullen, P. C., and M. L. Nelson. "Montanans and 'The Most Peculiar Disease': The Influenza Epidemic and Public Health, 1918–1919." *Montana* 37, no. 2 (1987): 50–61.

Murphy, Brian R., and Robert G. Webster. "Orthomyxoviruses." In *Fields' Virology,* third edition, Bernard Fields, editor in chief. Philadelphia: Lippincott-Raven, 1996.

Nicolle, Charles, and Charles LeBailly. "Recherches experimentales sur la grippe." *Annales de l'Institut Pasteur* 33 (1919): 395–402.

Nutton, Vivian. "Humoralism." In *Companion Encyclopedia to the History of Medicine,* edited by Bynum and Porter. London: Routledge, 1993.

Nuzum, J. W. et al. "1918 Pandemic Influenza and Pneumonia in a Large Civil Hospital." *Illinois Medical Journal* 150, no. 6 (Dec. 1976): 612–16.

Osler, William. "The Inner History of Johns Hopkins Hospital." Edited by D. Bates and E. Bensley. *Johns Hopkins Medical Journal* 125 (1969): 184–94.

"Outbreak of Influenza, Madagascar, July–August 2002." *Weekly Epidemiological Report 77*, no. 46 (2002): 381–87.

Oxford, J. S. "The So-Called Great Spanish Influenza Pandemic of 1918 May Have Originated in France in 1916." In *The Origin and Control of Pandemic Influenza*, edited by W. Laver and R. Webster, Philosophical Transactions of the Royal Society 356, no. 1416 (Dec. 2001).

Palmer, E., and G. W. Rice. "A Japanese Physician's Response to Pandemic Influenza: Ijiro Gomibuchi and the 'Spanish Flu' in Yaita-Cho, 1918–1919." *Bulletin of the History of Medicine* 66, no. 4 (winter 1992): 560–77.

Pandit, C. G. "Communicable Diseases in Twentieth-Century India." *American Journal of Tropical Medicine and Hygiene* 19, no. 3 (May 1970): 375–82.

Pankhurst, R. "The Great Ethiopian Influenza (Ye Hedar Beshita) Epidemic of 1918." *Ethiopian Medical Journal* 27, no. 4 (Oct. 1989): 235–42.

———. "A Historical Note on Influenza in Ethiopia." *Medical History* 21, no. 2 (April 1977): 195–200.

Park, William H. "Anti-influenza Vaccine as Prophylactic." *New York Medical Journal* 108, no. 15 (Oct. 12, 1918).

Park, William H. et al. "Introduction." *Journal of Immunology* 6, Jan. 1921: 2–8.

Patterson, K. D., and G. F. Pyle. "The Diffusion of Influenza in Sub-Saharan Africa During the 1918–1919 Pandemic." *Social Science and Medicine* 17, no. 17 (1983): 1299–1307.

———. "The Geography and Mortality of the 1918 Influenza Pandemic." *Bulletin of the History of Medicine* 65, no. 1 (spring 1991): 4–21.

Pennisi, E. "First Genes Isolated from the Deadly 1918 Flu Virus." *Science* 275, no. 5307 (March 21, 1997): 1739.

Persico, Joe. "The Great Spanish Flu Epidemic of 1918." *American Heritage* 27 (June 1976): 28–31, 80–85.

Polson, A. "Purification and Aggregation of Influenza Virus by Precipitation with Polyethylene Glycol." *Prep Biochemistry* 23, nos. 1–2 (Feb.–May 1993, originally published 1974): 207–25.

Porter, Katherine Anne. "Pale Horse, Pale Rider." *The Collected Stories of Katherine Anne Porter.* New York: Harcourt, 1965, 304–317.

Pusey, William Allen, M.D. "Handling of the Venereal Problem in the U.S. Army in Present Crisis." *JAMA* 71, no. 13 (Sept. 28, 1918): 1017–19.

Raff, M. J., P. A. Barnwell, and J. C. Melo. "Swine Influenza: History and Recommendations for Vaccination." *Journal of the Kentucky Medical Association* 74, no. 11 (Nov. 1976): 543–48.

Ranger, T. "The Influenza Pandemic in Southern Rhodesia: a Crisis of Comprehension." In *Imperial Medicine and Indigenous Societies,* edited by D. Arnold, 172–88. Manchester, England, and New York: Manchester University Press, 1988.

Ravenholt, R. T., and W. H. Foege. "1918 Influenza, Encephalitis Lethargica, Parkinsonism." *Lancet* 2, no. 8303 (Oct. 16, 1982): 860–64.

Redden, W. R., and L. W. McQuire. "The Use of Convalescent Human Serum in Influenza Pneumonia." *JAMA* 71, no. 16 (Oct. 19, 1918): 1311–12.

"Review of *Offensive Fighting* by Major Donald McRae." *Military Surgeon* 43 (Feb. 1919).

Rice, G. "Christchurch in the 1918 Influenza Epidemic: A Preliminary Study." *New Zealand Journal of History* 13 (1979): 109–37.

Richmond, Phyllis Allen. "American Attitudes Toward the Germ Theory of Disease, 1860–1880." *Journal of the History of Medicine and Allied Sciences* 9 (1954): 428–54.

———. "Some Variant Theories in Opposition to the Germ Theory of Disease." *Journal of the History of Medicine and Allied Sciences* 9 (1954): 290–303.

Rivers, Thomas. "The Biological and the Serological Reactions of Influenza Bacilli Producing Meningitis." *Journal of Experimental Medicine* 34, no. 5 (Nov. 1, 1921): 477–94.

———. "Influenzal Meningitis." *American Journal of Diseases of Children* 24 (Aug. 1922): 102–24.

Rivers, Thomas, and Stanhope Bayne-Jones. "Influenza-like Bacilli Isolated from Cats." *Journal of Experimental Medicine* 37, no. 2 (Feb. 1, 1923): 131–38.

Roberts, R. S. "A Consideration of the Nature of the English Sweating Sickness." *Medical History* 9, no. 4 (Oct. 1965): 385–89.

Robinson, K. R. "The Role of Nursing in the Influenza Epidemic of 1918–1919." *Nursing Forum* 25, no. 2 (1990): 19–26.

Rockafellar, N. "'In Gauze We Trust': Public Health and Spanish Influenza on the Home Front, Seattle, 1918–1919." *Pacific Northwest Quarterly* 77, no. 3 (1986): 104–13.

Rogers, F. B. "The Influenza Pandemic of 1918–1919 in the Perspective of a Half Century." *American Journal of Public Health and Nations Health* 58, no. 12 (Dec. 1968): 2192–94.

Rosenberg, Charles. "The Therapeutic Revolution." In *Explaining Epidemics and Other Studies in the History of Medicine.* Cambridge, England, and New York: Cambridge University Press, 1992.

———. "Toward an Ecology of Knowledge." In *The Organization of Knowledge in Modern America, 1860–1920.* Edited by A. Oleson and J. Voss. Baltimore: Johns Hopkins University Press, 1979.

Rosenberg, K. D. "Swine Flu: Play It Again, Uncle Sam." *Health/PAC Bulletin* 73 (Nov.–Dec. 1976): 1–6, 10–20.

Ross, Katherine. "Battling the Flu." *American Red Cross Magazine* (Jan. 1919): 11–15.

Sage, M. W. "Pittsburgh Plague—1918: An Oral History." *Home Health Nurse* 13, no. 1 (Jan.–Feb. 1995): 49–54.

Salk, J. "The Restless Spirit of Thomas Francis, Jr., Still Lives: The Unsolved Problems of Recurrent Influenza Epidemics." *Archives of Environmental Health* 21, no. 3 (Sept. 1970): 273–75.

Sartwell, P. E. "The Contributions of Wade Hampton Frost." *American Journal of Epidemiology* 104, no. 4 (Oct. 1976): 386–91.

Sattenspiel, L., and D. A. Herring. "Structured Epidemic Models and the Spread of Influenza in the Central Canadian Subarctic." *Human Biology* 70, no. 1 (Feb. 1998): 91–115.

Scott, K. A. "Plague on the Homefront: Arkansas and the Great Influenza Epidemic of 1918." *Arkansas Historical Quarterly* 47, no. 4 (1988): 311–44.

Shope, Richard E. "Influenza: History, Epidemiology, and Speculation." *Public Health Reports* 73, no. 165 (1958).

———. "Swine Influenza I. Experimental Transmission and Pathology." *Journal of Infectious Disease* 54, no. 3 (1931): 349–60.

———. "Swine Influenza III. Filtration Experiments and Etiology." *Journal of Infectious Disease* 54, no. 3 (1931): 373–390.

Shortt, S. E. D. "Physicians, Science, and Status: Issues in the Professionalization of Anglo-American Medicine in the 19th Century." *Medical History* 27 (1983): 53–68.

Shryock, Richard. "Women in American Medicine." *Journal of the American Medical Women's Association* 5 (Sept. 1950): 371.

Simon, Harvey, and Martin Swartz. "Pulmonary Infections." In *Scientific American's Medicine,* edited by Edward Rubinstein and Daniel Feldman, chapter 20. New York: Scientific American, 1994.

Smith, F. B. "The Russian Influenza in the United Kingdom, 1889–1894." *Social History of Medicine* 8, no. 1 (April 1995): 55–73.

Snape, W. J., and E. L. Wolfe. "Influenza Epidemic. Popular Reaction in Camden 1918–1919." *New Jersey Medicine* 84, no. 3 (March 1987): 173–76.

Soper, George, M.D. "Epidemic After Wars." *JAMA* 72, no. 14 (April 5, 1919): 988–90.

———. "The Influenza-Pneumonia Pandemic in the American Army Camps, September and October 1918." *Science,* Nov. 8, 1918.

Springer, J. K. "1918 Flu Epidemic in Hartford, Connecticut." *Connecticut Medicine* 55, no. 1 (Jan. 1991): 43–47.

Starr, Isaac. "Influenza in 1918: Recollections of the Epidemic in Philadelphia." *Annals of Internal Medicine* 85 (1976): 516–18.

Stephenson, J. "Flu on Ice." *JAMA* 279, no. 9 (March 4, 1998): 644.

Strauss, Ellen G., James H. Strauss, and Arnold J. Levine. "Viral Evolution." In *Fields' Virology,* Bernard Fields, editor in chief. Philadelphia: Lippincott-Raven, 1996.

Stuart-Harris, C. H. "Pandemic Influenza: An Unresolved Problem in Prevention." *Journal of Infectious Disease* 122, no. 1 (July–Aug. 1970): 108–15.

Sturdy, Steve. "War as Experiment: Physiology, Innovation and Administration in Britain, 1914–1918: The Case of Chemical Warfare." In *War, Medicine and Modernity,* edited by Roger Cooter, Mark Harrison, and Steve Sturdy. Stroud: Sutton, 1998.

"Sure Cures for Influenza." *Public Health Reports* 91, no. 4 (July–Aug. 1976): 378–80.

Symmers, Douglas, M.D. "Pathologic Similarity Between Pneumonia of Bubonic Plague and of Pandemic Influenza." *JAMA* 71, no. 18 (Nov. 2, 1918): 1482–83.

Taksa, Lucy. "The Masked Disease: Oral History, Memory, and the Influenza Pandemic." In *Memory and History in Twentieth Century Australia,* edited by Kate Darian-Smith and Paula Hamilton. Melbourne, Australia: Oxford Press, 1994.

Taubenberger, J. K. "Seeking the 1918 Spanish Influenza Virus." *ASM News* 65, no. 7, (July 1999).

Taubenberger, J. K. et al. "Initial Genetic Characterization of the 1918 'Spanish' Influenza Virus." *Science* 275, no. 5307 (March 21, 1997): 1793–96.

Terris, Milton. "Hermann Biggs' Contribution to the Modern Concept of the Health Center." *Bulletin of the History of Medicine* 20 (Oct. 1946): 387–412.

Thayer, W. S. "Discussion of Influenza," *Proceedings of the Royal Society of Medicine* 12, part 1 (Nov. 13, 1918).

Thomson, J. B. "The 1918 Influenza Epidemic in Nashville." *Journal of the Tennessee Medical Association* 71, no. 4 (April 1978): 261–70.

Tomes, Nancy. "American Attitudes Toward the Germ Theory of Disease: The Richmond Thesis Revisited." *Journal of the History of Medicine and Allied Sciences* 52, no. 1 (Jan. 1997): 17–50.

Tomes, Nancy, and Warner John Harley. "Introduction—Rethinking the Reception of the Germ Theory of Disease: Comparative Perspectives." *Journal of the History of Medicine and Allied Sciences* 52, no. 1 (Jan. 1997): 7–16.

Tomkins, S. M. "The Failure of Expertise: Public Health Policy in Britain During the 1918–19 Influenza Epidemic." *Social History of Medicine* 5, no. 3 (Dec. 1992): 435–54.

Turner, R. Steven et al. "The Growth of Professorial Research in Prussia—1818–1848, Causes and Context." *Historical Studies in the Physical Sciences* 3 (1972): 137–182.

Van Helvoort, T. "A Bacteriological Paradigm in Influenza Research in the First Half of the Twentieth Century." *History and Philosophy of the Life Sciences* 15, no. 1 (1993): 3–21.

Wallack, G. "The Waterbury Influenza Epidemic of 1918/1919." *Connecticut Medicine* 41, no. 6 (June 1977): 349–51.

Walters, J. H. "Influenza 1918: The Contemporary Perspective." *Bulletin of the New York Academy of Medicine* 54, no. 9 (Oct. 1978): 855–64.

Ware, Lorraine, and Michael Matthay. "The Acute Respiratory Distress Syndrome." *New England Journal of Medicine* 342, no. 18 (May 4, 2000): 1334–49.

Warner, John Harley. "The Fall and Rise of Professional Mystery." In *The Laboratory Revolution in Medicine,* edited by Andrew Cunningham and Perry Williams. Cambridge, England: Cambridge University Press, 1992.

"War Reports from the Influenza Front." *Literary Digest* 60 (Feb. 22, 1919).

Wasserman, I. M. "The Impact of Epidemic, War, Prohibition and Media on Suicide: United States, 1910–1920." *Suicide and Life Threatening Behavior* 22, no. 2 (summer 1992): 240–54.

Waters, Charles, and Bloomfield, Al. "The Correlation of X-ray Findings and Physical Signs in the Chest in Uncomplicated Influenza." *Johns Hopkins Hospital Bulletin* 30 (1919): 268–70.

Webb, G. F. "A Silent Bomb: The Risk of Anthrax as Weapon of Mass Destruction." *Proceedings of the National Academy of Sciences* 100 (2003): 4355–61.

Wein, L. M., D. L. Craft, and E. H. Kaplan. "Emergency Response to an Anthrax Attack." *Proceedings of the National Academy of Sciences* 100 (2003): 4346–51.

Weinstein, Edward. "Woodrow Wilson's Neurological Illness." *Journal of American History* 57 (1970–71): 324–51.

Weinstein, L. "Influenza—1918, A Revisit?" *New England Journal of Medicine* 294, no. 19 (May 1976): 1058–60.

Wetmore, F. H. "Treatment of Influenza." *Canadian Medical Association Journal* 145, no. 5 (Sept. 1991, originally published 1919): 482–85.

Whipple, George. "Current Comment, Vaccines in Influenza." *JAMA* 71, no. 16 (Oct. 19, 1918).

White, K. A. "Pittsburgh in the Great Epidemic of 1918." *West Pennsylvania History Magazine* 68, no. 3 (1985): 221–42.

"WHO Influenza Surveillance." *Weekly Epidemiological Record* 71, no. 47 (Nov. 22, 1996): 353–57.

Wilkinson, L., and A. P. Waterson. "The Development of the Virus Concept as Reflected in Corpora of Studies on Individual Pathogens, 2: The Agent of Fowl Plague—A Model Virus." *Medical History* 19, no. 1 (Jan. 1975): 52–72.

"Will the Flu Return?" *Literary Digest* (Oct. 11, 1919).

Wilton, P. "Spanish Flu Outdid WWI in Number of Lives Claimed." *Canadian Medical Association Journal* 148, no. 11 (June 1, 1993): 2036–37.

Winslow, Charles-Edward. "The Untilled Fields of Public Health." *Science* 51, (Jan. 9, 1920): 30.

Wise, John C. "The Medical Reserve Corps of the U.S. Navy." *Military Surgeon* 43 (July 1918): 68.

Wooley, Paul. "Epidemic of Influenza at Camp Devens, Mass." *Journal of Laboratory and Clinical Medicine* 4 (1919).

Wright, P., et al. "Maternal Influenza, Obstetric Complications, and Schizophrenia." *American Journal of Psychiatry* 152, no. 12 (Dec. 1995): 1714–20.

Yankauer, A. "Influenza: Some Swinish Reflections." *American Journal of Public Health* 66, no. 9 (Sept. 1976): 839–41.

BOOKS AND PAMPHLETS

Ackerknecht, Erwin. *Medicine at the Paris Hospital, 1794–1848.* Baltimore: Johns Hopkins University Press, 1967.

American Red Cross. "A History of Helping Others." 1989.

Andrewes, C. H. *Biological Memoirs: Richard E. Shope.* Washington, D.C.: National Academy of Sciences Press, 1979.

Baruch, Bernard. *Baruch: The Public Years.* New York: Holt Rinehart, 1960.

Benison, Saul. *Tom Rivers: Reflections on a Life in Medicine and Science: An Oral History Memoir.* Cambridge, Mass.: MIT Press, 1967.

Berliner, Howard. *A System of Scientific Medicine: Philanthropic Foundations in the Flexner Era.* New York: Tavistock, 1985.

Beveridge, W. I. B. *Influenza: The Last Great Plague: An Unfinished Story of Discovery.* New York: Prodist, 1977.

Bledstein, Burton J. *The Culture of Professionalism: The Middle Class and the Development of Higher Education in America.* New York: Norton, 1976.

Bliss, Michael. *William Osler: A Life in Medicine.* Oxford and New York: Oxford University Press, 1999.

Bonner, Thomas. *American Doctors and German Universities: A Chapter in International Intellectual Relations, 1870–1914.* Lincoln: University of Nebraska Press, 1963.

———. *The Kansas Doctor.* Lawrence: University of Kansas Press, 1959.

Brock, Thomas. *Robert Koch: A Life in Medicine.* Madison, Wisc.: Science Tech Publishers, 1988.

Brown, E. Richard. *Rockefeller's Medicine Men.* Berkeley: University of California, 1979.

Brown, Ezra, ed. *This Fabulous Century: The Roaring Twenties 1920–1930.* Alexandria, Va.: Time-Life Books, 1985.

Bulloch, W. *The History of Bacteriology.* London: Oxford University Press, 1938.

Burnet, F. M., and Ellen Clark. *Influenza: A Survey of the Last Fifty Years.* Melbourne: Macmillan, 1942.

Cannon, Walter. *The Way of an Investigator.* New York: Norton, 1945.

Cassedy, James. *Charles V. Chapin and the Public Health Movement.* Cambridge, Mass.: Harvard University Press, 1962.

———. *Medicine in America: A Short History.* Baltimore, Md.: Johns Hopkins University Press, 1991.

Chase, Marilyn. *The Barbary Plague.* New York: Random House, 2003.

Chesney, Alan. *The Johns Hopkins Hospital and the Johns Hopkins University School of Medicine.* Baltimore, Md.: Johns Hopkins University Press, 1943.

Clark, P. F. *Pioneer Microbiologists in America.* Madison: University of Wisconsin Press, 1961.

Cliff, A. D., J. K. Ord, and P. Haggett. *Spatial Aspects of Influenza Epidemics.* London: Pion Ltd., 1986.

Coleman, William, and Frederic Holmes, eds. *The Investigative Enterprise: Experimental Physiology in Nineteenth Century Medicine.* Berkeley: University of California Press, 1988.

Collier, R. *The Plague of the Spanish Lady: The Influenza Pandemic of 1918–1919.* New York: Atheneum, 1974.

Collins, Selwyn et al. *Mortality from Influenza and Pneumonia in 50 Largest Cities of the United States 1910–1929.* Washington, D.C.: U.S. Government Printing Office, 1930.

Corner, George A. *A History of the Rockefeller Institute: 1901–1953, Origins and Growth.* New York: Rockefeller Institute Press, 1964.

Creighton, Charles. *A History of Epidemics in Britain.* London: Cambridge University Press, 1894.

Crile, George. *George Crile, An Autobiography.* Philadelphia: Lippincott, 1947.

Crookshank, F. G. *Influenza: Essays by Several Authors.* London: Heinemann, 1922.

Crosby, Alfred W. *America's Forgotten Pandemic: The Influenza of 1918.* Cambridge, England, and New York: Cambridge University Press, 1989.

Cunningham, Andrew, and Perry Williams, eds. *The Laboratory Revolution in Medicine.* Cambridge, England: Cambridge University Press, 1992.

Cushing, Harvey. *A Surgeon's Journal 1915–18.* Boston: Little Brown, 1934.

Cushing, John, and Arthur Stone, eds. *Vermont and the World War, 1917–1919.* Burlington, Vt.: published by act of legislature, 1928.

Davis, Allen, and Mark Haller, eds. *The Peoples of Philadelphia: A History of Ethnic Groups and Lower-Class Life, 1790–1940.* Philadelphia: Temple University Press, 1973.

Davis, Kingsley. *The Population of India and Pakistan.* Princeton, N.J.: Princeton University Press, 1951.

De Kruif, Paul. *Microbe Hunters.* New York: Harcourt, Brace and Company, 1939.

———. *The Sweeping Wind, A Memoir.* New York: Harcourt, Brace & World, 1962.

Dechmann, Louis. *Spanish Influenza (Pan-asthenia): Its Cause and Cure.* Seattle, Wash.: The Washington Printing Company, 1919.

Dewey, John. *Characters and Events: Popular Essays in Social and Political Philosophy.* New York: Henry Holt, 1929.

Dock, Lavinia et al. *History of American Red Cross Nursing.* New York: Macmillan, 1922.

Dorland's Illustrated Medical Dictionary, 28th ed. Philadelphia: W.B. Saunders and Company, 1994.

Dubos, René. *The Professor, the Institute, and DNA.* New York: Rockefeller University Press, 1976.

Duffy, John. *Epidemics in Colonial America.* Baton Rouge: Louisiana State University Press, 1953.

———. *A History of Public Health in New York City 1866–1966.* New York: Russell Sage Foundation, 1974.

Eisenhower, John, and Joanne Eisenhower. *Yanks: The Epic Story of the American Army in World War I.* New York: Free Press, 2001.

Fee, Elizabeth. *Disease and Discovery: A History of the Johns Hopkins School of Hygiene and Public Health, 1916–1939.* Baltimore, Md.: Johns Hopkins University Press, 1987.

Fields, Bernard, editor in chief. *Fields' Virology,* third edition. Philadelphia: Lippincott-Raven, 1996.

Finkler, Dittmar. *Influenza in Twentieth Century Practice,* v. 15. London: Sampson Low, 1898.

Fishbein, Morris, M.D. *A History of the American Medical Association, 1847 to 1947.* Philadelphia: W.B. Saunders & Co., 1947.

Fitzgerald, F. Scott. *This Side of Paradise.* New York: Scribner's, 1920.

Fleming, Donald. *William Welch and the Rise of American Medicine.* Boston: Little, Brown, 1954.

Flexner, James Thomas. *An American Saga: The Story of Helen Thomas and Simon Flexner.* Boston: Little, Brown, 1984.

Flexner, Simon, and James Thomas Flexner. *William Henry Welch and the Heroic Age of American Medicine.* New York: Viking, 1941.

Foucault, Michel. *The Birth of the Clinic: An Archaeology of Medical Perception.* New York: Vintage Books, 1976.

Fox, R., and G. Weisz, eds. *The Organization of Science and Technology in France, 1808–1914.* Cambridge, England, and New York: Cambridge University Press, 1980.

Fulton, John. *Harvey Cushing.* Springfield, Ill.: Chas. Thomas, 1946.

Fye, W. Bruce. *The Development of American Physiology: Scientific Medicine in the Nineteenth Century.* Baltimore: Johns Hopkins University Press, 1987.

Garrison, F. H. *John Shaw Billings: A Memoir.* New York: Putnam, 1915.

Geison, Gerald, ed. *Physiology in the American Context. 1850–1940.* Bethesda, Md.: Williams and Wilkins, 1987.

George, Lloyd. *Memoirs of the Peace Conference.* New Haven: Yale University Press, 1939.

Gibson, John M. *Physician to the World: The Life of General William C. Gorgas.* Tuscaloosa: University of Alabama Press, 1989.

Goethe, Johann Wolfgang. *Faust, Part One.* New York: Penguin Classics, 1949.

Gordon, Richard, M.D. *Great Medical Disasters.* New York: Stein & Day, 1983.

Grayson, Cary. *Woodrow Wilson: An Intimate Memoir.* New York: Holt, Rinehart, & Winston, 1960.

Harries, Meirion, and Susie Harries. *The Last Days of Innocence: America at War, 1917–1918.* New York: Random House, 1997.

Hausler, William Jr., Max Sussman, and Leslie Collier. *Microbiology and Microbial Infections,* v. 3, *Bacterial Infections.* New York: Oxford University Press, 1998.

Hawley, Ellis. *The Great War and the Search for a Modern Order: A History of the American People and Their Institutions, 1917–1933.* New York: St. Martin's Press, 1979.

Hertzler, Arthur E. *The Horse and Buggy Doctor.* New York: Harper & Brothers, 1938.

Hirsch, August. *Handbook of Geographical Historical Pathology.* London: New Sydenham Society, 1883.

Hirst, L. Fabian. *The Conquest of Plague: A Study of the Evolution of Epidemiology.* London: Oxford University Press, 1953.

Hoehling, Adolph A. *The Great Epidemic.* Boston: Little, Brown, 1961.

Hoover, Herbert. *America's First Crusade.* New York: Scribner's, 1942.

Hoover, Irwin H. *Forty-two Years in the White House.* New York: Houghton Mifflin, 1934.

Hope-Simpson, R. E. *The Transmission of Epidemic Influenza.* New York: Plenum Press, 1992.

Ireland, Merritt W., ed. *Medical Department of the United States Army in the World War,* v. 9, *Communicable Diseases.* Washington, D.C.: U.S. Army, 1928.

———. *Medical Department of the United States Army in the World War,* v. 12, *Pathology of the Acute Respiratory Diseases, and of Gas Gangrene Following War Wounds.* Washington, D.C.: U.S. Army, 1929.

Jensen, Joan. *The Price of Vigilance.* New York: Rand McNally, 1968.

Johnson, Richard T., M.D. *Viral Infections of the Nervous System,* 2nd ed. Philadelphia: Lippincott-Raven, 1998.

Jordan, Edwin O. *Epidemic Influenza.* Chicago: American Medical Association, 1927.

Judson, Horace. *The Eighth Day of Creation: The Makers of the Revolution in Biology.* New York: Simon & Schuster, 1979.

Kansas and Kansans. Chicago: Lewis Publishing Co., 1919.

Kennedy, David. *Over Here: The First World War and American Society.* New York: Oxford University Press, 1980.

Keynes, John Maynard. *Economic Consequences of the Peace.* New York: Harcourt, Brace and Howe, 1920.

Kilbourne, E. D., M.D. *Influenza.* New York: Plenum Medical, 1987.

Layton, Edwin. *The Revolt of the Engineers: Social Responsibility and the American Engineering Profession.* Cleveland: Press of Case Western Reserve University, 1971.

Lereboullet, Pierre. *La grippe, clinique, prophylaxie, traitement.* Paris: 1926.

L'Etang, Hugh. *The Pathology of Leadership.* New York: Hawthorn Books, 1970.

Luckingham, B. *Epidemic in the Southwest, 1918–1919.* El Paso: Texas Western Press, 1984.

Ludmerer, Kenneth M. *Learning to Heal: The Development of American Medical Education.* New York: Basic Books, 1985.

McAdoo, William. *Crowded Years.* Boston and New York: Houghton Mifflin Company, 1931.

MacCallum, William G. *William Stewart Halsted.* Baltimore, Md.: Johns Hopkins University Press, 1930.

McCullough, David. *The Path Between the Seas: The Creation of the Panama Canal 1870–1914.* New York: Simon & Schuster, 1977.

Macmillan, Margaret. *Paris 1919, Six Months That Changed the World.* New York: Random House, 2002.

McNeill, William. *Plagues and Peoples.* New York: Anchor Press/Doubleday, 1976.

McRae, Major Donald. *Offensive Fighting.* Philadelphia: J.B. Lippincott, 1918.

Magner, Lois. *A History of Medicine.* New York: M. Dekker, 1992.

Mahy, Brian W. J., and Leslie Collier. *Microbiology and Microbial Infections,* v. 1, *Virology.* New York: Oxford University Press, 1998.

Martin, Franklin B. *Fifty Years of Medicine and Surgery.* Chicago: Surgical Publishing Company, 1934.

Marx, Rudolph. *The Health of the Presidents.* New York: Putnam, 1961.

Murray, Robert. *Red Scare: A Study in National Hysteria.* Minneapolis: University of Minnesota Press, 1955.

Nasar, Sylvia. *A Beautiful Mind.* New York: Simon & Schuster, 1998.

Nobelstifelsen. *Nobel, The Man, and His Prizes.* New York: Elsevier, 1962.

Noyes, William Raymond. *Influenza Epidemic 1918–1919: A Misplaced Chapter in United States Social and Institutional History.* Ann Arbor, Mich.: University Microfilms, 1971, c1969.

Nuland, Sherwin. *How We Die.* New York: Vintage, 1993.

Oliver, Wade. *The Man Who Lived for Tomorrow: A Biography of William Hallock Park, M.D.* New York: E. P. Dutton, 1941.

Osborn, June. E. *Influenza in America, 1918–1976: History, Science and Politics.* New York: Prodist, 1977.

Osler, William. *Osler's Textbook Revisited,* edited by A. McGehee Harvey and Victor A. McKusick. New York: Appleton Century Crofts, 1967.

Packard, Francis, M.D. *History of Medicine in the United States.* New York: Hafner, 1963.

Papers Relating to the Foreign Relations of the United States: The Paris Peace Conference, v. 11. Washington, D.C.: Government Printing Office, 1942–1947.

Parish, H. J. *A History of Immunization.* Edinburgh: Livingstone, 1965.

Park, William H. *Collected Reprints of Dr. William H. Park,* v. 3, *1910–1920.* City of New York.

Park, William H., and Anna Williams. *Pathogenic Microorganisms.* Philadelphia: Lea & Febiger, 1939.

Patterson, Archibald. *Personal Recollections of Woodrow Wilson.* Richmond, Va.: Whittet & Shepperson, 1929.

Patterson, K. D. *Pandemic Influenza, 1700–1900: A Study in Historical Epidemiology.* Totowa, N.J.: Rowan & Littlefield, 1986.

Peabody, F. W., G. Draper, and A. R. Dochez. *A Clinical Study of Acute Poliomyelitis.* New York: The Rockefeller Institute for Medical Research, 1912.

Pettigrew, E. *The Silent Enemy: Canada and the Deadly Flu of 1918.* Saskatoon, Sask.: Western Producer Prairie Books, 1983.

Porter, Roy. *The Greatest Benefit to Mankind: A Medical History of Humanity.* New York: Norton, 1998.

Pyle, Gerald F. *The Diffusion of Influenza: Patterns and Paradigms.* Totowa, N.J.: Rowman & Littlefield, 1986.

Ravenel, Mayzyk, ed. *A Half Century of Public Health.* New York: American Public Health Association, 1921.

Rice, G. *Black November: The 1918 Influenza Epidemic in New Zealand.* Wellington, New Zealand: Allen & Unwin, 1988.

Richman, Douglas, Richard Whitley, and Frederick Hayden, eds. *Clinical Virology.* New York: Churchill Livingstone, 1997.

Robertson, John Dill. "Report of An Epidemic of Influenza in Chicago Occurring During the Fall of 1918." City of Chicago.

Roosevelt, Eleanor. *This Is My Story.* New York, London: Harper & Brothers, 1937.

Rosenberg, Charles. *The Cholera Years: The United States in 1832, 1849, and 1866.* Chicago: University of Chicago Press, 1962.

———. *Explaining Epidemics and Other Studies in the History of Medicine.* Cambridge and New York: Cambridge University Press, 1992.

Rosenberg, Steven, and John Barry. *The Transformed Cell: Unlocking the Secrets of Cancer.* New York: Putnam, 1992.

Rosenkrantz, Barbara Gutmann. *Public Health and the State: Changing Views in Massachusetts, 1842–1936.* Cambridge, Mass: Harvard University Press, 1972.

Rubenstein, Edward, and Daniel Feldman. *Scientific American Medicine.* New York: Scientific American, 1995.

Sabin, Florence. *Franklin Paine Mall: The Story of a Mind.* Baltimore: Johns Hopkins University Press, 1934.

St. John, Robert. *This Was My World.* Garden City, N.Y.: Doubleday, 1953.

Schlesinger, Arthur. *The Age of Roosevelt,* v. 1, *Crisis of the Old Order 1919–1933.* Boston: Houghton Mifflin, 1957.

Sentz, Lilli, ed. *Medical History in Buffalo, 1846–1996, Collected Essays.* Buffalo: State University of New York at Buffalo, 1996.

Shryock, Richard. *American Medical Research Past and Present.* New York: Commonwealth Fund, 1947.

———. *The Development of Modern Medicine,* 2nd ed. New York: Knopf, 1947.

———. *The Unique Influence of the Johns Hopkins University on American Medicine.* Copenhagen: Ejnar Munksgaard Ltd., 1953.

Silverstein, Arthur. *Pure Politics and Impure Science: The Swine Flu Affair.* Baltimore, Md.: Johns Hopkins University Press, 1981.

Simon Flexner Memorial Pamphlet. New York: Rockefeller Institute for Medical Research, 1946.

Smith, Elbert. *When the Cheering Stopped: The Last Years of Woodrow Wilson.* New York: Morrow, 1964.

Starr, Paul. *The Social Transformation of American Medicine.* New York: Basic Books, 1982.

Steele, Richard W. *Free Speech in the Good War.* New York: St. Martin's Press, 1999.

Stent, Gunther. Introduction to *The Double Helix: A Norton Critical Edition,* by James Watson, edited by Gunther Stent. New York: Norton, 1980.

Sternberg, Martha. *George Sternberg: A Biography.* Chicago: American Medical Association, 1925.

Thompson, E. Symes. *Influenza.* London: Percival & Co., 1890.

Thomson, David, and Robert Thomson. *Annals of the Pickett-Thomson Research Laboratory,* vols. 9 and 10, *Influenza.* Baltimore: Williams and Wilkens, 1934.

U. S. Census Bureau. *Mortality Statistics 1919.* Washington, D.C.: General Printing Office.

U.S. Congress, Senate Committee on Appropriations. "Influenza in Alaska." Washington, D.C.: Government Printing Office, 1919.

Van Hartesveldt, Fred R., ed. *The 1918–1919 Pandemic of Influenza: The Urban Impact in the Western World.* Lewiston, N.Y.: E. Mellen Press, 1992.

Vaughan, Victor A. *A Doctor's Memories.* Indianapolis: Bobbs-Merrill, 1926.

Vaughn, Stephen. *Holding Fast the Inner Lines: Democracy, Nationalism, and the Committee on Public Information.* Chapel Hill: University of North Carolina Press, 1980.

Vogel, Morris, and Charles Rosenberg, eds. *The Therapeutic Revolution: Essays on the Social History of American Medicine.* Philadelphia: University of Pennsylvania Press, 1979.

Wade, Wyn Craig. *The Fiery Cross: The Ku Klux Klan in America.* New York: Simon & Schuster, 1987.

Walter, Richard. *S. Weir Mitchell, M.D., Neurologist: A Medical Biography.* Springfield, Ill: Chas. Thomas, 1970.

Walworth, Arthur. *Woodrow Wilson.* Boston: Houghton Mifflin, 1965.

Warner, John Harley. *Against the Spirit of System: The French Impulse in Nineteenth-Century American Medicine.* Princeton, N.J.: Princeton University Press, 1998.

Watson, James. *The Double Helix: A Norton Critical Edition,* edited by Gunther Stent. New York: Norton, 1980.

Weigley, Russell, ed. *Philadelphia: A 300 Year History.* New York: Norton, 1982.

Wilson, Edith. *My Memoir.* Indianapolis and New York: Bobbs-Merrill, 1939.

Wilson, Joan Hoff. *Herbert Hoover: Forgotten Progressive.* Boston: Little Brown, 1974.

Winslow, Charles-Edward Amory, *The Conquest of Epidemic Disease: A Chapter in the History of Ideas.* Princeton: Princeton University Press, 1943.

———. *The Evolution and Significance of the Modern Public Health Campaign.* New Haven: Yale University Press, 1923.

———. *Life of Hermann M. Biggs,* Philadelphia: Lea & Febiger, 1929.

Winternitz, Milton Charles. *The Pathology of Influenza.* New Haven: Yale University Press, 1920.

Young, James Harvey. *The Medical Messiahs: A Social History of Health Quackery in Twentieth Century America.* Princeton, N.J.: Princeton University Press, 1967.

———. *The Toadstool Millionaires: A Social History of Patent Medicines in America before Federal Regulation.* Princeton, N.J.: Princeton University Press, 1961.

Zinsser, Hans. *As I Remember Him: The Biography of R. S.* Gloucester, Mass.: Peter Smith, 1970.

———. *Rats, Lice, and History.* New York: Black Dog & Leventhal, 1963.

UNPUBLISHED MATERIALS

Allen, Phyllis. "Americans and the Germ Theory of Disease." Ph.D. diss., University of Pennsylvania, 1949.

Anderson, Jeffrey. "Influenza in Philadelphia, 1918." MA thesis, Rutgers University, Camden, 1998.

Fanning, Patricia J. "Disease and the Politics of Community: Norwood and the Great Flu Epidemic of 1918." Ph.D. diss., Boston College, 1995.

"Influenza 1918." *The American Experience,* Boston, Mass.: WGBH, 1998.

Ott, Katherine. "The Intellectual Origins and Cultural Form of Tuberculosis in the United States, 1870–1925." Ph.D. diss., Temple University, 1990.

Parsons, W. David, M.D. "The Spanish Lady and the Newfoundland Regiment." Paper presented at Newfoundland and the Great War Conference, Nov. 11, 1998.

Pettit, Dorothy Ann. "A Cruel Wind: America Experiences the Pandemic Influenza, 1918–1920, A Social History." Ph.D. diss., University of New Hampshire, 1976.

Smith, Soledad Mujica. "Nursing as Social Responsibility: Implications for Democracy from the Life Perspective of Lavinia Lloyd Dock (1858–1956)." Ph.D. diss., Louisiana State University, 2002.

Wolper, Gregg. "The Origins of Public Diplomacy: Woodrow Wilson, George Creel, and the Committee on Public Information." Ph.D. diss., University of Chicago, 1991.

Index

Photographic Credits

FOR THE BEST IN PAPERBACKS, LOOK FOR THE 🐧

In every corner of the world, on every subject under the sun, Penguin represents quality and variety—the very best in publishing today.

For complete information about books available from Penguin—including Penguin Classics, Penguin Compass, and Puffins—and how to order them, write to us at the appropriate address below. Please note that for copyright reasons the selection of books varies from country to country.

In the United States: Please write to *Penguin Group (USA), P.O. Box 12289 Dept. B, Newark, New Jersey 07101-5289* or call 1-800-788-6262.

In the United Kingdom: Please write to *Dept. EP, Penguin Books Ltd, Bath Road, Harmondsworth, West Drayton, Middlesex UB7 0DA.*

In Canada: Please write to *Penguin Books Canada Ltd, 90 Eglinton Avenue East, Suite 700, Toronto, Ontario M4P 2Y3.*

In Australia: Please write to *Penguin Books Australia Ltd, P.O. Box 257, Ringwood, Victoria 3134.*

In New Zealand: Please write to *Penguin Books (NZ) Ltd, Private Bag 102902, North Shore Mail Centre, Auckland 10.*

In India: Please write to *Penguin Books India Pvt Ltd, 11 Panchsheel Shopping Centre, Panchsheel Park, New Delhi 110 017.*

In the Netherlands: Please write to *Penguin Books Netherlands bv, Postbus 3507, NL-1001 AH Amsterdam.*

In Germany: Please write to *Penguin Books Deutschland GmbH, Metzlerstrasse 26, 60594 Frankfurt am Main.*

In Spain: Please write to *Penguin Books S. A., Bravo Murillo 19, 1° B, 28015 Madrid.*

In Italy: Please write to *Penguin Italia s.r.l., Via Benedetto Croce 2, 20094 Corsico, Milano.*

In France: Please write to *Penguin France, Le Carré Wilson, 62 rue Benjamin Baillaud, 31500 Toulouse.*

In Japan: Please write to *Penguin Books Japan Ltd, Kaneko Building, 2-3-25 Koraku, Bunkyo-Ku, Tokyo 112.*

In South Africa: Please write to *Penguin Books South Africa (Pty) Ltd, Private Bag X14, Parkview, 2122 Johannesburg.*